D1625700

book is due for return on or bef   last date shown bel

Anesthesia for Otolaryngologic Surgery

Anesthesia for Otolaryngologic Surgery

Edited by

Basem Abdelmalak, MD

Associate Professor of Anesthesiology, Cleveland Clinic Lerner College of Medicine, and Director of Anesthesia for Bronchoscopic Surgery,
Anesthesiology Institute, Cleveland Clinic, Cleveland, Ohio, USA

D. John Doyle, MD, PhD

Professor of Anesthesiology, Cleveland Clinic Lerner College of Medicine, and Staff Anesthesiologist,
Anesthesiology Institute, Cleveland Clinic, Cleveland, Ohio, USA

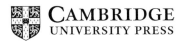

CAMBRIDGE
UNIVERSITY PRESS

CAMBRIDGE UNIVERSITY PRESS
Cambridge, New York, Melbourne, Madrid, Cape Town,
Singapore, São Paulo, Delhi, Mexico City

Cambridge University Press
The Edinburgh Building, Cambridge CB2 8RU, UK

Published in the United States of America
by Cambridge University Press, New York

www.cambridge.org
Information on this title: www.cambridge.org/9781107018679

First published 2013

Printed and bound in Great Britain by the MPG Books Group

A catalog record for this publication is available from the British Library

Library of Congress Cataloging in Publication data

Anesthesia for otolaryngologic surgery / edited by Basem Abdelmalak,
D. John Doyle.
    p.   cm.
    Includes index.
    ISBN 978-1-107-01867-9 (Hardback)
    1. Anesthesia in otolaryngology.   I. Abdelmalak, Basem.   II. Doyle,
D. John (Daniel John), 1951–
    RF52.A483 2013
    617.9′6751–dc23

                                                        2012020421

ISBN 978-1-107-01867-9 Hardback

We are particularly grateful for the wonderful support at home that we have despite having to give up family time for this endeavor. Special thanks should also go to the wonderful editorial team at Cambridge University Press, whose professionalism never ceased to amaze us. Finally, we are both grateful for the wonderful clinical environment provided by Cleveland Clinic that inspired us to produce this volume.

I am eternally grateful to my wife Lisa, my children David and Jeremy and my late parents for all they have done and the wonderful encouragement they have provided. Thanks also to all my mentors who have taught me so well, and my dear friend John Doyle; without his help this text book would not have existed.
Basem Abdelmalak

Special thanks to my wife of over three decades Dr. Jo-Anne Williams, my son Jonathan, my parents-in-law, and my late parents. I'm also grateful to the many residents who have kept me both young and humble. And finally, special thanks to Basem, who taught me that "good enough" is just not good enough.
John Doyle

Contents

Foreword by Prof. Hannenberg   ix
Foreword by Prof. Benninger   x
List of contributors   xi
Preface   xv

Section 1   Introduction

1   **Clinical head and neck anatomy for the anesthesiologist**   1
Nicole M. Fowler and Joseph Scharpf

2   **Otolaryngology instruments 101 for the anesthesiologist**   18
Paul C. Bryson and Michael S. Benninger

3   **Preoperative evaluation for ENT surgery**   26
Jie Zhou and Linda S. Aglio

4   **The difficult airway in otolaryngology**   36
D. John Doyle

5   **Preoperative endoscopic airway examination**   50
William H. Rosenblatt

6   **Awake intubation**   58
Carlos A. Artime and Carin A. Hagberg

7   **Anesthesia for ENT trauma**   83
Matthew R. Eng and Marshal B. Kaplan

8   **Anesthesia for ENT emergencies**   90
D. John Doyle

9   **Airway pathology in otolaryngology: anesthetic implications**   94
D. John Doyle

10   **Use of Heliox in managing stridor: an ENT perspective**   101
D. John Doyle

11   **Prevention and management of airway fires**   105
D. John Doyle

Section 2   Anesthesia for nasal, sinus and pituitary surgery

12   **Anesthesia for septoplasty and rhinoplasty**   113
Ursula Galway and Daniel Alam

13   **Anesthesia for endoscopic sinus surgery**   121
Paul Kempen

14   **Anesthesia for transsphenoidal pituitary surgery**   133
Gazanfar Rahmathulla, Robert Weil and David E. Traul

Section 3   Anesthesia for head and neck surgery

15   **Anesthesia for neck dissection and laryngectomy**   143
David W. Healy and Carol R. Bradford

16   **Anesthesia for head and neck flap reconstructive surgery**   151
Edward Noguera, Brian Burkey and Basem Abdelmalak

17   **Anesthesia for thyroid and parathyroid surgery**   163
Twain Russell and Richard M. Cooper

18   **Anesthesia for obstructive sleep apnea surgery**   175
Ursula Galway and Alan Kominsky

19   **Anesthesia for carotid body tumor resection**   186
Maged Argalious and Sivan Wexler

vii

20 **Anesthesia for Zenker's diverticulectomy** 195
Ashish Khanna, Benjamin Wood and
Basem Abdelmalak

21 **Anesthesia for parotid surgery** 203
Mauricio Perilla, Biao Lei and Daniel Alam

22 **Anesthesia for maxillary, salivary gland, mandibular and temporomandibular joint surgery** 210
Gail I. Randel and Tracey Straker

23 **Anesthesia for face transplantation** 220
Jacek B. Cywinski, Thomas Edrich and
D. John Doyle

24 **Anesthesia for airway panendoscopy** 228
Louise Ellard and David T. Wong

25 **Anesthesia for ENT laser surgery** 237
D. John Doyle

Section 4   Anesthesia for laryngotracheal surgery

26 **Anesthesia for laryngoplasty** 245
Michael S. Benninger and Tatyana Kopyeva

27 **Anesthesia for tracheotomy** 255
Onur Demirci and Marc Popovich

28 **Anesthesia for the management of subglottic stenosis and tracheal resection** 263
John George III and D. John Doyle

29 **Anesthesia for otologic and neurotologic surgery** 271
Vladimir Nekhendzy

Section 5   Anesthesia for bronchoscopic surgery

30 **Anesthesia for diagnostic bronchoscopic procedures** 297
Basem Abdelmalak and Mona Sarkiss

31 **Anesthesia for therapeutic bronchoscopic procedures** 309
Basem Abdelmalak and Mona Sarkiss

Section 6   Anesthesia for pediatric ENT surgery

32 **Anesthesia for pediatric otolaryngologic surgery** 321
Rahul G. Baijal and Emad B. Mossad

33 **Anesthesia for reconstructive airway surgery in pediatrics** 337
Megan Nolan and David S. Beebe

Index 346

Foreword

Medical historians enjoy a spirited debate about whether Dr. Crawford Long or Dr. William T.G. Morton deserves credit for introducing ether anesthesia. Long used the agent in 1842 in Georgia, but his work was largely unnoticed. In 1846, Dr. Morton made a public demonstration of ether anesthesia in Boston and quickly published his work, achieving widespread notice and revolutionizing medicine. Notably, it was head and neck surgery in both instances that was performed at the dawn of modern anesthesiology, forming a deep connection between otolaryngology and anesthesiology that carries on in this volume.

There may be no area of surgical specialization for which seamless coordination with the anesthesiologist is of such paramount importance. The shared, perhaps compromised, airway demands that each physician approach the patient with a deep understanding of each other's needs and abilities. More so than in many surgical fields, the ENT patient can be a newborn or a centenarian and the anesthesia knowledge base is correspondingly broad. The pace of innovation in ENT surgery has been relentless, with the introduction of advanced laser therapies, image guided procedures and endoscopic approaches. All these considerations demand an up-to-date reference for anesthesiologists involved in these procedures.

The editors have assembled a group of authors who have devoted their anesthesia careers to the highest level of care for patients undergoing the full range of otolaryngologic surgery. They come from institutions in which innovations in ENT surgery are developed and practiced. All of us now have the opportunity to benefit from their experience.

Alexander A. Hannenberg, MD
Boston, January 2012
Past President, American Society of Anesthesiologists
Clinical Professor of Anesthesiology,
Tufts University School of Medicine;
Associate Chair, Department of Anesthesiology,
Newton-Wellesley Hospital.

Foreword 2

The management of anesthesia for any surgical procedure is of the highest importance and is often fraught with difficulty and risk. This is particularly true for patients undergoing otolaryngology surgery. Compounding these issues is the pathology (tumor, infection, trauma, etc.) that prompted the need for surgery in the first place.

An otolaryngologic procedure case typically requires multiple exchanges of real-time clinical information between the surgeon and the anesthesia provider. There are few circumstances where preoperative planning and a formal "huddle" around the patient to discuss planned management are more critical than in an ENT patient. The roles of each member of the anesthesia, surgical and nursing team should be explicitly identified, and specific steps to ensure maximum safety should be articulated. All the necessary equipment should be available and ready. The group should also be prepared for unexpected problems that may necessitate the execution of a back-up plan.

Although this is not per se a textbook on clinical airway management, airway issues naturally arise on a regular basis in otolaryngology surgery. This is particularly true of upper airway surgery, which relies heavily on the coordinated efforts of both the anesthesia and surgical teams. In such cases these teams need to plan a coordinated approach to establishing a safe airway, must maintain that airway during the procedure and have to ensure that the airway is maintained as the procedure ends. There are many times throughout the procedure where the control of the airway needs to be shared or complete control relegated from one team to the other. This exchange requires not only knowledgeable team members and timely communication; it requires seamless transition and continuous vigilance.

This book will help to illustrate the complexities of anesthesia in the otolaryngology patient. It will help to identify the key procedures that are performed and the surgical and anesthesia set-up needed to protect the patient during the procedure. Besides airway management considerations, it details the other anesthetic considerations, systematically presented in the form of preoperative consideration, intraoperative management, as well as postoperative care and potential complications. Of great importance, the book highlights the significance of communication between the clinical teams and such a detailed "full picture" presentation of class of or individual procedures is expected to help greatly facilitate such communications. Only with an experienced and prepared combined effort can the procedures be performed in a safe and efficient manner.

Michael S. Benninger, MD
Chairman, Head and Neck Institute
Cleveland Clinic, President of the American Laryngological Association, and President of the International Association of Phonosurgery.

Contributors

Basem Abdelmalak, MD
Associate Professor of Anesthesiology, Departments of General Anesthesiology and Outcomes Research, Director, Anesthesia for Bronchoscopic Surgery, Director, Center for Sedation, Anesthesiology Institute, Cleveland Clinic, Cleveland, OH, USA

Linda S. Aglio, MD, MS
Director of Otorhinolaryngologic Anesthesia and Neuroanesthesia, Department of Anesthesiology, Perioperative and Pain Medicine, Brigham and Women's Hospital and Associate Professor of Anesthesia, Harvard Medical School, Boston, MA, USA

Daniel Alam, MD
Section Head Aesthetic & Reconstructive Surgery, Department of Otolaryngology, Head and Neck Institute, Cleveland Clinic, Cleveland, OH, USA

Maged Argalious, MD, MBA
Associate Professor of Anesthesiology, Medical Director, PACU and SDS, Cleveland Clinic, Cleveland, OH, USA

Carlos A. Artime, MD
Assistant Professor of Anesthesiology, Department of Anesthesiology, The University of Texas Medical School at Houston, TX, USA

Rahul G. Baijal, MD
Baylor College of Medicine, Texas Children's Hospital Department of Pediatrics and Anesthesiology, Houston, TX, USA

David Beebe, MD
Professor of Anesthesiology, Department of Anesthesiology, University of Minnesota Medical School, Minneapolis, MN, USA

Michael S. Benninger, MD
Chairman, Head and Neck Institute, Cleveland Clinic and Professor of Surgery, Cleveland Clinic Lerner College of Medicine of Case Western Reserve University, Cleveland, OH, USA

Carol R. Bradford, MD
Professor and Chair, University of Michigan Department of Otolaryngology, Ann Arbor, MI, USA

Paul C. Bryson
Staff Otolaryngologist, Department of Otolaryngology, Cleveland Clinic Foundation, Cleveland, OH, USA

Brian Burkey, MD
Adjunct Professor, Department of Otolaryngology, Vanderbilt University Medical Center and Staff Surgeon, Head and Neck Institute, Cleveland Clinic, Cleveland, OH, USA

Richard M. Cooper BSc, MSc, MD, FRCPC
Professor, Faculty of Medicine, University of Toronto and Toronto General Hospital, Department of Anesthesia and Pain Management, Toronto, Canada

Jacek B. Cywinski
Assistant Professor of Anesthesiology, Cleveland Clinic Lerner College of Medicine Department of General Anesthesiology, Cleveland Clinic Foundation, Cleveland, OH, USA

Onur Demirci, MD
Department of General Anesthesiology, Cleveland Clinic, Cleveland, OH, USA

D. John Doyle, MD, PhD
Professor of Anesthesiology and Staff Anesthesiologist, Department of General Anesthesiology, Cleveland Clinic, Cleveland, OH, USA

Thomas Edrich, MD, PhD
Department of Anesthesiology, Perioperative and Pain Medicine, Brigham and Women's Hospital, Boston, MA, USA

Louise Ellard, MBBS
Clinical fellow, Department of Anesthesia, University Health Network, University of Toronto, Toronto, Canada

Matthew R. Eng, MD
Department of Anesthesiology, Cedars-Sinai Medical Center, Los Angeles, CA, USA

Nicole M. Fowler, MD
Head and Neck Institute, Cleveland Clinic, Cleveland, OH, USA

Ursula Galway, MD
Assistant Professor of Anesthesiology, Cleveland Clinic Lerner College of Medicine, Staff Anesthesiologist, Department of General Anesthesiology, Cleveland Clinic, Cleveland, OH, USA

John George III, MD
Department of General Anesthesiology, Cleveland Clinic, Cleveland, OH, USA

Carin A. Hagberg, MD
Joseph C. Gabel Professor and Chair, Department of Anesthesiology, The University of Texas Medical School at Houston, TX, USA

David W. Healy, MD, MRCP, FRCA
Assistant Professor and Director, Head and Neck Anesthesiology, University of Michigan Department of Anesthesiology, Ann Arbor, MI, USA

Marshal B. Kaplan, MD
Attending Anesthesiologist, Cedars-Sinai Medical Center and Associate Clinical Professor, Department of Anesthesiology, UCLA David Geffen School of Medicine, Los Angeles, CA, USA

Paul Kempen, MD, PhD
Department of General Anesthesiology, Cleveland Clinic, Cleveland, OH, USA

Ashish Khanna, MD
Anesthesiology Resident, Anesthesiology Institute, Cleveland Clinic, Cleveland, OH, USA

Alan Kominsky, MD
Staff Surgeon, Department of otolaryngology, Head and Neck Institute, Cleveland Clinic, Cleveland, OH, USA

Tatyana Kopyeva MD
Staff Anesthesiologist, Department of General Anesthesiology, Anesthesiology Institute, Cleveland Clinic, Cleveland, OH, USA

Biao Lei, MD, PhD
Anesthesiology Resident, Anesthesiology Institute, Cleveland Clinic, Cleveland, OH, USA

Emad B. Mossad, MD
Professor of Anesthesiology, Baylor College of Medicine, Texas Children's Hospital Department of Pediatrics and Anesthesiology, Houston, TX, USA

Vladimir Nekhendzy, MD
Clinical Associate Professor of Anesthesia and Otolaryngology and Chief, ENT Anesthesia Division, Director, Difficult Airway Management Program, Stanford University School of Medicine, Stanford, CA, USA

Edward Noguera, MD
Attending Intensivist, Associate Instructor Case Western Reserve University Medical School, and Director, Surgical ICU, Louis Stokes Cleveland VA Medical Center, Cleveland, OH, USA

Megan Nolan, MD
Assistant Professor, Anesthesiology, Department of Anesthesiology, University of Minnesota Medical School, Minneapolis, MN, USA

Mauricio Perilla, MD
Staff Anesthesiologist, Section Head of Anesthesia, Glickman Urological Institute, Department of General Anesthesiology, Anesthesiology Institute, Cleveland Clinic, Cleveland, OH, USA

Marc Popovich, MD
Director of Surgical Intensive Care Unit, Department of General Anesthesiology, Cleveland Clinic, Cleveland, OH, USA

Gazanfar Rahmathulla, MD
Clinical Scholar, Neurosurgery Program, Burkhardt Brain Tumor & Neuro-Oncology Center, Department of Neurosurgery, Neurological Institute, Cleveland Clinic, Cleveland, OH, USA

Gail I. Randel, MD
Associate Clinical Professor, Northwestern Memorial Hospital, Feinberg School of Medicine, Chicago, IL, USA

William H. Rosenblatt, MD
Professor of Anesthesiology and Surgery, Yale University School of Medicine, New Haven, CT, USA

Twain Russell, MBBS, FRACGP, FANZCA
Anaesthesia Department, Sir Charles Gairdner Hospital, Hospital Ave, Nedlands, Western Australia, Australia

Mona Sarkiss, MD
Associate Professor of Anesthesiology, Department of Anesthesiology and Perioperative Medicine, Department of Pulmonary Medicine, University of Texas MD Anderson Cancer Center, Houston, TX, USA

Joseph Scharpf, MD
Staff Surgeon, Head and Neck Institute, Cleveland Clinic, Cleveland, OH, USA

Tracey Straker, MD, MPH
Associate Clinical Professor, Montefiore Medical Center, Albert Einstein College of Medicine, New York, NY, USA

David E. Traul, MD, PhD
Staff Anesthesiologist, Department of General Anesthesiology, Anesthesiology Institute, Cleveland Clinic, Cleveland, OH, USA

Robert Weil, MD
Staff Neurosurgeon, Burkhardt Brain Tumor & Neuro-Oncology Center, Department of Neurosurgery, Neurological Institute, Cleveland Clinic, Cleveland, OH, USA

Sivan Wexler, MD
Staff Anesthesiologist, Department of General Anesthesiology, Anesthesiology Institute, Cleveland Clinic, Cleveland, OH, USA

David T. Wong, MD
Associate Professor, Department of Anesthesia, University Health Network, University of Toronto, Toronto, Canada

Benjamin Wood, MD
Staff Surgeon, Head and Neck Institute, Cleveland Clinic, Cleveland, OH, USA

Jie Zhou, MD, MS, MBA
Staff Anesthesiologist, Department of Anesthesiology, Perioperative and Pain Medicine, Brigham and Women's Hospital, Harvard Medical School, Boston, MA, USA

Preface

This textbook was motivated by our discovery that there is a serious dearth of detailed information on the topic of anesthesia for ENT surgery in current anesthesiology texts. (For instance Kathryn E. McGoldrick's book *Anesthesia for Ophthalmic and Otolaryngologic Surgery* is now over 20 years old.) In most anesthesia books, anesthesia for ENT surgery shares a chapter with anesthesia for ophthalmologic procedures. However, because of size limitations, such chapters have barely enough information to begin to describe what it is like to provide safe, effective anesthesia for these often highly specialized procedures. In addition, anesthesia airway textbooks focus often on the management of the difficult airway, and airway devices, more so than discussing the broad spectrum of the anesthetic management options for otolaryngologic surgery. Thus, there is an information gap we seek to address.

This textbook is designed to provide an account of the currently available evidence in the field of anesthesia for ENT surgery. When rigorous scientific evidence is lacking (regretfully, this is still the case in many areas of medicine and surgery) expert opinion on the management of these often very complex procedures is offered. In addition, many new procedures have been introduced to the field, such as laryngoplasty, jaw and face reconstruction, and facial transplantation, which we cover in this volume. However, we have omitted some extremely rare procedures like laryngeal and tracheal transplantation. Also, the new expanding field of bronchoscopic surgery performed by ENT surgeons, pulmonologists, and thoracic surgeons is a one that only a specialized book like this would be able to discuss in detail.

In an attempt to make our textbook clinically relevant, we have ended many clinical chapters with clinical case descriptions where the concepts discussed in the chapter are applied to a clinical scenario. In addition, some especially important topics are covered briefly in early overview chapters and are covered in more detail later. We believe that this macro/micro approach has been helpful in our teaching and hope that it will also be successful here.

The diversity of the authors' institutions, background expertise, and geographical location was intentional, as it allows us to present different examples of clinical practice. For example, smooth emergence from anesthesia is one of the much sought after goals in the majority of otolaryngologic surgical procedures, and a number of chapters discuss completely different ways to accomplish that goal. Indeed, in many chapters, the presented anesthetic plan is not the editors' first choice, but is presented in the spirit of clinical diversity and clinical richness. It should similarly follow that this book is not intended as a resource to definitively state standards of clinical care so much as it aims to offer clinicians broad approaches to tackle difficult, sometimes unique, situations in ENT surgery.

Finally, we would like to point out that many chapters are intentionally co-authored by an anesthesiologist and a surgeon, to make sure that the chapter is providing an accurate account from both points of view.

We sincerely hope that this textbook will be of great value to both practicing clinicians and trainees, with the ultimate goal of improving patient safety and comfort.

Basem Abdelmalak
D. John Doyle
Cleveland, February 2012

Clinical head and neck anatomy for the anesthesiologist

Nicole M. Fowler and Joseph Scharpf

Introduction

An understanding of anatomy is paramount to the ability to safely anesthetize the head and neck surgery patient. In contrast to other patient populations, the head and neck surgery patient's pathology may obfuscate normal anatomy and impede or even prevent the anesthesiologist from being able to intubate the patient. Furthermore, recognized anatomic variations may complicate the anesthesiologist's management of the patient. Cooperation among the entire operating team is the key to a successful operation. The surgeon and anesthesiologist must discuss the particular patient's anatomy and specific procedural needs prior to each case. Potential airway management options such as routine oral intubation, nasotracheal intubation, awake fiberoptic intubation and even awake tracheotomy must be considered. Contemporary technological advances can enhance this discussion by including photography and videography. For example, computerized imaging systems in use in modern operating rooms can be synchronized to a server in the otolaryngology clinic to allow the review of both photographs and videos of patients' airways and the extent that they have been altered through disease progression. While the added dimension of visual review integrated into the discussion can be an invaluable adjunct to this team approach, always bear in mind that conditions could have worsened significantly since the imaging was performed.

Patient safety concerns continue to be increasingly recognized as a vital component of modern health care. At the authors' institution we perform both an operative "huddle" with the patient awake and a surgical "time-out" prior to performing any procedure. The huddle is an ideal time to review the intubation plan including the use or avoidance of long-acting muscle relaxants for the case. The huddle process also ensures that both the anesthesiologist and surgeon are present and ready to handle any potential perioperative complications. The head and neck surgeon should be considered an airway specialist and partner with the anesthesiologist.

Face anatomy

The basic underlying structure of the face is formed by the skull, facial bones and mandible (Figure 1.1). The skull is formed by a series of eight bones: paired parietal and temporal bones and single frontal, occipital, sphenoid and ethmoid bones [1]. The facial skeleton creates the anterior portion of the skull and includes the orbits, nares, maxilla and mandible. The face is formed by 12 uniquely shaped bones: paired lacrimal bones, nasal bones, maxillae, zygomatic and palatine bones and a single vomer and mandible. The maxillae and mandible support the teeth (Figure 1.1). The teeth are numbered from superior right to left and inferior left to right from 1 to 32 for adults and lettered A–T in the same order for pediatric primary dentition. Normal occlusion, also termed class I occlusion, is defined by the mesiobuccal cusp of the first maxillary molar impacting the mesiobuccal groove of the first mandibular molar [2]. Class II occlusion, commonly referred to as retrognathic, occurs when the mesiobuccal cusp of the first maxillary molar impacts mesial to the groove (overbite). Class III occlusion, commonly referred to as prognathic, occurs when the mesiobuccal cusp of the first maxillary molar impacts distal to the groove (underbite).

Trauma resulting in facial fractures can complicate intubation. Mandibular fractures are usually

Anesthesia for Otolaryngologic Surgery, ed. Basem Abdelmalak and D. John Doyle. Published by Cambridge University Press.
© Cambridge University Press 2013.

(A)

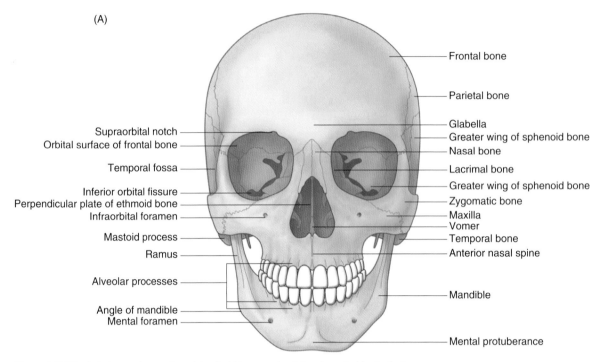

Frontal bone

Parietal bone

Glabella
Greater wing of sphenoid bone
Nasal bone

Lacrimal bone

Greater wing of sphenoid bone
Zygomatic bone
Maxilla
Vomer
Temporal bone
Anterior nasal spine

Mandible

Mental protuberance

Supraorbital notch
Orbital surface of frontal bone

Temporal fossa

Inferior orbital fissure
Perpendicular plate of ethmoid bone
Infraorbital foramen

Mastoid process
Ramus

Alveolar processes

Angle of mandible
Mental foramen

Figure 1.1 (A). Anterior cranium and overlying facial topography. Artwork created by Emily Evans.

paired and occur on opposite sides of the mandible. Fractures of the maxillae are commonly categorized based on the Le Fort classification [3]. Le Fort I fracture is a horizontal fracture of the maxilla superior to the alveolar process and the pterygoid plates of the sphenoid. Le Fort II fractures involve an oblique fracture of the maxillary sinus and horizontal fractures of the lacrimal and ethmoid bones across the nose resulting in an unstable midface where the hard palate is separated from the skull. Le Fort III fractures involve a horizontal fracture through the superior orbital fissure, the ethmoid and nasal bones through the greater wing of the sphenoid bone and frontozygomatic sutures. This may occur in conjunction with fractures of the zygomatic arches resulting in an unstable midface where the maxilla and zygomatic bones are no longer attached to the skull. If significant facial trauma has occurred the patient may have resulting skull and brain injuries which may supersede treatment of the facial injuries. Depending on the severity of the trauma, the airway may have been triaged in the field and an emergency cricothyroidotomy or tracheotomy may have already been performed if an oral intubation was not possible. When preparing to intubate a patient with a mandibular fracture carefully evaluate the teeth as the tooth roots are areas of bony weakness and may be involved in the fracture. Orbital fractures commonly of the inferior orbital rim may result in entrapment of the extraocular muscles; in particular, the inferior rectus can result in activation of the oculocardiac reflex [4]. This reflex between the trigeminal and vagus nerve can result in bradycardia, a junctional rhythm, asystole or even death. Treatment includes surgical release of the muscle, atropine or glycopyrrolate.

Face shape is determined by the bones, muscles and subcutaneous tissue (Figure 1.2). The muscles of facial expression lie within the subcutaneous tissue. The muscles of facial expression are innervated by the facial nerve. They generally attach to bone or fascia and act by pulling the skin to create facial expression. When performing surgery around the facial nerve or its branches, including otologic procedures, parotidectomy, submandibular gland excision and neck dissections, neuromuscular blockage is contraindicated and all or part of the ipsilateral face may need to be included in the surgical field for monitoring.

(B)

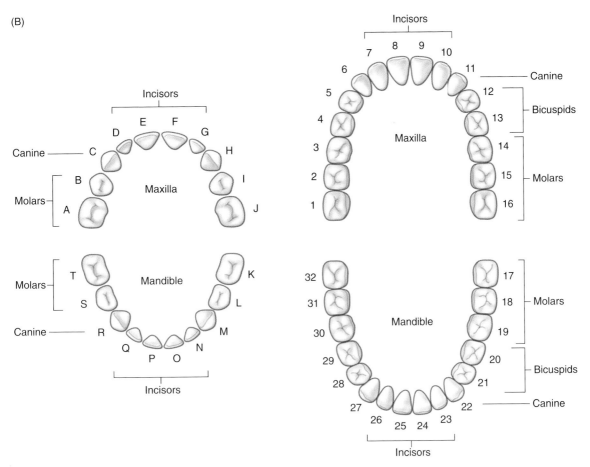

Figure 1.1 (B). The teeth are numbered from superior right to left and inferior left to right from 1 to 32 for adults and lettered A to T in the same order for pediatric primary dentition.

Ear anatomy

The ear is divided into three parts: the external, middle and internal. The external ear (Figure 1.3) includes the external auditory canal to the tympanic membrane. This is approximately 2–3 cm in length. The lateral one-third is cartilaginous and the inner two-thirds is composed of skin directly on the periosteum of the tympanic portion of the temporal bone. The middle ear is an air-filled cavity containing the three auricular ossicles – the malleus, incus, and stapes. The middle ear pressure is regulated by the eustachian tube, which opens into the nasopharynx. The inner ear is contained within the petrous portion of the temporal bone and includes the cochlea, vestibule and semicircular canals. The cochlear hair cells activate the cochlear nerve, resulting in hearing transmission. The vestibule is a small oval chamber containing the saccule and utricle, which along with the semicircular canals control balance. The labyrinthine and tympanic portions of the facial nerve lie in close proximity to these structures and may be dehiscent, necessitating lack of neuromuscular blockade and close monitoring of facial movements during certain otologic procedures.

Nose anatomy

The nose projects from the face largely based on the amount of cartilage. Extending from the nasal bone are the upper and lower lateral cartilages. Stability is provided from the underlying nasal septum which is also composed of both bone and cartilage. The posterior bony septum is formed from the perpendicular plate of the ethmoid and vomer but the majority of the septum, the anterior septum, is the quadrangular

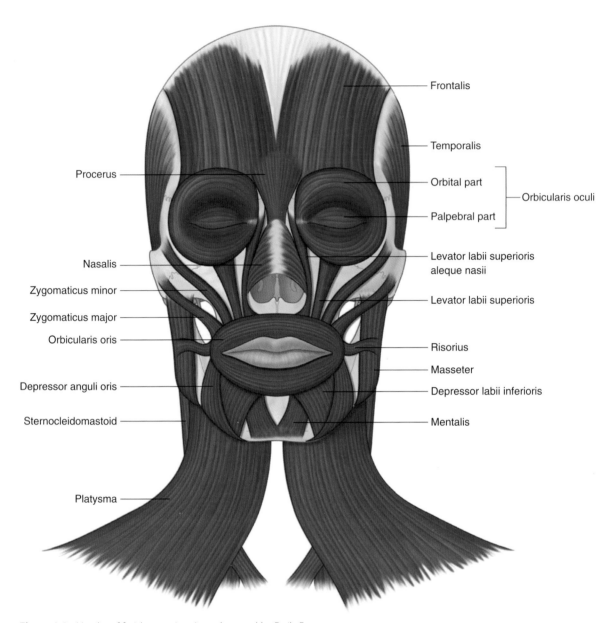

Figure 1.2. Muscles of facial expression. Artwork created by Emily Evans.

cartilage. The nasal ala are supported by U-shaped alar cartilage which is free and mobile, allowing the dilatation or constriction of each nostril. In preparation for a nasotracheal intubation or a fiberoptic intubation the nares should be examined for any septal deviation. The degree and site of deviation may help decide which nostril to use for the intubation. Care must be taken when placing any foreign object into the nose because of its robust blood supply. The anterior nasal septal area is referred to as Kiesselbach's plexus and is the site of a capillary anastomosis from the sphenopalatine artery, anterior and posterior ethmoid arteries, greater palatine artery and the superior labial artery. Any object placed into the nose should be directed along the floor of the nose, which is wider than the roof. In preparation for any nasal manipulation the nasal mucosa should be treated with a vasoconstrictor and anesthetic.

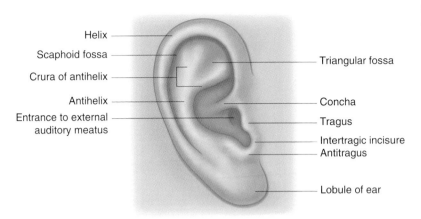

Figure 1.3. External ear structure. Artwork created by Emily Evans.

A vasoconstrictor such as phenylephrine or oxymetazoline will act on the erectile tissues of the nasal mucosa and result in decongestion and opening of the nasal passages. If profuse bleeding occurs pressure should be applied, and medications such as oxymetazoline (Afrin), phenylephrine or an epinephrine-soaked pledget can be placed into the nares. Following successful nasotracheal intubation extreme care must be taken to position the nasotracheal tube such that it is not applying pressure to the nasal alar skin. Even slight pressure can result in necrosis of the alar skin. Within each nostril are the three turbinates, inferior, middle and superior, which increase the surface area for humidification and warming of the inspired air. The paranasal sinuses are air-filled spaces extending into the frontal, ethmoid, sphenoid and maxillary bones. Since the advent of the endoscope much of rhinology has become endoscopic.

Mouth anatomy

The mouth is subdivided into the oral cavity and the oropharynx. The oral cavity begins at the skin–vermilion junction of the lips and extends posteriorly to the junction of the hard and soft palate superiorly and to the line of the circumvallate papillae on the tongue inferiorly. The oral cavity therefore includes the lips, buccal mucosa, maxillary and mandibular alveolar ridges/teeth/gingiva, floor of the mouth, hard palate, the retromolar trigone and the anterior oral tongue (Figure 1.4). The hard palate forms the roof of the mouth and separates the oral cavity from the anterior nasal vault. It is composed of the palatine

process of the maxilla and the horizontal plate of the palatine bone. Figure 1.5 shows a primary tonsillar cancer with extension to the soft palate. Tumors are very friable and will bleed easily so in this patient great care was taken to avoid any manipulation of the palate. The retromolar trigone is a triangular area just anterior to the ascending ramus of the mandible. A triangle is drawn with its medial aspect coinciding with the anterior tonsillar pillar, the base being across the mandibular alveolus posterior to the last molar and its apex being the coronoid process. In this area the mucosa is tightly adherent to the ascending ramus of the mandible. Carcinomas originating in this region tend to invade the mandibular periosteum and medial pterygoid muscle causing significant trismus. Referred otalgia is also a common symptom due to innervation by the mandibular branch of the trigeminal nerve, the lesser palatine nerve and the glossopharyngeal nerve. The circumvallate papillae and terminal sulcus divide the tongue into an anterior two-thirds and posterior one-third. The anterior two-thirds of the tongue can largely be easily visualized by the patient and clinician. Patients will routinely present with a small non-healing ulcer or sore lesion. The oral tongue is composed of three extrinsic tongue muscles: the genioglossus, hyoglossus and styloglossus muscles (Figure 1.6; Table 1.1a). In combination with the intrinsic tongue musculature these muscles assist with speech articulation and deglutition. The tongue musculature is innervated by the hypoglossal nerve (CN XII). Taste to the anterior oral tongue is supplied by the lingual nerve (CN V3) having received fibers from the chorda typani nerve. As these nerve fibers travel with those to the external ear, external

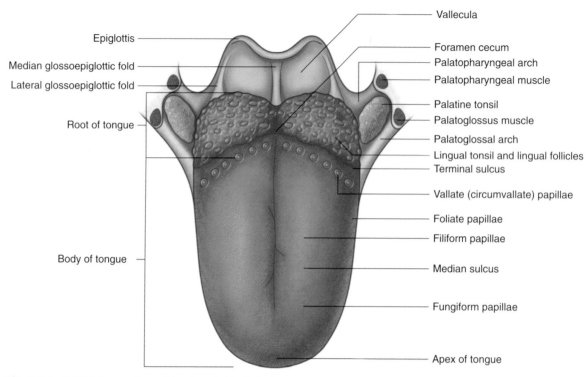

Vallecula
Epiglottis
Foramen cecum
Median glossoepiglottic fold
Palatopharyngeal arch
Lateral glossoepiglottic fold
Palatopharyngeal muscle
Palatine tonsil
Root of tongue
Palatoglossus muscle
Palatoglossal arch
Lingual tonsil and lingual follicles
Terminal sulcus
Vallate (circumvallate) papillae
Foliate papillae
Filiform papillae
Body of tongue
Median sulcus
Fungiform papillae
Apex of tongue

Figure 1.4. Dorsal tongue anatomy. Artwork created by Emily Evans.

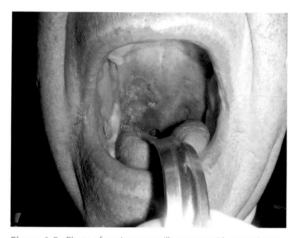

Figure 1.5. Photo of a primary tonsillar cancer with extension to the soft palate. Photo courtesy of Dr. Joseph Scharpf.

auditory canal and tympanic membrane referred otalgia is a common presenting symptom with tongue cancers. Lateral tongue cancers drain to the ipsilateral level IB or II nodes. The medial tongue may drain directly to level III. The tip of the tongue drains to level IA. The floor of the mouth is the mucosa lying between the mandibular alveolus and the oral tongue.

This area is pierced by the submandibular gland duct (Wharton's duct) bilaterally on either side of the lingual frenulum. The length and site of attachment of the lingual frenulum on the ventral surface of the tongue can affect tongue protrusion. Tethering of the tongue is termed ankyloglossus and can be surgically cut if it affects speech articulation or feeding as an infant. Odontogenic infections can become life-threatening if they spread into the submental or submandibular spaces. Ludwig's angina is a severe infection involving the floor of mouth. As the infection and swelling worsens the tongue is pushed posteriorly and superiorly, causing respiratory obstruction. The patient may have marked trismus in addition to odynophagia and may have dysphagia to the extent that they cannot tolerate their own secretions. Infections in this space are considered an airway emergency and may require an awake tracheotomy for management. Complete airway obstruction is the most frequent cause of death from this disease [2]. The oropharynx extends from an imaginary line extending back from the hard palate superiorly to the level of the hyoid bone inferiorly and includes the soft palate, tonsils, base of tongue and posterior pharyngeal wall. This

Table 1.1a. Muscles of the soft palate. Reproduced with permission from Olson TR, Pawlina W. *ADAM Student Atlas of Anatomy*. Cambridge University Press, 2008

Muscle	Superior attachment	Inferior attachment	Innervation	Main actions
Levator veli palatini	Cartilage of auditory tube and petrous part of temporal bone	Palatine aponeurosis	Pharyngeal br. of vagus n. via pharyngeal plexus (CN X)	Elevates soft palate during swallowing and yawning
Tensor veli palatini	Scaphoid fossa of medial pterygoid plate, spine of sphenoid bone & cartilage of auditory tube		Medial pterygoid n. (a br. of the mandibular n.) via otic ganglion (CN V3)	Tenses soft palate and opens cartilagenous part of auditory tube during swallowing and yawning
Palatoglossus	Palatine aponeurosis	Side of tongue	Pharyngeal br. of vagus n. (CN X) via pharyngeal plexus	Elevates posterior part of tongue and draws soft palate onto tongue
Palatopharyngeus	Hard palate and palatine aponeurosis	Lateral wall of pharynx		Tenses soft palate and pulls walls of pharynx superiorly, anteriorly, and medially during swallowing
Musculus uvulae	Posterior nasal spine and palatine aponeurosis	Mucosa of uvula		Shortens uvula and pulls it superiorly

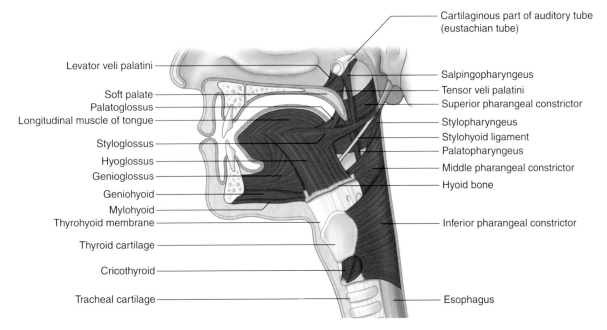

Figure 1.6. Sagittal view of the pharyngeal musculature. Artwork created by Emily Evans.

area is much more difficult to visualize for both the patient and the clinician. The pharyngeal walls are composed of mucosa, submucosa, pharyngobasilar fascia, the superior and upper middle constrictor muscle, and buccopharyngeal fascia (Figure 1.7; Table 1.1b and Table 1.2). Posterior to the buccopharyngeal fascia is the retropharyngeal space. This potential space exists between the buccopharyngeal fascia and the alar layer of the prevertebral fascia (Figure 1.7). This space extends from the skull base to the superior

Table 1.1b. Extrinsic muscles of the tongue. Reproduced with permission from Olson TR, Pawlina W. *ADAM Student Atlas of Anatomy.* Cambridge University Press, 2008

Muscle	Stable attachment	Mobile attachment	Innervation	Actions
Genioglossus	Sup. part of mental spine of mandible	Dorsum of tongue and body of hyoid bone	Hypoglossal n. CN XII	Protrudes, retracts and depresses tongue; its post. part protrudes tongue
Hyoglossus	Body and greater horn of hyoid bone	Side of tongue		Depresses and retracts tongue
Styloglossus	Styloid process and stylohyoid lig.	Side and inf. aspect of tongue		Retracts tongue and draws it up to create a trough for swallowing
Palatoglossus	Palatine aponeurosis of soft palate	Side of tongue	Pharyngeal br. CN X and pharyngeal plexus	Elevates post. part of tongue

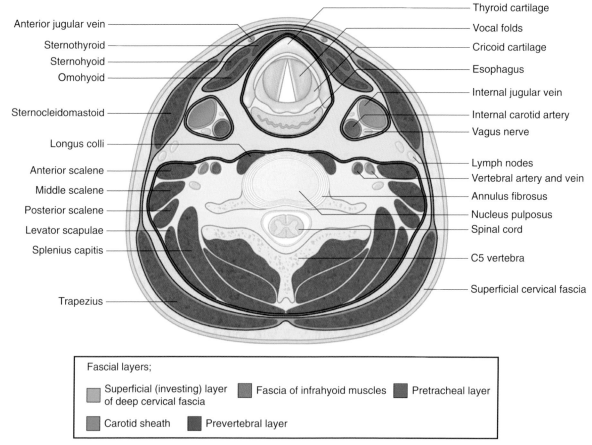

Figure 1.7. Divisions of the cervical fascia. Artwork created by Emily Evans.

Table 1.2. Pharyngeal muscles. Reproduced with permission from Olson TR, Pawlina W. *ADAM Student Atlas of Anatomy.* Cambridge University Press, 2008

Muscle	Lateral attachments	Medial attachments	Innervation	Main actions
Circular pharyngeal muscles				
Superior constrictor	Pterygoid hamulus, pterygomandibular raphe, post. end of mylohyoid line of mandible and side of tongue	Median raphe of pharynx and pharyngeal tubercle	Pharyngeal and sup. laryngeal brr. of vagus n. [CN X] through pharyngeal plexus	Constrict wall of pharynx during swallowing
Middle constrictor	Stylohyoid lig. and greater and lesser horns of hyoid bone			
Inferior constrictor	Oblique line of thyroid cartilage and side of cricoid cartilage	Median raphe of pharynx		Elevate pharynx and larynx during swallowing, speaking[a]
Longitudinal pharyngeal muscles				
Palatopharyngeus	Hard palate and palatine aponeurosis	Post. border of lamina of thyroid cartilage and side of pharynx and esophagus		
Salpingopharyngeus	Cartilaginous part of auditory tube	Blends with palatopharyngeus		
Stylopharyngeus	Styloid process of temporal bone	Post. and sup. borders of thyroid cartilage with palatopharyngeus m.	Glossopharyngeal n. [CN IX]	

[a] The salpingopharyngeus muscle also opens the auditory tube.

mediastinum. Contingent upon the patient, his or her clinical history, and the location of a retropharyngeal space abscess in relation to the great vessels (carotid artery, internal jugular vein), the abscess may be amenable to transoral drainage versus a more traditional transcervical drainage. The tonsils are housed within a fossa created by two muscles, the anterior tonsillar pillar formed from the palatoglossus muscle and the posterior tonsillar pillar by the palatopharyngeal muscle. A small primary tonsillar or base of tongue tumor may be asymptomatic and present with metastatic cervical lymphadenopathy. Careful examination of the oral excursion is advised in any patient with a tonsillar tumor as invasion into the lateral pterygoid muscle may result in trismus, which will not improve with muscular relaxation. The soft palate is composed of the levator veli palatini, tensor veli palatini, musculus uvulae and tonsillar pillars muscles as above. The base of the tongue extends from the circumvallate papillae to the glossoepiglottic fold. The lingual tonsils are found laterally and lie in a superficial plane creating an irregularity to the surface. Alternatively, base of tongue tumors may grow to very large sizes with minimal symptoms. Patients with a large base of tongue tumor may be able to maintain their airway but extreme caution should be taken prior to induction. An awake tracheotomy should be considered based on the anesthesiologist's experience and comfort with awake fiberoptic intubation.

The throat or pharynx is subdivided into the larynx and the hypopharynx. The larynx is further subdivided into three spaces: the supraglottis, glottis and subglottis. Furthermore the larynx is composed of nine cartilages joined by ligaments and membranes: three single cartilages: thyroid, cricoid and epiglottic; and three paired cartilages: arytenoid, corniculate and cuneiform (Figure 1.8). The largest of the cartilages, the thyroid cartilage, was so named from the Greek word thyreos, or shield, due to its shield-like appearance and its main function being that of protection of the vocal cords. It is composed

9

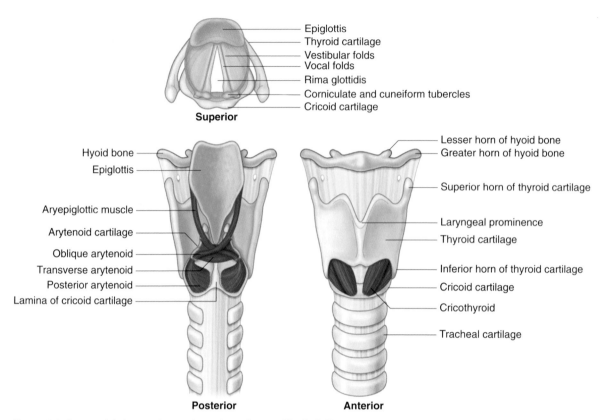

Figure 1.8. Laryngeal skeleton and musculature. Artwork created by Emily Evans.

of two large plate-like laminae which fuse in the midline forming a prominent V, which in men is termed the "Adam's apple". Inferior to the thyroid is the cricoid cartilage, which is shaped as a signet ring and is the only complete cartilaginous ring in the airway. In women the cricoid cartilage is the most prominent cartilaginous landmark. The cricothyroid membrane bridges the gap between the thyroid and cricoid cartilages. This cricothyroid space is easily palpable as a soft spot either inferior to the thyroid cartilage (in men) or immediately superior to the prominent cricoid cartilage (in women). This is the site of the most superficial aspect of the larynx that is externally accessible. An emergency cricothyroidotomy utilizes these critical features in an airway emergency. The two cartilages articulate at the cricothyroid joint. This joint allows rotation of the thyroid cartilage, resulting in changes in the vocal cord length and tension and ultimately changes in vocal pitch. Posteriorly the cricoid cartilage articulates with the arytenoid cartilage, forming the cricoarytenoid joint, which allows the arytenoids

to move medially and laterally, as well as tilt anteriorly and posteriorly. The vocal ligament is the skeleton on which the vocal cords form and extends from the thyroid cartilage to the arytenoid cartilages. The supraglottis extends from the top of the epiglottis to the ventricles. This includes the epiglottis (both lingual and laryngeal surfaces), arytenoids, aryepiglottic folds (AE folds) and false vocal cords. The epiglottis is a heart-shaped elastic cartilage which is pedicled off the thyroid cartilage extending superiorly. The epiglottis may be omega-shaped, retroflexed or floppy and may decrease the ability to visualize the vocal cords on intubation (depending on intubation technique). Sensation of the supraglottis is supplied by the internal branch of the superior laryngeal nerve. Figure 1.9A is a drawing of the laryngeal complex with a supraglottic mass centered in the epiglottis. Safe intubation techniques include an awake fiberoptic intubation. Figure 1.9B is a picture of an actual laryngeal complex having been removed as a total laryngectomy specimen for a patient with an extensive supraglottic tumor. The glottis includes each true

(A)

(B)

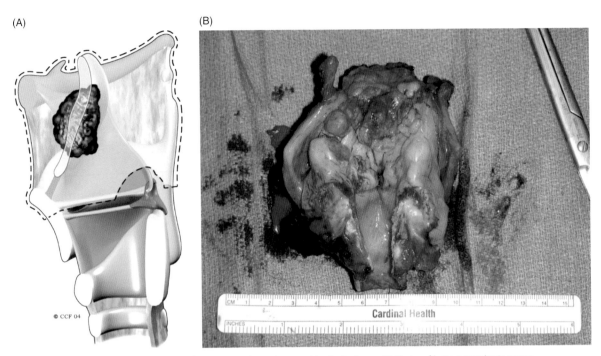

Figure 1.9. (A) Artist rendering of supraglottic tumor. Artwork created by Emily Evans. (B) Photo of large supraglottic tumor. Photo courtesy of Dr. Joseph Scharpf.

vocal cord, the anterior commissure and posterior intra-arytenoid area. The true vocal cords are instrumental in sound production and, more importantly, the prevention of aspiration and maintenance of a patent pathway for respiration. The true vocal cords are composed of the vocal ligament and the vocalis muscle (Figure 1.8). Figure 1.10A is of a large transglottic tumor and 10B is that of a very exophytic transglottic tumor. The intrinsic muscles of the larynx are all supplied by the recurrent laryngeal nerve off the vagus nerve (CN X) except for the cricothyroid muscle supplied by the external branch of the superior laryngeal nerve. There is only one main abductor of the true vocal cords; the posterior cricoarytenoid muscle. The other intrinsic laryngeal muscles (cricothyroid, lateral cricoarytenoid, thyroarytenoid, arytenoid muscles) adduct, tense or relax the vocal cords. The subglottis extends 5 mm (anteriorly) to 10 mm (posteriorly) inferior to the apex of the true vocal cords. A subglottic tumor is pictured in Figure 1.11.

Airway stenosis and particularly subglottic stenoses may result from trauma, systemic diseases (e.g. granulomatosis with polyangiitis, previously known as Wegener's granulomatosis) or without a recognizable etiology (idiopathic). It has been proposed that the subglottis is prone to stenosis due to the complete cricoid ring, lack of a direct vascular supply (it is a watershed area between two vascular beds), complex mechanical forces resulting from turbulent airflow, and exposure of the respiratory epithelium to gastric contents [5]. Due to the slowly progressive nature of the disease patients will accommodate their activity to match their breathing ability. In cases of tight airway stenosis the patient may need to be mask ventilated and jet ventilated until the stenosis has been lysed or dilated enough to accommodate an endotracheal tube. Figure 1.12A,B shows a subglottic stenosis pre- and postoperatively.

The hypopharynx extends from the level of the hyoid to the cricoid cartilage. The hypopharynx is divided into three subsites: the posterior pharyngeal wall, the post-cricoid area and the piriform sinuses. Laterally the pyriform sinuses are triangularly shaped. The base is located superiorly at the pharyngoepiglottic fold and the triangle extends to its apex at the level of the true vocal cords, medially is the larynx and laterally is the thyroid cartilage. The

11

(A)

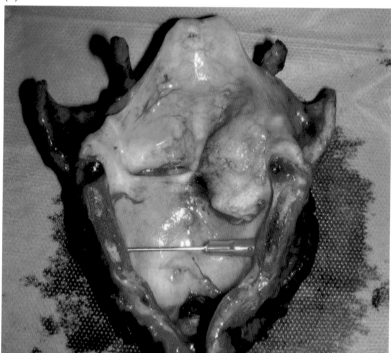

Figure 1.10. A and B; Two examples of transglottic tumors. Photos courtesy of Dr. Joseph Scharpf.

(B)

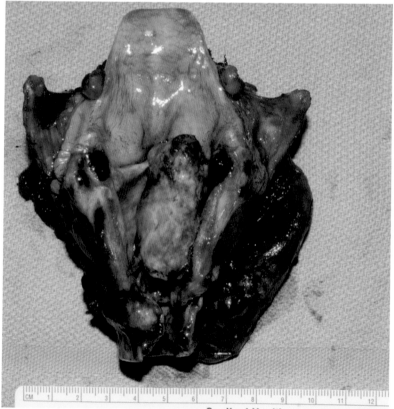

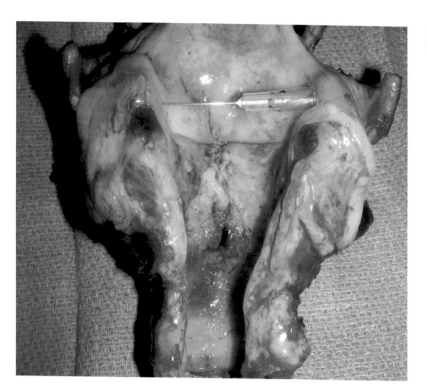

Figure 1.11. Photo of subglottic tumor. Photo courtesy of Dr. Joseph Scharpf.

(A)

(B)

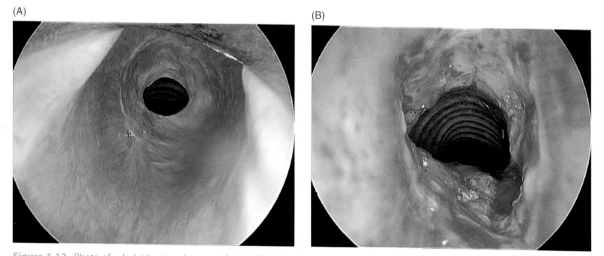

Figure 1.12. Photo of subglottic stenosis pre- and post-dilatation. Photos courtesy of Dr. Joseph Scharpf.

hypopharynx is in direct communication with the oropharynx superiorly and the cervical esophagus inferiorly. A large hypopharyngeal tumor is pictured in Figure 1.13. Inferior to the inferior constrictor is the cricopharyngeus muscle which acts as the upper esophageal sphincter. Normal resting tone prevents or reduces reflux of esophageal contents into the hypopharynx. The coordinated relaxation of the cricopharyngeus is critical for normal swallowing. The esophagus is lined by a layer of stratified squamous epithelium. The cervical esophagus is composed of voluntary striated muscle, in contrast to the lower esophagus, which is largely composed of involuntary smooth muscle.

Potential anatomy pitfalls exist for each of the categories within the oral cavity, nasopharynx,

13

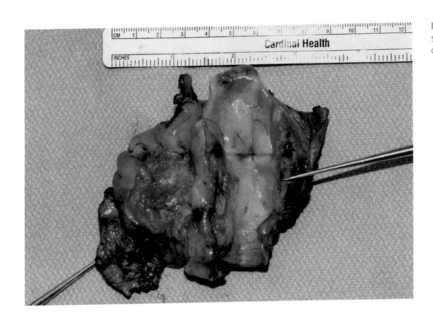

Figure 1.13. Photo of a large pyriform sinus hypopharyngeal tumor. Photo courtesy of Dr. Joseph Scharpf.

oropharynx, larynx, and hypopharynx. Within the oral cavity large masses can develop which will be readily visible and can therefore be appropriately considered prior to intubation planning. The more difficult cases occur with cancers of the retromolar trigone, tonsils or posterior oropharyngeal wall with accompanying trismus which decreases the ability to visualize the full extent of these lesions and limits the intubation options. In addition the surface overlying a cancerous growth may be ulcerated or friable and can result in significant bleeding with minimal manipulation. Base of tongue tumors may grow to a large size prior to detection or may hinder intubation not only by bulk effect but also by displacing the epiglottis posteriorly so that it overlies the vocal cords. Epiglottic tumors may cause a direct mass effect or may again overhang the vocal cords, hindering intubation. A glottic tumor or transglottic tumor may limit the glottic aperture by its bulk or may result in vocal cord immobility. The subglottic area may be stenosed, which needs to be considered when choosing the appropriate endotracheal tube size. The anesthesiologist must trust their otolaryngologist colleague regarding the size, extent and airway patency in cases of oropharyngeal, laryngeal and hypopharyngeal lesions as these are not able to be visualized prior to making the intubation plan unless the aforementioned photodocumentation strategies have been utilized to synchronize office evaluation pictures with the operating suite computers.

Neck anatomy

The neck is the connection between the head and the body. It includes several life-sustaining structures including the spine and associated nerves, blood vessels and glands. The cervical spine is composed of cervical vertebrae 1–7. Superiorly the neck extends from the inferior aspect of the mandible to the clavicles. Immediately beneath the skin and subcutaneous tissue lies the platysma muscle. This muscle serves as a protective landmark, demarcating a safe plane in which to raise both superior and inferior flaps in a variety of neck procedures. The next key cervical landmark is the sternocleidomastoid muscle (SCM) which divides the neck into anterior and posterior triangles. This muscle has two heads, the sternal and clavicular heads, which attach to the sternum and clavicle respectively.

Anatomical levels of the neck

The neck is further divided into levels (Figure 1.14; see Figure 15.2). Levels IA and IB are located superior to the hyoid bone. Level IA is the triangle of space formed between the midline medially, anterior belly of the digastric muscle laterally and hyoid inferiorly. Level IA dissections are usually performed bilaterally and therefore include all fibroadipose tissue between the anterior bellies of the

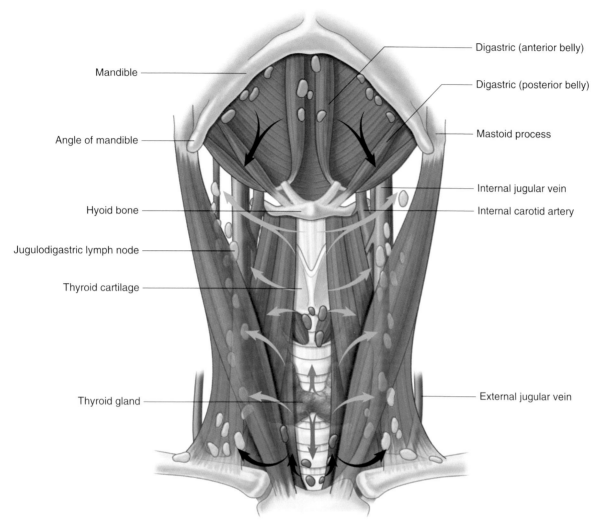

Mandible

Angle of mandible

Hyoid bone

Jugulodigastric lymph node

Thyroid cartilage

Thyroid gland

Digastric (anterior belly)

Digastric (posterior belly)

Mastoid process

Internal jugular vein

Internal carotid artery

External jugular vein

Figure 1.14. Cervical lymphatic levels. Artwork created by Emily Evans.

digastric muscle from the mandible to the hyoid bone. This region is also termed the submentum. Laterally level IB is composed of the submandibular triangle, which is found between the anterior and posterior bellies of the digastric muscle. Level II extends superiorly from the skull base to the hyoid inferior and from the sternohyoid muscle anteromedially to the SCM muscle posterolaterally. This level is divided into level IIA and level IIB by the accessory nerve (CN XI), with level IIA being anteromedial to the nerve and level IIB being postolateral to the nerve. Level III extends from the hyoid bone superiorly to the cricoid cartilage inferiorly and from the sternohyoid muscle anteromedially

to the SCM muscle posterolaterally. Level IV extends from the cricoid cartilage superiorly to the clavicle inferiorly and from the sternohyoid muscle anteromedially to the SCM muscle posterolaterally. Levels II, III, and IV comprise the anterior cervical triangle. Level V extends superiorly between the skull base superiorly and clavicle inferiorly and between the SCM anteromedially and trapezius muscle posterolaterally and is also referred to as the posterior triangle. Level VI extends from the hyoid bone superiorly to the sternal notch or innominate artery inferiorly and laterally extends from carotid artery to carotid artery. This is also termed the central compartment. The goal of a neck

15

dissection is to remove all the fibroadipose tissue contained within each respective compartment and in doing so remove all lymph nodes which may be harboring metastatic disease.

The thyroid and parathyroid glands

The thyroid gland lies beneath the sternohyoid and sternothyroid muscles at approximately C5–T1. It consists of two lobes, the left and right, with a central isthmus usually found anterior to the second and third tracheal rings. The thyroid gland is very vascular and is supplied by the superior and inferior thyroid arteries, which enter the gland laterally at the superior and inferior pedicles respectively. It is important to recognize an enlarged thyroid gland or goiter as this may cause pressure on the trachea or tracheal deviation to occur. Even more importantly, thyroid cancers may invade the trachea or the recurrent laryngeal nerves, causing vocal cord paralysis. Not only may thyroid disorders make intubation difficult but a surgical airway may be extremely difficult in the setting of a large thyroid goiter or thyroid cancer. Posterior to the thyroid gland lies the parathyroid glands which are usually a total of four paired glands (two superior and two inferior). These glands control calcium levels through the action of parathyroid hormone.

Neck anatomy after neck dissection surgery

Neck anatomy can be significantly altered by cancer or cancer treatments including surgery and radiation or chemoradiation therapy. Cancers may invade or compress vital structures including the internal jugular vein or carotid artery. The radical neck dissection pioneered in 1906 by Dr. Crile of the Cleveland Clinic includes the removal of three structures: the SCM muscle, the accessory nerve (CN XI) and the internal jugular vein. Patients who have undergone this surgery are easily recognized by the resultant neck deformity. Routinely otolaryngologists are now able to perform selective neck dissections or modified radical neck dissections which allow preservation of these structures and selective removal of the neck levels at highest risk of metastasis. It is very important to investigate any neck scars to determine previous cervical procedures prior to intubation.

Altered anatomy following laryngectomy surgery

An important example of altered cervical anatomy occurs after total laryngectomy. After removal of the larynx a permanent tracheocutaneous stoma will be created. The result of this procedure is the permanent separation of the nares, nasopharynx, oral cavity and oropharynx from the lungs and pulmonary system. Therefore a total laryngectomy patient can only be intubated through their stoma. Any attempt to instrument their nose or oral cavity can only result in communication with the esophagus and stomach. Vocal rehabilitation after a total laryngectomy is obtained through placement of a voice prosthesis through a transesophageal puncture. A puncture is placed in the posterior tracheal wall through the anterior esophageal wall. A one-way valve is then placed in this tract allowing air to travel from the lungs into the esophagus and out of the mouth, providing a modified version of esophageal speech. When preparing to intubate a total laryngectomy patient an endotracheal tube can be passed directly into the stoma, taking care not to dislodge their voice prosthesis (if present) and being especially cognizant of the fact that the tube can be easily advanced into the right mainstem due to the shortened distance of the trachea. The endotracheal tube should not be advanced beyond the first mark so that the cuff is located immediately distal to the stoma site.

Summary

In conclusion, knowledge of the anatomical background pertaining to head and neck surgery as well as the details of the pathologic processes involved and the expected post-surgical changes will assist the anesthesiologist to better communicate with his or her surgical colleagues and to devise a safe plan for general anesthesia and airway management.

Clinical pearls

- Knowledge of the anatomical background for head and neck surgery as well as the details of the pathologic processes involved and the expected post-surgical changes will assist the anesthesiologist to better communicate with his or her surgical colleagues and to devise a safe plan for anesthesia and airway management.

- Cooperation among the entire operating team is the key to a successful operation. The surgeon and anesthesiologist must discuss the particular patient's anatomy, pathology and specific procedural needs prior to each case.

- If significant facial trauma has occurred, the patient may have resulting skull and brain injuries which may supersede the treatment of the facial injuries.

- Orbital fractures commonly of the inferior orbital rim may result in entrapment of the extraocular muscles, particularly the inferior rectus, which can result in activation of the oculocardiac reflex. This reflex involving the trigeminal and vagus nerves can result in bradycardia, a junctional rhythm, and even asystole. Treatment includes surgical release of the muscle, and the administration of atropine or glycopyrrolate.

- Care must be taken when placing any foreign object into the nose because of its robust blood supply. The anterior nasal septal area is referred to as Kiesselbach's plexus and is the site of a capillary anastomosis from the sphenopalatine artery, anterior and posterior ethmoid arteries, greater palatine artery and the superior labial artery. Any object placed into the nose should be directed along the floor of the nose, which is wider than the roof.

- Ludwig's angina is a severe infection involving the floor of the mouth. As the infection and swelling worsen, the tongue is pushed posteriorly and superiorly, causing respiratory obstruction. The patient may have marked trismus. Infections in this space are considered an airway emergency.

- It has been proposed that the subglottis is prone to stenosis due to the complete cricoid ring, lack of a direct vascular supply (it is a watershed area between two vascular beds), complex mechanical forces resulting from turbulent airflow, and exposure of the respiratory epithelium to gastric contents.

- Cancers of the retromolar trigone (a band of mucosa situated behind the mandibular molars and covering the ascending ramus), tonsils or posterior oropharyngeal wall are often accompanied by trismus, which impairs the ability to visualize the full extent of these lesions and limits the intubation options.

- Not only may thyroid disorders make intubation difficult but a surgical airway may be extremely difficult in the setting of a large thyroid goiter or thyroid cancer.

References

1. Moore K, Dalley A. *Clinically Oriented Anatomy*, 4th edn. Philadelphia: Lippincott Williams & Wilkins; 1999.

2. Bailey B, Johnson J, Newlands S. *Head & Neck Surgery – Otolaryngology*, 4th edn. Philadelphia: Lippincott Williams & Wilkins; 2006.

3. Allsop D, Kennett K. Skull and facial bone trauma. In Nahum AM, Melvin J, eds. *Accidental Injury: Biomechanics and Prevention*. Berlin: Springer; 2002.

4. Paton J, Boscan P, Pickering AE, Nalivaiko E. The yin and yang of cardiac autonomic control: vago-sympathetic interactions revisited. *Brain Res Rev* 2005; **49**(3):555–65.

5. Gluth MB, Shinners PA, Kasperbauer JL. Subglottic stenosis associated with Wegener's granulomatosis. *Laryngoscope* 2003;**113**(8):1304–7.

2

Otolaryngology instruments 101 for the anesthesiologist

Paul C. Bryson and Michael S. Benninger

Introduction

The anesthesiologist and otolaryngologist share the airway. The surgeon requires adequate visualization of the pathology to perform surgery and the anesthesiologist requires adequate oxygenation and ventilation. While communication between the anesthesiologist and the otolaryngologist is crucial, it is also prudent for the anesthesiologist to become familiar with the equipment used by the otolaryngologist, particularly when the surgical procedure involves the upper aerodigestive tract. This chapter will introduce and discuss some of the more common equipment used during procedures involving the larynx, trachea, cervical esophagus, pharynx, and paranasal sinuses.

Surgery of the larynx and trachea

Surgery of the larynx, pharynx, and trachea begins with securing the airway with an appropriate device that will allow for adequate ventilation. Often, a smaller-sized endotracheal tube or an endotracheal tube that is safe for laser surgery is selected (Figure 2.1). There are also occasions where the patient's pathology may preclude the use of an endotracheal tube and require the use of jet ventilation. Jet ventilation is typically employed via a subglottic Hunsaker catheter, via supraglottic attachment to the laryngoscope (Figure 2.2), or via jet laryngoscope. Both techniques have been found to be useful and safe for microlaryngeal surgery [1–3]. For certain tracheal pathology, the use of a rigid bronchoscope (Figure 2.3) may be necessary. In this situation, the anesthesiologist can connect the breathing circuit to the rigid bronchoscope's side port. For airway obstructive pathology, the surgeon may also employ dilatational balloons and powered instrumentation,

such as a micro-debrider, to increase the airway diameter (Figure 2.4).

For microlaryngeal surgery, the surgeon will typically use a tubular laryngoscope that allows him or her to visualize the pathology of interest. Once the pathology is visualized, the surgeon must suspend the laryngoscope to allow for a stable, motion-free operative field. There are many surgical laryngoscopes, but the more common operative laryngoscopes include the Dedo laryngoscope (Teleflex-Pilling, Research Triangle Park, NC, USA) and the Universal Modular Glottiscope (Endocraft, LLC, Providence, Rhode Island, USA) [4]. To achieve a motion free operative field, there are two suspension devices/systems employed by most otolaryngologists – a chest anchored, torsion-fulcrum device and an elevated vector suspension device (Figure 2.5) [5]. Once in suspension, the surgeon will bring the operating microscope into the field and use a variety of microlaryngeal instruments to manage the pathology of interest (Figure 2.6).

Surgery of the pharynx and cervical esophagus

Airway management for endoscopic surgery of the pharynx and cervical esophagus is similar to that of the larynx and trachea in that a smaller-sized endotracheal tube or laser-safe endotracheal tube is typically used. Typical pathology treated by the otolaryngologist includes cancer, Zenker's diverticulum, cricopharyngeal hypertrophy or achalasia, and pharyngo-esophageal stenosis. Surgery in this area can employ a number of unique scopes including a Weerda-type distending diverticuloscope, A Feyh-Kastenbauer (FK) laryngo-pharyngoscope, Dohlman/Kashima diverticuloscope, and a rigid esophagoscope

Anesthesia for Otolaryngologic Surgery, ed. Basem Abdelmalak and D. John Doyle. Published by Cambridge University Press.
© Cambridge University Press 2013.

(A)

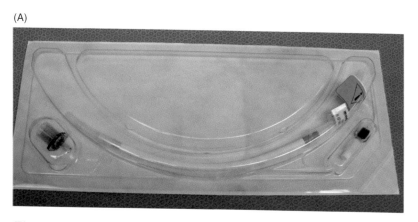

Figure 2.1. Two types of laser-safe endotracheal tubes. The cuffs of both tubes are typically filled with saline. Care should be taken to remove all of the fluid prior to extubation.

(B)

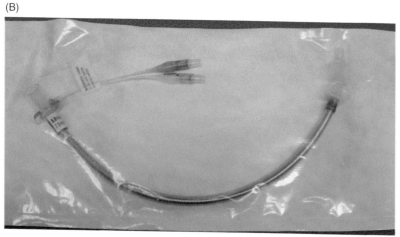

(A)

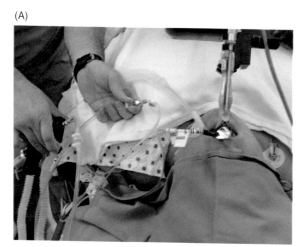

(B)

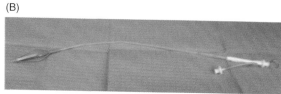

Figure 2.2. Jet ventilation systems; (A) supraglottic system; (B) subglottic Hunsaker catheter. The supraglottic ventilation system is typically attached to the laryngoscope.

(Figure 2.7). All of these devices allow for wide exposure of pathology and allow room for necessary instrumentation. The FK retractor has become more common as trans-oral robotic surgery has become more widespread. Serial dilatation systems for stenosis include Maloney-type and Savory-type dilatation systems (Figure 2.8).

Surgery of the nose and paranasal sinuses

Surgery in the nose and paranasal sinuses can present unique challenges to the anesthesia team. These are

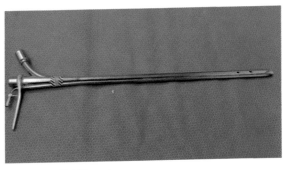

Figure 2.3. Rigid bronchoscope.

primarily related to the anesthesia access to the airway during the procedure. Since the nose opens inferiorly above the mouth, the position of access to the nose by the nasal surgeon generally requires them to be positioned at the side of patient below the head. This can obstruct continuous access to the airway and a clear separation of the anesthesiologist from the endotracheal tube.

Many cases of septoplasty and rhinoplasty are performed under local anesthesia with varying degrees of sedation. In such cases, there are two issues that need to be considered by the anesthesiologist. Does the patient require supplemental oxygen? This can be delivered with a nasal cannula placed in the mouth. Will the surgeons be utilizing a device like an electrocautery or a surgical laser, where care must be taken to avoid high oxygen levels which might lead to a fire?

Endoscopic sinus surgery (ESS) is a particularly complicated set-up. If performed under local anesthesia the set-up and airway issues are similar to those which are considered with septoplasty and rhinoplasty. Most endoscopic sinus surgeries and many functional and cosmetic operations are performed under general anesthesia, usually with the head

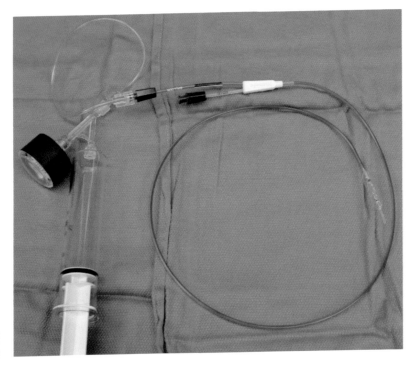

Figure 2.4. Radial dilatation balloon. These balloons come in a variety of sizes and will require a period of apnea while inflated.

(A)

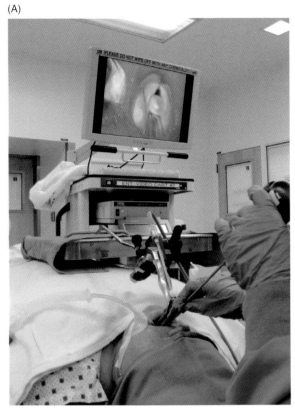

(B)

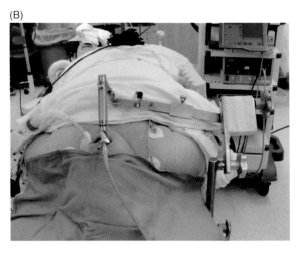

Figure 2.5. Laryngeal suspension devices (A, chest support; B, elevated vector). The choice of device is largely surgeon-dependent.

Figure 2.6. Microlaryngeal instruments.

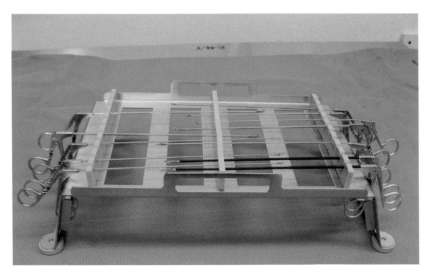

elevated above the body or in a reverse Trendelenburg position. Since most surgeons are right-handed, they will need to stand (or sit) on the right side of the patient's body. There may be an assistant on the left side for septoplasty, rhinoplasty, or nasal reconstruction.

With ESS, only one surgeon typically operates at any given time, so they will remain on one side of the patient. In such cases, the endotracheal tube should be brought out through the opposite side of the mouth and the anesthesia team and machine should be on the opposite side of the body. In many cases, an image

(A)

(B)

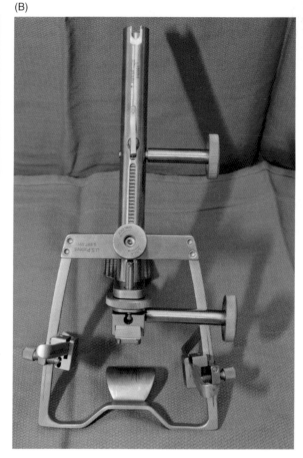

(C)

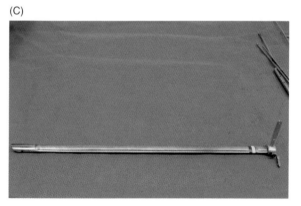

Figure 2.7. (A) Weerda diverticuloscope, (B) FK retractor, (C) rigid esophagoscope. The Weerda diverticuloscope is a large, extended length proximally and distally extending scope used to endoscopically treat Zenker's diverticulum. Given the size of the scope, a smaller endotracheal tube should be used to help facilitate scope placement. The FK retractor is a specialized scope used in trans-oral robotic surgery as well as in sleep surgery. It is a larger scope and has the capability to attach blades of varied length and cheek retractors. A smaller endotracheal tube is typically helpful with this scope as well.

guidance system is used to assist with important endonasal and skull base landmarks. Some image guidance systems run off a headpiece and others use optical systems which are a short distance from the patient, but where the line of the optics has to be free from obstruction. This may become important when a bispectral index (BIS) monitoring system (Covedien Inc., Dublin, Ireland) is used. In these cases, the BIS monitor may need to be placed higher on the forehead with the attachment cable running underneath the operative table, keeping in mind that it may also result in some interference with the imaging system,

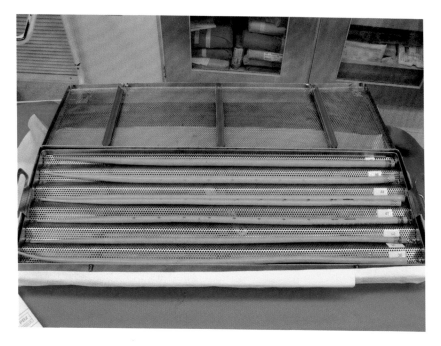

Figure 2.8. Esophageal dilatation system. The dilatation system shown in this figure is mercury-weighted and soft. Other dilatation systems include dilators that are placed over a guide wire and balloon dilatation systems.

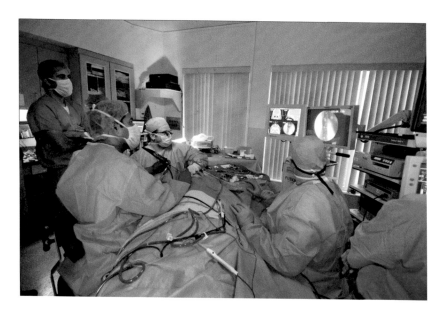

Figure 2.9. Typical set-up for endoscopic sinus surgery. The surgeon is positioned on the right side of the body and is able to view both the navigation equipment and monitor. The surgical nurse/assistant will be on the opposite side of the patient. The endotracheal tube and circuit are on the left side of the body and the anesthesiologist is on the left side behind the nurse.

prohibiting its use all together. In all cases, the surgeons will be utilizing telescopes and video monitors, and therefore the anesthesia team needs to be positioned to avoid obstructing their view. Finally, to facilitate the passing of instruments, the scrub nurse will need to be on the opposite side of the body from the surgeon. This will place the anesthesia machine farther away from the patient, behind the surgical assistant. With this in mind, there will be a need to use a longer breathing circuit (Figure 2.9).

The last important issue with nasal and sinus surgery has to do with the growth of intranasal approaches to the skull base. These techniques are used to repair CSF leaks as well as resection of skull base or brain lesions where the surgery may result in a CSF leak. In such cases it is optimal to have a smooth and gentle emergence from anesthesia to avoid coughing or bucking, which may increase intracranial pressure and break down the skull base repair.

Transoral robotic surgery

Transoral robotic surgery is an emerging technology that is becoming more common at tertiary care centers. Specially trained head and neck surgeons are using this technology to surgically resect tumors and masses from the oropharynx, larynx, and hypopharynx. There are several considerations that must be kept in mind when providing anesthesia for these patients. Airway management may involve standard transoral intubation with care to avoid the pathology or the lesion may require a flexible fiberoptic approach. Preoperative discussions with the operating surgeon are imperative. Additionally, laser assistance and electrocautery are frequently used. Appropriate laser-safe endotracheal tubes, laser precautions for the patient and staff, and open communication are necessary throughout the procedure. Finally, the current size of the surgical robots requires a large operating room with enough space for the robot (Figure 2.10), operating team, and the anesthesiology team. As this technology becomes more common and refined, instrumentation and size are expected to decrease.

Summary

Surgery of the upper aerodigestive tract deals with diverse pathology that requires a variety of special surgical instrumentation. Given the demands of the surgeon and anesthesiologist, it is crucial for optimal patient care that open communication before, during, and after the procedure be standard operating protocol. Basic understanding of otolaryngologic instrumentation as described in this chapter will hopefully allow for mutual understanding between the surgical and anesthesia teams.

Clinical pearls

- Given the demands on the surgeon and anesthesiologist, it is crucial that open

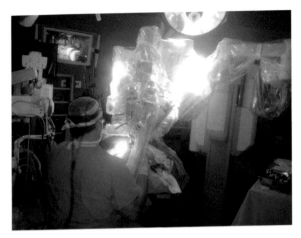

Figure 2.10.

communication before, during, and after the procedure be standard operating protocol. A basic understanding of the otolaryngologic instrumentation will help allow for mutual understanding between the surgical and anesthesia teams.

- For certain tracheal pathologies, the use of a rigid bronchoscope may be necessary. In this situation, the anesthesiologist can connect the breathing circuit to the rigid bronchoscope's side port, or utilize a special adapter to deliver jet ventilation through the same side port.

- To achieve a motion-free operative field with direct laryngoscopy, there are two suspension devices/systems employed by most otolaryngologists – a chest-anchored, torsion-fulcrum device and an elevated vector suspension device.

- Some image guidance systems for sinus endoscopy surgery employ a headpiece while others use an optical system located a short distance from the patient, but where the line of sight has to be free of obstructions. This may become important when a bispectral index (BIS) monitoring system is desired to be used. In these cases, the BIS monitor may need to be placed higher on the forehead with the attachment cable running underneath the operative table. In addition, the BIS monitor may interfere with the imaging system, prohibiting its use all together.

References

1. Davies JM, Hillel AD, Maronian NC, Posner KL. The Hunsaker Mon-Jet tube with jet ventilation is effective for microlaryngeal surgery. *Can J Anaesthes* 2009;**56**(4):284–90.

2. Orloff LA, Parhizkar N, Ortiz E. The Hunsaker Mon-Jet ventilation tube for microlaryngeal surgery: optimal laryngeal exposure. *Ear Nose Throat J* 2002;**81**(6): 390–4.

3. Rezaie-Majd A, Bigenzahn W, Denk DM, *et al.* Superimposed high-frequency jet ventilation (SHFJV) for endoscopic laryngotracheal surgery in more than 1500 patients. *Br J Anaesth* 2006;**96**(5):650–9.

4. Zeitels SM. Universal modular glottiscope system: the evolution of a century of design and technique for direct laryngoscopy. *Ann Otol Rhinol Laryngol Suppl* 1999;**179**:2–24.

5. Zeitels SM, Burns JA, Dailey SH. Suspension laryngoscopy revisited. *Ann Otol Rhinol Laryngol* 2004; **113**(1):16–22.

Chapter

3

Preoperative evaluation for ENT surgery

Jie Zhou and Linda S. Aglio

The first public demonstration of ether on October 16, 1846 was administered for ENT surgery. Dr. William Morton anesthetized patient Edward Gilbert Abbott for removal of a tumor from Abbott's neck by Dr. John Warren [1]. Since then, significant advances in both ENT anesthesia and ENT surgery have been made. The relationship between ENT anesthesia and ENT surgery has never been stronger than it is today, and there is probably no other subspecialty of anesthesia that has such close ties with a subspecialty of surgery. ENT surgical procedures require that anesthesiologists share the airway with the ENT surgeons. A good ENT anesthesiologist should not only understand the condition of the patient preoperatively, but should also be able to anticipate the effects of surgery on the patient.

Traditionally, ENT operations consist of relatively short procedures, ranging from tonsillectomies, to tympanostomies, to tracheostomies. However, some of the most dreaded anesthesia tragedies occur in this setting. For instance, Bishop documented that anesthesia-related intraoperative death accompanying tonsillectomy and adenoidectomy ranged from 12% to 17% of the entire intraoperative mortality during the 1920s and 1930s in the United States [2]. Both anesthesiologists and surgeons should realize that nothing is trivial just because the procedure is small and short. Improvements in both anesthesia and surgery have been made to ensure the safety of the patients.

One of the standards implemented was proper preoperative evaluation. The information acquired during preoperative evaluation is pertinent to determining the anesthetic and the surgical techniques. Essentially, it is also a risk assessment process. In addition, it also, in part, predicts the postoperative course of the patient.

A thorough preoperative evaluation will provide both anesthesiologist and surgeon valuable information which may alter the course of patient care. Anesthetic preoperative evaluation is composed of four components: patient history, physical examination, laboratory studies, and anesthetic plan.

Patient history

It is important for the clinician to spend time with the patient or proxy and the patient's family. Some of the generic information related to patient history includes: patient's demographic information, height and weight, presence of systemic conditions, previous hospitalizations and operations, previous anesthetic issues, family history of any relevant conditions, allergies, medications, social history, recreational agent or tobacco consumption, and the patient's fasting status.

For the patient preparing for an ENT surgery, some of the pertinent information is crucial for the anesthesiologist. For example, for pediatric patients undergoing tonsillectomy, it is useful to obtain information on signs and symptoms of sleep apnea. Specific considerations during preoperative evaluation with each surgical condition will be discussed in depth in its respective chapter.

Physical examination

Physical examination is a very important step for anesthesiologists to appreciate the patient and his/her condition. The examination usually starts with baseline vital signs. A review of systems examination is usually a useful approach; this includes assessment of cardiac, pulmonary, renal, hepatic, neurological, gastrointestinal, endocrinological/metabolic, musculoskeletal, psychiatric, gynecological and obstetric organ systems. When assessing a pediatric patient, attention should be paid to clinically significant inherited conditions, such as muscular dystrophies, which may carry serious clinical consequences. The majority of pediatric patients have never had previous anesthesia.

Cardiac anomalies

Anesthesiologists should be informed if adult patients have a history of congenital anomaly. Likewise, anesthesiologists should pay attention to pediatric patients with congenital anomalies. Some of these conditions are associated with cardiac, respiratory and other systemic problems. For example, a significant portion of the patients with the Pierre Robin syndrome also have cardiac anomalies. Ventricular septal defect, patent ductus arteriosus, and atrial septal defect are the most common congenital cardiac anomalies in this syndrome [3].

Pulmonary system

Pulmonary assessment is crucial to anesthesiologists caring for patients scheduled for ENT procedures. Patients with preexisting pulmonary conditions may benefit from receiving preoperative testing before elective procedures. Some of the acute changes (in the clinical presentation and/or test results) may require immediate attention, which may result in deferral of the elective ENT procedure. A patient who suffers from chronic airway obstruction may develop pulmonary hypertension or even right-sided heart failure (cor pulmonale).

Neurological system

ENT procedures can directly affect central and peripheral nervous systems. Preoperative evaluation should check for any preexisting neurological deficit if indicated. Review of systems should include history of seizures and other neurological symptoms.

Psychological evaluation and preparation

Psychological preparation for patients undergoing ENT operations is imperative, especially in the pediatric population. Patients may express fear and anxiety towards having surgery. One of the reasons for anxiety is the lack of adequate information and good communication. Hatava *et al.* rated children's anxiety and satisfaction with information and care, which demonstrated that intramuscular injection of premedication and induction of anesthesia were the most negative procedures reported independently by children and

parents, respectively [4]. Adult patients undergoing laryngectomy may experience very intrusive, life-changing impact from loss of speech. A preoperative preparation program and counseling have been shown to alleviate anxiety in not only patients of all ages, but also parents of the children [5,6].

Anesthetic-specific elements

During the past three decades, the anesthesia-related mortality rate has decreased 10-fold [7]. As a result, anesthesia is often cited as the only specialty in health care to have reached the six sigma defect rate [7]. However, recent retrospective studies showed that the incidence of dental injury, most commonly involving upper incisors, was still reported to be around 0.05% [8] to 0.36% [9] in the developed world. While the airway is often shared between anesthesia and surgical personnel, a thorough preoperative inspection of the patient's dental condition is critical. The authors are in favor of utilizing the standardized tooth numbering system beginning with the right maxillary molar tooth in both pediatric and adult patients (Figure 3.1). At Brigham and Women's Hospital in Boston, the authors raised the awareness of dental injury through departmental educational conferences. Documentation of dental injuries should at least include descriptions of enamel damage, loose or missing teeth, and other preexisting conditions.

Airway assessment should include examination of voice quality, respiratory rate, auscultation for breath sounds to detect stridor and wheezing, testing for ability to handle secretions, and checking for dysphagia. A history of radiation to the head and neck could imply airway fragility. Assessment of visible anatomic landmarks, including the Mallampati scale, may be of value in predicting difficult intubation. However, lingual tonsil hyperplasia may interfere with face-mask ventilation and rigid laryngoscopic intubation, despite a promising examination on the Mallampati scale [10]. In children with obstructive sleep apnea syndrome, the maximal upper airway narrowing is located in the region where the adenoids and tonsils overlap [11]. The size of the palatine tonsil may indicate the potential for airway obstruction, which may have a greater impact in overweight patients [12]. A history of snoring should alert the practitioner that the patient is at risk for sleep apnea. Pediatric patients with congenital syndromes often have associated difficult airways, which need extra attention. For

27

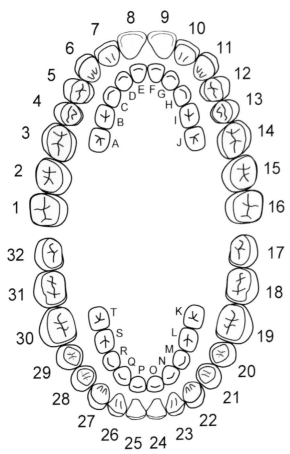

Figure 3.1. Illustration of standard numbering of primary and permanent teeth.

example, patients with trisomy 21 (Down syndrome) often have a large tongue with relative hypotonia; a curved Macintosh blade may provide a better view for intubation in such an instance. Concerns about possible atlanto-axial instability in Down's patients may require radiological evaluation. The anesthesia plan should be tailored towards the findings of the individual patient.

Laboratory evaluation

The use of preoperative laboratory study may be divided into two categories: routine or "screening" and indicated or "diagnostic". The American Society of Anesthesiologists (ASA) task force on preanesthesia evaluation defines a routine test as a test ordered in the absence of a specific clinical indication or purpose. An indicated test is defined as a test that is ordered for a specific clinical indication or purpose [13]. The use of routine preoperative laboratory studies is pervasive, partially due to the misconception that it provides medicolegal protection against liability [14]. The ASA practice advisory on preanesthesia evaluation concluded that there was not sufficiently rigorous literature to permit an unambiguous assessment of the clinical benefits or harms associated with routine testing or testing in the presence of specific clinical characteristics. The decision-making parameters for a specific preoperative test or timing of the test cannot be unequivocally determined from the available scientific literature [13]. Indicated or diagnostic studies are for diagnosis of individual conditions. For example, the American Academy of Pediatrics recommended polysomnography as the gold standard for establishing the presence and severity of sleep-disordered breathing in children [15].

With the implementation of anesthesiologist-led preoperative clinics, there have been substantial changes in clinical practice in the past two decades [16]. It is now the general consensus that tests should be obtained only for specific clinical indications. The authors advocate a reasonable consideration of the five elements of the intended laboratory tests, including relevance, normal value, sensitivity and specificity, cost, and risk/benefit analysis, before determining the usefulness and interpretation of laboratory test results [14].

A recent survey of 793 US board-certified otolaryngologists demonstrated that most physicians (69.9%) do not order routine laboratory tests prior to tonsillectomy; of interest, private-practice otolaryngologists ordered more tests than did those in academia [17]. Nevertheless, pediatric surgeons and academic surgeons were significantly more likely to admit patients postoperatively [17]. In 1999, the American Academy of Otolaryngology – Head and Neck Surgery issued a consensus statement entitled the "Clinical Indicators Compendium", which stated that the performance of coagulation and bleeding work-up was appropriate only if there was an abnormality suspected or genetic information was unavailable [18].

Anesthesia assessment and plan

In 1963, the American Society of Anesthesiologists (ASA) adopted a five-category classification system to summarize patient physical status. A sixth category for brain-dead patients was added later (Table 3.1). In

Table 3.1. ASA Physical Status Classification System, reproduced with permission of the American Society of Anesthesiologists

Class 1	A normal healthy patient
Class 2	A patient with mild systemic disease
Class 3	A patient with severe systemic disease
Class 4	A patient with severe systemic disease that is a constant threat to life
Class 5	A moribund patient who is not expected to survive with or without the operation
Class 6	A declared brain-dead patient whose organs are being removed for donor purposes

the case of an emergency, a letter "E" is designated to follow the physical status classification.

The ASA physical status classification has been used to dictate the care plan for patients. Patients with low risk (ASA I and II) undergoing minor ENT surgery are often cared for in an outpatient setting. There are benefits to patients, especially the pediatric population, if the operations are performed in a day surgery fashion. It usually involves much less behavioral change, which may hasten the recovery process of the children [19–21]. However, on most occasions, it is to the anesthesiologist's disadvantage. There is often less certainty on patient fasting status. In addition, the entire team is under time pressure for preoperative evaluation, surgical time and postoperative discharge.

Patient selection becomes a crucial process to balance clinical efficiency and patient safety. Although some studies showed no statistical difference in complication rate of ASA class III patients compared with that of ASA classes I and II, most of the clinical guidelines for outpatient patient selection consist of only ASA classes I and II patients. There is controversy regarding the age limit of children for outpatient procedures. Premature infants have a series of potential problems due to prematurity, including but not limited to pulmonary dysplasia, hypothermia and anemia. There is also a reported 25% incidence of apnea within the first 12 hours postoperatively, resulting from immature brain stem function [22]. Positive findings on patient history, physical examination and laboratory study may require further workup.

The ASA recently updated its practice guidelines for preoperative fasting and use of pharmacological agents to reduce the risk of pulmonary aspiration based on scientific and opinion-based evidence [23]. The current recommended minimal fasting periods for clear liquid, breast milk, infant formula,

nonhuman milk, light meal and fatty food are 2 h, 4 h, 6 h, 6 h, 6 h and 8 h, respectively. Although the guidelines above apply to patients of all ages, they do not guarantee complete gastric emptying. Acceptable clear liquid drinks include water, fruit juices without pulp, carbonated beverages, clear tea, and black coffee. Minimal fasting time of 8 h or more may be needed for meals that include fried or fatty foods or meat. While they recognize the effectiveness of the combined use of histamine-2 receptor antagonists and gastrointestinal stimulants in reducing both gastric volume and acidity, the new guidelines do not recommend routine use of any gastrointestinal stimulants, gastric acid secretion blockers, antacids, antiemetics, anticholinergics, or combinations of the medications above. The 2011 ASA fasting guidelines may not apply to, or may need to be modified for, (1) patients with coexisting diseases or conditions that can affect gastric emptying or fluid volume (e.g., pregnancy, obesity, diabetes, hiatal hernia, gastroesophageal reflux disease, ileus or bowel obstruction, emergency care, external tube feeding) and (2) patients in whom airway management might be difficult [23].

Indications for surgery postponement and cancellation

With the implementation of preoperative evaluation clinics, the rate of cancellation for outpatient surgery has decreased. For ENT surgery, most of the time, anesthetic-related reasons for cancellation are due to recent upper respiratory infection or non-compliance with preoperative fasting guidelines. Cancellation of cases because of upper respiratory infection remains controversial. The decision whether or not to proceed with the operation should be an individualized decision based on discussion involving the patient, anesthesiologist and surgeon.

Informed consent

Modern medical ethics respects the concepts of autonomy, beneficence, nonmaleficence, and justice. The 1957 landmark case of Salgo v Leland Stanford etc. Bd. Trustees emphasized the need to discuss with patients the nature of the procedure, potential risks and complications, anticipated benefits, and therapeutic alternatives [24].

Naturally, this crucial task should be achieved by honest, knowledgeable and responsible individuals with good communication skills. The process of informed consent consists of seven elements: (1) establishing the decision-making capacity or competency of the patient, (2) establishing freedom or voluntariness in decision-making, including absence of over-riding legal or state interests, (3) ensuring that adequate disclosure of material information has occurred, (4) offering a clinical plan recommendation, (5) ensuring an understanding of the above by the patient, (6) a decision by the patient in favor of the recommended plan, and (7) authorization of that plan [24].

A recent study of the role of informed consent in patient recall of perioperative risk showed that ENT patients who received written summaries had a higher recall of the risk discussion [25,26]. There was a tendency for patients to remember serious complications, such as facial nerve paralysis (88%) and hearing loss (85%), compared to anesthesia reactions (4%) and hoarseness (2%) [25].

Although it has been a routine practice to obtain informed consent for clinical research protocols to be conducted at least 24 hours before the intervention to allow enough time for the patient's consideration, it is generally acceptable for day surgery ENT patients to give consent on the same day as the surgery. However, in the United Kingdom, there were a number of medicolegal cases in which the plaintiffs argued that they were not given enough time to consider the risks of surgery. Berry *et al.* conducted a prospective audit for ENT patients concerning policy changes for written consent to be done prior to the day of surgery; they concluded that such a policy change not only protects the hospital but also provides a smooth journey for the patients [27].

Informed consent for minors is not always a simple issue. For example, problems can arise when the parents are divorced. In such circumstances, legal custody, but not physical custody, empowers the right to consent. With regard to informed consent in the case of medical care for a minor, most states allow it when a specified age, e.g. 12, 14 or 17, is reached. One should seek counsel for individual state's minors' consent law. In case of a medical emergency, the situation can become very difficult. Generally speaking, one should inform the institutional legal counsel and risk management teams, while proceeding under the legal doctrine of "implied consent". Note that in some emergency situations health care providers may still be required to inform the minor's parent(s) or guardian.

Refusal of care

As with treatment consent, competent adult patients also have the right to refuse treatment, even if necessary to save life or limb. This concept is rooted in the fundamental legal tradition of self-determination. One of the examples of such is the refusal, on religious grounds, of a clinically necessary blood transfusion in Jehovah's Witness patients.

Preoperative evaluation for pediatric patients

Pediatric patients are unique in many ways for anesthesiologists. To better serve this special population, one should understand that there are a number of important physiological and anatomical differences between pediatric and adult airways [28].

(1) Oxygen consumption is 6 ml/kg/min in neonates, which gradually approaches that of 3 ml/kg/min in adults.

(2) The foramen ovale closes over in a few months, but may remain patent in 15%–25% of adults.

(3) The sympathetic nervous system matures more slowly than the parasympathetic system, resulting in an exaggerated vagal response to stimuli, e.g., during airway instrumentation.

(4) Infants possess a relatively large occiput; a shoulder roll may help in extending the head and opening of the mouth.

(5) The pediatric larynx (cricoid cartilage at C4) is located cephalad compared to that of adult (cricoid cartilage at C7). It may take until age 13 years for the adult position of the cricoid cartilage to be assumed.

(6) The narrowest portion of the infant airway is the cricoid cartilage vs. the vocal cords in an adult. This

is because the shape of the adult larynx is cylindrical, while it is funnel-shaped in infants. This is why uncuffed endotracheal tubes can be sealed successfully in pediatric patients.

(7) The infant epiglottis is often relatively larger and stiffer than that in an adult. Lifting of the epiglottis with the tip of the laryngoscope is often needed to visualize vocal cords during laryngoscopy.

(8) The nares of infants are much smaller, and so are prone to obstruction by secretions, edema, bleeding or an improperly placed face mask.

Premedication should be considered in children older than the age of 6 to 9 months when separation anxiety has developed. Psychological preparation is also important [4,29]. Doll-play has been recognized as an excellent way to communicate with the child [30]. The anesthesiologist should always have a good understanding of the surgical plan, because it not only improves collaboration with the surgeons intraoperatively, but also facilitates in alleviating the anxiety of the parents during the preoperative evaluation process.

Preoperative evaluation for geriatric patients

The geriatric label usually applies to patients who are 65 years old or older. While age itself is not a surgical contraindication, increased age is associated with multiple systemic comorbidities. In addition, advanced age also places the patient at higher risk for postoperative delirium and cognitive dysfunction [31–33]. Therefore, geriatric patients require a thorough preoperative evaluation before any procedure.

Preoperative evaluation of comorbidity, functional status and pharmacological status is critical to the safety of geriatric surgery [34]. Preoperative mental status assessment of the elderly provides a reference for postoperative delirium or alteration, which should be carefully documented. This information may be helpful in determining the intraoperative anesthetic approach [35]. Preoperative laboratory testing should be considered based on the history and the physical examination. While most of the ENT procedures are in the low surgical risk category, some of the large elective ENT operations are considered intermediate surgical risk. According to the 2009 American College of Cardiology Foundation

and American Heart Association (ACC/AHA) perioperative guidelines, head and neck surgery is rated intermediate risk with a reported cardiac risk generally of 1%–5% [36]. A preoperative resting 12-lead ECG is recommended for patients with known coronary heart disease, peripheral arterial disease, or cerebrovascular disease who are undergoing intermediate-risk surgical procedures. It is also reasonable for patients with at least one clinical risk factor, which includes a history of ischemic heart disease, a history of compensated or prior heart failure, a history of cerebrovascular disease, diabetes mellitus, or renal failure, who are undergoing intermediate-risk operative procedures. Preoperative ECG testing is not indicated in asymptomatic persons undergoing low-risk surgical procedures [36].

According to the 2009 ACC/AHA perioperative guidelines, the cardiac evaluation and care algorithm for noncardiac surgery should follow a five-step process based on active clinical conditions, known cardiovascular disease, or cardiac risk for patients 50 years of age or greater [27].

Step 1: evaluate the need for emergency noncardiac surgery: if needed, proceed to the operating room with perioperative surveillance and postoperative risk stratification and risk factor management.

Step 2: assess whether the patient has active cardiac conditions: if so, consider surgery after evaluation and treatment per ACC/AHA guidelines.

Step 3: determine whether the procedure is of low risk: if so, proceed with the planned surgery.

Step 4: assess whether the patient's functional capacity is greater than or equal to 4 metabolic equivalents (METs) without symptoms: if so, proceed with planned surgery.

Step 5: if all of above are inapplicable and the patient has 1–3 or more clinical risk factors, surgical procedure should still be able to proceed with heart rate control. Consider noninvasive testing if it will change management.

The 2009 ACC/AHA guidelines also provided a detailed recommendation regarding the application, withdrawal, risk, and caveats of the perioperative administration of beta-blockers [36].

Evaluation of patient capacity sometimes enters into the process of informed consent or refusal in the elderly. Clinicians often face difficulty in determining decision-making capacity in such cases;

for example, the diagnosis of mild dementia does not preclude capacity for medical decision-making. In general, decision-making capacity requires three basic elements: (1) the capacity to understand and communicate; (2) the capacity to reason and deliberate; and (3) possession of a set of values and goals [37]. Contrary to the legal term of competency, medical decision-making capacity is not an all-or-none property.

Advance directives and do-not-resuscitate (DNR) order

All patients undergoing anesthesia and surgical procedures should be given an opportunity for producing advance directives, which are decisions that the patient makes while he/she still retains the capacity for making such decisions. The advance directives assume power when the patient loses capacity. The living will and proxy directive are the two forms of advance directive [37]. Advance directives are recognized by the US Federal Patient Self-Determination Act, which is legally binding in all 50 states.

A DNR order, also known as DNAR order (do-not-attempt-resuscitation), is a medical decision made by patients in preparation for possible life-terminating cardiac/pulmonary events. Traditionally, anesthesiologists often consider perioperative cardiac and pulmonary events relatively controlled and easily reversible. Therefore, some institutions require automatic suspension of DNR status during the immediate perioperative period. However, ASA ethical guidelines affirmed in 2008 advised that such practices may not sufficiently address a patient's rights to self-determination. Such directives should be clarified and modified based on institutional guidelines and the preferences of the patient [38].

Safe surgery checklist and teamwork

As anesthesia and ENT personnel sometimes share the airway, teamwork is extremely important. Close communication is crucial to safe, smooth patient care. Use of the World Health Organization (WHO) Safe Surgery Checklist is highly recommended [39]. The checklist identifies three phases of an operation, each corresponding to a specific period in the normal flow of work: before the induction of anesthesia ("sign in"), before the incision of the skin ("time out"), and before the patient leaves the operating room ("sign out"). At each phase, the surgery team

should complete specified tasks before proceeding with the operation. In addition, all operating room personnel, including anesthesia providers, ENT surgeons and nurses, should have a clear plan and role designation for potential emergencies, such as airway fires and difficult airway problems.

Case study
Case description

The patient is a 68-year-old male, 5'9" (175 cm) in height and weighing 86 kg, with a history of anaplastic thyroid cancer metastatic to lungs and liver. He refused surgery on his thyroid cancer; since then the size of his thyroid mass has been increasing. He had been on adriamycin for chemotherapy and was placed on sorafenib 2 weeks prior to admission. He now presents to an outside hospital with acute respiratory distress, progressive stridor, hemoptysis, and difficulty clearing secretions. He is scheduled for an urgent tracheostomy.

Past medical history: hypertension, type II diabetes, hypercholesterolemia, severe chronic obstructive pulmonary disease, 40 pack year smoking history.

Past surgical history: percutanous endoscopic gastrostomy tube placement (tube feedings stopped 8 hours ago).

Other medication: metformin, atorvastatin, coumadin.

Code status: DNR, DNI.

Preoperative evaluation

Comorbidities: hypertension and diabetes.

Airway: Mallampati Class 4 airway, thyromental distance of 2 finger breadths, no overbite. Large thyroid mass.

Psychological: patient is awake, alert and oriented. He is capable of decision-making.

CT scan of the neck revealed a 6.4 cm × 7.1 cm neck mass compressing the airway (Figure 3.2).

Laboratory study: International Normalized Ratio (INR) was 1.0; partial thromboplastin time was 33.6 seconds.

The patient understood the risks and benefits of anesthesia and the proposed operation. He was consented for awake fiberoptic intubation for tracheostomy. He would like to suspend the DNR and DNI orders during the perioperative period.

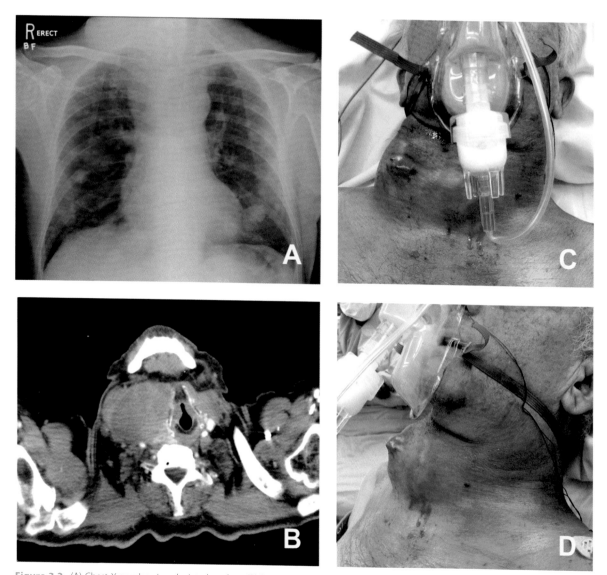

Figure 3.2. (A) Chest X-ray showing deviated trachea. (B) Preoperative CT scan of the neck showing the thyroid mass compressing the trachea. (C and D) Photo of the patient with a large thyroid mass in the semi-sitting position before an awake fiberoptic intubation.

Induction of anesthesia

The patient had been NPO for more than 8 hours. The anesthesia team and the surgical team discussed the procedure and airway management plans. The plan for anesthesia is an awake fiberoptic intubation approach based on the preoperative evaluation.

After transporting the patient onto the operating table, he was placed in a semi-sitting position with the back up at 70 degrees. After applying standard monitors, the patient was premedicated with intravenous administration of 50 μg of fentanyl. The patient was then pre-oxygenated with a face mask and albuterol nebulizer.

Awake fiberoptic intubation was achieved with spontaneous breathing maintained. Airway was secured with a #5.5 cuffed endotracheal tube. Positioning of the ET tube was confirmed by chest rise, the presence of bilateral breath sounds and capnography. Fiberoptic bronchoscopy was performed to confirm the depth of the tube and to rule out other intrapulmonary processes. The patient was maintained on helium (79%)/oxygen (21%) mix and sevoflorane. Tracheostomy was performed smoothly without difficulty. Potential complications of acute airway, bleeding (including endobronchial bleeding), pneumomediastinum, pneumothorax, laryngospasm, and bronchospasm, were avoided.

Clinical pearls

- A good ENT anesthesiologist should not only understand the condition of the patient preoperatively, but should also be able to anticipate the effects of surgery on the patient.
- The assessment of pediatric patients should pay attention to clinically significant inherited conditions, such as muscular dystrophies, which may carry serious clinical consequences.
- A thorough preoperative inspection of the patient's dental condition is critical. Documentation of dental injuries should include descriptions of enamel damage, loose or missing teeth and other preexisting conditions.
- Airway assessment should include examination of voice quality, respiratory rate, auscultation for

breath sounds to detect stridor and wheezing, testing for ability to handle secretions, and checking for dysphagia. A history of radiation to the head and neck could imply airway fragility.

- Routine preoperative testing is no longer utilized; it is now the general consensus that tests should be obtained only for specific clinical indications.
- The 2011 ASA fasting guidelines may not apply to, or may need to be modified for, patients in whom airway management might be difficult.
- Cancellation of surgery because of upper respiratory infection remains controversial. The decision whether or not to proceed with the operation should be an individualized decision based on a discussion involving the patient, anesthesiologist and surgeon.
- While most of the ENT procedures are in the low surgical risk category, some of the large elective ENT operations are considered intermediate-risk surgery.

References

1. Edward Gilbert Abbott. 2011 April 8, 2011 [cited 2011 July 31, 2011]; Available from: http://en.wikipedia.org/wiki/Edward_Gilbert_Abbott

2. Bishop HF. Operating room deaths. *Anesthesiology* 1946;**7**(6): p. 651–62.

3. Pearl W. Congenital heart disease in the Pierre Robin syndrome. *Pediatr Cardiol* 1982;**2**(4):307–9.

4. Hatava P, Olsson GL, Lagerkranser M. Preoperative psychological preparation for children undergoing ENT operations: a comparison of two methods. *Paediatr Anaesth* 2000;**10**(5):477–86.

5. Fincher W, Shaw J, Ramelet AS. The effectiveness of a standardised preoperative preparation in reducing child and parent anxiety: a single-blind randomised controlled trial. *J Clin Nurs* 2012;**21**(7–8):946–55.

6. Cady J. Laryngectomy: beyond loss of voice – caring for the

patient as a whole. *Clin J Oncol Nurs* 2002;**6**(6):347–51.

7. Haller G, Laroche T, Clergue F. Morbidity in anaesthesia: today and tomorrow. *Best Pract Res Clin Anaesthesiol* 2011;**25**(2): 123–32.

8. Newland MC, Ellis SJ, Peters KR, et al. Dental injury associated with anesthesia: a report of 161,687 anesthetics given over 14 years. *J Clin Anesth* 2007;**19**(5):339–45.

9. Ueda N, Kirita T, Imai Y, et al. [Dental injury associated with general anesthesia and the preventive measures]. *Masui* 2010;**59**(5):597–603.

10. Ovassapian A, Glassenberg R, Randel GI, et al. The unexpected difficult airway and lingual tonsil hyperplasia: a case series and a review of the literature. *Anesthesiology* 2002;**97**(1): 124–32.

11. Arens R, McDonough JM, Corbin AM, et al. Upper airway size analysis by magnetic resonance imaging of children with obstructive sleep apnea syndrome.

Am J Respir Crit Care Med 2003;**167**(1):65–70.

12. Wang JH, Chung YS, Cho YW, et al. Palatine tonsil size in obese, overweight, and normal-weight children with sleep-disordered breathing. *Otolaryngol Head Neck Surg* 2010;**142**(4):516–9.

13. Practice advisory for preanesthesia evaluation: a report by the American Society of Anesthesiologists Task Force on Preanesthesia Evaluation. *Anesthesiology* 2002;**96**(2):485–96.

14. Kumar A, Srivastava U. Role of routine laboratory investigations in preoperative evaluation. *J Anaesthesiol Clin Pharmacol* 2011;**27**(2):174–9.

15. Clinical practice guideline: diagnosis and management of childhood obstructive sleep apnea syndrome. *Pediatrics* 2002;**109** (4):704–12.

16. Power LM, Thackray NM. Reduction of preoperative investigations with the introduction of an anaesthetist-led preoperative assessment clinic.

Anaesth Intensive Care 1999;
27(5):481–8.

17. Setabutr D, Adil EA, Adil TK, Carr MM. Emerging trends in tonsillectomy. *Otolaryngol Head Neck Surg* 2011;**145**(2): 223–9.

18. Wieland A, Belden L, Cunningham M. Preoperative coagulation screening for adenotonsillectomy: a review and comparison of current physician practices. *Otolaryngol Head Neck Surg* 2009;**140**(4):542–7.

19. Bong CL, Ng AS. Evaluation of emergence delirium in Asian children using the Pediatric Anesthesia Emergence Delirium Scale. *Paediatr Anaesth* 2009;**19**(6):593–600.

20. Fishkin S, Litman RS. Current issues in pediatric ambulatory anesthesia. *Anesthesiol Clin North America* 2003;**21**(2):305–11, ix.

21. Zuckerberg AL. Perioperative approach to children. *Pediatr Clin North Am* 1994;**41**(1):15–29.

22. Stenger MM. Anesthesia for outpatient ear, nose, and throat procedures. In McGoldick K, ed. *Anesthesia for Ophthalmic and Otolaryngologic Surgery.* Philadelphia: W.B. Sauders; 1992. pp. 144–55.

23. Practice guidelines for preoperative fasting and the use of pharmacologic agents to reduce the risk of pulmonary aspiration: application to healthy patients undergoing elective procedures: an updated report by the American Society of Anesthesiologists Committee on Standards and Practice Parameters. *Anesthesiology* 2011;**114**(3):495–511.

24. Hoehner PJ. Ethical aspects of informed consent in obstetric anesthesia – new challenges and solutions. *J Clin Anesth* 2003;**15**(8):587–600.

25. Aremu SK, Alabi BS, Segun-Busari S. The role of informed consent in risks recall in otorhinolaryngology surgeries: verbal (nonintervention) vs written (intervention) summaries of risks. *Am J Otolaryngol,* 2011;**32**(6):485–9.

26. Henney S, Rakhra S. Patient information in otorhinolaryngology: a prospective audit. *JRSM Short Rep* 2011;**2**(5):37.

27. Berry NH, Phillips JS, Salam MA. Written consent – a prospective audit of practices for ENT patients. *Ann R Coll Surg Engl* 2008;**90**(2):150–2.

28. Infosino A. Pediatric upper airway and congenital anomalies. *Anesthesiol Clin North America* 2002;**20**(4):747–66.

29. Tanaka K, Oikawa N, Terao R, *et al.* Evaluations of psychological preparation for children undergoing endoscopy. *J Pediatr Gastroenterol Nutr* 2011; **52**(2):227–9.

30. Letts M, Stevens L, Coleman J, Kettner R. Puppetry and doll play as an adjunct to pediatric orthopaedics. *J Pediatr Orthop* 1983;**3**(5):605–9.

31. Rathier MO, Baker WL. A review of recent clinical trials and guidelines on the prevention and management of delirium in hospitalized older patients. *Hosp Pract (Minneap)* 2011;**39**(4):96–106.

32. Steiner LA, Postoperative delirium. Part 1: pathophysiology

and risk factors. *Eur J Anaesthesiol* 2011;**28**(9):628–36.

33. Steiner LA. Postoperative delirium. part 2: detection, prevention and treatment. *Eur J Anaesthesiol* 2011;**28**(10): 723–32.

34. Bettelli G. Preoperative evaluation in geriatric surgery: comorbidity, functional status and pharmacological history. *Minerva Anestesiol,* 2011;**77**(6):637–46.

35. Muravchick S, Grichnik K. Evaluation of the geriatric patient. In Longnecker DE, *et al.*, eds. *Anesthesiology* New York: McGraw-Hall; 2008. pp. 341–57.

36. Fleischmann KE, Beckman JA, Buller CE, *et al.* 2009 ACCF/AHA focused update on perioperative beta blockade. *J Am Coll Cardiol* 2009;**54**(22):2102–28.

37. Hoehner PJ. Ethical decisions in perioperative elder care. *Anesthesiol Clin North America* 2000;**18** (1):159–81, vii–viii.

38. Ethical guidelines for the anesthesia care of patients with do-not-resuscitate orders or other directives that limit treatment. October 22, 2008; available from: http://www.asahq.org/For-Healthcare-Professionals/~/media/For%20Members/documents/Standards%20Guidelines%20Stmts/Ethical%20Guidelines%20for%20the%20Anesthesia%20Care%20of%20Patients.ashx. Accessed August 23, 2011.

39. Haynes AB, Weiser TG, Berry WR, *et al.* A surgical safety checklist to reduce morbidity and mortality in a global population. *N Engl J Med* 2009;**360**(5): 491–9.

The difficult airway in otolaryngology

4

D. John Doyle

Introduction

This chapter is concerned with difficult airway management in the context of otolaryngologic surgery. (A related chapter, Chapter 9, is concerned with some specific otolaryngologic tumors and infections.) While the focus here is on otolaryngologic surgery, most of the principles discussed herein apply to clinical airway management in general, regardless of the surgical procedure. In particular, the American Society of Anesthesiologists' difficult airway algorithm (or similar algorithm), briefly outlined in this chapter and shown in Figure 4.1, should ordinarily be a starting point for nearly all aspects of clinical airway management.

To a large extent, the airway management technique for otolaryngologic surgery will depend on clinical circumstances (Table 4.1) as well as the airway management skills of the anesthesiologist and the available equipment (Tables 4.2 and 4.3).

The following general options exist: (1) general endotracheal anesthesia, (2) general anesthesia using a supraglottic airway device such as a laryngeal mask airway, (3) general anesthesia using an ENT laryngoscope (to expose the airway) in conjunction with jet ventilation, (4) employing intermittent apnea, (5) general anesthesia using the patient's natural airway, with or without adjuncts such as jaw-positioning devices or nasopharyngeal airways, and (6) local anesthesia in conjunction with IV sedation in some form, with the patient breathing spontaneously. The first option is doubtless the most popular, but the technique chosen, as well as the method of implementing the technique chosen, will depend on factors such as the perceived difficulty of intubating the patient using ordinary methods. Evaluation of the airway in this particular respect is discussed elsewhere in this book (Chapters 3 and 5).

The obstructed airway

A patient's airway can become obstructed for many reasons. Examples include aspirated foreign bodies; infections such as epiglottitis, diphtheria or Ludwig's angina; laryngospasm; tumors and hematomas impinging on the airway; trauma to the airway; obstructive sleep apnea; tonsillar hypertrophy; airway edema (for example, due to anaphylaxis, prolonged laryngoscopy or smoke inhalation burn injury), as well as many other causes.

Although tracheal intubation is the "gold standard" means of managing the obstructed airway, in many cases the airway may be opened with a simple jaw thrust, the use of a nasopharyngeal airway or an oropharyngeal airway, or the use of a supraglottic airway device such as the laryngeal mask airway (LMA). Ordinary mask ventilation is frequently employed where positive-pressure ventilation is desired.

Mask ventilation

Mask ventilation is an important clinical skill to master, but can sometimes be difficult [1–3]. In most resuscitation settings a self-reinflating bag with non-rebreathing valves is used to provide positive-pressure ventilation, usually using 100% oxygen. This bag fills spontaneously after being squeezed and can be used even when oxygen is unavailable. Ventilation is often made much easier when the "jaw thrust maneuver" is carried out. Oropharyngeal or nasopharyngeal airways can also be helpful. Following prolonged bag and mask ventilation, a nasogastric tube may be used to vent any air that may have been forced into the stomach.

Ordinarily, should intubation be difficult, clinicians can still provide ventilation and oxygenation

Anesthesia for Otolaryngologic Surgery, ed. Basem Abdelmalak and D. John Doyle. Published by Cambridge University Press. © Cambridge University Press 2013.

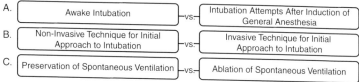

AMERICAN SOCIETY
OF ANESTHESIOLOGISTS

DIFFICULT AIRWAY ALGORITHM

1. Assess the likelihood and clinical impact of basic management problems:
   A. Difficult Ventilation
   B. Difficult Intubation
   C. Difficulty with Patient Cooperation or Consent
   D. Difficult Tracheostomy

2. Actively pursue opportunities to deliver supplemental oxygen throughout the process of difficult airway management

3. Consider the relative merits and feasibility of basic management choices:

   A. Awake Intubation —vs— Intubation Attempts After Induction of General Anesthesia
   B. Non-Invasive Technique for Initial Approach to Intubation —vs— Invasive Technique for Initial Approach to Intubation
   C. Preservation of Spontaneous Ventilation —vs— Ablation of Spontaneous Ventilation

4. Develop primary and alternative strategies:

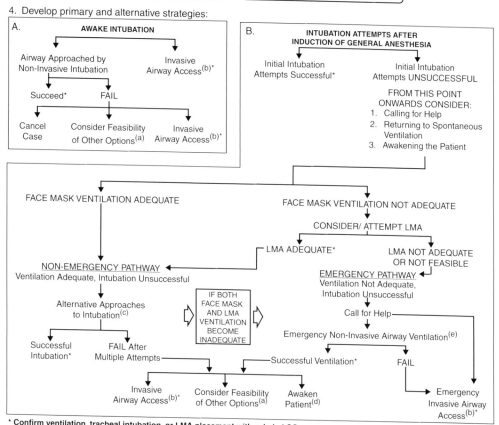

* Confirm ventilation, tracheal intubation, or LMA placement with exhaled CO_2

a. Other options include (but are not limited to): surgery utilizing face mask or LMA anesthesia, local anesthesia infiltration or regional nerve blockade. Pursuit of these options usually implies that mask ventilation will not be problematic. Therefore, these options may be of limited value if this step in the algorithm has been reached via the Emergency Pathway.

b. Invasive airway access includes surgical or percutaneous tracheostomy or cricothyrotomy.

c. Alternative non-invasive approaches to difficult intubation include (but are not limited to): use of different laryngoscope blades, LMA as an intubation conduit (with or without fiberoptic guidance), fiberoptic intubation, intubating stylet or tube changer, light wand, retrograde intubation, and blind oral or nasal intubation.

d. Consider re-preparation of the patient for awake intubation or canceling surgery.

e. Options for emergency non-invasive airway ventilation include (but are not limited to): rigid bronchoscope, esophageal–tracheal combitube ventilation, or transtracheal jet ventilation.

Figure 4.1. Synopsis of the 2003 ASA difficult airway algorithm. It is expected that future editions of the algorithm will place special emphasis on the use of videolaryngoscopy for those situations where direct laryngoscopy produces an unsatisfactory view of the glottic structures. Reproduced with permission from the American Society of Anesthesiologists.

Table 4.1. Some ENT diseases and conditions associated with difficult airway management

Infection-related

- Abscess of upper airway
- Epiglottitis
- Ludwig's angina
- Quinsy
- Retropharyngeal abscess

Tumor-related

- Supraglottic and glottic tumors
- Tumors of base of tongue
- Oral malignancies
- Previous head and neck surgery
- Previous radiation treatment to head and neck

Trauma-related

- Facial smash
- Fractured larynx
- Maxillofacial trauma
- Cervical spine trauma
- Trismus
- Temporomandibular joint injury

Other conditions

- Externally fixed head (eg. halo traction)
- Wired jaws or teeth
- Congenital malformation
- Very anterior larynx
- Fused cervical-spine (e.g. ankylosing spondylitis)
- Supraglottic or subglottic edema

Table 4.2. Popular supraglottic airway devices

- LMA family of products
  - Disposable LMA (LMA Unique)
  - Flexible LMA
  - Intubating LMA (LMA Fastrach)
  - LMA Proseal
- Combitube
- Laryngeal tube and variants
- i-gel family of supraglottic airways
- Air-Q family of supraglottic airways
- King tube

Table 4.3. Popular and specialty laryngoscopes

"Conventional" laryngoscopes

- Macintosh-type laryngoscopes
- Miller-type laryngoscopes and other straight-blade designs
- McCoy laryngoscope and variants

Rigid fiberoptic laryngoscopes

- Bullard laryngoscope
- Upsher laryngoscope
- Wu laryngoscope

Video laryngoscopes

- GlideScope video laryngoscope
- Storz video laryngoscope
- McGrath video laryngoscope
- KingVision video laryngoscope
- Clarus family of laryngoscopes

via face-mask ventilation. However, in some cases, mask ventilation can be difficult. Obviously, being able to accurately predict difficult mask ventilation may improve the safety of airway management. In a study of this matter by Langeron *et al.* [1], difficult mask ventilation (DMV) was defined as the inability of an unassisted anesthesiologist to maintain the oxygen saturation over 92% or to prevent or reverse signs of inadequate ventilation during positive-pressure mask ventilation under general anesthesia. With this definition, DMV was found in 75 of 1502

patients studied (5%), with one case of impossible ventilation. Of particular interest, DMV was anticipated by the anesthesiologist in only 13 patients, or 17% of the DMV cases. Using multivariate analysis, five criteria were identified as independent factors for DMV. These are listed in Table 4.4. The presence of two factors was found to indicate an especially high likelihood of DMV (sensitivity, 0.72; specificity, 0.73).

In a study conducted at the University of Michigan [2], the authors studied the incidence and predictors of difficult and impossible mask ventilation

Table 4.4. Predictors of difficult mask ventilation. From Langeron O, Masso E, Huraux C, *et al.* Prediction of difficult mask ventilation. *Anesthesiology* 2000;**92**:1229–36

- Age over 55 yr
- Body mass index exceeding 26 kg/m^2
- Presence of a beard
- Lack of teeth
- History of snoring

Table 4.5. Grading scale for difficulty of mask ventilation developed by Han *et al.* (2004)

Classification	Description/ definition
Grade 0	Ventilation by mask not attempted
Grade 1	Ventilated by mask
Grade 2	Ventilated by mask with oral airway or other adjuvant
Grade 3	Difficult mask ventilation (inadequate, unstable, or requiring two practioners)
Grade 4	Unable to mask ventilate

(MV) using the grading scale developed by Han *et al.* [3] (Table 4.5). This scale consists of five categories (grades 0–4), with grades 3 and 4 representing difficult and impossible mask ventilation respectively. The authors summarize their findings as follows: "Body mass index of 30 kg/m^2 or greater, a beard, Mallampati classification III or IV, age of 57 yr or older, severely limited jaw protrusion, and snoring were identified as independent predictors for grade 3 MV. Snoring and thyromental distance of less than 6 cm were independent predictors for grade 4 MV. Limited or severely limited mandibular protrusion, abnormal neck anatomy, sleep apnea, snoring, and body mass index of 30 kg/m^2 or greater were independent predictors of grade 3 or 4 MV and difficult intubation." These findings emphasize the importance played by a large neck size (e.g., such as may be found in obesity) or by abnormal neck anatomy (e.g., such as may be found following radiation treatment to the neck.)

Tracheal intubation in patients undergoing otolaryngologic surgery

Most patients undergoing otolaryngologic surgery have their airway managed via tracheal intubation. Under ordinary circumstances, tracheal intubation is straightforward and ordinary laryngoscopic techniques work well. From time to time, patients who are expected to be difficult to intubate are encountered, and these patients are usually managed using techniques such as videolaryngoscopy or fiberoptic intubation (Figure 4.2). A key decision in such cases is whether or not the intubation should be carried out awake or following the induction of general anesthesia. Another important decision is what tools/interventions to employ in the event that difficulty with ventilation or with intubation is encountered.

Patients for otolaryngologic surgery are often intubated using an ordinary polyvinyl chloride

(PVC) endotracheal tube, but microlaryngeal, laser tubes and reinforced tubes are frequently employed. In the case of reinforced tubes, their principal advantages are that they are very unlikely to kink and that they fit especially well into tracheostomy stomas because of their excellent flexibility. Laser tubes are discussed in Chapter 25.

The usual considerations in this situation start with the fact that the tube must be adequately secured using tape or by other means (some maxillofacial surgeons prefer to tie the tube to the side of the mouth or to tie the tube to the teeth with wire). One should also ensure that the tube tip is not too close to the carina (or worse, positioned endobronchially), that the tube cuff is positioned appropriately deep past the vocal cords, and that the tube not be situated so that kinking is likely to occur with head movement or so that it exerts pressure onto the posterior pharyngeal wall.

In addition, it is important that the cuff pressures in the endotracheal tube ordinarily be kept less than 25 mmHg to avoid damage to the tracheal mucosa. With respect to this last issue, it should be remembered that in cases where nitrous oxide is used the cuff pressures will gradually increase over time as nitrous oxide enters the cuff by diffusion. This is of particular concern in surgical procedures of long duration, such as free-flap surgery.

Role of the ASA difficult airway algorithm

The American Society of Anesthesiologists (ASA) has issued guidelines for management of the difficult airway. This began with an algorithm initially published in 1993 [4], followed by a revision in 2003 [5], These guidelines, as well as similar guidelines from

(A)

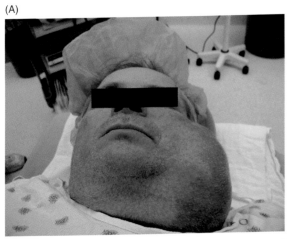

(B)

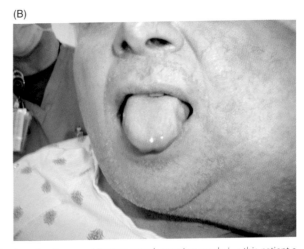

Figure 4.2. This is a patient with a massive parotid tumor, encroaching into the airway and limiting mouth opening, rendering this patient a difficult airway that required awake intubation. Image courtesy of Dr. B. Abdelmalak. Reprinted with permission, Cleveland Clinic Center for Medical Art & Photography © 2012. All rights reserved.

other sources [6–28], offer considerable useful advice to the clinician facing potentially difficult airway challenges. Such advice includes (1) the importance of performing an airway evaluation prior to inducing anesthesia, (2) the importance of providing oxygen at every opportunity, (3) the potential value of awake intubation, (4) the value of supraglottic airway devices such as the laryngeal mask airway (LMA™) as a possible airway rescue maneuver should failure occur, and so on. Figure 4.1 summarizes the 2003 ASA difficult airway algorithm.

Prediction of intubation difficulty: intubation difficulty scale

Before attempting tracheal intubation it is very helpful to have a means to predict which patients will be difficult to intubate using direct laryngoscopy. While a number of studies and reviews on the topic are available [24–28], most clinicians will be satisfied with the 11-point airway assessment tool included with the 2003 ASA difficult airway algorithm. This is summarized in Table 4.6, while Table 4.7 lists some techniques useful in clinical airway management. In addition, following the completion of tracheal intubation, it can sometimes be helpful to summarize the difficulty (if any) encountered. Here, the Intubation Difficulty Scale (IDS) introduced by Adnet *et al.* [28] can be useful. It is a numerical score indicating overall intubation difficulty based on seven descriptors associated with intubation difficulty:

number of supplementary intubation attempts, number of supplementary operators, alternative techniques used, laryngoscopic grade, subjective lifting force, the use of external laryngeal manipulation, and the characteristics of the vocal cords.

Laryngoscopes

Most intubations are achieved using traditional Macintosh and Miller laryngoscopes, although a number of alternative laryngoscopes have been advocated. Where the view at laryngoscopy is suboptimal, the use of introducers such as the Eschman stylet ("gum elastic bougie") can sometimes be very helpful [29–31]. It is used as follows: when a poor laryngoscopic view of the glottic structures is obtained, the intubator places the introducer into the patient's mouth and gently advances it through the glottic opening (in the case of a Grade II view) or anteriorly under the epiglottis (in the case of a Grade III view). Subtle clicks resulting from the introducer passing over the tracheal rings help confirm proper placement of the introducer. With the introducer held steady, one then railroads a tracheal tube over the introducer into the glottis. Some clinicians preload the introducer with a tracheal tube as shown in Figure 4.3.

Special devices such as the McCoy laryngoscope and the Bullard laryngoscope are also popular in some centers. In recent years, however, video laryngoscopes such as the GlideScope, the McGrath video laryngoscope, the Storz video laryngoscope and the

Table 4.6. Components of the preoperative airway physical examination as recommended in the ASA difficult airway algorithm (2003 edition). In ordinary clinical practice, special emphasis is usually placed on the visibility of the oropharyngeal structures with the tongue protruded when the patient is in the sitting position (Mallampati classification)

Airway examination component	Nonreassuring findings
1. Length of upper incisors	Relatively long
2. Relation of maxillary and mandibular incisors during normal jaw closure	Prominent "overbite" (maxillary incisors anterior to mandibular incisors)
3. Relation of maxillary and mandibular incisors during voluntary protrusion of mandible	Patient cannot bring mandibular incisor anterior to (in front of) maxillary incisors
4. Interincisor distance	Under 3 cm
5. Visibility of uvula	Not visible when tongue is protruded with patient in sitting position (e.g., Mallampati class greater than class II)
6. Shape of palate	Highly arched or very narrow
7. Compliance of mandibular space	Stiff, indurated, occupied by mass, or nonresilient
8. Thyromental distance	Less than 3 ordinary finger breadths
9. Length of neck	Short
10. Thickness of neck	Thick
11. Range of motion of head and neck	Patient cannot touch tip of chin to chest or cannot extend neck

Table 4.7. Techniques for difficult airway management. This table from the 2003 ASA difficult airway algorithm lists some commonly cited techniques. Since the time of publication the use of video laryngoscopy (e.g., GlideScope, McGrath video laryngoscope, Storz video laryngoscope, Pentax AWS) has become commonplace and should be added to the left-hand column. Naturally, the tools used in any particular situation will depend on the specific circumstances

Techniques for difficult intubation	Techniques for difficult ventilation
Alternative laryngoscope blades	Esophageal tracheal Combitube
Awake intubation	Intratracheal jet stylet
Blind intubation (oral or nasal)	Laryngeal mask airway (LMA)
Fiberoptic intubation	Oral and nasopharyngeal airways
Intubating stylet or tube changer	Rigid ventilating bronchoscope
Intubation via LMA	Invasive airway access
Light wand	Transtracheal jet ventilation
Retrograde intubation	Two-person mask ventilation
Invasive airway access	

Pentax AWS have proven to be particularly valuable, especially in patients with an "anterior" larynx or in patients with cervical spine immobilization. Among the available videolaryngoscopes, the GlideScope (Figure 4.4) has the largest market share. Figure 4.5 shows a typical view of the glottis during intubation with the GlideScope. Figure 4.6 shows a sample "difficult airway letter" that may be included in the patient's chart and given to the patient.

Fiberoptic intubation: awake intubation

Awake intubation involves endotracheal tube insertion in a conscious or lightly sedated patient and is usually performed because intubation under general anesthesia is judged to be too risky because of concerns about possible difficulties with ventilation or intubation or concerns about aspiration. While fiberoptic intubation under topical anesthesia is the most common means of carrying out awake intubation, other methods include awake blind nasal intubation using an Endotrol® (or similar) endotracheal tube, or using a Macintosh, Miller, GlideScope or other laryngoscope under topical anesthesia. A number of airway blocks can be used in addition to topical anesthesia. These are discussed in Chapter 6.

41

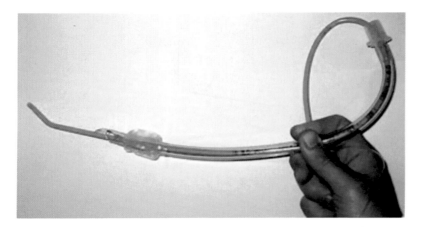

Figure 4.3. Photograph showing a tracheal tube with a preloaded introducer containing a Coude tip. Intended for situations where the laryngoscopic view is suboptimal, the upturned distal Coude tip is placed under the epiglottis or, if visible, above the interarytenoid notch, followed by advancement of the tracheal tube into the trachea. Image credit: http://www.airwaycam.com/images/bougieKiwiGrip_01.gif.

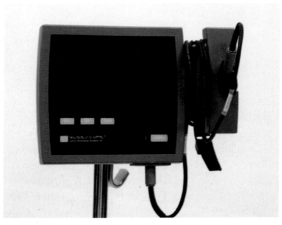

Figure 4.4. The GlideScope videolaryngoscope utilizes a color CMOS video camera and LED light source embedded into a plastic laryngoscope blade. The standard (adult) blade is 14.5 mm at its maximum width, and bends 60° at the mid-line. This configuration provides a view that is frequently superior to that obtained by direct laryngoscopy. The video image is displayed on a liquid crystal display (LCD) monitor, and can also be recorded electronically. An anti-fog mechanism helps ensure that a quality image is obtained. In addition to the standard blade, a mid-sized (pediatric) blade and a neonatal blade are also available.

The use of fiberoptic intubation for the airway management of patients undergoing otolaryngologic surgery is popular because this technique works well in the presence of many kinds of airway pathology. While fiberoptic intubation can often be safely performed under complete general anesthesia [32] many clinicians opt to perform this technique under topical anesthesia with the patient only lightly sedated ("awake fiberoptic intubation"), depending on the skill level of the anesthesiologist, the cooperation of the patient,

and the severity of the pathology. A central consideration behind the choice of "awake" versus "asleep" fiberoptic intubation is the safety margin an awake technique allows: if intubation is not successfully accomplished, the patient's ability to maintain his or her own airway remains intact. In addition, during awake intubation, airway reflexes are generally maintained sufficiently to guard against pulmonary aspiration, an important point in patients with high aspiration risk such as full stomach trauma patients.

It should also be emphasized that awake intubation is not synonymous with fiberoptic intubation. Awake intubation can be accomplished safely utilizing many other airway devices. Other possible options for awake intubation include but are not limited to: direct laryngoscopy with Macintosh and Miller laryngoscopes, blind nasal intubation, use of a GlideScope or other video laryngscope, use of a lighted stylette, etc.

Typically, with awake intubation the airway is anesthetized with gargled and atomized 4% lidocaine. Superior laryngeal and transtracheal blocks are occasionally also employed. In addition, judicious sedation is usually administered. Midazolam, fentanyl, remifentanil, ketamine, propofol and clonidine have all been used in this setting. Recently, the use of dexmedetomidine, a selective α_2 agonist with sedative, analgesic, amnestic, and antisialagogue properties, has been reported [33]. A key advantage of this agent is that it maintains spontaneous respiration with minimal respiratory depression. Patients under dexmedetomidine sedation are generally easy to arouse. However, this advantage, along with that of

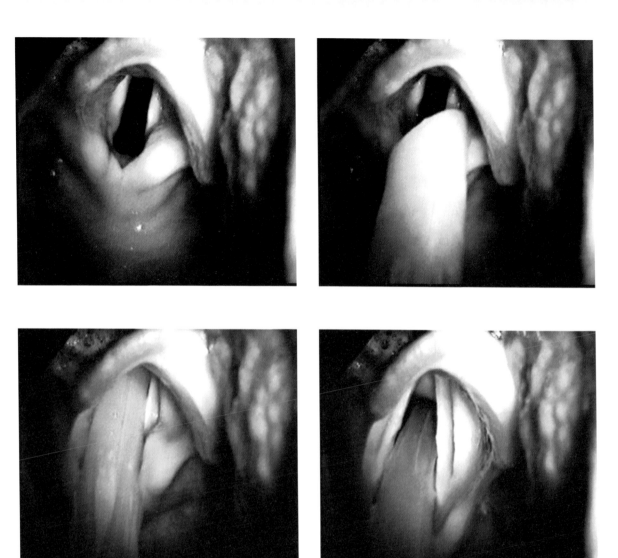

Figure 4.5. Close-up views from the GlideScope, as the endotracheal tube (ETT) passes through the vocal cords. Note that during ETT placement the tube tip often tends to hit against the anterior tracheal wall. This problem is easily handled by pulling back the stylette by about 3 cm and then advancing the ETT. Sometimes it also helps to rotate the ETT 180° to direct the ETT tip more posteriorly (once the stylette has been removed). From case 112 of the author's unpublished series.

maintaining spontaneous respiration, may not hold under very large doses.

Doyle [34] has described the successful use of the GlideScope in four cases of awake intubation. The following potential advantages are worthy of note. First, the view is generally excellent. Second, the method appears to be less affected by the presence of secretions or blood as compared to the use of fiberoptic intubation. Third, there are no special restrictions on the type of ETT that can be placed when using the GlideScope, while this is not the case

for fiberoptic methods. Fourth, the GlideScope is much more rugged than a fiberoptic bronchoscope, and is far less likely to be damaged with use. It should also be noted that while it is well known that advancing the ETT into the trachea over the fiberoptic bronchoscope often fails as a result of the ETT impinging on the arytenoid cartilages, this is generally not a problem with the GlideScope.

In the end, however, the use of awake fiberoptic intubation in the setting of the patient with airway pathology remains steadfastly popular, because it is

***IMPORTANT ***

To the physician: This person was found to be a DIFFICULT INTUBATION on

__ __/__ __ __/__ __ __   at _____ (Hospital),

Tel: _____

Reasons for difficulty included (circle all that apply):

1) Poor neck mobility

2) Poor jaw mobility

3) Prominent teeth

4) Large/stiff tongue

5) Anterior larynx

6) Limited mouth opening

7) Other (specify)

Ventilation with bag and mask was:

1) Easy

2) Difficult

3) Impossible

Ventilation adjuncts used included (circle all that apply):

1) Oropharyngeal airway

2) Nasopharyngeal airway

3) Other (specify)

Success was achieved:

1) Unconscious / paralyzed

2) Awake

using (circle all that apply):

1) Alternate blade (specify)

2) Video laryngoscope (specify)

3) Fiberoptic bronchoscope

4) Light wand / transillumination

5) Blind nasal intubation

6) Other (specify)

44

Figure 4.6. Model difficult airway form. This is a model difficult airway form you can adapt for your clinical practice. It is suggested that you keep these forms readily available in the anesthesia lounge to report difficult airway information to the patient and to his or her physician. It is provided courtesy of John R. Davidson MD FRCPC.

For future anesthetics in fasted patients I recommend:

1) Long pre-oxygenation, short acting agents, early wake-up if success not forthcoming.
2) Awake intubation.

I hope this information is helpful to you.

— — — — — —— —— —— — —— —— — — — —— — — —— —— —— —— — —— —— — — — —

*** IMPORTANT ***

To The Patient:

During general anesthesia (sleep for surgery) an oxygen tube is usually placed in the patient's throat. This assures an adequate supply of oxygen to the lungs, heart, brain and other vital organs.

At the time of your recent anesthetic there was difficulty getting this tube into position. Such difficulties arise because of the relative position of a patient's mouth, teeth, and windpipe.

The attached form describes the problem in detail for the benefit of any anesthesiologist taking care of you in the future. Please keep this form and show it to your anesthesiologist if you ever have surgery in the future. It will warn the anesthesiologist and will enable him or her to take better care of you.

You should also get a Medic Alert bracelet to warn of this problem. The bracelet should say: "DIFFICULT INTUBATION". The address information for the MedicAlert Foundation is as follows:

MedicAlert Foundation International
2323 Colorado Avenue
Turlock, California, USA 95382
http://www.medicalert.org

By phone, 24 hours a day:
888-633-4298
209-668-3333 from outside the U.S.

This is IMPORTANT! Knowing you are a "Difficult Intubation" could save your life in an emergency.

Figure 4.6. *(cont.)*

gentle to the airway, is generally well tolerated, and does not require the application of force to obtain glottic exposure.

In addition, concerns about injuries associated with the use of the GlideScope have added to some individuals' reluctance to use the device on a routine basis [35].

Can't intubate – what now?

Occasionally one encounters patients who cannot be intubated by direct laryngoscopy either due to poor judgment or from unexpected difficulty. Depending on the clinical circumstances, one may choose one of the following options.

Always remember to call for help when needed

[Option 1] Ventilate the patient and allow them to wake up. If ventilation is also difficult, utilize a two-person technique whereby one person manages the mask and holds the jaw in position using both hands, while the other ventilates the patient by hand using the rebreathing bag. Insertion of an airway of some kind, such as an oral airway or a nasopharyngeal airway, can be helpful. Alternately, ventilation can be assisted with the use of a supraglottic airway, although this may be of limited value in some patients with abnormal airways. Then one can either cancel the case, proceed with awake intubation or proceed with regional anesthesia, as appropriate. The regional anesthesia option suffers from the disadvantage that the airway will be in jeopardy should local anesthetic toxicity be a problem.

[Option 2] While the patient is still under general anesthesia, proceed to intubate using a video laryngoscope, a lighted stylette or a fiberoptic bronchoscope.

[Option 3] Keep the patient asleep and insert a supraglottic airway of some kind. Then either do the case using a supraglottic airway or use the supraglottic airway as a conduit for tracheal intubation. However, performing the case using a supraglottic airway may not be a satisfactory option in many cases, such as in prone cases or patients at substantial risk of aspiration.

[Option 4] Allow an otolaryngologist to attempt intubation using specialized equipment such as a Dedo laryngoscope, an anterior commissure laryngoscope or a rigid bronchoscope.

[Option 5] In patients where neither intubation nor ventilation is possible despite everyone's best efforts, a surgical airway will be needed.

Airway edema in ENT cases

Airway edema is a frequent accompaniment to prolonged surgery of any kind, especially when vigorous fluid resuscitation has been carried out, or in patients with some forms of airway pathology, such as some infections. Many clinicians have used the leak test to determine readiness for extubation, despite its recognized limitations. (The presence of a leak around the endotracheal tube when the cuff is down is said to imply that the airway is not overly edematous.)

Difficult extubation

Extubation, removing an endotracheal tube (ETT) from the patient's trachea, should ordinarily only be done with the patient awake enough to obey verbal commands. Even under such conditions, however, catastrophes following extubation can occur, such as total collapse of the airway in a patient with tracheomalacia. Sometimes it is wise to extubate over an ETT exchange catheter, such as any patient who would be very difficult to reintubate or where delayed edema following laser airway surgery is expected.

Such an exchange catheter can be left in place and later used to facilitate reintubation should a trial of extubation end in failure. If reintubation becomes necessary the exchange catheter can then be used as a far-from-foolproof guide to direct the new ETT through the cords. Some exchange catheters can also be used to administer low-flow oxygen deep into the lungs (e.g. 2–4 liters/min flow rate) as well as for capnography or even emergency jet ventilation in a manner similar to transtracheal jet ventilation (TTJV).

Patients may be at high risk following extubation either because of an inability to tolerate extubation or because of potential difficulties in reestablishing the airway. Examples of the former include tracheomalacia, vocal cord palsy, bilateral recurrent laryngeal nerve injury, etc. Difficulty reestablishing the airway may occur with major head or neck surgery, previous intubation difficulties, maxillomandibular fixation and many other situations.

Summary

Difficult airway management for otolaryngologic surgery relies heavily on the American Society of Anesthesiologists difficult airway algorithm and, particularly, on the use of awake intubation in the spontaneously breathing patient. In addition, one must always have at hand a plan for the situation where the patient cannot easily be intubated by direct laryngoscopy.

Case study

A 55-yr-old, 59-kg man was admitted to hospital with an acute exacerbation of COPD/emphysema requiring intubation and mechanical ventilation. While breathing room air, his PaO_2 was 50 mmHg and $PaCO_2$ was 63 mmHg. He was known to be difficult to intubate as a result of extensive radiation for head and neck cancer. Intravenous sedation with dexmedetomidine was started with a loading dose of 1 μg/kg followed by an infusion of 0.7 μg/kg/h while oxygen was delivered by nasal cannula. Following this, oxygen saturation measured by pulse oximeter stayed above 90% and the respiratory rate declined from 32 breaths/min to 18 breaths/min. Topicalization of the airway was achieved with gargled 2% viscous lidocaine and 4% lidocaine spray. A Williams airway was used to facilitate orotracheal intubation. Once the cords were in view, additional 4% lidocaine was administered under direct vision via an epidural catheter introduced into the biopsy channel of the bronchoscope. Once the tube was advanced into the trachea and the correct position established clinically, fiberoptically and capnographically, additional sedation using propofol was used to facilitate positive-pressure ventilation.

Clinical pearls

- To a large extent, the airway management technique for otolaryngologic surgery will depend on specific clinical circumstances as well as the airway management skills of the anesthesiologist.

- Should intubation be difficult, clinicians can still provide ventilation and oxygenation via face-mask ventilation. However, it some cases, mask ventilation can be difficult.
- Body mass index of ≥ 30 kg/m^2, a beard, Mallampati classification III or IV, age of ≥ 57 yr, severely limited jaw protrusion, thyromental distance of less than 6 cm and snoring were identified as independent predictors of difficult mask ventilation.
- Although patients for otolaryngologic surgery are often intubated using an ordinary polyvinyl chloride (PVC) endotracheal tube, microlaryngeal, laser-safe and wire-reinforced tubes are frequently employed.
- Awake intubation is usually performed because intubation under general anesthesia is judged to be too risky (difficulties with ventilation or intubation or concerns about aspiration). A central consideration behind the choice of "awake" versus "asleep" fiberoptic intubation is the safety margin an awake technique allows.
- The use of fiberoptic intubation for the airway management of patients undergoing otolaryngologic surgery is popular because this technique works well in the presence of many kinds of airway pathology. Moreover, it is gentle to the airway, generally well tolerated, and does not require the application of force to obtain glottic exposure.
- Awake intubation is not synonymous with fiberoptic intubation, as awake intubation can be accomplished safely using many other airway devices, such as direct laryngoscopy with Macintosh and Miller laryngoscopes, blind nasal intubation, use of a GlideScope or other video laryngscopes, use of a lighted stylette, etc.
- In patients where neither intubation nor ventilation is possible despite everyone's best efforts, a surgical airway will be needed.

References

1. Langeron O, Masso E, Huraux C, et al. Prediction of difficult mask ventilation. *Anesthesiology* 2000;**92**:1229–36.

2. Kheterpal S, Han R, Tremper KK, et al. Incidence and predictors of difficult and impossible mask ventilation. *Anesthesiology* 2006;**105**(5):885–91.

3. Han R, Tremper KK, Kheterpal S, O'Reilly M. Grading scale for mask ventilation. *Anesthesiology* 2004;**101**:267

4. Practice guidelines for management of the difficult airway. A report by the American Society of Anesthesiologists Task Force on Management of the Difficult Airway. *Anesthesiology* 1993;**78**:597–602.

5. Practice guidelines for management of the difficult airway: an updated report by the

American Society of Anesthesiologists Task Force on Management of the Difficult Airway. *Anesthesiology* 2003;**98**:1269–77.

6. Frova G, Sorbello M. Algorithms for difficult airway management: a review. *Minerva Anestesiol* 2009;**75**(4):201–9.

7. Cook TM. Difficult Airway Society guidelines. *Anaesthesia* 2004;**59**:1243–4; author reply 1247.

8. Crosby ET, Cooper RM, Douglas MJ, *et al.* The unanticipated difficult airway with recommendations for management. *Can J Anaesth* 1998;**45**(8):757–76.

9. Combes X, Jabre P, Margenet A, *et al.* Unanticipated difficult airway management in the prehospital emergency setting: prospective validation of an algorithm. *Anesthesiology* 2011;**114**(1):105–10.

10. Amathieu R, Combes X, Abdi W, *et al.* An algorithm for difficult airway management, modified for modern optical devices (Airtraq laryngoscope; LMA CTrach™): a 2-year prospective validation in patients for elective abdominal, gynecologic, and thyroid surgery. *Anesthesiology* 2011;**114**(1):25–33.

11. Weiss M, Engelhardt T. Proposal for the management of the unexpected difficult pediatric airway. *Paediatr Anaesth* 2010;**20**(5):454–64. Epub 2010 Mar 22.

12. Dupanovic M, Fox H, Kovac A. Management of the airway in multitrauma. *Curr Opin Anaesthesiol* 2010;**23**(2):276–82.

13. Vaida SJ, Pott LM, Budde AO, Gaitini LA. Suggested algorithm for management of the unexpected difficult airway in obstetric anesthesia. *J Clin Anesth* 2009;**21**(5):385–6. Epub 2009 Aug 22.

14. Heard AM, Green RJ, Eakins P. The formulation and introduction of a 'can't intubate, can't ventilate' algorithm into clinical practice. *Anaesthesia* 2009;**64**(6):601–8.

15. Saxena S. The ASA difficult airway algorithm: is it time to include video laryngoscopy and discourage blind and multiple intubation attempts in the nonemergency pathway? *Anesth Analg* 2009;**108**(3):1052.

16. Boseley ME, Hartnick CJ. A useful algorithm for managing the difficult pediatric airway. *Int J Pediatr Otorhinolaryngol* 2007;**71**(8):1317–20.

17. Heidegger T, Gerig HJ. Algorithms for management of the difficult airway. *Curr Opin Anaesthesiol* 2004;**17**(6):483–4.

18. Petrini F, Accorsi A, Adrario E, *et al.* Gruppo di Studio SIAARTI "Vie Aeree Difficili"; IRC e SARNePI; Task Force. Recommendations for airway control and difficult airway management. *Minerva Anestesiol* 2005;**71**(11):617–57.

19. Segal R. A response to 'Difficult Airway Society guidelines for management of the unanticipated difficult intubation', Henderson JJ, Popat MT, Latto IP and Pearce AC, *Anaesthesia* 2004;**59**:675–94. *Anaesthesia* 2004;**59**(11):1150–1.

20. Rosenblatt WH. The Airway Approach Algorithm: a decision tree for organizing preoperative airway information. *J Clin Anesth* 2004;**16**(4):312–6.

21. Henderson JJ, Popat MT, Latto IP, Pearce AC; Difficult Airway Society. Difficult Airway Society guidelines for management of the unanticipated difficult intubation. *Anaesthesia* 2004;**59**(7):675–94.

22. Combes X, Le Roux B, Suen P, *et al.* Unanticipated difficult airway in anesthetized patients: prospective validation of a management algorithm. *Anesthesiology* 2004;**100**(5):1146–50.

23. Rosenblatt WH, Whipple J. The difficult airway algorithm of the American Society of Anesthesiologists. *Anesth Analg* 2003;**96**(4):1233.

24. Randell T: Prediction of difficult intubation. *Acta Anaesthesiol Scand* 1996;**40**:1016–23.

25. Iohom G, Ronayne M, Cunningham AJ. Prediction of difficult tracheal intubation. *Eur J Anaesthesiol* 2003;**20**:31–6.

26. Honarmand A, Safavi MR. Prediction of difficult laryngoscopy in obstetric patients scheduled for Caesarean delivery. *Eur J Anaesthesiol* 2008;**25**:714–20.

27. Khan ZH, Mohammadi M, Rasouli MR, Farrokhnia F, Khan RH. The diagnostic value of the upper lip bite test combined with sternomental distance, thyromental distance, and interincisor distance for prediction of easy laryngoscopy and intubation: a prospective study. *Anesth Analg* 2009;**109**:822–4.

28. Adnet F, Borron SW, Racine SX, *et al.* The intubation difficulty scale (IDS): proposal and evaluation of a new score characterizing the complexity of endotracheal intubation. *Anesthesiology* 1997;**87**:1290–7.

29. Shah KH, Kwong BM, Hazan A, Newman DH, Wiener D. Success of the gum elastic bougie as a rescue airway in the emergency department. *J Emerg Med* 2011;**40**(1):1–6.

30. Boedeker BH, Bernhagen M, Miller DJ, Murray WB. Comparison of a disposable bougie versus a newly designed malleable bougie in the intubation of a difficult manikin airway. *Stud Health Technol Inform.* 2011;**163**:65–7.

31. Combes X, Dumerat M, Dhonneur G. Emergency gum elastic bougie-assisted tracheal intubation in four patients

with upper airway distortion. *Can J Anaesth* 2004;**51**(10): 1022–4.

32. Abdelmalak BB, Bernstein E, Egan C, *et al.* GlideScope® vs flexible fibreoptic scope for elective intubation in obese patients. *Anaesthesia* 2011;**66** (7): 550–5. PubMed PMID: 21564041.

33. Abdelmalak B, Marcanthony N, Abdelmalak J, *et al.* Dexmedetomidine for anesthetic management of anterior mediastinal mass. *J Anesth* 2010;**24**(4):607–10. PubMed PMID: 20454810.

34. Doyle DJ. Awake intubation using the GlideScope video laryngoscope: initial experience in four cases. *Can J Anaesth* 2004;**51** (5):520–1. PubMed PMID: 15128649.

35. Cooper RM. Complications associated with the use of the GlideScope videolaryngoscope. *Can J Anaesth* 2007; **54**(1):54–7. PubMed PMID: 17197469.

Chapter

5

Preoperative endoscopic airway examination

William H. Rosenblatt

Patients presenting to the operating room must be evaluated for the presence of anatomic or functional issues which may affect safe airway control, regardless of the need to employ general anesthesia. If monitored anesthesia care with sedation or infiltrative or regional anesthesia is anticipated, an airway plan is still needed [1].

All patients fall into one of three broad categories: the patient with no known or suspected airway abnormalities, the patient with obvious airway distortion, and the patient with "unknown" airway disease, i.e., presenting with a diagnosis of pathology affecting some part of the airway. Using the American Society of Anesthesiologist (ASA) difficult airway algorithm as a benchmark, the first group of patients is managed via the routine induction root point (Figure 5.1, box B) that includes the control of the airway after the induction of anesthesia [2].

On occasion, problems with noninvasive ventilation or tracheal intubation (by one or any means) may occur. The ASA algorithm provides for these occurrences with guidelines for the use of alternative ventilation/intubation techniques, returning to spontaneous ventilation and, eventually, invasive airways. The large majority of patients presenting to the operating room will enter the ASA algorithm at this root point.

The other two patient groups, the known and "unknown" difficult airway patients, provide a conundrum in the era of modern airway management. Prior to the development of the sophisticated armamentarium of the modern airway manager, the patient who presented with obvious difficulty for laryngoscopy (e.g., fixed trismus) or the patient presenting with a significant airway mass was often managed with awake intubation [3]. Though successful airway management was readily accomplished, application to

patients who did not truly require this intensity of care represented an overutilization of resources, and often produced undue patient and staff stress. Because the need for this what is considered by some as an aggressive approach could not be ruled in or out, a priori, this choice was made in the pursuit of safety and represented, at times, a "mis-diagnosis". This is akin to the now out-dated adage that unless a general surgeon had a 10% false-positive diagnosis rate for acute appendicitis, he or she was under-diagnosing this condition [4]. In the era of ubiquitous CT scans and ultrasounds, the "negative appendectomy" is much less common.

The goal of this chapter is to highlight a technique of airway evaluation which is readily available to the anesthesiologist, is minimally invasive and may provide enough information to reduce the use of awake intubation by providing improved clinical information. Preoperative endoscopic airway examination (PEAE), uses the commonly available flexible intubation scope, and unlike use of the same instrument for awake intubation, requires minimal time and patient preparation because it is well tolerated by patients, mimicking an ordinary office ENT laryngoscopic examination.

The transnasal endoscopic exam was first introduced into the practice of otolaryngologic evaluation in 1968 [5]. It is considered an ideal method of airway evaluation because it does not interfere with pharyngeal and laryngeal function, which can therefore be observed [6]. Its use has been adopted by many medical specialties including pulmonary and emergency medicine. Anesthesiologists have employed the transnasal endoscopic approach for tracheal intubation, but until the work by Moorthy et al. it had not been described in an objective fashion for diagnostic use [7].

The idea of applying flexible endoscopic evaluation of the airway in the practice of anesthesiology

Anesthesia for Otolaryngologic Surgery, ed. Basem Abdelmalak and D. John Doyle. Published by Cambridge University Press.
© Cambridge University Press 2013.

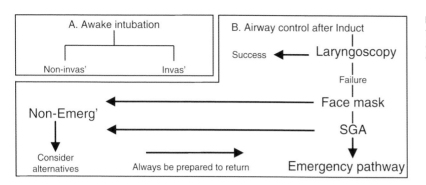

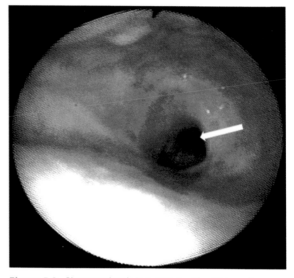

was first proposed Williams *et al.*, in the otolaryngology literature [8]. These authors described a series of patients who failed indirect mirror laryngoscopy, but who could be successfully examined with a nasal fiberscope, and suggested that anesthesiologists might glean important airway information about the achievability of direct laryngoscopy via the same assessment. These authors also described how the superior diagnostic view afforded by the fiberscope resulted in fewer patients requiring general anesthesia for direct laryngoscopy and biopsy.

Flexible nasal endoscopy was first applied to evaluation for intubation in an objective manner by Moorthy *et al.* [7] in a non-randomized series of patients who presented with a surgical diagnosis of papillomas, carcinomas, sarcomas, chondromas, hemangiomas, webs and cysts of the airway (Figure 5.2). These lesions, invisible on the anesthesiologist's routine physical exam of the airway, have the potential to cause both airflow obstruction and impediment to tracheal intubation after the induction of anesthesia. Other signs and symptoms (e.g., dysphagia, stridor, loss of voice quality) may not be illuminating as to the extent of the pathology and its bearing on the success of airway control [7]. Moorthy *et al.* performed indirect laryngoscopy of the airway using a 6 mm flexible bronchoscope. This procedure was undertaken in the operating room, and included the thorough use of topical anesthetics (4 ml of 4% lidocaine, Cetacain spray ™ and 0–4 ml of 4% lidocaine via the flexible scope). Patients were assigned an airway grade based upon both their symptoms and the degree to which the laryngeal inlet could be visualized. The plan to control the airway was based upon the assigned grade (Table 5.1).

Moorthy *et al.* applied an endoscopic technique familiar to most anesthesiologists to the internal

Figure 5.2. Pharyngeal web in a patient with a history of pharyngeal radiation therapy. The patient complained of mild dysphagia and no other symptoms. The vocal folds can be seen (arrow) beyond the hypopharyngeal web.

evaluation of the airway, hitherto limited to an external exam. This group's approach potentially avoided catastrophic outcomes (e.g., avoided anesthetic induction and failed airway control of group 2b patients with few subjective signs of airway compromise) as well as reduced the use of an at best time-consuming (at least for the infrequent practitioner of awake intubation), and at worst uncomfortable and stressful procedure (e.g., avoided awake intubation in the group 1 or 2a patient).

Rosenblatt *et al.* tested the hypothesis that the information gleaned from PEAE could change the clinical approach to airway management in a high-risk population, reducing the need for awake

Table 5.1. Airway grades based on respiratory symptoms and degree of the laryngeal inlet visualization

Grade	Symptoms	Airway mass	Laryngeal view	Root point of ASA-DAA[a]
0	None	No lesion	Complete view	B
1	Hx smoking, no hoarseness	Small lesion	Complete view	B
2a	Hoarse voice, no difficulty in breathing	Laryngeal or supraglottic lesion	Clear view of vocal folds partial of fully	B
2b	Hoarse voice, no difficulty in breathing	Large laryngeal or supraglottic lesion	Partial view of parts of the vocal folds	A
3	Hoarse voice, some difficulty in breathing	Large laryngeal or supraglottic lesion	Difficult to view vocal folds. May be seen only on inspiration	A
4		Large mass	Vocal folds cannot be visualized	A[b]

[a] Root points of the ASA difficult airway algorithm include Box A: awake intubation and Box B: airway control after the induction of anesthesia.
[b] Awake tracheostomy.

intubation, and detecting patients with unsuspected significant disease [9]. One hundred and thirty-eight patients presenting for diagnostic and therapeutic procedures underwent a routine airway history and physical exam. After a clinical airway plan was recorded, PEAE was performed, and the clinician was allowed to make a change in the airway plan based upon his or her findings.

Though 68% of this high-risk group were slated to have routine anesthetic induction and airway control based on routine exam alone, 74% were managed in this manner after PEAE. The net result of PEAE appears to be a reduction in the use of awake intubation, as clinicians' concerns about the airway architecture were allayed. PEAE therefore had the effect of reducing unnecessary awake intubations, and consequently anesthesia care time. Conversely, a closer look at Figure 5.3 reveals that eight patients, whose standard assessment suggested that routine anesthetic induction prior to airway control was a safe course, underwent awake intubation following PEAE. These eight patients represent the population that PEAE serves best: those whose clinical exam belies the true extent of their disease. Based on the low incidence of complete airway failure even in high-risk populations, it is uncertain how many of these patients would have required invasive airway intervention had routine induction been undertaken.

Neither study by Moorthy *et al.* or Rosenblatt *et al.* employed a randomized controlled protocol [7,9]. In an ideal study, all patients would undergo

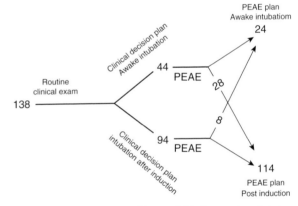

Figure 5.3. Data from Rosenblatt *et al.* [9]. After routine clinical examination 44 of 138 patients with known airway disease were to undergo awake intubation. Following subsequent PEAE this number was reduced to 24 patients, representing crossover in both directions.

PEAE, and only a subset have their airway plan affected by the results of the endoscopy. Additionally, careful logging of procedure time could attest to the efficiency of one approach over another [10].

Patients presenting to the operating room under the care of an otolaryngologist for management (diagnostic or therapeutic) of an airway lesions have, in most cases, undergone a flexible endoscopy in the surgeon's office. Though communication between specialties is no more important than among those who share the airway, relying solely on the otolaryngologist's assessment may be at best immaterial, and

Table 5.2. Information sought during PEAE

Surgeon's exam	Anesthesiologists' exam
Extent and location of disease	Sagittal-plane access to the larynx
Preservation of function	Presence of lesions which might interfere with supraglottic airway placement
Immediacy of intervention required	Presence of anterior lesions which might be damaged by traditional laryngoscopy

at worst misleading. The exam of the otolaryngologist is focused on three matters (Table 5.2) of less importance to the anesthesiologist: (1) location and extent of disease, (2) preservation of laryngeal function and (3) urgency of proceeding to the operating room for corrective or debulking procedures [8]. The surgeon's exam does not concern itself with the ease of direct laryngoscopy, the potential for difficult or impossible mask ventilation, or likelihood of visual obstruction with the induction of anesthesia. For example, the otolaryngologist is unlikely to comment on findings such as lingual tonsil hyperplasia, which is a common finding in a normal population, but might have severe implications for the laryngoscopist [11]. Lastly, some lesions described during the surgeon's preoperative exam may have progressed significantly if that exam occurred more than a few days prior to presentation to the operating room.

To the uninitiated, PEAE may appear to duplicate the exam of the otolaryngologist. Apart from giving the anesthesiologist a first-hand view of what may have been appreciated by the surgeon, the endoscopist explores three other aspects of the airway (Table 5.2).

Apart from the flexible intubating scope (fiberoptic or digital), conventional as well as innovative intubating devices are primarily dependent on movement in a sagittal plane from the mouth or nose to the larynx. Direct laryngoscopes, video laryngoscopes, optical stylets, channeled scopes, and intubating laryngeal masks may produce or facilitate the creation of a spatial conduit from the operator to the larynx, but only in a single plane which follows the airway axes (Figure 5.4).

Masses which occupy the airway or deform native tissues and distort this plane have the potential to render these devices ineffective. PEAE affords the laryngoscopist information about this sagittal plane access – information not available through routine, visible anatomy examination (e.g., Mallampati class, thyromental distance, interincisor gap, etc.). In cases where sagittal-plane access does not exist based on

PEAE, the clinician might consider the use of a flexible intubation scope after the induction of anesthesia, but risks not knowing the complexity of anatomy beyond the obstruction. Once appreciating the loss of the sagittal-plane access, most experienced anesthesiologists would pursue awake intubation. In cases where the sagittal-plane access appears present on PEAE, the clinician must be competent to manage any unexpected findings. For example, as described by Moorthy et al., a patient may have a partially visible larynx [7]. The induction of anesthesia and onset of neuromuscular relaxation may result in the anteroposterior movement of the larynx relative to the plane of the pharynx, converting from a grade 2 to a grade 3 or 4 in the asleep patient [12].

Modern airway resuscitation was buoyed significantly by the advent of supraglottic ventilation. The introduction of the laryngeal mask airway resulted in hundreds of case reports of airway rescue and spurred the American Society of Anesthesiologists and the American Heart Association to include supraglottic ventilation in their resuscitation guidelines [2,13]. Newer supraglottic airways have also been reported in airway salvage [14]. Because all supraglottic devices rely on positioning within or below the inferior cricopharyngeus muscle (or upper esophageal sphincter), PEAE can be used to evaluate anatomy in this region. Large lesions occupying the hypopharynx posterior to the laryngeal inlet, or pharyngeal wall osteophytes and other masses seen on PEAE may herald difficult or impossible SGA placement [15]. Conversely, the absence of such lesions as well as the lack of sagittal-plane deformity could encourage the routine induction of anesthesia and airway management in the patient who has external airway exam findings consistent with difficult laryngoscopy, but who might be accessed with an alternative instrument.

Lastly PEAE can be used to evaluate lesions which might preclude or be damaged by airway instruments which rely on anterior anatomic positioning. The finding of lingual tonsil hyperplasia, epiglottic

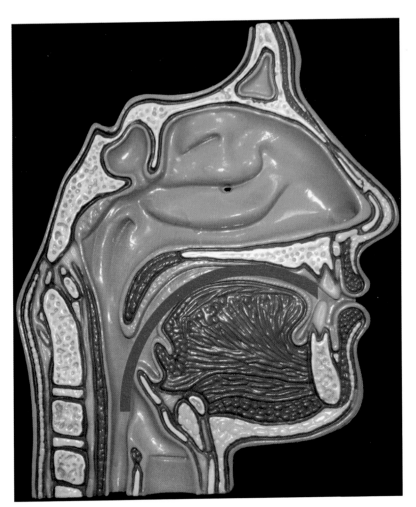

Figure 5.4. The airways sagittal plane arch.

hemangiomas or friable papillomas may influence the clinician to either avoid those instruments which might be traumatic or might fail due to increased base of tongue size (e.g., direct laryngoscopy).

Routine PEAE

PEAE may be performed in the preoperative clinic setting, holding area or operating room. Once the proper equipment has been assembled, the procedure will require less than 5 minutes (with good time management an experienced endoscopist will require less than 1 minute). Even a 5 or more minute delay in the holding area will be balanced by the avoidance of a longer awake intubation procedure in the operating room. The otolaryngology service will soon appreciate these time savings [9]. It is important to pay close attention to patient comfort during the endoscopy – this will often

be the first procedural interaction between anesthesiologist and patient and building trust is paramount. It is likely that the patient has undergone prior nasal endoscopies, and will be comparing your technique to their cumulative experience. If, based on the endoscopy findings, an awake intubation procedure is chosen, a good PEAE experience will result in a cooperative patient.

Unless there are unusual circumstances, the nasal route is chosen over an oral approach for PEAE. As will be discussed, minimal nasal mucosa analgesia will be required, and there is rarely a need to blunt the gag reflex. If the oral route is chosen, the flexible scope is likely to have more contact with the posterior pharyngeal wall, eliciting gag. Because of the risk of biting as well as patients' innate tendency to "hump up" the tongue, an intubating oral airway will probably be necessary, provoking gag and requiring more significant airway analgesia [8].

Risks of nasal PEAE include epistaxis, laryngospasm, local anesthetic allergic reaction, and pain. Unique untoward events will be addressed. Identical to the office exam routinely performed by otolaryngologists, PEAE requires no monitoring, desiccation or intravenous access. Because it is not a sterile procedure, it does not require gowning or a change from street clothes for either the patient or clinician. Gloves and eye protection are appropriate as the flexible scope will be in contact with the patient's mucosa. Though not required, nasal vasoconstriction and the application of a local anesthetic are recommended for the prevention of epistaxis and for patient comfort. Commercial vasoconstrictors or a preparation of 1% phenylephrine is applied to the nose. Because the anatomy on the right or left may be more accommodating of the fiberscope, both nasal passages should be prepared unless there is a contraindication. Any local anesthetic agent and preparation may be used. Historically, cocaine was employed by the otolaryngologist because of its vasoconstricting actions [8]. The anesthetic may be applied to the nasal passage on soaked pledgets or via a non-needle catheter. Only a minimal amount of local anesthetic is needed: no airway analgesia beyond the nasal passages is required. It is unnecessary to anesthetize the tongue, fauces, pharynx or larynx [8]. If there is a strong suspicion that the PEAE will be followed by an awake intubation, a desiccant can be given. This is otherwise unnecessary for the PEAE and can be unpleasant for the patient. Guiding the flexible scope tangential to the posterior oropharygeal wall and avoiding direct contact with the epiglottis and structures of the laryngeal inlet minimizes pain, gag, and cough.

Once the local anesthetic has been applied, the patient is asked to extend the head on the neck comfortably to encourage posterior drainage. A flexible intubation scope or a dedicated nasopharyngosocpe can be used. Scopes 2.5 to 3.5 mm are ideal, being less likely to cause trauma and pain than larger instruments (e.g., 5 mm or larger) which are often preferred for tracheal intubation. Though helpful, suction or oxygen need not be applied if the flexible scope includes a working channel. This may not be an option in smaller-diameter scopes.

The patient may be in a sitting or recumbent position. A right-handed clinician typically stands facing the patient, on their right side. If a video system is available, it is best placed close to the left side of the patient's head. The patient is asked to keep their head in a neutral position and to keep their eyes open. A surgical lubricant or local anesthetic preparation may be applied to the distal 15 cm of the flexible scope. Using his or her dominant hand, the scope's distal end is placed into the nasal cavity (left or right), the back of the hand resting on the patients nose, avoiding pressure on the eyes. Slow advancement whilst gauging the patient's discomfort is advised. The flexible scope should skirt the nasal floor, traveling below the large inferior turbinate. Unrelenting pain or obstruction to advancement typically implies a rostral migration of the flexible scope or a blocked passage. Significant pain may also dictate a change to the contralateral nostril, or reapplication of the anesthetic agent. The nasopharygeal wall is typically encountered in 4 to 6 cm. At this juncture gentle contact of the objective lens with the nasopharyngeal wall will clear secretions and moisture, without causing undue discomfort. A caudad deflection of the flexible scope's articulating tip will direct it towards the oral pharynx. As the insertion continues, the epiglottis and base of tongue will come into view. Masses, mass effects, papillomas, lingual tonsil hyperplasia and other lesions should be noted. Often secretions or moisture on the objective lens are encountered. Asking the patient to swallow or deflecting the objective lens against tissue will "clean" it. Barring the existence of a large mass, the structures of the larynx should be visible beyond the epiglottis. To improve the view, the fiberscope can be gently inserted deeper, with care to avoid touching the epiglottis. Asking the patient to "pant" or produce a prolonged "i" sound may reveal the larynx from behind the epiglottis. During this phonation, the symmetry and movement of the vocal folds can be observed, and pathologic findings noted. Because only minimal local anesthetic has been used, touching the vocal folds will probably result in cough or laryngospasm. Despite this, views of the larynx as far as the cricoid cartilage may be possible (Figure 5.5). With the fiberscope objective lens repositioned above the epiglottis, side-to-side rotation will allow evaluation of the pyriform sinuses. Having the patient "blow" against closed lips and pinched nares may improve visualization. Once the exam has been completed the flexible scope is withdrawn. Pain is not unusual during removal, and the patient should be reassured. Care should be taken to ensure that the flexible scope's articulating segment is in the neutral position during withdrawal. This is best accomplished by

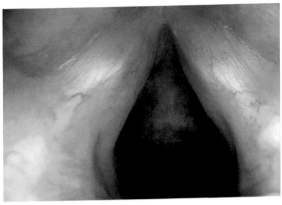

Figure 5.5. The cricoid cartilage as well as a tracheal web can be visualized distal to the vocal folds during a PEAE.

removing the operator's fingers from the control lever.

Mention should be made of the use of the "awake look" technique whereby the airway is examined using conventional laryngoscopy under topical anesthesia. The belief is that if the glottic aperture is visible in this setting, it is safe to induce anesthesia in such a patient. Unfortunately, a number of individuals have stories of patients in whom the view while awake was good but with the introduction of anesthesia and muscle relaxation changes in the glottic architecture made intubation unexpectedly difficult.

Finally, there are other exciting technologies that may be useful in this context. In particular, the use of 3D radiologic imaging (virtual laryngoscopy) can provide insights into the airway not readily available by classic means. Advantages include its noninvasive and painless characteristics; disadvantages include radiation exposure and the cost of the procedure [16]. Unlike PEAE, these exams are not available at the immediate pre-procedure bedside, which makes them impractical for most outpatients unless reliably coordinated with the surgical staff.

Summary

Preoperative endoscopic airway exam extends the anesthesiologist's ability to evaluate the patient's airway beyond the bounds of the naked eye and

palpation, using instruments and techniques familiar to him or her. Patients who present with "invisible" airway pathology (e.g., papillomas, supraglottic masses), which may compromise the clinician's ability to control the airway, can be more thoroughly assessed. This evaluation can be rapidly performed at the time of presentation to the operating room. Because awake intubation is often the safest course of action in these cases, but may not be necessary, PEAE can clarify the airway architecture prior to entering the operating room. Similarly, patients who present with obvious airway deformity, whether congenital, iatrogenic or traumatic, may have benign "invisible" anatomy. In these cases, though direct laryngoscopy and similar devices may not be effective, the clinician can glean from the PEAE information allowing routine anesthetic induction and the use of alternative airway control devices.

Clinical pearls

- PEAE extends the anesthesiologist's ability to evaluate the patient's airway beyond the bounds of the naked eye and palpation; the population that PEAE serves best are those whose clinical exam belies the true extent of their disease.
- The information gleaned from a preoperative endoscopic airway exam (PEAE) could change the clinical approach to airway management in high-risk patients, as pathology having the potential to cause airflow obstruction or serve as an impediment to tracheal intubation is sometimes identified.
- Large lesions occupying the hypopharynx posterior to the laryngeal inlet or pharyngeal wall osteophytes and other masses seen on PEAE may herald difficult or impossible SGA placement.
- The induction of anesthesia and onset of neuromuscular relaxation may result in the anteroposterior movement of the larynx relative to the plane of the pharynx, converting the airway view from a grade 2 to a grade 3 or 4 in the asleep patient.

References

1. Peterson GN, Domino KB, Caplan RA, *et al.* Management of the difficult airway: closed claims database. *Anesthesiology* 2005;**102**:33–9.

2. Practice guidelines for management of the difficult airway. An updated report by the American Society of Anesthesiologists Task Force on Management of the Difficult Airway. *Anesthesiology* 2003;**98**:1269–77.

3. Benumof JL. Management of the difficult adult airway. *Anesthesiology* 1991; **75**; 1087–110.

4. Storer EH. Appendix. In Schwartz SI, Shires GT, Spencer FC, Storer EH, eds. *Principles of Surgery, 4th edn.* New York: McGraw-Hill; 1983. pp. 1245–56.

5. Sawashima M, Hirose H. New laryngoscope technique by use of fiberoptics. *J Acoust Soc Am* 1968; **43**:168–9.

6. Leder SB, Ross DA, Briskin KB, *et al.* A prospective, double-blind, randomized study on the use of a topical anesthetic, vasoconstrictor, and placebo during transnasal flexible fiberoptic endoscopy. *J Speech Lang Hear Res* 1997; **40**:1352–7.

7. Moorthy SS, Gupta S, Laurent B, *et al.* Management of airway in patients with laryngeal tumors. *J Clin Anesth* 2005; **17**:604–9.

8. Williams GT, Farquharson IM, Anthony J. Fibreoptic laryngoscopy in the assessment of laryngeal disorders. *J Laryngol Otol* 1975;**89**:299–316.

9. Rosenblatt WH, Ianus AI, Sukhupragarn W, *et al.* Preoperative endoscopic airway examination (PEAE) provides superior airway information and may reduce the use of unnecessary awake intubation. *Anesth Analg* 2011;**112**:602–7.

10. Akça O, Lenhardt R, Heine M, *et al.* Can transnasal flexible fiberoptic laryngoscopy contribute to airway management decisions? *Anesth Analg* 2011;**112**:519–20.

11. Ovassapian A, Glassenberg R, Randel G, *et al.* The unexpected difficult airway and lingual tonsil hyperplasia. *Anesth Analg* 2002;**97**:124–32.

12. Sivarajan M, Joy JV. Effects of general anesthesia and paralysis on upper airway changes due to head position in humans. *Anesthesiology* 1996;**85**:787–93.

13. Neumar RW, Otto CW, Link MS. Adult advanced cardiovascular life support: 2010 American Heart Association Guidelines for Cardiopulmonary Resuscitation and Emergency Cardiovascular Care (Part 8). *Circulation* 2010;**122**:S729–67.

14. Cook TM, Hommers C. New airways for resuscitation? *Resuscitation* 2006;**69**:371–87.

15. Cesur M, Alici HA, Erdem AF. An unusual cause of difficult intubation in a patient with a large cervical anterior osteophyte: a case report. *Acta Anaesthesiol Scand* 2005;**49**:264–6.

16. Osorio F, Perilla M, Doyle DJ, Palomo JM. Cone beam computed tomography: an innovative tool for airway assessment. *Anesth Analg* 2008;**106**(6):1803–7. PubMed PMID: 18499613.

Chapter

6

Awake intubation

Carlos A. Artime and Carin A. Hagberg

Introduction

The incidence of difficult airway is higher in patients undergoing ENT surgery and, specifically, in patients undergoing ENT cancer surgery [1]. Airway management of the patient with a known or predicted difficult airway undergoing ENT surgery requires a thorough preoperative evaluation, a discussion with the ENT surgeon regarding the patient's airway and surgery-specific issues, and a detailed plan of action.

The American Society of Anesthesiologists (ASA) formed a Task Force on Difficult Airway Management in 1992, and sought to establish a "difficult airway algorithm" to facilitate the management of the difficult airway and reduce the likelihood of adverse outcomes [2]. In this algorithm, which was updated in 2002, one of the primary management choices for the anesthesiologist is the decision of whether or not to perform awake intubation or attempt intubation after induction of general anesthesia [2,3]. The ASA algorithm stresses the concept that formulation of a strategy for intubation should include the feasibility of three basic options: awake intubation vs. intubation after induction of general anesthesia, noninvasive vs. invasive (surgical) techniques, and preservation vs. ablation of spontaneous ventilation [7]. It is well-accepted that the safest method for a patient who requires endotracheal intubation and has a difficult airway is for that patient to undergo awake intubation for the following reasons [2–8].

1. Patency of the airway is maintained through upper pharyngeal muscle tone.
2. Spontaneous ventilation is maintained.
3. A patient who is awake and well topicalized is easier to intubate, as the larynx moves to a more anterior position after induction of anesthesia, as compared to while awake.

4. The patient can still protect his or her airway from aspiration.
5. The patient is able to monitor his or her own neurologic symptoms to guard against disruption of the integrity of their own neurologic system (for example, the patient with cervical spine pathology).

General indications for awake intubation are presented in Table 6.1 [4,6,9]. There are no absolute contraindications to awake intubation other than patient's refusal, a patient who is unable to cooperate (such as a child, a patient with an intellectual disability, or an intoxicated, combative patient), or a patient with a documented true allergy to all local anesthetics [7].

Extreme caution should be taken in the patient with critical airway obstruction. Even the process of topicalization with local anesthetic can precipitate loss of the airway, as can some of the complications associated with awake intubation (e.g., airway bleeding and laryngospasm) [10]. These patients require coordination of their care with the ENT surgeon and one must consider the feasibility and appropriateness of an awake surgical airway.

Preoperative preparations

Chart review

Whenever possible, previous anesthetic records should be examined, especially those involving airway management [3,11]. One should note the degree of difficulty of prior intubations, the position used for laryngoscopy, and the equipment used. Other records documenting ease of mask ventilation and tolerance of drugs are also valuable. One should be alert for evidence of reactions to local anesthetics and of apnea with minimal doses of opioids.

Anesthesia for Otolaryngologic Surgery, ed. Basem Abdelmalak and D. John Doyle. Published by Cambridge University Press. © Cambridge University Press 2013.

Table 6.1. Indications for awake intubation [4,6,9]

1. Previous history of difficult intubation

2. Anticipated difficult airway based on physical examination:
   Small mouth opening
   Receding mandible/micrognathia
   Macroglossia
   Short, muscular neck
   Limited range of motion of the neck (rheumatoid arthritis, ankylosing spondylitis, prior cervical fusion)
   Congenital airway anomalies
   Morbid obesity
   Pathology involving the airway (tracheomalacia)
   Airway masses (malignancy of the tongue, tonsils, or larynx; large goiter; mediastinal mass)
   Upper airway obstruction

3. Unstable cervical spine

4. Trauma to the face or upper airway

5. Anticipated difficult mask ventilation

6. Severe risk of aspiration

7. Severe hemodynamic instability

8. Respiratory failure

Adapted from Hagberg CA, ed. *Benumof's Airway Management*, 2nd edn. St. Louis: Mosby; 2007. p. 257.

The ENT surgeon's notes should also be reviewed in detail, with specific attention to characterizations of the patient's airway, as well as any results of nasopharyngeal laryngoscopy performed beforehand. Computed tomography (CT) of the airway, if performed, should also be examined prior to formalizing an airway management plan.

The patient interview

After the medical records have been reviewed, a careful patient history should be obtained, including a review of symptoms that may indicate airway obstruction, such as stridor or paroxysmal nocturnal dyspnea [10]. The preoperative interview should also address the possibility of events having occurred since the last anesthetic such as weight gain, laryngeal stenosis from previous airway intervention, airway radiation, facial cosmetic surgery, and worsening temporomandibular joint disorder or rheumatoid arthritis.

Once the anesthesia practitioner and surgeon have made the decision that awake intubation is necessary,

communication with the patient and psychological preparation is of the utmost importance in order to maximize the odds for a successful awake intubation [7]. In a careful, unhurried manner, the anesthesiologist should describe conventional intubation contrasted with awake intubation to the patient and focus on the fact that, while the former is easier and less time-consuming, the latter is safer in light of the patient's own anatomy or condition. The anesthesiologist should present his or herself as a knowledgeable, caring physician who is willing to take extra measures to ensure the patient's safety. Recommendations should be presented to the patient with conviction, and if the patient is skeptical about proceeding as such, help from the surgeon may be enlisted. Since the patient has an established relationship with their surgeon, the surgeon's reinforcement of the anesthesiologist's opinion may be quite helpful [8].

Complications of awake intubation should also be presented, including local anesthetic toxicity, airway trauma, discomfort, recall, and failure to secure the airway. Patients' recall after awake intubation using different methods of sedation, analgesia, or local anesthetics has not been studied in a controlled fashion. Although episodes of explicit awareness during general anesthesia are rare, it is anticipated that the incidence of recall during awake intubation with minimal levels of sedation would be higher [12].

Staff, monitors, and equipment

Per the ASA difficult airway guidelines, there should be "at least one additional individual who is immediately available to serve as an assistant in difficult airway management" [3]. Preferred, whenever possible, is a second member of the anesthesia care team who can assist in the monitoring, ventilation, and pharmacotherapy of the patient, as well as provide an extra set of hands during fiberoptic intubation (FOI). In the case of a patient in extremis or with a critically obstructed airway, the ENT surgeon should be available with the appropriate equipment to perform an emergency surgical airway, if necessary.

During awake intubation, the routine use of ECG, pulse oximetry, NIBP, and capnography is required as part of standard basic intraoperative monitoring. Depending on the complexity of the surgery and the patient's condition, invasive hemodynamic monitoring (i.e., arterial line) may be necessary prior to awake intubation. Indications for this include hemodynamic instability, severe ischemic or valvular heart disease,

Table 6.2. Pharmacologic characteristics of anticholinergic drugs

	Tachycardia	Antisialagogue effect	Sedation
Atropine	+++	++	+
Glycopyrrolate	++	+++	0
Scopolamine	+	+++	+++

0, no effect; +, minimal effect; ++, moderate effect; +++, marked effect.
Adapted from Morgan GE Jr, Mikhail MS, Murray MJ. *Clinical Anesthesiology*, 3rd edn. New York: McGraw-Hill; 2002. p. 208.

and patients for whom hypertension and tachycardia are potentially dangerous (e.g., the patient with aortic dissection or intracerebral aneurysm).

Adequate preoxygenation and the use of supplemental O_2 throughout airway management (including sedation, topicalization, intubation, and extubation) is encouraged in all patients undergoing awake intubation [3]. In addition to the standard methods of supplemental O_2 delivery (nasal cannula or face mask), other opportunities include, but are not limited to: delivering O_2 through the suction port of the fiberoptic broncho-scope (FOB) [7], through the atomizer or nebulizer during topicalization, or by elective transtracheal jet ventilation (TTJV) in the patient in extremis [7,13,14].

There are many techniques that can be used to secure the airway in the awake patient. Direct laryngoscopy, video laryngoscopy, intubating LMAs, flexible fiberoptic bronchoscopy, rigid fiberoptic laryngoscopy, retrograde intubation, lighted stylets, and blind nasal intubation have all been used successfully in performing awake intubation [4,15–20]. No matter which technique is selected, all necessary equipment should be prepared ahead of time and be readily available, when needed. The practitioner should also have several back-up modalities in mind, and the required equipment available, in case the initial technique used is ineffective (i.e., Plan B, C, etc.).

Premedication

Prior to awake intubation, premedication is commonly used to reduce secretions, enable adequate topicalization of the airway, reduce the risk of epistaxis, and protect against the risk of aspiration.

Antisialagogues

One of the most important goals of premedication for awake intubation is drying of the airway. Secretions can obscure the view of the glottis, especially when using flexible fiberoptic bronchoscopy or videolaryngoscopy. In addition, secretions can prevent local anesthetics from reaching intended areas, resulting in failed topicalization, or can wash away and dilute local anesthetics, diminishing their potency and duration of action.

The medications most often used for their antisialagogic properties are the anticholinergics, which inhibit salivary and bronchial secretions by way of their antimuscarinic effects. They should be administered as early as possible for maximal effect (at least 30 minutes in advance), as they do not eliminate existing secretions but rather prevent new secretion formation. The anticholinergics most often used in clinical practice are glycopyrrolate, scopolamine, and atropine [21]. A summary of their pharmacologic properties is presented in Table 6.2. Glycopyrrolate (0.1–0.3 mg IV) is the anticholinergic of choice for most clinical circumstances due to its marked antisialagogue effect and rapid onset of 1 to 2 minutes after IV dosing. It is moderately vagolytic and is devoid of CNS effects, as its quaternary amine structure prevents passage through the blood–brain barrier. Scopolamine (0.4 mg IV) is the least vagolytic of the anticholinergics in clinical use and, as a result, may be the drug of choice for patients in whom tachycardia is undesirable (e.g., a patient with advanced coronary artery disease in whom the use of glycopyrrolate would be relatively contraindicated). Scopolamine has an onset of 5 to 10 minutes after IV bolusing. In addition to being a very effective antisialagogue, scopolamine has potent CNS effects, with sedative and amnestic properties. In some patients, this may lead to restlessness, delirium, and difficulty waking after short procedures. Atropine (0.4–0.6 mg IV) produces only a mild antisialagogic effect, but causes significant tachycardia due to its potent vagolytic effects. As such, it is not an ideal drug for use in drying the airway [21].

Table 6.3. Drugs used for aspiration prophylaxis

	Route	Adult dose	Pediatric dose	Onset	Effect on gastric volume	Effect on gastric pH
Bicitra	PO	15–30 ml	0.4 ml/kg	5 min	↑	↑
Metoclopramide	IV	10 mg	0.15 mg/kg	1–3 min	↓	–
H$_2$ antagonists						
Cimetidine	IV	300mg	5–10 mg/kg	45–60 min	↓	↑
Ranitidine	IV	50 mg	0.25–1 mg/kg	30–60 min		
Famotidine	IV	20 mg	0.15 mg/kg	60–120 min		

Nasal mucosal vasoconstrictors

The nasal mucosa and nasopharynx are highly vascular. When a patient requires nasotracheal intubation, adequate vasoconstriction is essential, as bleeding can make visualization of the larynx extremely difficult, especially during nasal FOI. Nasal mucosal vasoconstrictors should be applied 15 minutes prior to nasal intubation. One commonly used agent is 4% cocaine, which has both vasoconstrictive and local anesthetic effects. It can be applied to the nasal mucosa using cotton-tipped applicators. The maximum dose is 1.5–3 mg/kg. Caution should be taken in patients with hypertension, coronary artery disease, hyperthyroidism, pseudocholinesterase deficiency or preeclampsia, and in patients taking MAOIs. Alternatively, a mixture of lidocaine 3% and phenylephrine 0.25% can be made by combining lidocaine 4% and phenylephrine 1% in a 3:1 ratio [22]. This combination has similar anesthetic and vasoconstrictive properties to cocaine and can be used as a substitute. This mixture can be either sprayed intranasally or applied with cotton-tipped applicators. Commercially available nasal decongestants containing either oxymetazoline 0.05% (Afrin) or phenylephrine 0.5% (Neo-Synephrine) may also be applied to nasal mucosa. The usual dose is two sprays in each nostril. Pediatric patients are especially sensitive to these drugs and require lower concentrations.

Aspiration prophylaxis

Routine prophylaxis against aspiration pneumonitis is not recommended, but may be beneficial in patients with risk factors for aspiration such as a full stomach, symptomatic gastroesophageal reflux disease, hiatal hernia, presence of a nasogastric tube, morbid obesity, diabetic gastroparesis, s/p esophagectomy with stomach pull through, or pregnancy [23,24]. The goal of aspiration prophylaxis is two-fold: to decrease gastric volume and to increase gastric fluid pH. Commonly used agents include non-particulate antacids (e.g., Bicitra), pro-motility agents (e.g., metoclopramide), and H$_2$-receptor antagonists. These drugs may be used alone or in combination. See Table 6.3 for dosing and pharmacology.

Sedation

Depending on the clinical circumstance, intravenous sedation may be useful in allowing the patient to tolerate awake intubation by providing anxiolysis, amnesia, and analgesia. Benzodiazepines, opioids, hypnotics, α_2 agonists, and neuroleptics can be used alone or in combination [15]. It is important that these agents be carefully titrated to effect, as over-sedation can render a patient uncooperative and make awake intubation more difficult and unsafe [7]. Spontaneous respiration with adequate oxygenation and ventilation should always be maintained [15]. Extreme caution should be taken in patients with critical airway obstruction, as awake muscle tone is sometimes necessary in these patients to maintain airway patency [25]. In these situations, sedation should be used sparingly or avoided altogether. Avoidance of over-sedation is also important in the patient with a full stomach, as an awake patient can protect his or her own airway in the event of aspiration [7].

Benzodiazepines

Benzodiazepines, via their action at the γ-aminobutyric acid (GABA)-benzodiazepine receptor complex, have hypnotic, sedative, anxiolytic, and amnestic properties [26]. They have also been shown to depress

61

upper airway reflex sensitivity [27], a property that is desirable for awake intubation. Benzodiazepines are frequently used to achieve sedation for awake intubation in combination with opioids [28], or are used for their amnestic and anxiolytic effects when any of the other sedatives (e.g., dexmedetomidine, ketamine, or remifentanil) is chosen as the primary agent [29,30]. Three benzodiazepine receptor agonists are commonly used in anesthesia practice: midazolam, diazepam, and lorazepam [26]. Due to its more rapid onset and relatively short duration of action, midazolam is the more commonly used agent.

Sedation with midazolam is achieved with doses of 1 to 2 mg IV repeated until the desired level of sedation is achieved. The IM dose is 0.07 to 0.1 mg/kg. Onset is rapid, with peak effect usually achieved within 2 to 3 minutes of IV administration. Duration of action is 20 to 30 minutes, with termination of effect primarily as a result of redistribution. Although recovery is rapid, the elimination half-life is 1.7 to 3.6 hours, with prolongation noted in cirrhosis, congestive heart failure, obesity, the elderly, and patients with renal failure [26,31].

The primary effects of benzodiazepines are amnesia, sedation, a decrease in respiratory rate and tidal volume, and a mild decrease in systemic vascular resistance and cardiac output. These effects are augmented synergistically by other medications used for sedation, including opioids, propofol, and α_2 agonists [32,33]. Systemic absorption of local anesthetics used for airway topicalization may also lead to potentiation of the sedative/hypnotic effects of midazolam [34].

Oversedation with benzodiazepines can cause respiratory depression, which may lead to hypoxemia or apnea [26]. Flumazenil, a specific benzodiazepine antagonist, may be used to reverse the sedative and respiratory effects of benzodiazepines if a patient becomes too heavily sedated. It is administered in incremental IV doses of 0.2 mg, repeated as needed to a maximum dose of 3 mg. Because it has a half-life of 0.7 to 1.8 hours, resedation can be a problem if it is being used to reverse high doses or longer-acting agents and patients should be monitored carefully in those circumstances. Flumazenil is generally safe and devoid of major side effects [35,36].

Opioids

Opioids, by way of their agonist effect on opioid receptors in the brain and spinal cord, provide analgesia, depress airway reflexes, and prevent hyperventilation associated with pain or anxiety. These properties make them a useful addition to the sedation regimen for awake intubation. While any opioid receptor agonist could theoretically be used for this purpose, fentanyl, alfentanil, and remifentanil are particularly useful due to their rapid onset, relatively short duration of action, and ease of titration [37].

Fentanyl is widely used in anesthetic practice, and is the most commonly used opioid for awake intubation. The sedative dose ranges from 0.5 to 2 µg/kg IV. Onset is rapid, within 2 to 3 minutes. The relatively short duration of action (30 to 45 minutes) is due to redistribution of fentanyl to a large peripheral compartment rather than rapid elimination; hence the duration of action after cessation of a prolonged infusion is markedly longer, due to redistribution to the central compartment from the peripheral compartment. [28,38].

Alfentanil has an even quicker onset (1.5 to 2 minutes) and a more rapid recovery after a single bolus dose (10 to 15 minutes) than fentanyl. This potentially makes alfentanil the drug of choice when a transient peak effect after a single bolus is desired, as in awake intubation [39,40]. The sedative dose ranges from 10 to 30 µg/kg IV, administered in 3–5 µg/kg aliquots [37].

Remifentanil is an ultrashort-acting opioid that is unique compared with the other short-acting agents in that it is metabolized by nonspecific plasma esterases, with a half-life of 3 minutes. It undergoes no redistribution and, therefore, has no context-sensitivity. Its potency approximates that of fentanyl [41]. Several studies have shown the effectiveness and safety of remifentanil sedation for awake intubation as a single agent [29,30,42], as well as in combination with midazolam [43–46] or propofol [47]. Remifentanil is usually administered as a weight-based infusion. A bolus of 0.5 µg/kg followed by an infusion of 0.1 µg/kg/min, as described by Atkins and Mirza [41], achieves a plasma concentration that provides adequate sedation with preservation of spontaneous ventilation in most patients. The infusion can subsequently be titrated by 0.025 to 0.05 µg/kg/min increments in 5-minute intervals to effect. Lower doses may be required when remifentanil is combined with other agents.

The most serious adverse effect of opioids is respiratory depression leading to overt apnea. Factors that increase the susceptibility to opioid-induced respiratory depression include old age, obstructive sleep apnea, and concomitant administration of central nervous system depressants. Naloxone, an opioid antagonist, can be used to restore spontaneous ventilation in patients after an opioid overdose. Onset after IV administration is rapid, within 1–2 minutes, and duration of action is 30–60 minutes. Naloxone should be administered in 0.04–0.08 μg IV boluses every 2 to 3 minutes. Doses of 1–2 μg/kg will restore adequate spontaneous ventilation in most cases while preserving adequate analgesia. Potential complications of naloxone administration are reversal of analgesia, tachycardia, hypertension, and in severe cases, pulmonary edema or myocardial ischemia [37].

Chest wall rigidity leading to ineffectual bag-mask ventilation is commonly cited as a potential adverse effect of opioids, particularly fentanyl, alfentanil, and remifentanil. Clinically significant rigidity usually occurs after an opioid dose sufficient to cause apnea, as a patient loses consciousness [37]. Careful titration to prevent overdose is perhaps the best way to prevent rigidity-associated difficult ventilation. Should it occur, however, treatment with naloxone or neuromuscular blocking agents is effective [48,49].

Propofol

Propofol is the most frequently used intravenous anesthetic today. Its primary effect is hypnosis as a result of an unclear mechanism; however, there is evidence that a significant portion of this hypnotic effect is mediated by interaction with GABA receptors. After an induction dose of 1.5 to 2.5 mg/kg IV, propofol has a quick onset (60 to 90 s) with recovery in 4 to 5 minutes as a result of both rapid elimination and redistribution. It attenuates airway responses and provides a smooth induction with few excitatory effects [26]. For awake intubation, intermittent doses of 0.25 mg/kg IV or a continuous IV infusion of 25 to 75 μg/kg/min provide an easily titratable level of sedation with rapid recovery. The use of propofol in awake intubation is well described both as a single agent [16,44] and in combination with remifentanil [47]. Care should be taken in the patient with a critical airway, as propofol causes reduction of tidal volumes and an increase in respiratory frequency at sedative doses. At sufficiently elevated plasma concentrations, propofol can lead to apnea. Other common adverse effects are a decrease in arterial blood pressure and pain on injection.

Dexmedetomidine

Dexmedetomidine is a centrally acting, highly selective α_2-adrenoreceptor agonist with several properties that make it well suited for use in awake intubation. It has sedative, analgesic, anxiolytic, antitussive, and antisialagogue effects while causing minimal respiratory impairment, even at high doses. Dexmedetomidine sedation provides unique conditions in which the patient is asleep, but is easily arousable and cooperative when stimulated [50–52]. There are several reports of dexmedetomidine sedation in awake FOI, both in combination with other sedatives or as a sole agent in conjunction with airway topicalization by local anesthetics [53–57]. Dosing for awake intubation is a 1 μg/kg load over 10 minutes (loading dose), followed by a continuous infusion of 0.2 to 1 μg/kg/h. A reduced dose should be considered in the elderly, in patients with depressed systolic function, and in patients with hepatic or renal impairment [58]. Dexmedetomidine is not a reliable amnestic [59] and is frequently combined with midazolam to decrease the incidence of recall [55]. Adverse hemodynamic effects include bradycardia, hypotension, and hypertension. During the loading dose, hypertension and bradycardia can occur due to stimulation of peripheral postsynaptic α_{2B}-adrenergic receptors resulting in vasoconstriction. Central α_{2A}-mediated sympatholysis eventually leads to bradycardia, hypotension, and decreased cardiac output [60]. The bradycardic effect can be mitigated by pretreatment with an anticholinergic (e.g., glycopyrrolate) [55].

Ketamine

Ketamine is an N-methyl-D-aspartate (NMDA) antagonist that produces dissociative anesthesia, which manifests clinically as a cataleptic state with many reflexes intact, including the corneal, cough, and swallow reflexes. Ketamine-induced anesthesia is associated with amnesia, nystagmus, and the potential for hallucinations and other undesirable psychological reactions; benzodiazepines are commonly administered to attenuate or treat these effects. Usual doses for sedation range from 0.2 to 0.8 mg/kg IV, with onset in 1 to 2 minutes and a duration of hypnosis of 5 to 10 minutes. At these doses, minute ventilation, tidal volume, functional residual capacity, and the minute ventilation response to CO_2 are maintained [26]. Ketamine increases blood pressure, heart rate, cardiac

63

output, and myocardial oxygen consumption via a centrally mediated stimulation of the sympathetic nervous system. Ketamine is a direct myocardial depressant, however, and in patients with depleted catecholamine stores (e.g., the patient in shock) it may cause hypotension [61]. Its use in awake intubation has been described in combination with benzodiazepines [4] and dexmedetomidine [62,63]. Patients receiving ketamine sedation should always be pretreated with an antisialagogue, as ketamine causes increased airway secretions that can lead to upper airway obstruction or make FOI difficult.

Droperidol

Droperidol is a neuroleptic medication occasionally used in anesthesia practice for its sedative and antiemetic properties. Its mechanism of action is antagonism of dopamine receptors in the central nervous system; it also interferes with GABA-, norepinephrine-, and serotonin-mediated neuronal activity. In combination with opioids, it produces a state of hypnosis, analgesia, and immobility classically referred to as neuroleptanalgesia [8,26]. This combination has been used for awake intubation with favorable results [4,64,65]. In this state, patients may experience extreme fear and apprehension despite appearing outwardly calm; droperidol is also a poor amnestic. For this reason, benzodiazepines should be administered for anxiolysis and amnesia. Doses for neuroleptanalgesia range from 2.5 to 5 mg IV; the antiemetic dose is 0.625 to 1.25 mg. Onset is in 20 minutes, with a half-life of approximately 2 hours. Side effects include mild hypotension due to peripheral α-adrenergic blockade, dysphoria, and extrapyramidal symptoms. Droperidol can also cause QT prolongation, especially in larger doses. This has led to an FDA "black box" warning concerning the risk of potentially fatal torsades de pointes. As a result, droperidol should not be administered to patients with a prolonged QT interval (>440 ms for males, >450 ms for females) and ECG monitoring should be performed during and for 2 to 3 hours following treatment [66].

Topicalization

Topicalization of the airway with local anesthetics should, in most cases, be the primary anesthetic for awake intubation; many times, it is all that is needed [7]. While intubation of a topicalized, non-sedated patient is considered the safest method of difficult airway management, it is not without risk. Total airway obstruction during topical anesthesia in a non-sedated patient with a critical airway has been reported. This was postulated to have been caused by dynamic airway obstruction related to loss of upper airway tone as a result of topicalization [67]. In addition, local anesthetic toxicity is a real concern; death due to lidocaine toxicity of a healthy volunteer undergoing bronchoscopy has occurred [68,69].

Local anesthetics

When using local anesthetics, it is important to be familiar with the speed of onset, duration of action, optimal concentration, signs and symptoms of toxicity, and the maximum recommended dosage of the drug chosen [70]. The rate and amount of topical local anesthetic absorption vary depending on the site of application, the concentration and total dose of local anesthetic applied, the hemodynamic status of the patient, and individual patient variation [71]. Early symptoms of local anesthetic toxicity include euphoria, dizziness, tinnitus, confusion, perioral numbness, and metallic taste. Higher plasma levels can lead to seizures, respiratory failure, loss of consciousness, and circulatory collapse [15]. The most commonly used agents for topical anesthesia of the airway are lidocaine and cocaine.

Lidocaine, an amide local anesthetic, is an excellent choice for airway anesthesia due to a rapid onset of 2 to 5 minutes and a wide therapeutic index [72,73]. Its duration of action is 30 to 60 minutes after topical application or infiltration. It is available in various concentrations (1% to 10%) and preparations including aqueous and viscous solutions, ointments, gels, and creams. For infiltration and minor nerve blocks, 1% to 2% is commonly used; for topical anesthesia the concentration utilized is 2% to 4%. The maximum recommended dosage for infiltration of lidocaine without epinephrine is 4–5 mg/kg of lean body mass. For topicalization of the airway, the maximum dose is less well-established. The British Thoracic Society recommends a maximum dose of 8.2 mg/kg [74], based on a study by Langmack et al. [75]. Other studies of peak lidocaine plasma concentration after topicalization have shown significant variability between patients with regard to absorption [76,77]. Some authors, therefore, recommend using the lower limit of 4–5 mg/kg and encourage the use of 2% lidocaine for airway topicalization [78].

Cocaine, a naturally occurring ester anesthetic, is used primarily for anesthesia of the nasal mucosa when the nasal route is planned for awake intubation [79]. It has a vasoconstrictor property that makes it particularly useful for this application, as the nose is highly vascularized and bleeding can make FOI impossible. It is available commercially as a 4% solution (each drop contains 3 mg), and can be applied to the nasal mucosa using cotton pledgets or cotton-tipped swabs. The maximum recommended dosage for intranasal application is 100 mg (1.5 mg/kg). Cocaine is primarily metabolized by plasma pseudocholinesterase; it also undergoes slow hepatic metabolism and is excreted unchanged by the kidney. The signs and symptoms of cocaine toxicity include tachycardia, cardiac dysrhythmia, hypertension, and fever. Severe complications include convulsions, respiratory failure, coronary spasm, cardiac arrest, stroke, and death. It must be used with caution in patients with hypertension, coronary artery disease, hyperthyroidism, pseudocholinesterase deficiency, preeclampsia, and in those patients taking monoamine oxidase inhibitors [79].

Other local anesthetics that have been used for airway topicalization include benzocaine and tetracaine. Benzocaine, available as a 20% spray, is an ester-type local anesthetic agent that is mainly useful for topical application. It has a rapid onset (<1 minute) with an effective duration of 5 to 10 minutes. Its primary limitation is the significant risk of methemoglobinemia, which can occur with as little as 1 to 2 seconds of spraying [73,80]. Cetacaine is a topical application spray containing 14% benzocaine, 2% tetracaine, and 2% butyl aminobenzoate (a local anesthetic similar to benzocaine). Like 20% benzocaine spray, this combination produces rapid airway anesthesia, but with a prolonged duration of action compared to benzocaine alone. The risk of methemoglobinemia is still a consideration, and cases of severe toxicity have been reported [81,82]. Tetracaine, a long-acting amide local anesthetic, is infrequently used due to the fact that it is rapidly absorbed through the respiratory tract, increasing the risk of toxicity [15].

Application techniques

Local anesthetic may be directly applied to the airway mucosa by several different methods. It is helpful to differentiate the airway into three distinct areas: the nasal cavity and nasopharynx; the oral cavity and oropharynx; and the larynx, trachea, and oropharynx. The basis for this distinction involves the innervation of these different areas and is explained in more detail later on in this chapter.

Regardless of which technique is used to anesthetize the nasal cavity, the nares should be inspected for patency using a nasal speculum or an FOB. Alternatively, the patient can be asked to breathe deeply through each individual nare while occluding the opposite nare; the nare through which the patient breathes more freely should be chosen as the route for nasotracheal intubation. Nasal anesthesia can be achieved by placing cotton pledgets or cotton-tipped swabs soaked in cocaine 4%, lidocaine 4% with epinephrine 1:200 000, or a 3:1 mixture of lidocaine 4% and phenylephrine 1% in the nares. A similar preparation using viscous 4% lidocaine can be applied using a syringe attached to a 14G angiocatheter [73].

Oral cavity topicalization is not necessary for awake intubation per se. The gag reflex and the posterior oropharynx, however, do require anesthesia, particularly if the airway management technique chosen will be stimulating these areas. A 2% to 4% solution of lidocaine can be used to "swish, gargle, and spit" [83]. This technique adequately anesthetizes the oral and pharyngeal mucosa, although the larynx and trachea may require additional topicalization.

Laryngeal anesthesia can be achieved via the aspiration of local anesthetic. There are several methods to achieve this. A "lidocaine lollipop" can be made by placing lidocaine 5% ointment or viscous lidocaine 2–4% on the end of a tongue depressor. This is then placed lidocaine-side-down onto the posterior tongue. The patient is encouraged not to swallow, but rather allow the lidocaine to "melt" and run down the base of the tongue and pool above the glottis, where it is then aspirated. The "toothpaste method" is a similar concept that involves placing a line of lidocaine 5% ointment down the middle of the tongue. The patient is instructed to place the tongue against the roof of the mouth and is encouraged not to swallow.

Aspiration of liquid lidocaine can be achieved by slowly trickling 10–12 ml of lidocaine 2% onto the back of the tongue, while the tongue is held by the operator between two pieces of gauze. This prevents the patient from swallowing and results in aspiration of the lidocaine, resulting in adequate laryngotracheal anesthesia [84].

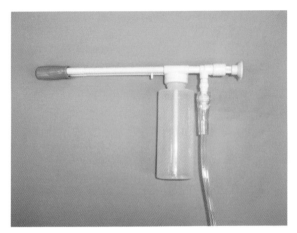

Figure 6.1. Typical disposable atomizer (from Hagberg CA, ed. Benumof's Airway Management, 3rd edn., St. Louis; Mosby 2012).

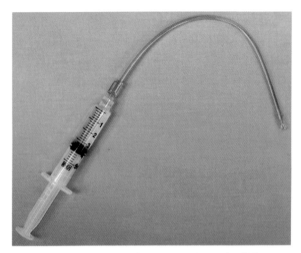

Figure 6.2. MADgic Mucosal Atomization Device (Wolfe Tory Medical, Inc., Salt Lake City, UT).

The "spray-as-you-go" technique involves injecting local anesthetics through the suction port of an FOB or other airway device. One method requires attaching a triple stopcock to the proximal portion of the suction port in order to connect oxygen tubing from a regulated oxygen tank set to flow at 2–4 l/min. Under direct vision through the bronchoscope, targeted areas are sprayed with aliquots of 0.2 to 1.0 ml of 2% to 4% lidocaine. The physician then waits 30 to 60 seconds before advancing to deeper structures and repeating the maneuver. The flow of oxygen allows higher FiO_2 delivery, keeps the FOB lens clean, disperses mucous secretions away from the lens, and aids in nebulizing the local anesthetic [73]. A second method involves passing a multiorifice epidural catheter (internal diameter of 0.5 to 1.0 mm) through the suction port of an adult FOB and intermittently administering aliquots of 0.2 to 1.0 ml of 2% to 4% lidocaine [85].

These techniques are especially useful in patients who are at risk of aspirating gastric contents, because the topical anesthetic is applied only seconds before the intubation is accomplished and allows the patient to maintain his or her airway reflexes as long as possible.

Atomization is a common method of local anesthetic application to the airway. Disposable plastic atomizers are available for this purpose (Figure 6.1). The atomizer reservoir is filled with 2% to 4% lidocaine and tubing is connected from the atomizer to an oxygen cylinder with a flow rate of 8 to 10 l/min. The phalange is depressed and the spray of local anesthetic solution is directed towards the soft palate and posterior pharynx to topicalize the mucosa. A disadvantage with this method is the difficulty in controlling the exact amount of local anesthetic administered. Alternatively, the MADgic® Mucosal Atomization Device (Wolfe Tory Medical, Inc., Salt Lake City, UT) is a disposable, latex-free device that, when attached to a Luer fitted syringe containing local anesthetic, can be used to dispense a fine mist to the oropharyngeal or nasal mucosa (Figure 6.2). The tubing is malleable, allowing for delivery of local anesthetic to deeper pharyngeal structures and the glottis. Because a syringe is used, a known amount of local anesthetic can be administered. The primary disadvantage of this device is that smaller particle sizes are not achieved, limiting the amount of local anesthetic that reaches the trachea.

Nebulizers may also be used to apply local anesthetic to the airway. A standard mouthpiece-type nebulizer (Figure 6.3) can topicalize the oropharynx and trachea. If nasal cavity anesthesia is needed, a face-mask-type nebulizer (Figure 6.4) can be used; the patient is instructed to breathe in through the nose. This approach is especially advantageous in patients with increased ICP, open eye injury, and severe coronary artery disease, due to a decreased incidence of coughing [86]. A typical dose of lidocaine used in a standard nebulizer is 4 ml of 4% lidocaine. This results in a total dose of 160 mg of lidocaine, which is well within the safe dosage range.

Nerve blocks

Although topicalization of the mucosa can supply adequate anesthesia to the entire airway in many circumstances, clinical scenarios may arise where the

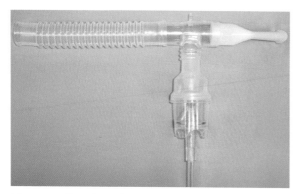

Figure 6.3. Typical mouthpiece-type nebulizer.

denser anesthesia provided by airway nerve blocks is preferable. Some studies have shown superior patient comfort and hemodynamic stability when a combined regional block technique is used in comparison to nebulized local anesthetic [87]. The nerve blocks presented in this section are notable for their ease of performance, their minimal risk to the patient, and their fast onset.

Airway sensory innervations

The anatomy of the airway as it relates to sensory innervations [7,11,15,73,88,89] can be generally divided into three regions (Figure 6.5): the nasal cavity and nasopharynx, innervated by branches of the trigeminal nerve (cranial nerve [CN] V); the oropharynx and posterior third of the tongue, innervated by branches of the glossopharyngeal nerve (CN IX); and the larynx and trachea, innervated by branches of the vagus nerve (CN X).

Sensory input from the nasal cavity and nasopharynx is supplied by the greater and lesser palatine nerves and the anterior ethmoidal nerve. The palatine nerves are derived from branches of the maxillary nerve (CN V_2) and arise from the sphenopalatine ganglion (also known as the pterygopalatine or Meckel's ganglion). They provide sensory innervation to the nasal turbinates and most of the nasal septum, as well as the roof of the mouth, soft palate, and tonsils. The anterior ethmoidal nerve is derived from a branch of the ophthalmic nerve (CN V_1). It provides sensory innervation to the anterior portion of the nasal cavity.

The glossopharyngeal nerve (GPN) supplies sensory innervation to the posterior and lateral walls of the pharynx, the vallecula, the anterior surface of the

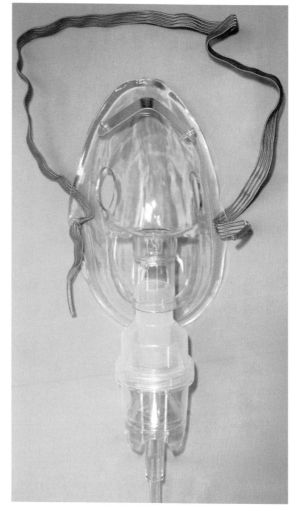

Figure 6.4. Typical facemask-type nebulizer (from Hagberg CA, ed. Benumof's Airway Management, 3rd edn., St. Louis; Mosby 2012).

epiglottis, and the tonsillar pillars. By way of its lingual branch, the GPN also innervates the posterior third of the tongue and acts as the afferent limb of the gag reflex. It emerges from the skull through the jugular foramen and passes anteriorly between the internal jugular and carotid vessels, traveling along the lateral wall of the pharynx.

Sensory innervation of the larynx is supplied by the superior laryngeal nerve (SLN), a branch of the vagus nerve. The internal branch of the SLN contains sensory fibers that are distributed to the base of the tongue, epiglottis, aryepiglottic folds, arytenoids, and the glottis down to the level of the vocal cords. It passes medially between the greater cornu of the hyoid bone and the superior cornu of the thyroid

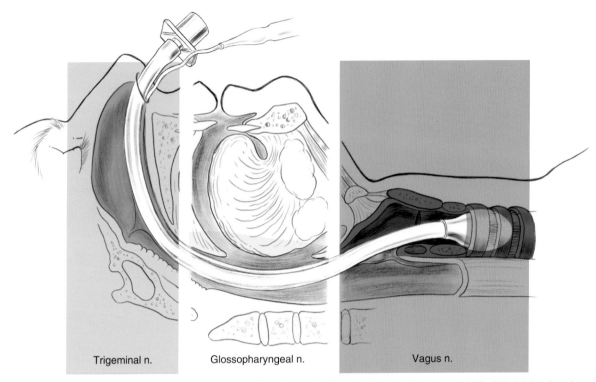

| Trigeminal n. | Glossopharyngeal n. | Vagus n. |

Figure 6.5. Innervation of the upper airway. (Reproduced from Brown D, ed. *Atlas of Regional Anesthesia*, 2nd edn. Philadelphia: Saunders; 1999, with permission from Elsevier.)

cartilage and pierces the thyrohyoid membrane along with the superior laryngeal artery and vein. The nerve then lies in a closed space bounded by the thyrohyoid membrane laterally and the laryngeal mucosa medially, termed the paraglottic space, where it ramifies. The recurrent laryngeal nerves, also branches of the vagus nerve, supply sensory innervation to the tracheobronchial tree up to and including the vocal cords, as well as supplying motor nerve fibers to the intrinsic muscles of the larynx (except the cricothyroid).

Sphenopalatine ganglion block

The sphenopalatine ganglion block provides anesthesia to portions of the airway innervated by the greater and lesser palatine nerves, including the posterior two-thirds of the nasal cavity. It also blocks sensation from the roof of the mouth, soft palate, and tonsils, making it useful even when a transoral intubation is planned [85,89,90].

The sphenopalatine ganglion lies in the pterygopalatine fossa, posterior to the middle turbinate, just under the nasopharyngeal mucosa. Long cotton-

tipped applicators soaked in either 4% cocaine or 4% lidocaine with epinephrine 1:200 000 are passed along the upper border of the middle turbinate at approximately a 45° angle to the hard palate and directed posteriorly until the upper posterior wall of the nasopharynx is reached. The sphenopalatine ganglion underlies the mucosal surface at this point (Figure 6.6A). The applicator is then left in place for approximately 5 minutes. Alternatively, cotton pledgets soaked in local anesthetic solution may be used and applied to the nasal cavity in the same manner using bayonet forceps [85,89,90].

Anterior ethmoidal nerve block

The anterior third of the nasal cavity can usually be sufficiently anesthetized by either topical or nebulized local anesthetic; however, selective blockade of the anterior ethmoidal nerve can also be performed. A long cotton-tipped applicator, soaked in either 4% cocaine or 4% lidocaine with epinephrine 1:200 000, is inserted parallel to the dorsal surface of the nose until it meets the anterior surface of the cribriform plate

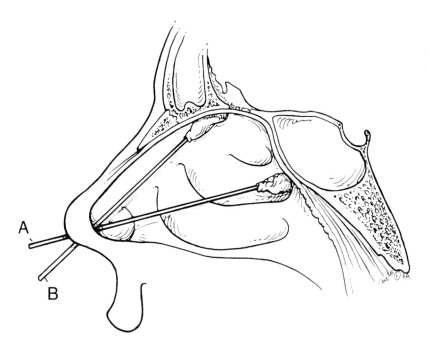

A

B

Figure 6.6. Left lateral view of the right nasal cavity, showing long cotton-tipped applicators soaked in local anesthetic. A, applicator angled at 45° to the hard palate with cotton swab over mucosal surface overlying the sphenopalatine ganglion. B, applicator placed parallel to the dorsal surface of the nose, blocking anterior ethmoidal nerve. (From University of California, Irvine, Department of Anesthesia, D.A. Teaching Aids; reprinted with permission from Hagberg CA, ed. *Benumof's Airway Management*, 2nd edn. St. Louis: Mosby; 2007.)

(Figure 6.6B). The applicator is held in position for 5 minutes [90].

Glossopharyngeal nerve block: intraoral approach

The afferent limb of the gag reflex, mediated by the lingual branch of the GPN, arises from stimulation of deep pressure receptors found in the posterior third of the tongue, which many times cannot be reached by the diffusion of local anesthetics through the mucosa. In situations where blunting of a prominent gag reflex is desired, selective blockade of the lingual branch of the GPN may be performed [7,91–93].

The patient is placed in the sitting position with the physician facing the patient on the contralateral side of the nerve to be blocked. The patient's mouth is opened wide with the tongue protruded. With the non-dominant hand, a tongue blade is used to displace the tongue medially, forming a gutter or trough along the floor of the mouth between the tongue and the teeth. The gutter ends in a cul-de-sac formed by the base of the palatoglossal arch (also known as the anterior tonsillar pillar), which is a U- or J-shaped structure starting at the soft palate and running along the lateral aspect of the pharynx. A 25-gauge spinal needle is inserted 0.25 to 0.5 cm deep at the base of the palatoglossal arch, just lateral to the base of the

tongue, and an aspiration test is performed (Figure 6.7). If air is aspirated, the needle has been advanced too deeply (the tip has advanced all the way through the palatoglossal arch) and should be withdrawn until no air can be aspirated; if blood is aspirated, the needle should be redirected more medially. Two milliliters of 1% to 2% lidocaine are injected, and the procedure is repeated on the contralateral side. The same procedure can be performed noninvasively with cotton-tipped swabs soaked in 4% lidocaine; the swab is held in place for 5 to 10 minutes [7,91–93].

Glossopharyngeal nerve block: external approach (peristyloid)

This approach is most useful when the patient's mouth opening is insufficient to allow adequate visualization to perform an intraoral block. The patient is placed supine with the head in a neutral position. The styloid process is located by identifying the midpoint of the line between the mastoid process and the angle of the jaw. A skin wheal with local anesthetic is made at this location and a 22-gauge spinal needle is advanced perpendicularly to the skin until the styloid process is contacted. Depending on the patient's habitus, this should occur at a depth of 1 to 2 cm. The needle is then redirected posteriorly and as soon as contact is lost with the styloid process, 5 to 7 ml of

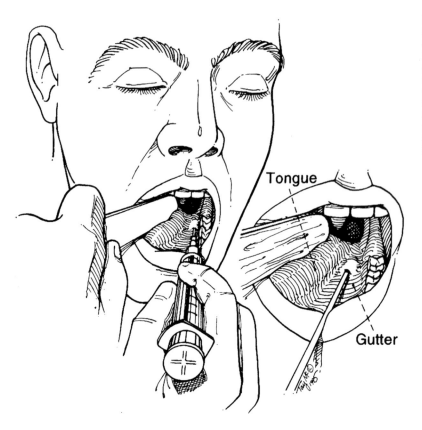

Tongue

Gutter

Figure 6.7. Glossopharyngeal nerve block, anterior approach. Tongue displaced medially forming a gutter (glossogingival groove), which ends distally in a cul-de-sac. A 25-gauge spinal needle is placed at the base of the palatoglossal fold. (From University of California, Irvine, Department of Anesthesia, D.A. Teaching Aids; Reprinted with permission from Hagberg CA, ed. *Benumof's Airway Management*, 2nd edn. St. Louis: Mosby; 2007.)

0.5% to 1% lidocaine is injected after a negative aspiration for blood (Figure 6.8). The procedure is then repeated on the opposite side [73].

Because of the proximity of the GPN at this location to the internal carotid artery, care must taken to avoid intraarterial injection, which could result in headache or seizure. If blood is aspirated or the patient complains of headache during injection, the needle should be removed and repositioned. Tachycardia may result from blockade of the afferent nerve fibers of the GPN that arise from the carotid sinus [94].

Superior laryngeal nerve block

Blockade of the SLN produces dense anesthesia of the hypopharynx and upper glottis, including the vallecula and the laryngeal surface of the epiglottis. In combination with oropharyngeal topical anesthesia with or without a glossopharyngeal nerve block, this allows adequate airway anesthesia for a variety of awake intubation techniques, including direct laryngoscopy [6,73,88,95–97]. In this approach, local

anesthetic is injected into the paraglottic or preepiglottic space, targeting the nerve soon after it pierces the thyrohyoid ligament. Using lidocaine 1% to 2%, satisfactory sensory blockade is achieved within 5 minutes, with a success rate of 92% to 100% [97].

The patient is placed in the supine position, head slightly extended, with the physician standing on the side to be blocked. Several different landmarks may be used: the greater cornu of the hyoid, the superior cornu of the thyroid, and the thyroid notch [6,73,88,95–97].

The greater cornu of the hyoid is the most lateral aspect of the hyoid bone that can be palpated. One side can be made more prominent by displacing the contralateral side toward the side being blocked. A 25-gauge needle is "walked off" the cornu of the hyoid bone in an anterior–inferior direction aiming toward the middle of the thyrohyoid membrane (Figure 6.9A). A slight resistance is felt as the needle is advanced through the membrane usually at a depth of 1 to 2 cm (2 to 3 mm deep to the hyoid bone). The needle at this point has entered the preepiglottic space. Aspiration through the needle should be

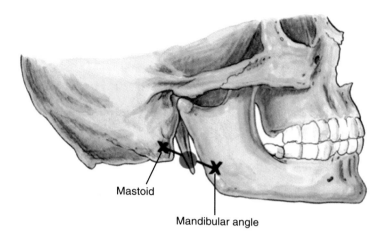

Figure 6.8. Glossopharyngeal nerve block, peristyloid approach. A 22-gauge spinal needle is contacted with the styloid process. It is then redirected posteriorly, putting the tip of the needle in proximity to the glossopharyngeal nerve. (Reproduced from Brown D, ed. *Atlas of Regional Anesthesia*, 2nd edn. Philadelphia: Saunders; 1999, with permission from Elsevier.)

Mastoid

Mandibular angle

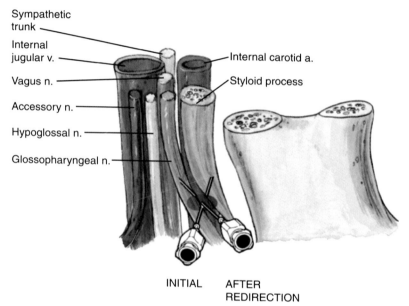

Sympathetic trunk

Internal jugular v.

Vagus n.

Accessory n.

Hypoglossal n.

Glossopharyngeal n.

Internal carotid a.

Styloid process

INITIAL   AFTER REDIRECTION

attempted. If air is aspirated, the needle has gone too deep and may have entered the pharynx, and it should be withdrawn until no air can be aspirated. If blood is aspirated, the needle has cannulated either the superior laryngeal artery or vein or has cannulated the carotid artery; the needle should be directed more anteriorly. When satisfactory needle placement is achieved, 2 to 3 ml of local anesthetic is injected as the needle is withdrawn. The block is repeated on the opposite side. An ultrasound-guided technique to this approach has been described, and may be beneficial in patients with abnormal neck anatomy [98].

The superior lateral cornu of the thyroid cartilage can be identified by palpating the superior thyroid notch ("Adam's apple") and tracing the upper edge of the thyroid cartilage laterally until the most lateral aspect is identified. In many patients, this structure is easier and less painful to palpate than the hyoid bone. A 25-gauge needle is walked off the cornu of the thyroid cartilage in a superior–anterior direction aiming toward the lower third of the thyroid membrane (Figure 6.9B); the same precautions as before are taken and the local anesthetic solution is injected as the needle is withdrawn. The block is repeated on the opposite side.

The easiest landmark to identify in many patients, especially in the morbidly obese, is the thyroid notch (Adam's apple), the most medial and superficial

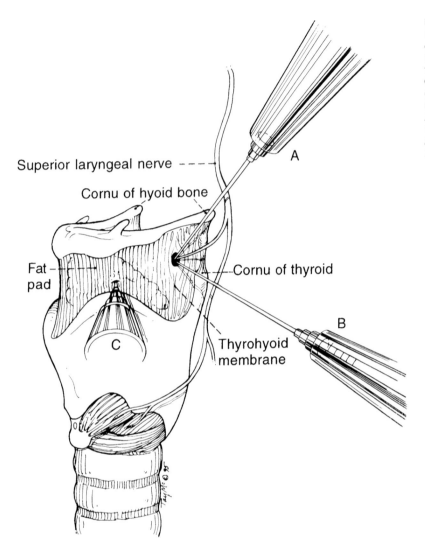

Superior laryngeal nerve ---

Cornu of hyoid bone

Fat
pad

Cornu of thyroid

A

B

C

Thyrohyoid
membrane

Figure 6.9. Superior laryngeal nerve
block, external approach. A, using the
greater cornu of the hyoid bone as
landmark; B, using the superior cornu of
the thyroid cartilage as landmark; and
C, using the thyroid notch as landmark.
(From University of California, Irvine,
Department of Anesthesia, D.A. Teaching
Aids; Reprinted with permission from
Hagberg CA, ed. *Benumof's Airway
Management*, 2nd edn. St. Louis: Mosby;
2007.)

aspect of the thyroid cartilage. The thyroid notch is palpated, and the upper border of the thyroid cartilage is traced laterally for approximately 2 cm. Using a 25-gauge needle, the thyrohyoid ligament is pierced just above the thyroid cartilage at this location and the needle is advanced in a posterior and cephalad direction to a depth of 1 to 2 cm from the skin (Figure 6.9C). After an aspiration test, the 2 to 3 ml of local anesthetic is injected before the needle is withdrawn. The block is repeated on the opposite side. An added benefit of this approach is the decreased likelihood of blocking the motor branch of the SLN.

When performing a SLN block, care should be taken to avoid insertion of the needle into the thyroid cartilage to avoid the possibility of injecting the local anesthetic at the level of the vocal cords, which could cause laryngeal edema and airway obstruction. The carotid artery should be identified and displaced posteriorly to minimize the risk of intravascular injection; even small amounts (0.25 to 0.5 ml) of local anesthetic injected into the carotid artery can induce seizures. Hypotension and bradycardia have also been associated with SLN blockade. A number of possible causes of this reaction have been postulated: (1) vasovagal reaction related to painful stimulation, (2) digital pressure on the carotid sinus, (3) excessive manipulation of the larynx causing vasovagal reaction, (4) large doses of or accidental intravascular administration of local anesthetic drugs, and (5) direct neural stimulation of the branch of the vagus

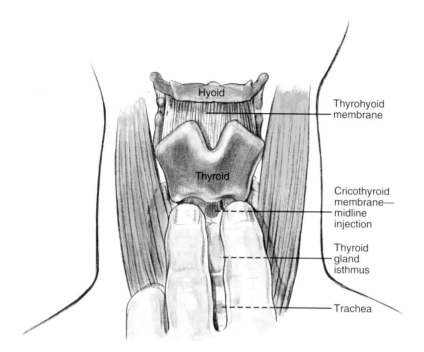

Figure 6.10. Translaryngeal anesthesia, anatomic landmarks. (Reproduced from Brown D, ed. *Atlas of Regional Anesthesia*, 2nd edn. Philadelphia: Saunders; 1999, with permission from Elsevier)

Figure labels: Hyoid, Thyrohyoid membrane, Thyroid, Cricothyroid membrane—midline injection, Thyroid gland isthmus, Trachea

nerve by the needle [99]. It is recommended that anticholinergics be administered before the block is performed. Contraindications to the external approach include local infection, local tumor growth, and coagulopathy. Although not universally accepted, some have advocated avoidance of SLN anesthesia in patients at high risk of aspiration [100].

Transtracheal anesthesia

As both the sensory and motor fibers of the recurrent laryngeal nerves run together, bilateral recurrent laryngeal nerve blocks cannot be performed because they would result in bilateral vocal cord paralysis and complete airway obstruction. The alternative is topicalization of the tracheal mucosa by transtracheal injection. While not a nerve block in the strictest sense, this technique is invasive and bears similar risks to other airway nerve blocks. Tracheal topicalization is of particular benefit in cases where a neurologic exam is required after intubation, as it makes the presence of an endotracheal tube more tolerable.

The patient should be positioned supine with the neck in extension. The thyroid cartilage (Adam's apple) is palpated at midline and followed caudally until a depression and a firm ring of tissue are identified. These are the cricothyroid groove and the cricoid cartilage, respectively. Overlying the cricoid groove is the cricothyroid membrane.

The physician should stand at the side of the patient with the dominant hand closest to the patient. The patient is asked not to talk, swallow, or cough until instructed. The midline of the cricothyroid membrane is identified as the needle insertion site. The index and middle finger of the nondominant hand can be used to mark this spot and stabilize the trachea (Figure 6.10). Using a tuberculin syringe or a 25-gauge needle, a small skin wheal is raised. A 20-gauge angiocatheter attached to a 5 to 10-ml syringe containing 3 to 5 ml saline is used. The needle is advanced through the skin perpendicularly or slightly caudally while aspirating. When air is freely aspirated, the sheath of the angiocatheter is advanced slightly, the needle is removed, and a syringe containing 3 to 5 ml of 2% to 4% lidocaine is carefully administered using the catheter sheath that has been left in place. Aspiration of air is reconfirmed, the patient is warned to expect vigorous coughing, and the local anesthetic is injected rapidly during inspiration (Figure 6.11). The sheath of the angiocatheter may be left in place until the intubation is complete in case more local anesthetic is needed and to decrease the likelihood of subcutaneous emphysema. Coughing helps to nebulize the local anesthetic so that the inferior and

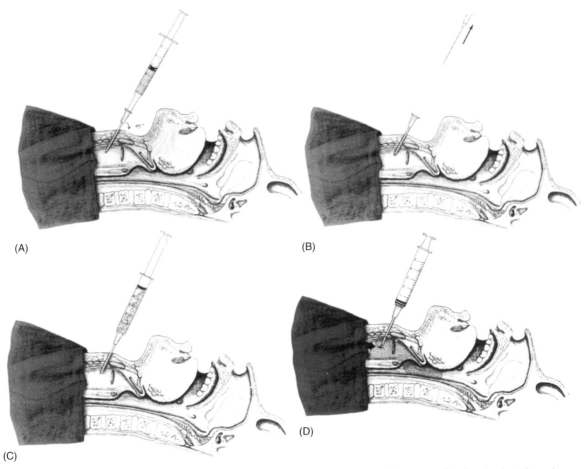

(A)

(B)

(C)

(D)

Figure 6.11. Translaryngeal anesthesia (midsagittal view of the head and neck). (A) Angiocatheter inserted at the cricothyroid membrane, aimed caudally. Aspiration test performed to verify position of tip of needle in tracheal lumen. (B) Needle is removed from angiocatheter. (C) Syringe containing local anesthetic attached. Aspiration test repeated. (D) Local anesthetic is injected, resulting in coughing and nebulization of the local anesthetic (shaded area). (From University of California, Irvine, Department of Anesthesia, D.A. Teaching Aids; Reprinted with permission from Hagberg CA, ed. *Benumof's Airway Management*, 2nd edn. St. Louis: Mosby; 2007.)

superior surfaces of the vocal cords can be anesthetized along with the tracheobronchial tree and inferior larynx. Anesthesia of the epiglottis, vallecula, tongue, and posterior pharyngeal wall are possible, but unreliable [11,15,73,88,101]. The success of translaryngeal anesthesia has been found to be as high as 95% and is attributed to both topicalization of the airway and systemic absorption.

This technique may also be performed using a standard 20- or 22-gauge needle without the placement of an angiocatheter. This may, however, increase the risk of airway injury by way of the sharp metal bevel as the patient coughs. If this technique is utilized, care should be taken to remove the needle immediately after injection of the local anesthetic.

Smaller-gauge needles should not be used due to the risk of breakage [101].

The tip of the needle should never be aimed in a cephalad direction in order to avoid laryngeal trauma and to ensure adequate local anesthetic spread below the vocal cords. Because this procedure may potentially eliminate the patient's ability to protect his/her own airway from aspiration, it should not be performed in patients at high risk of aspiration. Transtracheal injection should be avoided in patients with local tumor or large goiter. Potential complications include bleeding (subcutaneous and intratracheal), infection, subcutaneous emphysema [102], pneumomediastinum, pneumothorax, vocal cord trauma, and esophageal perforation [101].

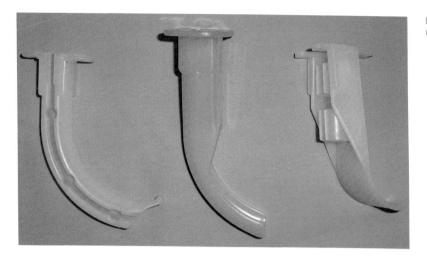

Figure 6.12. Berman, Williams, and Ovassapian airways.

Awake intubation techniques

While flexible fiberoptic bronchoscopy is the most common technique for awake intubation, numerous other methods have been described. The decision of which technique to use should depend on the route chosen (orotracheal vs. nasotracheal), the patient's airway conditions, and the familiarity of the anesthesiologist with specific modalities. The latter is an important point – the difficult airway is not an appropriate setting during which to experiment with a new technique!

Orotracheal vs. nasotracheal intubation

The decision of whether to proceed with intubation via the oral or nasal route should be made before deciding which airway management technique will be utilized. Many times in ENT surgery, the intubation route is dictated by the needs of the surgeon for a particular procedure. When the surgery allows for either route, however, the benefits and disadvantages of each route should be taken into account.

The orotracheal route has several advantages. It is potentially less traumatic and presents a lower risk of bleeding compared to the nasotracheal route, it usually allows for placement of a larger endotracheal tube (ETT), and it provides for more options in terms of airway management techniques. The major disadvantage is that orotracheal techniques usually result in stimulation of the gag reflex, requiring denser airway anesthesia and potentially being less comfortable for the patient. Nasotracheal intubation, on the other hand, bypasses the gag reflex and is usually more easily tolerated by the awake patient. However, the risks of epistaxis, trauma to the nasal turbinates, and submucosal tunneling in the nasopharynx must be taken into account [7].

Flexible fiberoptic bronchoscopy

FOI using an FOB is currently the most commonly used and well-described airway management technique used in the awake patient. FOI provides several advantages: it allows for visual examination of the airway prior to intubation, it provides confirmation of tube placement, avoiding esophageal and endobronchial intubation, it is well tolerated in awake patients, it has less potential for airway and dental trauma, and it can be performed in multiple positions. FOI is a useful technique for both orotracheal and nasotracheal intubation [7,8,25,103].

For orotracheal FOI, one major challenge is navigating the FOB around the base of the tongue to achieve a satisfactory view of the larynx. To facilitate this, specialized intubating oral airways are commonly used. There are several types available, each with unique design differences; they include the Ovassapian, Berman, and Williams airways (Figure 6.12). In addition to providing a conduit for the FOB, these airways protect the FOB from damage by biting. A disadvantage of these devices is that they place pressure on the base of the tongue, potentially causing gagging in awake patients. ROTIGS (Hanu Surgical Devices; Honolulu, HI) is a novel device that has been developed to replace the intubating oral airway during awake oral FOI. ROTIGS (Rapid OroTracheal Intubation Guidance

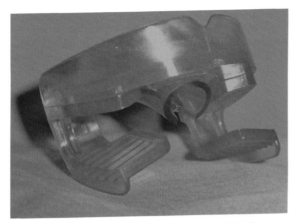

Figure 6.13. ROTIGS (Hanu Surgical Devices, Honolulu, HI).

System) is composed of a mouthpiece, bite block, and guidance tube (Figure 6.13). The mouthpiece and bite blocks keep the device centered and allow a midline approach to the larynx. Because the device does not rest on the tongue, it does not cause gagging, making it well-suited for use in awake and minimally sedated patients.

For nasotracheal FOI, the challenge is usually related to placement of the ETT through the nasal passage into the nasopharynx. There are several steps that can be taken to increase the chances of success: (1) administering a nasal mucosal vasoconstrictor, (2) gauging the degree of patency of the nasal passage using soft plastic nasopharyngeal airways (nasal trumpets), (3) placing the ETT into the nares first, as a conduit for the FOB, and (4) using a smaller ETT, a rotating ETT going counter-clockwise as the ETT enters the glottis, so the bevel is positioned anteriorly, and the use of a specially designed ETT, such as the Parker Flex-Tip™ Tube (Parker Medical, Highlands Ranch, CO, USA). Items 4–6 can also be useful for orotracheal fiberoptic intubation.

There are limitations to the use of FOI in certain situations. Severe airway bleeding can obscure anatomical landmarks and soil the tip of the FOB with blood, making visualization of the larynx extremely difficult. Obstruction or severe stenosis of the airway, such that an FOB cannot be passed, can also make FOI impossible.

Video laryngoscopy

Videolaryngoscopes are novel intubation devices containing a miniature video camera, allowing indirect visualization of the glottis. They provide superior views of the glottis compared to standard direct laryngoscopes in patients with both normal and difficult airways. The use of videolaryngoscopy has been well described as a technique for awake intubation. Video laryngoscopy provides several advantages compared to a standard FOI: a faster and easier glottic view, equipment that is simpler to set up and less prone to breakage, and less training required to develop proficiency in its use [104]. One of the first devices using similar technology described for use in awake intubation was the Bullard® laryngoscope (Gyrus ACMI, Southborough, MA, USA) [7,19]. More recently, the GlideScope® (Verathon Medical, Bothell, WA, USA), the Pentax-AWS® (Pentax Corporation, Tokyo, Japan), and the McGrath® video laryngoscope (Aircraft Medical, Edinburgh, UK) have been used for awake intubation [106,117,118].

Video laryngoscopes that incorporate an angulated blade, such as the GlideScope® and the McGrath® videolaryngoscope, eliminate the necessity for three-axis alignment and facilitate visualization of the glottis. There have been several case series published describing their use for awake intubation of the difficult airway, including patients with upper airway neoplasm and signs of airway obstruction [18,105–107]. The blades are relatively small and, because of the angulated blade, minimal pressure is placed on the tongue, allowing for minimal discomfort to the awake, topicalized patient.

The Pentax-AWS® is a rigid videolaryngoscope that incorporates two channels: a main channel is used to guide the ETT, while a side channel can accommodate a suction catheter. This side channel can be used in awake intubation, however, as a means to administer topical anesthesia with a catheter such as the MADgic® mucosal atomization device. Suction and supplemental oxygen can then be administered through the ETT by using a suction catheter via a Bodai connector and the breathing circuit [104, 108,109]. Limitations of this technique are the necessity for at least a 25 mm mouth opening and the necessity to lift once the tip of the video laryngoscope is in the vallecula, potentially requiring a greater degree of airway anesthesia than other techniques. The Pentax-AWS® has been used successfully to facilitate awake nasotracheal intubations, as well [110,111].

Optical stylets

Another class of devices that can be used for awake intubation is the rigid optical stylet. The Bonfils Retromolar Intubating Fiberscope™ (Karl Storz GmbH, Tuttlingen, Germany) is a rigid fiberscope with a fixed anterior tip curvature of 40°. The rigid shaft allows for greater facility in navigating through soft tissues and around airway structures. A 1.2 mm working channel can be used for applying local anesthetic either directly, or with the aid of an epidural catheter [112–115]. The Sensascope™ (Acutronic Medial Systems AG, Hirzel, Switzerland) is a similar device that incorporates an S-shaped curve and a steerable, flexible distal tip. It has also been used successfully for awake intubation [116].

Other techniques

Essentially, any technique that can be used to intubate the patient under general anesthesia can be used to perform awake intubation. Conventional direct laryngoscopy with a standard laryngoscope was commonly used prior to the advent of the FOB [4]. Of all the techniques, however, it is the most stimulating and requires dense airway anesthesia [7]. Blind techniques, such as a blind nasotracheal intubation or a blind orotracheal intubation through an intubating oral airway, have been shown to have high success rates. The risk of upper airway bleeding, however, should be taken into consideration as this may make subsequent fiberoptic attempts more difficult [4]. Blind techniques should not be attempted in the setting of airway neoplasm. Other techniques that have successfully been used for awake intubations and may be indicated in specific circumstances include lightwand-guided intubation, the intubating LMA, and retrograde intubation [16,17,20].

Case study

The patient is a 56 kg, 73-year-old male with a past history of laryngeal cancer treated with radiation monotherapy 2 years ago. He has noticed a progressive shortness of breath, worsening stridor, and a change in voice over the past 2 months. During an outpatient ENT clinic visit 2 weeks ago, diagnostic nasopharyngeal laryngoscopy (NPL) was performed, revealing an edematous larynx with obstruction of the supraglottis by an enlarged, prolapsed right arytenoid and right aryepiglottic fold. The vocal cords were not fully visualized. A PET scan was performed which showed evidence of local recurrent neoplasm. Other medical history is significant for controlled hypertension and malnutrition. He now presents for elective tracheostomy, direct laryngoscopy, and biopsy. He has been NPO for 12 hours.

Clinical management

The patient's history, clinical status, and imaging were reviewed. The recent NPL findings and airway plan were discussed in detail with the attending ENT surgeon. The decision was made to attempt awake nasotracheal FOI. The patient was brought into the operating room and placed in a seated position. Premedication with glycopyrrolate 0.2 mg IV and midazolam 1 mg IV was administered. Airway topicalization was initiated with 5 ml of nebulized 4% lidocaine. Sedation was achieved with a dexmedetomidine IV load of 0.5 µg/kg over 5 minutes, followed by an infusion of 0.5 µg/kg/h.

The nasal passage was prepared with cotton swabs soaked in a solution of lidocaine 3% with 0.25% phenylephrine. Once the back of the nasopharynx could be reached, a sphenopalatine block was performed by holding the soaked cotton swabs in place for 5 minutes. The decision was made not to attempt any further topicalization of the larynx to avoid coughing and potential airway compromise. The patient at this point was comfortable, following commands, and reporting numbness of the back of the throat.

A 6.0 ETT was placed in the right nostril and a lubricated FOB was advanced through the tube, into the nasopharynx until a view of the glottis was possible. The findings were similar to those seen 2 weeks previously. The fiberoptic scope was navigated down towards the larynx and maneuvered around the right aryepiglottic mass into the subglottic space, which showed no stenosis or mass. The ETT was advanced over the fiberoptic scope into the trachea; there was minimal resistance noted. Once the ETT was in place, bilateral breath sounds and positive end-tidal carbon dioxide were confirmed, general anesthesia was induced with propofol 100 mg IV, and muscle relaxation was achieved with 30 mg of rocuronium. Mechanical ventilation was initiated, and the tube was secured.

Clinical pearls

- When faced with an anticipated difficult airway, awake intubation is the gold standard for airway management.
- Special caution should be taken for the patient with a critical airway obstruction; awake surgical airway may be preferred in these circumstances.

- Preparation begins with a careful history and physical examination, a review of pertinent imaging, and a detailed discussion of the plan with the ENT surgeon.
- The goals of premedication are to alleviate anxiety, provide a clear and dry airway, protect against the risk of aspiration, and enable adequate topicalization.
- Many times, airway topicalization with local anesthetic is sufficient to perform awake intubation; sedation is not always necessary.
- Sedation, if needed, may be accomplished with benzodiazepines, opioids, or intravenous hypnotics either alone or in combination; these agents must be titrated carefully so as to maintain cooperation and adequate ventilation.
- When airway topicalization is insufficient, airway nerve blocks may be employed to supplement airway anesthesia.
- There are many choices involved when preparing for awake intubation. Safety should be the primary consideration.
- The incidence of difficult airways is higher in patients undergoing ENT surgery and, specifically, in patients undergoing ENT cancer surgery.
- There are no absolute contraindications to awake intubation other than patient's refusal, a patient who is unable to cooperate (such as a child, a patient with an intellectual disability, or an intoxicated, combative patient), or a patient with a documented true allergy to all known local anesthetics.
- Potential complications of awake intubation include local anesthetic toxicity, airway trauma, discomfort, recall, and failure to secure the airway.
- No matter which device is selected, all necessary equipment should be prepared ahead of time and be readily available, when needed. The practitioner should also have several back-up modalities in mind, and the required equipment available, in case the initial technique used is ineffective.
- The nasal mucosa and nasopharynx are highly vascular. When a patient requires nasotracheal intubation, adequate vasoconstriction is essential, as bleeding can make visualization of the larynx extremely difficult.
- When using local anesthetics for awake intubation, it is important to be familiar with the speed of onset, duration of action, optimal concentration, signs and symptoms of toxicity, and the maximum recommended dosage of the drug chosen.

References

1. Arne J, Descoins P, Fusciardi J, et al. Preoperative assessment for difficult intubation in general and ENT surgery: predictive value of a clinical multivariate risk index. *Br J Anaesth* 1998;**80**:140–6.

2. Practice guidelines for management of the difficult airway: a report by the American Society of Anesthesiologists Task Force on Management of the Difficult Airway. *Anesthesiology* 1993;**78**:596–602.

3. Practice guidelines for management of the difficult airway: an updated report by the American Society of Anesthesiologists Task Force on Management of the Difficult Airway. *Anesthesiology* 2003;**98**:1269–77.

4. Kopman AF, Wollman SB, Ross K, et al. Awake endotracheal intubation: a review of 267 cases. *Anesth Analg* 1975;**54**:323–27.

5. Meschino A, Devitt JH, Koch P, et al. The safety of awake tracheal intubation in cervical spine injury. *Can J Anaesth* 1992;**39**: 114–7.

6. Thomas JL. Awake intubation: Indications, techniques and a review of 25 patients. *Anaesthesia* 1969;**24**:28–35.

7. Benumof JL. Management of the difficult adult airway, with special emphasis on awake tracheal intubation. *Anesthesiology* 1991;**75**:1086–110.

8. Reed AP, Han DG. Preparation of the patient for awake fiberoptic intubation. *Anesthesiol Clin North Am* 1991;**9**:69–81.

9. Bailenson G, Turbin J, Berman R. Awake intubation – indications and technique. *Anesth Prog* 1967;**14**:272–8.

10. Mason RA, Fielder CP. The obstructed airway in head and neck surgery. *Anaesthesia* 1999;**54**:625–8.

11. Barash PG, Cullen BF, Stoelting RK, et al. *Clinical Anesthesia*, 6th edn. Philadelphia: Lippincott Williams & Wilkins; 2009.

12. Miller RD, ed. *Miller's Anesthesia*, 7th edn. Philadelphia: Elsevier Churchill Livingstone; 2009.

13. Benumof JL, Scheller MS. The importance of transtracheal jet ventilation in the management of the difficult airway. *Anesthesiology* 1989;**71**:769–78.

14. Boucek CD, Gunnerson HB, Tullock WC. Percutaneous

transtracheal high-frequency jet ventilation as an aid to fiberoptic intubation. *Anesthesiology* 1987;**67**:246–9.

15. Reed AP. Preparation of the patient for awake flexible fiberoptic bronchoscopy. *Chest* 1992;**101**:244–53.

16. Hamard F, Ferrandiere M, Sauvagnac X, *et al.* Propofol sedation allows intubation of the difficult airway with the Fastrach LMA. *Can J Anesth* 2005; **52**:421–7.

17. Xue F, He N, Liao X, *et al.* Clinical assessment of awake endotracheal intubation using the lightwand technique alone in patients with difficult airways. *Chin Med J* 2009;**122**: 408–15.

18. Doyle DJ. Awake intubation using the GlideScope video laryngoscope: initial experience in four cases. *Can J Anaesth* 2004;**51**:520–1.

19. Cohn AI, McGraw SR, King WH. Awake intubation of the adult trachea using the Bullard laryngoscope. *Can J Anaesth* 1995;**42**:246–8.

20. Raval C, Patel H, Patel P, *et al.* Retrograde intubation in a case of ankylosing spondylitis posted for correction of deformity of the spine. *Saudi J Anaesth* 2010; **4**:38–41.

21. Stoelting RK. Anticholinergic drugs. In *Pharmacology and Physiology in Anesthetic Practice*, 3rd edn. Philadelphia: Lippincott Williams & Wilkins; 2005.

22. Gross JB, Hartigan ML, Schaffer DW. A suitable substitute for 4% cocaine before blind nasotracheal intubation: 3% lidocaine-0.25% phenylephrine nasal spray. *Anesth Analg* 1984;**63**:915–8.

23. Kallar SK, Everett LL. Potential risks and preventive measures for pulmonary aspiration: new concepts in preoperative fasting guidelines. *Anesth Analg* 1993;**77**:171–82.

24. White PF, Recart Friere A. Ambulatory outpatient anesthesia. In Miller RD, ed. *Miller's Anesthesia,* 6th edn. Philadelphia: Elsevier Churchill Livingstone; 2005. pp. 2589–636.

25. Walsh M, Shorten G. Preparing to perform an awake fiberoptic intubation. *Yale J Biol Med* 1998;**71**:536–49.

26. Reves JG, Glass PSA, Lubarsky DA, *et al.* Intravenous nonopioid anesthetics. In Miller RD, ed. *Miller's Anesthesia,* 6th edn. Philadelphia: Elsevier Churchill Livingstone; 2005. pp. 316–78.

27. Murphy PJ, Erskine R, Langton JA. The effect of intravenously administered diazepam, midazolam and flumazenil on the sensitivity of upper airway reflexes. *Anaesthesia* 1994;**49**: 105–10.

28. Reed AP. Preparation for intubation of the awake patient. *Mt Sinai J Med* 1995;**62**:10–20.

29. Puchner W, Egger P, Löckinger A, *et al.* Evaluation of remifentanil as single drug for awake fiberoptic intubation. *Acta Anaesthesiol Scand* 2002; **46**:350–4.

30. Lee MC, Absalom AR, Menon DK, *et al.* Awake insertion of the laryngeal mask airway using topical lidocaine and intravenous remifentanil. *Anaesthesia* 2006;**61**:32–5.

31. Reves JG, Fragen RJ, Vinik HR, *et al.* Midazolam: pharmacology and uses. *Anesthesiology* 1985;**62**:310–24.

32. Hendrickx JF, Eger EI 2nd, Sonner JM, *et al.* Is synergy the rule? A review of anesthetic interactions producing hypnosis and immobility. *Anesth Analg* 2008;**107**:494–506.

33. Lichtenbelt BJ, Olofsen E, Daha A, *et al.* Propofol reduces the distribution and clearance of midazolam. *Anesth Analg* 2010;**110**:1596–606.

34. Ben-Shlomo I, Tverskoy M, Fleyshman G, *et al.* Intramuscular administration of lidocaine or bupivacaine alters the effect of midazolam from sedation to hypnosis in a dose-dependent manner. *J Basic Clin Physiol Pharmacol* 2003;**14**:256–63.

35. White PF, Shafer A, Boyle WA 3rd, *et al.* Benzodiazepine antagonism does not provoke a stress response. *Anesthesiology* 1989;**70**:636–9.

36. Amrein R, Hetzel W. Clinical pharmacology of flumazenil. *Eur J Anaesthesiol Suppl* 1988;**2**: 15–24.

37. Fukuda K. Intravenous opioid anesthetics. In Miller RD, ed. *Miller's Anesthesia,* 6th edn. Philadelphia: Elsevier Churchill Livingstone; 2005. pp. 379–438.

38. Machata AM, Gonano C, Holzer A, *et al.* Awake nasotracheal fiberoptic intubation: patient comfort, intubating conditions, and hemodynamic stability during conscious sedation with remifentanil. *Anesth Analg* 2003;**97**:904–8.

39. Shafer SL, Varvel JR. Pharmacokinetics, pharmacodynamics, and rational opioid selection. *Anesthesiology* 1991;**74**:53–63.

40. Randell T, Valli H, Lindgren L. Effects of alfentanil on the responses to awake fiberoptic nasotracheal intubation. *Acta Anaesthesiol Scand* 1990;**34**: 59–62.

41. Atkins JH, Mirza N. Anesthetic considerations and surgical caveats for awake airway surgery. *Anesthesiol Clin* 2010;**28**:555–75.

42. Mingo OH, Ashpole KJ, Irving CJ, *et al.* Remifentanil sedation

for awake fibreoptic intubation with limited application of local anesthetic in patients for elective head and neck surgery. *Anaesthesia* 2008;**63**:1065–9.

43. Machata AM, Gonano C, Holxer A, *et al.* Awake nasotracheal fiberoptic intubation: patient comfort, intubating conditions, and hemodynamic stability during conscious sedation with remifentanil. *Anesth Analg* 2003;**97**:904–8.

44. Rai MR, Parry TM, Dombrovskis A, *et al.* Remifentanil target-controlled infusion vs propofol target-controlled infusion for conscious sedation for awake fibreoptic intubation: a double-blinded randomized controlled trial. *Br J Anaesth* 2008;**100**: 125–30.

45. Teganeh N, Roshani B, Azizi B, *et al.* Target-controlled infusion of remifentanil to provide analgesia for awake nasotracheal fiberoptic intubations in cervical trauma patients. *J Trauma* 2010;**69**: 1185–90.

46. Xu YC, Xue FS, Luo MP, *et al.* Median effective dose of remifentanil for awake laryngoscopy and intubation. *Chin Med J (Engl)* 2009;**122**: 1506–12.

47. Cafiero T, Esposito F, Fraioli G, *et al.* Remifentanil-TCI and propofol-TCI for conscious sedation during fibreoptic intubation in the acromegalic patient. *Eur J Anaesth* 2008;**25**:670–4.

48. Ackerman WE, Phero JC, Theodore GT. Ineffective ventilation during conscious sedation due to chest wall rigidity after intravenous midazolam and fentanyl. *Anesth Prog* 1990;**37**: 46–8.

49. Jaffe TB, Ramsey FM. Alleviation of fentanyl-induced truncal rigidity. *Anesthesiology* 1983;**58**:562–4.

50. Belleville JP, Ward DS, Bloor BC, *et al.* Effects of intravenous dexmedetomidine in humans, I: sedation, ventilation, and metabolic rate. *Anesthesiology* 1992;**77**:1125–33.

51. Coursin DB, Coursin DB, Maccioli GA. Dexmedetomidine. *Curr Opin Crit Care* 2001;7:221–6.

52. Ebert TJ, Hall JE, Barney JA, *et al.* The effect of increasing plasma concentrations of dexmedetomidine in humans. *Anesthesiology* 2000;**93**:382–94.

53. Abdelmalak B, Makary L, Hoban J, *et al.* Dexmedetomidine as sole sedative for awake intubation in management of the critical airway. *J Clin Anesth* 2007;**19**:370–3.

54. Bergese SD, Khabiri B, Roberts WD, *et al.* Dexmedetomidine for conscious sedation in difficult awake fiberoptic intubation cases. *J Clin Anesth* 2007;**19**:141–4.

55. Bergese SD, Bender SP, McSweeney TD, *et al.* A comparative study of dexmedetomidine with midazolam and midazolam alone for sedation during elective awake fiberoptic intubation. *J Clin Anesth* 2010;**22**:35–40.

56. Avitsian R, Lin J, Lotto M, *et al.* Dexmedetomidine and awake fiberoptic intubation for possible cervical spine myelopathy. *J Neurosurg Anesthesiol* 2005;**17**:96–9.

57. Bergese SD, Candiotti KA, Bokesch PM, *et al.* A Phase IIIb, randomized, double-blind, placebo-controlled, multicenter study evaluating the safety and efficacy of dexmedetomidine for sedation during awake fiberoptic intubation. *Am J Ther* 2010;**17**:586–95.

58. *Precedex [package insert].* Lake Forest, IL: Hospira, Inc.; 2008.

59. Ustün Y, Gündüz M, Erdogan O, *et al.* Dexmedetomidine vs.

midazolam in outpatient third molar surgery. *J Oral Maxillofac Surg* 2006;**64**:1353–8.

60. Bloor BC, Ward DS, Belleville JP, *et al.* Effects of intravenous dexmedetomidine in humans, II: hemodynamic changes. *Anesthesiology* 1992;**77**:1134–42.

61. Perouansky MA, Hemmings HC Jr. Intravenous anesthetic agents. In Hemmings HC Jr, Hopkins PM, eds. *Foundations of Anesthesia, Basic and Clinical Sciences,* 2nd edn. St. Louis: Mosby; 2006. pp. 295–310.

62. Iravani M, Wald SH. Dexmedetomidine and ketamine for fiberoptic intubation in a child with severe mandibular hypoplasia. *J Clin Anesth* 2008;**20**:455–7.

63. Scher CS, Gitlin MC. Dexmedetomidine and low-dose ketamine provide adequate sedation for awake fiberoptic intubation. *Can J Anaesth* 2003;**50**:606–10.

64. Coppen JE, Fox JWC. Endobronchial intubation under neuroleptanalgesia for a patient with severe hemoptysis. *Anesth Analg* 1968;**47**:70–1.

65. Redden RL, Biery KA, Campbell RL. Arterial oxygen desaturation during awake endotracheal intubation. *Anesth Prog* 1990;**37**:201–4.

66. *Droperidol [package insert].* Lake Forest, IL: Hospira, Inc.; 2004.

67. Ho AMH, Chung DC, To EWH, *et al.* Total airway obstruction during local anesthesia in a non-sedated patient with a compromised airway. *Can J Anesth* 2004;**51**:838–41.

68. Day RO, Chalmers DRC, Williams KM, *et al.* Death of a healthy volunteer in a human research project: implications for Australian clinical research. *Med J Aust* 1998;**168**:449–51.

69. Case report on death of University of Rochester student

issued; available at: http://www.
health.state.ny.us/press/releases/
1996/wan.htm. Accessed January
2012.

70. Adriani J, Zepernick R, Arens J,
    et al. The comparative potency
    and effectiveness of topical
    anesthetics in man. Clin
    Pharmacol Ther 1964;5:
    49–62.

71. Perry LB. Topical anesthesia for
    bronchoscopy. Chest
    1978;73:691–3.

72. Strichartz GR, Berde CB. Local
    anesthetics. In Miller RD, ed.
    Miller's Anesthesia, 6th edn.
    Philadelphia: Elsevier Churchill
    Livingstone; 2005. pp. 573–604.

73. Simmons ST, Schleich AR.
    Airway regional anesthesia for
    awake fiberoptic intubation. Reg
    Anesth Pain Med 2002;27:180–92.

74. British Thoracic Society
    guidelines on diagnostic flexible
    laryngoscopy. Thorax 2001;
    56:1–21.

75. Langmack EL, Martin RJ, Pak J,
    et al. Serum lignocaine
    concentrations in asthmatics
    undergoing research
    bronchoscopy. Chest
    2000;117:1055–60.

76. Parkes SB, Butler CS, Muller R.
    Plasma lignocaine concentration
    following nebulization for awake
    intubation. Anaesth Intensive
    Care 1997;25:369–71.

77. Wieczorek PM, Schricker T,
    Vinet B, et al. Airway
    topicalization in morbidly obese
    patients using atomized lidocaine:
    2% compared with 4%.
    Anaesthesia 2007;62:984–8.

78. Xue FS, Liu HP, He N, et al.
    Spray-as-you-go airway topical
    anesthesia in patients with a
    difficult airway: a randomized,
    double-blind comparison of 2%
    and 4% lidocaine. Anesth Analg
    2009;108:536–43.

79. Donlon JV Jr, Doyle DJ, Feldman
    MA. Anesthesia for eye, ear, nose,
    and throat surgery. In Miller RD,

ed. Miller's Anesthesia, 6th edn.
    Philadelphia, Elsevier Churchill
    Livingstone, 2005; 2526–56.

80. Novaro GM, Aronow HD,
    Militello MA, et al. Benzocaine-
    induced methemoglobinemia:
    experience from a high-volume
    transesophageal
    echocardiography laboratory.
    J Am Soc Echocardiogr
    2003;16:170–5.

81. Douglas WW, Fairbanks VF.
    Methemoglobinemia induced by
    a topical anesthetic spray
    (cetacaine). Chest 1977;71:
    586–91.

82. Sandza JG Jr, Roberts RW, Shaw
    RC, et al. Symptomatic
    methemoglobinemia with a
    commonly used topical
    anesthetic, cetacaine. Ann Thorac
    Surg 1980;30:186–90.

83. Murphy MF. Sedation and
    anesthesia for awake intubation.
    In Walls RM, Murphy MF, eds.
    Manual of Emergency Airway
    Management, 3rd edn.
    Philadelphia: Lippincott Williams
    and Wilkins; 2008. pp. 94–103.

84. Chung DC, Mainland PA, Kong
    AS. Anesthesia of the airway by
    aspiration of lidocaine. Can
    J Anaesth 1999;46:215–9.

85. Ovassapian A. Fiberoptic Airway
    Endoscopy in Anesthesia and
    Critical Care. New York: Raven
    Press; 1990.

86. Bourke DL, Katz J, Tonneson A.
    Nebulized anesthesia for awake
    endotracheal intubation.
    Anesthesiology 1985;63:690–2.

87. Kundra P, Kutralam S,
    Ravishankar M. Local anesthesia
    for awake fiberoptic nasotracheal
    intubation. Acta Anaesthesiol
    Scand 2000;44:511–6.

88. Roberts JT. Anatomy and patient
    positioning for fiberoptic
    laryngoscopy. Anesthesiol Clin
    North Am 1991;9:53.

89. Standring S. Gray's Anatomy, the
    Anatomical Basis of Clinical

Practice, 40th edn. Philadelphia:
    Churchill Livingstone; 2009.

90. Hagberg CA. Airway blocks. In
    Chelly JE, ed. Peripheral Nerve
    Blocks: A Color Atlas, 3rd edn.
    Philadelphia: Lippincott Williams
    & Wilkins; 2008. pp. 176–84.

91. Mulroy MF. Regional Anesthesia,
    An Illustrated Procedural Guide,
    4th edition. Philadelphia,
    Lippincott Williams & Wilkins,
    2008.

92. Henthorn RW, Amayem A,
    Ganta R. Which method for
    intraoral glossopharyngeal nerve
    block is better? Anesth Analg
    1995;81:1113–4.

93. Saliba DL, McCutchen TA,
    Laxton MJ, et al. Reliable block of
    the gag reflex in one minute or
    less. J Clin Anesth 2009;21:463.

94. Kodama K, Seo N, Murayama T,
    et al. Glossopharyngeal nerve
    block for carotid sinus syndrome.
    Anesth Analg 1992;75:1036–7.

95. DeMeester TR, Skinner DB,
    Evans RH, et al. Local nerve
    block anesthesia for peroral
    endoscopy. Ann Thorac Surg
    1977;24:278–83.

96. Gotta AW, Sullivan CA.
    Anaesthesia of the upper airway
    using topical anaesthetic and
    superior laryngeal nerve block.
    Br J Anaesth 1981;53:1055–8.

97. Furlan JC. Anatomical study
    applied to anesthetic block
    technique of the superior
    laryngeal nerve. Acta Anaesthesiol
    Scand 2002;46:199–202.

98. Manikandan S, Neema PK,
    Rathod RC. Ultrasound-guided
    bilateral superior laryngeal nerve
    block to aid awake endotracheal
    intubation in a patient with
    cervical spine disease for
    emergency surgery. Anaesth
    Intensive Care 2010;38:946–8.

99. Wiles JR, Kelly J, Mostafa SM.
    Hypotension and bradycardia
    following superior laryngeal
    nerve block. Br J Anaesth
    1989;63:125–7.

100. Walts LF, Kassity KJ. Spread of local anesthesia after upper airway block. *Arch Otolaryngol* 1965;**81**:76–9.

101. Gold MI, Buechel DR. Translaryngeal anesthesia: a review. *Anesthesiology* 1959;**20**:181–5.

102. Wong DT, McGuire GP. Subcutaneous emphysema following trans-cricothyroid membrane injection of local anesthetic. *Can J Anaesth* 2000;**47**:165–8.

103. Ovassapian A, Krejcie TC, Yelich SJ, *et al.* Awake fibreoptic intubation in the patient at high risk of aspiration. *Br J Anaesth* 1989;**62**:13–6.

104. Jarvi K, Hillermann C, Danha, *et al.* Awake intubation with the Pentax Airway Scope. *Anaesthesia* 2011;**66**:314.

105. Xue FS, Li CW, Zhang GH, *et al.* GlideScope®-assisted awake fibreoptic intubation: initial experience in 13 patients. *Anaesthesia* 2006;**61**:1014–5.

106. McGuire BE. Use of the McGrath video laryngoscope in awake patients. *Anaesthesia* 2009;**64**:912–4.

107. Uslu B, Damgaard Nielsen R, Kristensen BB. McGrath® videolaryngoscope for awake tracheal intubation in a patient with severe ankylosing spondylitis. *Br J Anaesth* 2010;**104**:118–9.

108. Suzuki A, Kunisawa T, Takahata O, *et al.* Pentax-AWS (Airway Scope®) for awake tracheal intubation. *J Clin Anesth* 2007;**19**:642–6.

109. Hirabayashi Y, Seo N. Awake intubation using the Airway Scope. *J Anesth* 2007;**21**:529–30.

110. Asai T. Pentax-AWS videolaryngoscope for awake nasal intubation in patients with unstable necks. *Br J Anaesth* 2010;**104**:108–11.

111. Xue FS, Xiong J, Yuan YJ, *et al.* Pentax-AWS videolaryngoscope for awake nasotracheal intubation in patients with a difficult airway. *Br J Anaesth* 2010;**104**:505.

112. Mazères JE, Lefranc A, Cropet C, *et al.* Evaluation of the Bonfils intubating fibrescope for predicted difficult intubation in awake patients with ear, nose, and throat cancer. *Eur J Anaesth* 2011;**28**:646–50.

113. Corbanese U, Possamai C. Awake intubation with the Bonfils fibrescope in patients with difficult airway. *Eur J Anaesth* 2009;**26**:836–41.

114. Xue FS, Luo MP, Liao X, *et al.* Airway topical anesthesia using the Bonfils fiberscope. *J Clin Anesth* 2009;**21**:154–5.

115. Abramson SI, Holmes AA, Hagberg CA. Awake insertion of the Bonfils retromolar intubation fiberscope in five patients with anticipated difficult airways. *Anesth Analg* 2008;**106**:1215–7.

116. Greif R, Kleine-Brueggeney M, Theiler L. Awake tracheal intubation using the Sensascope™ in 13 patients with an anticipated difficult airway. *Anaesthesia* 2010;**65**:525–8.

117. Choi GS, Park SI, Lee EH, Yoon SH. Awake Glidescope® intubation in a patient with a huge and fixed supraglottic mass – a case report. *Korean J Anesthesiol* 2010;**59**:S26–9.

118. Jeyadoss J, Nanjappa N, Nemeth D. Awake intubation using Pentax AWS videolaryngoscope after failed fibreoptic intubation in a morbidly obese patient with a massive thyroid tumour and tracheal compression. *Anaesth Intensive Care* 2011;**39**(2):311–12.

Anesthesia for ENT trauma

Matthew R. Eng and Marshal B. Kaplan

Introduction

Head trauma accounts for 10 to 15% (approximately 230000) of trauma hospitalizations in the United States per year, resulting in the second leading cause of trauma hospitalizations [1]. Further, trauma is the leading cause of death and disability in Americans younger than 40 years of age [2]. Although motor vehicle accidents and falls account for the majority of head trauma in the United States, such injuries often occur with sporting accidents or assaults.

Maxillofacial trauma poses a difficult challenge for the anesthesiologist with regard to the patient's airway. Injuries to the head and neck may result in airway obstruction from disrupted or distorted anatomy, tissue edema, foreign debris, vomitus, or bleeding. Craniofacial injuries may distort the anatomy of the tongue or pharynx to such an extent that airway patency is compromised. Traumatic brain injury may result in loss of central mechanisms of airway protection. Trauma to the neck may additionally cause direct airway obstruction when there is injury to the larynx. While airway management will be discussed in this chapter, the overriding principle in the event of an inability to quickly establish an airway should be to perform a surgical airway. In a report of patients with laryngeal fractures, 74% required advanced airway techniques [3].

Cervical spine injury has been reported to occur in up to 6% of patients with maxillofacial trauma [4–6]. Significant cervical injury should be presumed until definitively "ruled out" on clinical grounds and by radiographic imaging.

The general principles for the anesthetic management of other trauma surgery must be applied to ENT trauma operations. The anesthesiologist must act as the primary resuscitator and principal manager of the airway.

Primary survey: ABCDE

The advanced trauma life support (ATLS) course describes a series of surveys in which the prioritization of resuscitation and assessment actions is defined. The trauma life support training program for physicians is the most widely recognized program available. In the primary survey, lasting 2 to 5 minutes, the ABCDE sequence of trauma should be performed – **A**irway, **B**reathing, **C**irculation, **D**isability and neurologic status, and **E**xposure and overall evaluation for other injuries. Appropriate intervention should be performed immediately by specialized trauma medical providers. Following the primary survey, more comprehensive secondary and tertiary surveys are performed.

Airway management

Ventilation and oxygenation are the greatest priorities in a trauma patient, and management of the airway in patients with trauma to the head and neck requires a skilled practitioner. Knowledge of injury patterns, anatomy, and a timely strategy allows for optimal airway management. The failure of oxygenation and ventilation may occur secondary to shock states, anatomical injury, or CNS injury.

In all trauma cases, the physician should administer high-flow oxygen and employ a pulse oximeter monitor. Also, a high-volume suction should be available since these patients are at an increased risk of vomiting. These patients should also be placed in a rigid cervical collar to avoid further injury in patients with possible cervical spine injury. Although placing the patient in a "sniffing" position is often utilized for improved visualization of the airway during laryngoscopy, this technique is contraindicated in patients

---

Anesthesia for Otolaryngologic Surgery, ed. Basem Abdelmalak and D. John Doyle. Published by Cambridge University Press.
© Cambridge University Press 2013.

with a suspected cervical spine injury. While not contraindicated, jaw thrust and chin lift may be more difficult in the presence of a cervical collar or in comminuted fractures of the mandible. These maneuvers have also been associated with movement of the cervical spine, and must be performed with appropriate support of the head to prevent spinal injury [7].

The use of oropharyngeal and nasopharyngeal airways requires careful consideration in the patient with midface injuries. Oropharyngeal airways may be poorly tolerated in a patient with an intact gag reflex or may cause airway obstruction with improper sizing or improper placement [8]. Inserting a nasopharyngeal airway may exacerbate nasopharyngeal bleeding (or produce epistaxis in patients without midface injuries.) There is also a concern regarding insertion of nasogastric tubes in patients with midface injuries or suspected anterior skull base fractures following a series of reports of these devices entering the cranium [9–11]. Therefore, blind insertion of nasogastric tubes in a patient with these injuries should be avoided.

Tracheal intubation or surgical cricothyroidotomy may be used to provide a definitive airway by experienced clinicians. A definitive airway should be secured by intubation when any of the following criteria are present:

(1) inability to oxygenate and ventilate
(2) inability to maintain an adequate airway
(3) underlying injury and physiology of the patient that may lead to a failure to maintain an adequate airway, oxygenate, or ventilate.

Practice management guidelines established by ATLS and The Eastern Association for the Surgery of Trauma include the following indications for tracheal intubation [12]:

(1) bilateral mandibular fractures
(2) copious bleeding into the mouth
(3) loss of protective laryngeal reflexes
(4) severe cognitive impairment with GCS < 8 or > 2-point fall
(5) seizures
(6) deteriorating blood gases
(7) acute airway obstruction
(8) hypoventilation
(9) severe hypoxemia despite supplemental oxygen
(10) severe hemorrhagic shock
(11) cardiac arrest.

Oral endotracheal intubation with cervical in-line immobilization may be effective in patients with suspected cervical spine injury. In a series of cadaveric studies and clinical studies, cervical in-line immobilization has been shown to be safe without any reports of associated myelopathy [13–15]. Less cervical manipulation has been reported in the use of a McCoy laryngoscope blade and bougie [16]. However, there remains a significant concern in obtaining an optimal view of the vocal cords with restricted neck extension and positioning in the "sniffing" positioning. For this reason, many clinicians favor other techniques.

Oral intubation utilizing the GlideScope [17], intubating LMA [18], video Macintosh laryngoscope, lightwand [17], or the Bullard laryngoscope [18] has been shown to provide intubating conditions with less cervical spine manipulation compared to direct laryngoscopy. These methods, however, can be more time-consuming and equipment access may be limited in emergency situations.

Oral and nasal intubations with fiberoptic technique have been suggested to minimize manipulation of the cervical spine as compared to direct laryngoscopy [13,14]. Nasal intubations should not be attempted in the presence of severe trauma to the midface or basilar skull fractures since the intubation could breach the cranial vault [19–22]. Basilar skull fractures present clinically with Battle's sign (retroauricular hematoma) and raccoon eyes (periorbital hematoma). Using a fiberoptic scope, even by skilled practitioners, can still be challenging since visualization can easily become obscured by a single drop of blood or secretions on the tip of the scope [23]. Awake fiberoptic intubation may be appropriate to reduce the possibility of losing the patent airway during the induction of anesthesia and possible gastric aspiration. Intoxicated or agitated patients may be poor candidates for an awake fiberoptic intubation since patients should ideally be calm and cooperative during the intubation. The oral mucosa should be anesthetized by application of a local anesthetic spray, injection, or nebulizer to the oral/nasal pharyngeal mucosa.

Retrograde intubation is another potential technique that may facilitate tracheal intubation in a patient with suspected cervical spine injury. First described in 1960, the retrograde intubation is usually performed by needle cannulation through the cricothyroid membrane with passage of a flexible guidewire or epidural catheter to the oropharynx. The guidewire or epidural catheter is then retrieved through the mouth and affixed to the Murphy's eye of an endotracheal tube. In a review of 24 patients undergoing retrograde intubation, the anesthesiologists were 100% successful in using this method, with an 88% success of intubating on the first attempt [24]. The technique is cited in the ASA difficult airway algorithm [25], but the experience of this technique in trauma settings is extremely limited [24].

In the event of a difficult airway that cannot be secured using an endotracheal tube, a supraglottic airway device or esophageal obturator airway should be utilized as described in the ASA difficult airway algorithm [25] in the event of an unable to intubate, unable to ventilate situation, a Classic LMA may facilitate rescue ventilation, but should not be considered a definitive airway, and it should be kept in mind that the patient is still at risk of aspiration. The LMA Supreme, introduced in late 2007, has a built-in drain tube which may be used for gastric access and an anatomic curve which facilitates a blind placement [26]. Again, the LMA Supreme does not completely ensure a definitively protected airway, but may serve as a better rescue ventilation option as compared to the Classic LMA.

Surgical airways

An advanced surgical airway is necessary when it is not possible to secure a definitive airway in a timely fashion by any other method. Acute obstruction from upper airway trauma (laryngotracheal trauma) or failed intubations may necessitate a cricothyroidotomy or tracheostomy. Surgical airway preparations should be made prior to any planned intubation attempt in a patient with ENT trauma in the event that intubation is not successful. In these circumstances, a needle or surgical cricothyroidotomy may be the preferred airway because it is relatively superficial, less vascular, and accomplished with success of greater than 90% [27]. The complication rate of a cricothyroidotomy is reported to be 28.7% [12], and includes pneumothorax, failed procedure, hemorrhage, misplaced tube, and development of tracheal stenosis. In children, oxygenation and ventilation are best accomplished by a needle cricothyroidotomy. A needle cricothyroidotomy may be used to temporize the patient until a more formal surgical airway is established.

Types of injury
Laryngeal trauma

Airway management for a patient with laryngeal trauma is controversial, and attempting intubation can be very difficult. It is essential to gather any clues regarding the diagnosis of the laryngeal injury, including the presence of pain or bruising across the anterior neck, hoarseness or stridor, or the presence of crepitus or subcutaneous emphysema. In a recent review of 19 patients presenting with injury to the upper aerodigestive tract, 100% were found to have subcutaneous emphysema, 21% had dysphagia, and 63% had stridor or hoarseness [28]. Attempts at intubating a patient with laryngeal trauma may result in further iatrogenic injury or loss of a tenuous airway. If any intubation attempt is to be made, it should be done carefully using a fiberoptic bronchoscope with a small endotracheal tube. If difficulty is encountered, the intubation should be abandoned, and a surgical airway established. Supraglottic devices should not be used in a traumatized larynx since these devices may worsen the subcutaneous emphysema with positive-pressure ventilation.

Mandibular fractures

The mandible is the second most commonly fractured facial bone after the nose. While any injury to the mandible may pose a risk to the airway, a bilateral mandibular fracture is of grave concern. Bilateral fractures of the mandible can result in a "flail mandible" and may lead to an oral cavity collapse on the posterior pharynx. This acute obstruction of the airway necessitates immediate intubation or a surgical airway. The otolaryngologist can improve the airway by placing "bridle wires" in a dentate patient to obviate the emergent airway intervention. Mandibular fractures are also associated with vascular damage with injury to the internal carotid artery and vascular injury to the inferior alveolar artery within the mandibular canal. Adequate lighting and suctioning are essential in the event of severe bleeding. While bleeding can be controlled by packing the wound or pressure, the definitive control is sometimes only attained by angiography and embolization.

Maxillary fractures

Maxillary fractures often produce severe bleeding and the risk of aspiration of broken teeth, blood, and fragments of soft tissue. Rene Le Fort defined a classification of maxillary fractures based on his study of cadaver experiments [29]. A Le Fort Level I fracture is a horizontal fracture that involves the inferior nasal aperture, separating the maxillary alveolus from the rest of the midfacial skeleton. This fracture typically occurs as a result of force directed to the lower midface. Le Fort Level II fractures may result from a blow to the lower or mid maxilla and involve the inferior orbital rim. These fractures are pyramidal-shaped nasalmaxillary fractures that break from the upper craniofacial skeleton. Le Fort Level III fractures are more rare, and usually result from blunt force to the nasal bridge or upper maxilla. The fractures may result in separation of facial skeleton from the skull base.

Patients with facial injuries may additionally present with difficult mouth opening because of pain or trismus. Induction of anesthesia can provide relaxation to facilitate an endotracheal intubation.

Spine injuries

Standard practice dictates that all blunt trauma victims be assumed to have an unstable cervical spine until this condition is ruled out. Cervical spine injury has a reported incidence of 5–10% in trauma patients [30] and up to 6% in maxillofacial trauma patients [4–6].

"Clearing" the cervical spine should occur as soon as possible because of the issues related to neck immobilization [31]. The cervical spine may be protected by manual stabilization, rigid collar, or lateral restraints and tape until the spine has been cleared.

The cervical spine may be "cleared" without imaging in many cases, and immobilization can be removed safely based on clinical criteria alone. The following clinical criteria should be met for clearance of the cervical spine:

1. Fully awake, i.e. GCS 14 or 15.
2. No alcohol or intoxicants (in the patient).
3. No (painful) distracting injuries.
4. No pain or tenderness of the spine on deep palpation.
5. Active movement without pain or neurological change.

Nevertheless, many practitioners feel that the neck must remain stabilized pending definitive imaging studies. In the unconscious patient or a patient with multiple injuries or brain injury, the clinical assessment for cervical spine clearance may be unfeasible. In these situations, clearance requires imaging options including CT, MRI, and direct fluoroscopy [32]. Plain radiographs do not adequately identify all cervical spine injuries [33] and result in false negatives in 10% of cases [34,35].

In considering plain radiographs the three standard ATLS views (lateral, anteroposterior and open-mouth odontoid peg) should now be regarded as inadequate [36], identifying only approximately 90% of cervical spine injuries [33]. In the presence of brain injury and an abnormal brain CT scan the false-negative rate of plain radiographs at the craniocervical junction is approximately 10% [34,35]. The false-negative rate for a helical CT of the cervical spine is less than 0.5% [32,37]. In these instances, isolated ligamentous injuries may be missed and the patient's cervical spine may still be at risk.

For definitive clearance, the practitioner may elect to allow the patient to recover for a proper clinical assessment. However, the prolonged spinal immobilization carries increased morbidity and mortality. The imaging modality of choice for spinal immobilization clearance is MRI, which may detect up to 25% of ligamentous and soft tissue injuries missed by radiographs and CT. Dynamic fluoroscopy is another technique used to identify cervical spine injury. This requires a specialist and continuous fluoroscopy during dynamic manipulation of the cervical spine. There are few data to support a significant advantage of dynamic fluoroscopy compared to combined radiographs and CT imaging [31].

Inhalational injuries

As with all other trauma injuries, the airway should be assessed first in the event of an inhalational injury to the nasopharynx. The patient should be administered 100% oxygen and monitored with pulse oximetry. Impending airway obstruction may occur in the presence of stridor, hoarseness, wheezing, or tachypnea, and a patent airway should be established immediately.

The inhalational damage is primarily from the inhaled toxins and chemicals which exert injury at the bronchi and alveoli. Heat is mostly dispersed throughout the upper airway. With bronchoscopy, the chemical mucosal damage is evident with neutrophil-mediated inflammatory changes including erythema, edema, and carbonaceous exudates. Frequent suctioning should be performed to clear exudates that may plug bronchioles and cause shunting.

Summary

Anesthesia for head and neck trauma should be approached utilizing the basic principles of ATLS. Airway management is best performed with knowledge of airway anatomy, an understanding of the impact of the trauma on the airway, and a thoughtful approach to the deployment of different airway devices. Ultimately, patients with difficult airways and distorted anatomy may require a surgical airway without delay.

Case study

Not surprisingly, emergency providers around the world tremble at the thought of having to manage the emergency patient with respiratory distress following severe head and neck trauma. In airway circles the following semi-mythical story sometimes circulates as a sort of cautionary tale. So here goes the story.

An otherwise healthy young man ran his outdoor ATV into a suspended cable and was severely injured. His companion called for help. The arriving "light flight" doctor instantly filled with complete dread as he saw a battered, bloody, gurgling face deeply cut by some sort of wire. The patient was barely breathing, and possibly partially decapitated. "Now there was an impossible airway", thought the paramedic.

As feared, even with the best field suction, there was no way that the patient was able to be intubated orally. Nasal intubation looked hopeless too. There was blood everywhere, and secretions to deal with as well. And a failed attempt at intubation. The flight doctor switched back to mask ventilation, but it wasn't satisfactory either, even with an oral airway and a nasopharyngeal airway placed in what looked like where the nose was. Then he remembered a maxim his mentor always emphasized: "If you can't intubate and can't ventilate, then it's time to heal with steel." He grabbed a scalpel with a size 15 blade with a

view to opening up the airway, but when he got close and suctioned, he could see that the trachea had been almost completely transected by the wire. In fact, the inside of the trachea was clearly visible after suctioning. Intubation then became as easy as simply identifying the distal tracheal section and passing an ETT in the direction of the carina.

Clinical pearls

- Injuries to the head and neck may result in airway obstruction from disrupted or distorted anatomy, tissue edema, foreign debris, vomitus, or bleeding. Traumatic brain injury may result in loss of central mechanisms of airway protection.
- Insertion of nasogastric tubes in patients with midface injuries or suspected anterior skull base fractures may result in their entering the cranium.
- Attempts at intubating a patient with laryngeal trauma may result in further iatrogenic injury or loss of a tenuous airway. If any intubation attempt is to be made, it should be done carefully using a fiberoptic bronchoscope with a small endotracheal tube.
- Supraglottic devices should not ordinarily be used in a traumatized larynx since these devices may worsen the subcutaneous emphysema with positive-pressure ventilation.
- An inability to quickly establish an airway should lead to consideration of a surgical airway.
- The imaging modality of choice for spinal immobilization clearance is MRI, which may detect up to 25% of ligamentous and soft tissue injuries missed by radiographs using CT.
- The following clinical criteria should be met for clearance of the cervical spine:
  - Fully awake, i.e. GCS 14 or 15.
  - No alcohol or intoxicants (in the patient).
  - No (painful) distracting injuries.
  - No pain or tenderness of the spine on deep palpation.
  - Active movement without pain or neurological change.

References

1. Thurman D, Guerrero J. Trends in hospitalization associated with traumatic brain injury. *JAMA* 1999;**282**:954–7.

2. Web-Based Injury Statistics Query and Reporting System (WISQARS). *National Center for Injury Prevention and Control*; 2007.

3. Verschueren DS, Bell RB, Bagheri SC, Dierks EJ, Potter BE. Management of laryngo-tracheal injuries associated with craniomaxillofacial trauma. *J Oral Maxillofac Surg* 2006;**64**:203–14.

4. Beirne JC, Butler PE, Brady FA. Cervical spine injuries in patients with facial fractures: a 1-year prospective study. *Int J Oral Maxillofac Surg* 1995;**24**: 26–9.

5. Davidson JS, Birdsell DC. Cervical spine injury in patients with facial skeletal trauma. *J Trauma* 1989;**29**:1276–8.

6. Sinclair D, Schwartz M, Gruss J, McLellan B. A retrospective review of the relationship between facial fractures, head injuries, and cervical spine injuries. *J Emerg Med* 1988;**6**:109–12.

7. Donaldson WF 3rd, Heil BV, Donaldson VP, Silvaggio VJ. The effect of airway maneuvers on the unstable C1-C2 segment. A cadaver study. *Spine (Phila Pa 1976)* 1997;**22**:1215–8.

8. Greenberg RS. Facemask, nasal, and oral airway devices. *Anesthesiol Clin North America* 2002;**20**:833–61.

9. Hanna AS, Grindle CR, Patel AA, Rosen MR, Evans JJ. Inadvertent insertion of nasogastric tube into the brain stem and spinal cord after endoscopic skull base surgery. *Am J Otolaryngol* 2011.

10. Chandra R, Kumar P. Intracranial introduction of a nasogastric tube in a patient with severe craniofacial trauma. *Neurol India* 2010;**58**:804–5.

11. Spurrier EJ, Johnston AM. Use of nasogastric tubes in trauma patients – a review. *J R Army Med Corps* 2008;**154**:10–3.

12. Dunham CM, Barraco RD, Clark DE, *et al.* Guidelines for emergency tracheal intubation immediately after traumatic injury. *J Trauma* 2003;**55**: 162–79.

13. Lennarson PJ, Smith D, Todd MM, *et al.* Segmental cervical spine motion during orotracheal intubation of the intact and injured spine with and without external stabilization. *J Neurosurg* 2000;**92**:201–6.

14. Majernick TG, Bieniek R, Houston JB, Hughes HG. Cervical spine movement during orotracheal intubation. *Ann Emerg Med* 1986;**15**: 417–20.

15. McGuire G, el-Beheiry H. Complete upper airway obstruction during awake fibreoptic intubation in patients with unstable cervical spine fractures. *Can J Anaesth* 1999;**46**:176–8.

16. Gabbott DA. Laryngoscopy using the McCoy laryngoscope after application of a cervical collar. *Anaesthesia* 1996;**51**:812–4.

17. Turkstra TP, Craen RA, Pelz DM, Gelb AW. Cervical spine motion: a fluoroscopic comparison during intubation with lighted stylet, GlideScope, and Macintosh laryngoscope. *Anesth Analg* 2005;**101**:910–5, table of contents.

18. Wahlen BM, Gercek E. Three-dimensional cervical spine movement during intubation using the Macintosh and Bullard laryngoscopes, the bonfils fibrescope and the intubating laryngeal mask airway. *Eur J Anaesthesiol* 2004;**21**:907–13.

19. Bahr W, Stoll P. Nasal intubation in the presence of frontobasal fractures: a retrospective study. *J Oral Maxillofac Surg* 1992;**50**:445–7.

20. Goodisson DW, Shaw GM, Snape L. Intracranial intubation in patients with maxillofacial injuries associated with base of skull fractures? *J Trauma* 2001;**50**: 363–6.

21. Zmyslowski WP, Maloney PL. Nasotracheal intubation in the presence of facial fractures. *JAMA* 1989;**262**:1327–8.

22. Junsanto T, Chira T. Perimortem intracranial orogastric tube insertion in a pediatric trauma patient with a basilar skull fracture. *J Trauma* 1997;**42**:746–7.

23. Mason RA, Fielder CP. The obstructed airway in head and neck surgery. *Anaesthesia* 1999;**54**:625–8.

24. Gill M, Madden MJ, Green SM. Retrograde endotracheal intubation: an investigation of indications, complications, and patient outcomes. *Am J Emerg Med* 2005;**23**:123–6.

25. Caplan RA, Benumof JL, Berry FA. Practice guidelines for management of the difficult airway. An updated report by the American Society of Anesthesiologist Task Force on management of the difficult airway. *Anesthesiology* 2003;**98**:1269.

26. Timmermann A, Cremer S, Eich C, *et al.* Prospective clinical and fiberoptic evaluation of the Supreme laryngeal mask airway. *Anesthesiology* 2009;**110**:262–5.

27. Wright MJ, Greenberg DE, Hunt JP, Madan AK, McSwain NE Jr. Surgical cricothyroidotomy in trauma patients. *South Med J* 2003;**96**:465–7.

28. Goudy SL, Miller FB, Bumpous JM. Neck crepitance: evaluation and management of suspected upper aerodigestive tract injury. *Laryngoscope* 2002;**112**:791–5.

29. Le Fort R. Etude experimentale sur les fractures de la machoire superieure. *Rev Chir* 1901: 479–507.

30. Chiu WC, Haan JM, Cushing BM, Kramer ME, Scalea TM. Ligamentous injuries of the cervical spine in unreliable blunt trauma patients: incidence, evaluation, and outcome. *J Trauma* 2001;**50**:457–63; discussion 64.

31. Morris CG, McCoy E. Clearing the cervical spine in unconscious polytrauma victims, balancing risks and effective screening. *Anaesthesia* 2004;**59**:464–82.

32. Griffen MM, Frykberg ER, Kerwin AJ, *et al*. Radiographic clearance of blunt cervical spine injury: plain radiograph or computed tomography scan? *J Trauma* 2003;**55**:222–6; discussion 6–7.

33. Stiell IG, Clement CM, McKnight RD, *et al*. The Canadian C-spine rule versus the NEXUS low-risk criteria in patients with trauma. *N Engl J Med* 2003;**349**:2510–8.

34. Cusmano F, Ferrozzi F, Uccelli M, Bassi S. [Upper cervical spine fracture: sources of misdiagnosis]. *Radiol Med* 1999;**98**:230–5.

35. Link TM, Schuierer G, Hufendiek A, Horch C, Peters PE. Substantial head trauma: value of routine CT examination of the cervicocranium. *Radiology* 1995;**196**:741–5.

36. Kreipke DL, Gillespie KR, McCarthy MC, *et al*. Reliability of indications for cervical spine films in trauma patients. *J Trauma* 1989;**29**:1438–9.

37. Hogan GJ, Mirvis SE, Shanmuganathan K, Scalea TM. Exclusion of unstable cervical spine injury in obtunded patients with blunt trauma: is MR imaging needed when multi-detector row CT findings are normal? *Radiology* 2005;**237**:106–13.

Anesthesia for ENT emergencies

D. John Doyle

Introduction

Writing a short chapter on ENT emergencies (Table 8.1) is seemingly oxymoronic given that the topic could easily be the subject of entire textbooks. This fact notwithstanding, it is the intent of this chapter to offer a brief overview of otolaryngologic emergencies, covering the topic in broad strokes. In this sense the chapter can be envisioned as an overview that links to more detailed discussions in more specialized chapters to follow.

Equipment

A special effort should be made to ensure adequate preparation for ENT emergencies [1], especially in terms of airway equipment (Table 8.2). In addition to these airway gadgets and unlisted items favored by individual practitioners, ENT surgeons will want ready access to an emergency tracheotomy tray as well as to some form of suspension laryngoscope or rigid bronchoscope (see Chapter 2). Special attention to the maintenance and cleaning of fiberoptic bronchoscopes is also important given that they must always be easily accessible and reliable when needed. In the case of electronic fiberscopes incorporating a video display, establishing that illumination settings and white balancing have been done correctly prior to use is particularly important.

Airway obstruction

Complete or partial airway obstruction is not uncommon in ENT practice and anesthesiologists are familiar with a variety of measures, such as tracheal intubation, to deal with this event. Table 8.3 lists some causes of airway obstruction.

Table 8.1. A sampling of otolaryngologic emergencies

Bleeding after tonsillectomy, UVPP (uvulopalatopharyngoplasty) or similar procedure

Bleeding after carotid artery surgery, leading to pressure on airway structures

The patient exhibiting stridor, reflecting a state of almost complete airway obstruction

The patient with an obstructed airway (See Table 8.3. Some causes of airway obstruction)

The patient with head and neck infection, abscess, or inflammation

The patient with severe epistaxis

Table 8.2. Possible components for ENT airway emergencies cart

Bag-valve mask ("Ambu") bag

Oropharyngeal and nasopharyngeal airways

Supraglottic airways

Endotracheal tubes, including "Microlaryngeal" tubes

Malleable stylets

Topical anesthesia, with syringes, and atomizers

Laryngoscope collection with extra batteries

McGill forceps (useful for nasal intubation)

Airway introducer ("gum elastic bougie")

Tube exchange catheters

Carbon dioxide detection system

Video laryngoscope (e.g., GlideScope, McGrath, Pentax-AWS, etc.)

Surgical airway kit (e.g., Melker cricothyrotomy kit)

Fiberoptic broncohoscope

Anesthesia for Otolaryngologic Surgery, ed. Basem Abdelmalak and D. John Doyle. Published by Cambridge University Press.
© Cambridge University Press 2013.

Table 8.3. Some causes of airway obstruction

Tumors compressing the airway from the outside

Tumors invading the airway from the inside

Airway obstruction from inflamed/edematous airway structures

Obstructive sleep apnea/obstruction from altered oropharyngeal muscle tone

Buildup of airway secretions

Angioedema

Angioedema (old term: angioneurotic edema) is the rapid swelling of the dermis, subcutaneous tissue, mucosa and submucosal tissues, usually from an allergic reaction to either a food or medication [2–4]. This process is mediated via the release of histamine and other inflammatory mediators. Hereditary angioedema is a variant existing in three forms caused by an autosomal dominant genetic mutation. All forms involve anomalous activation of the complement system.

Although very often angioedema is harmless and does not affect breathing, dysphonia, dysphagia, and dyspnea can all occur, including the possibility of complete and irrevocable loss of the airway. Just as with anaphylaxis, epinephrine may be lifesaving when the angioedema is allergic in cause, but treatment with epinephrine has not been shown to be helpful in cases of hereditary angioedema. Intubation is often needed in cases of angioedema; this will usually be performed under topical anesthesia with the patient awake or lightly sedated.

Airway infections

Airway-related infections such as epiglottitis, retropharyngeal abscess and Ludwig's angina are covered in Chapter 9. One approach commonly taken in such cases is awake intubation, especially in conjunction with a fiberscope.

Bleeding

Airway-related bleeding may occur spontaneously, as with a bleeding tumor, as a consequence of anticoagulation (e.g., for atrial fibrillation), or following surgery (e.g., after UVPP surgery). Chapter 32 discusses the management of bleeding after tonsillectomy surgery. Such cases offer a number of special challenges, such as the presence of blood impairing the view at laryngoscopy, the need for suction to remove blood and secretions, the possibility of aspirating oropharyngeal blood and the possibility of the patient going into hypovolemic shock in the case of extreme blood loss. Assuming that any coagulation issues are corrected, attention will be directed at finding the bleeding source and stopping it with cautery, using a ligature or by other means. This will very often require reintubation of the patient.

Bleeding after carotid artery surgery may similarly require intubation of the patient. Both edema secondary to venous and lymphatic obstruction and direct compression of the trachea from an expanding hematoma serve to make intubation more difficult. Awake intubation is a popular choice in this situation [5,6].

Epistaxis

Epistaxis is bleeding from the nose [7]. While it is usually benign and self-limiting, it can every now and then be life-threatening. Epistaxis is divided into two types, anterior bleeds (90% of cases) and posterior bleeds (10% of cases), on the basis of the site where the bleeding originates. Anterior nasal packing for bleeding may be undertaken should direct pressure, topical agents, or silver nitrate cauterization fail. Posterior epistaxis may be more severe, may be accompanied by hematemesis or melena and may require general anesthesia and intubation as part of the treatment. Bleeding diatheses such as hereditary hemorrhagic telangiectasia (Osler–Weber–Rendu syndrome) or (more ordinarily) the use of anticoagulants like aspirin or warfarin should also be ruled out.

Stridor

One of the most potentially serious ENT emergencies is dealing with the stridorous patient. Stridor is noisy inspiration from upper airway turbulent gas flow resulting from breathing through a partly obstructed airway. Stridor should always command immediate attention. The first issue of clinical concern in the setting of stridor is whether or not intubation or a surgical airway is immediately needed. If intubation can be delayed for a period of time, a number of other options can be considered; these are presented in the chapter on Heliox. (Patients who are stridorous are sometimes helped with the administration of Heliox; this and more information on stridor is discussed in Chapter 10.) Finally, attempts should be made to determine the cause of the stridor (e.g., foreign body, glottic edema, etc.).

Case study

Ludwig's angina

The patient was a 66-year-old male, 5'6″ in height and weighing 76 kg, with a recent history of an infected tooth. He had been taking antibiotics for a week for a sore throat that had developed after the offending tooth was removed. Recently, his symptoms had worsened with the onset of fever and dyspnea.

When seen in the emergency department he presented with a "gurgling" sound while breathing. He drooled saliva. Trismus was present and he was not able to protrude his tongue. Vital signs were: temperature 38.9°C, pulse 120/min, blood pressure 185/95 and a respiratory rate of 25/min. His oxygen saturation was 92% on room air and 99% on 10 l/min oxygen delivered by face mask. The patient was seated in an upright sitting posture, given 6 mg of intravenous dexamethasone while the on-call anesthesia and ENT teams were paged. Ludwig's angina was suspected.

A decision was made to bring the patient to the operating theater for an emergency intubation and drainage of the infection. The plan was awake fiberoptic intubation with tracheostomy under local anesthesia as a backup.

Preoperative evaluation

Past medical history: hypertension, hypercholesterolemia, chronic bronchitis.

Past surgical history: appendectomy at age 39.

Medications: atenalol, atorvastatin, aspirin.

Comorbidities: hypertension and hypercholesterolemia.

Airway: Mallampati Class 4 airway, thyromental distance of 4 cm, mouth opening 2 cm.

Laboratory studies: Hct 48%. ECG shows only nonspecific T wave changes. Normal echo.

NPO: the patient has been NPO for more than 8 hours.

Patient education: the patient was explained the risks, benefits and alternatives of both the proposed operation and the anesthetic plan.

Management

The anesthesia team and the surgical team reviewed various airway management plans. The chosen plan was for placing a size 6.0 mm ID MLT tube via fiberoptic intubation. After transporting the patient onto the operating table, he was placed in the supine position, with the head resting on a foam pillow. After ensuring adequate IV access and applying standard monitors, the patient was premedicated with glycopyrrolate but was not given any sedatives. The airway was topicalized using gargled and sprayed lidocaine as best as could be achieved with limited mouth opening. After some difficulty a size 9 Williams airway was placed. The fiberscope was then advanced and used to deliver additional topical anesthesia on the glottis. Copious secretions had to be suctioned, making the process difficult. After several attempts the glottis was finally visualized and the fiberscope passed into the trachea, followed by placement of the ETT. After clinical and capnographic confirmation of correct tube placement, the patient was induced with midazolam, fentanyl, and propofol and relaxed using rocuronium. The surgeons then drained the lesion, sent pus for microbial studies and placed a surgical drain. The patient was then brought to the ICU, where he was ventilated until the next day. He was then extubated over a tube exchanger, in case reintubation became necessary.

Clinical pearls

- A special effort should be made to ensure adequate preparation for ENT emergencies, especially in terms of airway equipment. Ready access to an emergency tracheotomy tray is especially important.
- Special attention to the maintenance and cleaning of fiberoptic bronchoscopes is important given that they must always be easily accessible and reliable when needed.
- Epinephrine may be lifesaving when the cause of angioedema is allergic in cause, but treatment with epinephrine has not been shown to be helpful in cases of hereditary angioedema. Intubation is often needed when angioedema strikes.
- Posterior epistaxis may be particularly severe, may be accompanied by hematemesis or melena, and may require general anesthesia and intubation as part of the treatment.
- Airway-related infections such as epiglottitis, retropharyngeal abscess and Ludwig's angina constitute an emergency airway. One approach commonly taken in such cases is awake intubation, especially in conjunction with a fiberscope.

References

1. Banga R, Thirlwall A, Corbridge R. How well equipped are ENT wards for airway emergencies? *Ann R Coll Surg Engl* 2006;**88** (2):157–60. PubMed PMID: 16551407; PubMed Central PMCID: PMC1964098.

2. Weis M. Clinical review of hereditary angioedema: diagnosis and management. *Postgrad Med* 2009;**121**(6):113–20. Review. PubMed PMID: 19940422.

3. Gompels MM, Lock RJ, Abinun M, *et al.* C1 inhibitor deficiency: consensus document. *Clin Exp Immunol* 2005;**139**(3): 379–94.

4. Lipozencić J, Wolf R. Life-threatening severe allergic reactions: urticaria, angioedema, and anaphylaxis. *Clin Dermatol* 2005;**23**(2):193–205. PubMed PMID: 15802213.

5. Beamish D. Airway problems after carotid endarterectomy.

Br J Anaesth 1997;**78**(6):776. PubMed PMID: 9215043.

6. Munro FJ, Makin AP, Reid J. Airway problems after carotid endarterectomy. *Br J Anaesth* 1996;**76**(1):156–9. PubMed PMID: 8672360.

7. Pope LE, Hobbs CG. Epistaxis: an update on current management. *Postgrad Med J* 2005;**81**(955): 309–14. PubMed PMID: 15879044; PubMed Central PMCID: PMC1743269.

Chapter

9

Airway pathology in otolaryngology: anesthetic implications

D. John Doyle

Introduction

This chapter is intended as a minimal synopsis of selected airway pathology in terms of associated anesthetic and airway implications. The case types covered in the following discussion are those where awake intubation by some means (e.g., by fiberoptic methods) is often the method of choice. Where awake intubation is impractical (e.g., inadequate equipment or experience) tracheostomy under local anesthesia (with minimal or no sedation in extreme cases) is often advocated as the best means of managing the airway.

In all the conditions discussed herein, complete airway obstruction is the outcome that is most feared, and this can easily occur when sedating agents such as propofol are used, as they lower the tone of the airway musculature, thereby changing the airway architecture.

Our selection of pathologic conditions herein is a rather limited sampling of only the most commonly encountered pathologic conditions in clinical practice; for more unusual pathologic entities that impact on the airway, more information is available from other chapters of this book and recourse to the abundant ENT literature is encouraged.

Acute epiglottitis

Epiglottitis is among the most dreaded of airway infections, especially in children [1–7]. Pediatric victims are usually children aged 2 to 6, often infected with *Haemophilus influenzae*. Fortunately, an available vaccine against *H. influenzae* has greatly reduced the frequency of this tragic affliction. Infected children may appear to be systemically ill ("toxic") possibly with a fever and/or assuming a "tripod" position. Drooling from the mouth related to difficulty with swallowing is common. Examining the child's airway

Table 9.1. Some pathologic conditions in otolaryngology with airway implications, some of which are covered in this chapter

Airway infections

    Abscess in the upper airway

    Epiglottitis

    Ludwig's angina

    Quinsy

    Retropharyngeal abscess

Airway tumors

    Tumors of upper airway

    Anterior mediastinal mass

    Oral malignancies/tongue malignancies

    Glottic tumors

    Previous head and neck tumor surgery

    Previous radiation treatment to head and neck

Other conditions

    Congenital malformation (e.g., Pierre Robin sequence)

    Periglottic edema (e.g., following rigid bronchoscopy)

    Recurrent laryngeal nerve injury

    Jaw wired shut following maxillofacial surgery

    Maxillofacial trauma (covered in Chapter 7)

    Zenker's diverticulum (covered in Chapter 20)

    Obstructive sleep apnea (OSA) (covered in Chapter 18)

    Laryngospasm (covered in Chapter 8)

may exacerbate the problem (by increasing airway edema) so tongue depressors and laryngoscopy are usually not good options in the initial management. Anything that might bring the child to cry (for

Anesthesia for Otolaryngologic Surgery, ed. Basem Abdelmalak and D. John Doyle. Published by Cambridge University Press. © Cambridge University Press 2013.

example, needles) should be avoided where possible. Consequently (and for other reasons), the usual approach to management involves a careful inhalational induction with the child sitting in the anesthetist's lap and intubation of the child while he or she is breathing spontaneously under deep sevoflurane anesthesia. If at laryngoscopy the orifice through the epiglottis can't be identified, one trick is to have someone compress the child's chest, thus generating a small air bubble in the glottis that the intubator can aim for. In the past patients were often managed by emergency tracheostomy; however, contemporary management of children includes short-term nasal intubation and intravenous antibiotic therapy. For further details the reader is directed to Chapter 32, dealing with pediatric otolaryngologic issues.

Epiglottitis can occur in adults too (George Washington is said to have died of it) but the situation is less dreadful here because the adult airway is larger. Most clinicians would use awake fiberoptic laryngoscopy to secure the airway where necessary in this situation. Although there is considerable disagreement concerning optimal airway management in the adult with epiglottitis, there seems to be a growing consensus that most adults are adequately treated in an intensive care unit with inhaled mist, antibiotics and corticosteroids, and that tracheal intubation is necessary only if symptoms of respiratory distress develop.

Retropharyngeal abscess

Retropharyngeal abscess formation may occur from bacterial infection of the retropharyngeal space secondary to tonsillar or dental infections [8–15]. Untreated, the posterior pharyngeal wall may advance anteriorly into the oropharynx, resulting in a dyspnea and airway obstruction. Other clinical findings may include difficulty in swallowing, trismus and a fluctuant posterior pharyngeal mass. An abscess cavity may be evident on lateral neck X-rays with anterior displacement of the esophagus and upper pharynx. Airway management may be complicated by trismus or airway obstruction. Because abscess rupture can lead to soiling of the trachea, contact with the posterior pharyngeal wall during laryngoscopy and intubation should be minimized. Incision and drainage are the mainstay of treatment. Tracheostomy is often, but not always, required.

Ludwig's angina

Ludwig's angina is a multispace infection of the floor of the mouth [16–25]. The infection starts with infected mandibular molars and spreads to sublingual, submental, buccal and submandibular spaces. The tongue becomes elevated and displaced posteriorly, which may lead to loss of the airway, especially when the patient is placed in the supine position. As with a retropharyngeal abscess, an additional concern is the potential for abscess rupture into the hypopharynx (with possible lung soiling) either spontaneously or with attempts at laryngoscopy and intubation. Airway management options will depend on clinical severity, surgical preferences, and other factors (e.g., CT or MRI findings), but elective tracheostomy prior to incision and drainage remains the classic, if arguably dated, treatment modality. Most experts advocate fiberoptic intubation if at all possible. In addition, since Ludwig's angina is often associated with trismus, nasal fiberoptic intubation is frequently needed.

Airway tumors

Airway tumors (Figure 9.1) can be benign or malignant, but regardless of type, suffocation from airway obstruction is always a potential concern [26–32]. Discussion with the surgical team concerning the expected type of pathology and the size and location of the tumor will help determine whether awake intubation is appropriate. Videos of any previously recorded nasopharyngoscopic examinations can also be helpful in establishing whether encountering tumor during laryngoscopy and intubation might be a problem.

Airway polyps

Polyps may be found throughout the airway [33–37]. Nasal polyps and polyps elsewhere in the airway can lead to partial or complete airway obstruction. Vocal cord granulomas and polyps may occur as a result of traumatic intubation, cord irritation from ETT movement or lubricant chemicals, and other causes. The problem occurs more frequently in women. Pedunculated granulomas or polyps detected following the investigation of hoarseness are usually removed surgically as they can sometimes lead to airway obstruction. Remember also the potential exacerbation of bronchial asthma in patients with nasal polyps who receive aspirin, ketorolac (Toradol) and other NSAIDs.

(A)

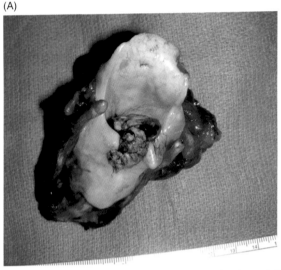

(B)

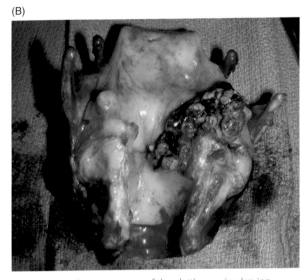

Figure 9.1. (A) This is a post-laryngectomy image showing a glottic mass that was obstructing most of the glottic opening leaving essentially a slit to permit the introduction of the a size 5.0 MLT endotracheal tube loaded over a 4.00 mm flexible fiberoptic scope. The patient was stridorous and was intubated awake. Image courtesy Drs. B. Abdelmalak and J. Scharpf. (B) The tissue sample in A with the larynx split open to show the pathology. Image courtesy Drs. B. Abdelmalak and J. Scharpf. Reprinted with permission, Cleveland Clinic Center for Medical Art & Photography © 2012. All rights reserved.

Laryngeal papillomatosis

Patients with laryngeal papillomatosis caused by a HPV infection may require frequent application of laser treatment for attempted eradication of the papillomas [38–42]. Prior to treatment the airway may be close to obstruction from an overgrowth of lesions. During laser treatment, inspired oxygen concentration should be kept to the minimum practical amount, with the avoidance of nitrous oxide, to reduce the chance of an airway fire (see Chapter 11). After treatment the airway will be raw and edematous. Laryngotracheomalacia may occasionally also be present, sometimes leading to complete upper airway collapse after extubation.

Anterior mediastinal mass

Patients with an anterior mediastinal mass may need anesthesia and surgery either to obtain a tumor biopsy with a view to obtaining a tissue diagnosis or for the relief of acute airway obstruction [43–52]. In the latter case, rigid bronchoscopy is frequently employed as a means of relieving the obstruction and establishing the location and extent of any airway compression. Should the airway become "lost" under anesthesia, with the patient unable to be ventilated, placing the patient in the lateral decubitus position or

prone position sometimes helps relieve the obstruction.

The position of an anterior mediastinal mass within the thorax can predispose patients to severe respiratory and/or cardiovascular complications during anesthesia, especially in the supine position and following the administration of muscle relaxants. Potential clinical challenges include airway obstruction, compression of cardiac chambers, and/or compression of the pulmonary artery.

Intraoperative management can be particularly difficult in these patients. In many cases the patient should be intubated awake (for example, via an awake fiberoptic technique) with judicious sedation administered while the patient is placed in the least symptomatic position.

Some experts suggest that cardiopulmonary bypass should be available on stand-by basis with femoral vessel cannulation achieved prior to induction for severe cases (e.g., over 50% reduction in airway diameter as estimated on a computed tomography scan). Even with such an arrangement, however, the time needed to achieve adequate cerebral oxygenation following complete airway obstruction may be too long to avoid a substantial degree of brain injury.

Althrough maintaining spontaneous breathing and performing an inhalational induction with sevoflurane directly or following awake intubation is often advocated as a means to provide anesthesia in some cases, others have described the option of maintaining spontaneous ventilation with dexmedetomidine as the near sole anesthetic, arguing that it could be very helpful in reducing the risk of complete airway obstruction in the anesthetic management of an anterior mediastinal mass.

Finally, obstruction of the superior vena cava by tumor (SVC syndrome) may occur in patients with an anterior mediastinal mass. This may lead to cyanosis, engorged upper body veins and edema of the head and neck, with risks of airway obstruction (from airway compression by tumor), hypotension (from impaired venous return to the heart) and bleeding from engorged veins. Such patients may also benefit from a semi-upright position to reduce airway edema.

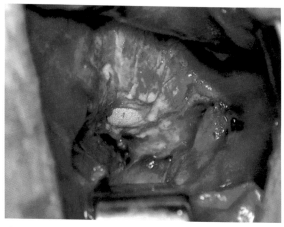

Figure 9.2. Photograph of a hole in the trachea sealed by the cuff on an ETT (see text). Image courtesy of Basem Abdelmalak, MD. Reprinted with permission, Cleveland Clinic Center for Medical Art & Photography © 2012. All Rights Reserved.

Case study 1

Carol and Saunders [53] describe a case of a young woman who collapsed following a sudden onset of dyspnea. When assessed in the emergency department she was unresponsive and cyanotic, with a pulse oximeter reading of 60%. A severe asthmatic attack was initially suspected. After attempts at conventional mask ventilation proved to be unsuccessful, the patient was administered etomidate and succinylcholine with a plan to intubate the trachea. While the view at laryngoscopy was excellent (Cormack Lehane Grade 1), the attempt at intubation was complicated by the presence of a polypoid mass situated above the right vocal cord and extending over the glottic aperture. As this lesion prevented the passage of a size 8 ETT into the trachea, a second attempt at intubation was made using a size 6 tube in conjunction with a tracheal introducer ("bougie"). Following this successful attempt, oxygenation and ventilation improved dramatically, and she was taken to the ICU. She then went to the operating room, where extensive papillomatous tissue was removed. She was then ventilated overnight, and extubated without difficulty the following day. She developed no neurological sequelae, and was discharged home 4 days after her original difficulties. Further history was eventually obtained that the patient suffered from respiratory papillomatosis and had an appointment for treatment the day following the incident.

Case study 2

Figure 9.2 shows a fascinating picture of a hole in the trachea sealed by the cuff on an ETT. The day prior the surgeons did a meticulous job shaving malignant tumor from the tracheal wall, being very careful to remove as much as possible without damaging the overall integrity of the tracheal wall. Unfortunately, the patient presented the next morning with subcutaneous neck emphysema, making the surgical team suspicious of the presence of a hole in the trachea. When brought back to the operating room (OR) the following image was obtained after careful dissection. Because of the loss of airway integrity that made positive-pressure ventilation dangerous (the risk being that of worsening the emphysema and compressing the airway), the second anesthetic was performed using an awake intubation technique done while maintaining spontaneous ventilation.

Clinical pearls

- In epiglottitis management, if at laryngoscopy the orifice through the epiglottis can't be identified, one trick is to have someone compress the child's chest, thus generating a small air bubble in the glottis that the intubator can aim for.
- Most clinicians would use awake fiberoptic laryngoscopy to secure the airway in adult epiglottitis. Although there is still substantial disagreement, there seems to be a growing consensus that most adults with epiglottitis can be

adequately treated in an intensive care unit with inhaled mist, antibiotics and corticosteroids, and that tracheal intubation is necessary only if symptoms of respiratory distress develop.

- Because retropharyngeal abscess rupture can lead to soiling of the trachea, contact with the posterior pharyngeal wall during laryngoscopy and intubation should be avoided.
- Since Ludwig's angina is often associated with trismus, nasal fiberoptic intubation is frequently needed.
- Should the airway become "lost" under anesthesia in patients with anterior mediastinal masses, with

the patient unable to be ventilated, placing the patient in the lateral decubitus position or prone position sometimes helps relieve the obstruction.

- Some experts suggest that cardiopulmonary bypass should be available on stand-by basis with femoral vessel cannulation achieved prior to induction for severe cases of an anterior mediastinal mass. Even with such an arrangement, however, the time needed to achieve adequate cerebral oxygenation following complete airway obstruction may be too long to avoid a substantial degree of brain injury.

References

Acute epiglottitis

1. Syed I, Odutoye T, Lee MS, Wong P. Management of acute epiglottitis in adults. *Br J Hosp Med (Lond)* 2011;**72**(5):M74–6. PubMed PMID: 21647034.

2. Tibballs J, Watson T. Symptoms and signs differentiating croup and epiglottitis. *J Paediatr Child Health* 2011;**47**(3):77–82. doi: 10.1111/j.1440–1754.2010.01892. x. Epub 2010 Nov 21. PubMed PMID: 21091577.

3. Ito K, Chitose H, Koganemaru M. Four cases of acute epiglottitis with a peritonsillar abscess. *Auris Nasus Larynx* 2011;**38**(2):284–8. Epub 2010 Aug 25. PubMed PMID: 20800396.

4. Al-Qudah M, Shetty S, Alomari M, Alqdah M. Acute adult supraglottitis: current management and treatment. *South Med J* 2010;**103**(8):800–4. Review. PubMed PMID: 20622745.

5. Cheatham ML. The death of George Washington: an end to the controversy? *Am Surg* 2008;**74** (8):770–4. PubMed PMID: 18705585.

6. Glynn F, Fenton JE. Diagnosis and management of supraglottitis (epiglottitis). *Curr Infect Dis Rep* 2008;**10**(3):200–4. PubMed PMID: 18510881.

7. Guldfred LA, Lyhne D, Becker BC. Acute epiglottitis: epidemiology, clinical presentation, management and outcome. *J Laryngol Otol* 2008;**122** (8):818–23. Epub 2007 Sep 25. PubMed PMID: 17892608.

Retropharyngeal abscess

8. Christoforidou A, Metallidis S, Kollaras P, *et al*. Tuberculous retropharyngeal abscess as a cause of oropharyngeal dysphagia. *Am J Otolaryngol* 2011 Aug 24. [Epub ahead of print] PubMed PMID: 21871690.

9. Afolabi OA, Fadare JO, Oyewole EO, Ogah SA. Fish bone foreign body presenting with an acute fulminating retropharyngeal abscess in a resource-challenged center: a case report. *J Med Case Reports* 2011;**5**(1):165. PubMed PMID: 21524286; PubMed Central PMCID: PMC3098805.

10. Hoang JK, Branstetter BF 4th, Eastwood JD, Glastonbury CM. Multiplanar CT and MRI of collections in the retropharyngeal space: is it an abscess? *AJR Am J Roentgenol* 2011;**196**(4): W426–32. Review. PubMed PMID: 21427307.

11. Rizk NN, Spalla TC, Al-Khudari S, Ghanem TA. Case report: mediastinal hematoma secondary to hypertension, presenting as a

retropharyngeal space abscess. *Laryngoscope* 2010;**120** Suppl 4: S179. PubMed PMID: 21225777.

12. Lee S, Joo KB, Lee KH, Uhm WS. Acute retropharyngeal calcific tendinitis in an unusual location: a case report in a patient with rheumatoid arthritis and atlantoaxial subluxation. *Korean J Radiol* 2011;**12**(4): 504–9. Epub 2011 Jul 22. PubMed PMID: 21852912; PubMed Central PMCID: PMC3150679.

13. Kakarala K, Durand ML, Emerick KS. Retropharyngeal abscess in the setting of immune modulation for rheumatoid arthritis. *Laryngoscope* 2010;**120** Suppl 4: S131. Review. PubMed PMID: 21225729.

14. Choi SH, Kim HJ. A case of Kawasaki disease with coexistence of a parapharyngeal abscess requiring incision and drainage. *Korean J Pediatr* 2010;**53**(9): 855–8. Epub 2010 Sep 13. PubMed PMID: 21189972; PubMed Central PMCID: PMC3005218.

15. Rao MS, Linga Raju Y, Vishwanathan P. Anaesthetic management of difficult airway due to retropharyngeal abscess. *Indian J Anaesth* 2010;**54**(3): 246–8. PubMed PMID: 20885875; PubMed Central PMCID: PMC2933487.

Ludwig's angina

16. Hasan W, Leonard D, Russell J. Ludwig's angina - a controversial surgical emergency: how we do it. *Int J Otolaryngol* 2011;**2011**:231816. Epub 2011 Jul 6. PubMed PMID: 21760800; PubMed Central PMCID: PMC3133010.

17. Greenberg SL, Huang J, Chang RS, Ananda SN. Surgical management of Ludwig's angina. *ANZ J Surg* 2007;**77**(7): 540–3. PubMed PMID: 17610689.

18. Loughnan TE, Allen DE. Ludwig's angina. The anaesthetic management of nine cases. *Anaesthesia* 1985;**40**(3):295–7. PubMed PMID: 3993888.

19. Allen D, Loughnan TE, Ord RA. A re-evaluation of the role of tracheostomy in Ludwig's angina. *J Oral Maxillofac Surg* 1985;**43** (6):436–9. PubMed PMID: 3858480.

20. Iwu CO. Ludwig's angina: report of seven cases and review of current concepts in management. *Br J Oral Maxillofac Surg* 1990;**28** (3):189–93. Review. PubMed PMID: 2135660.

21. Infante-Cossío P, Fernández-Hinojosa E, Mangas-Cruz MA, González-Pérez LM. Ludwig's angina and ketoacidosis as a first manifestation of diabetes mellitus. *Med Oral Patol Oral Cir Bucal* 2010;**15**(4):e624–7. PubMed PMID: 20173723.

22. Moreland LW, Corey J, McKenzie R. Ludwig's angina. Report of a case and review of the literature. *Arch Intern Med* 1988;**148**(2):461–6. Review. PubMed PMID: 3277567.

23. Ovassapian A, Tuncbilek M, Weitzel EK, Joshi CW. Airway management in adult patients with deep neck infections: a case series and review of the literature. *Anesth Analg* 2005; **100**(2):585–9. PubMed PMID: 15673898.

24. Saifeldeen K, Evans R. Ludwig's angina. *Emerg Med J* 2004;**21** (2):242–3. Review. PubMed PMID: 14988363; PubMed Central PMCID: PMC1726306.

25. Abramowicz S, Abramowicz JS, Dolwick MF. Severe life threatening maxillofacial infection in pregnancy presented as Ludwig's angina. *Infect Dis Obstet Gynecol* 2006;**2006**:51931. PubMed PMID: 17485803; PubMed Central PMCID: PMC1581466.

Airway tumors

26. Jung B, Murgu S, Colt H. Rigid bronchoscopy for malignant central airway obstruction from small cell lung cancer complicated by SVC syndrome. *Ann Thorac Cardiovasc Surg* 2011;**17**(1):53–7. PubMed PMID: 21587130.

27. Abdel Rahman AR. Bronchoplasty for primary broncho-pulmonary tumors. *J Egypt Natl Canc Inst* 2010;**22**(1):73–8. PubMed PMID: 21503009.

28. Blessing M, Schwartz D, Krellenstein D, Cohen E. Management of a patient with an unexpected obstructing carinal mass. *Minerva Anestesiol* 2010;**76** (9):761–4. Epub 2010 Jul 1. PubMed PMID: 20820156.

29. Manganaris C, Wittlin S, Xu H, et al. Metastatic papillary thyroid carcinoma and severe airflow obstruction. *Chest* 2010;**138** (3):738–42. PubMed PMID: 20822998; PubMed Central PMCID: PMC2950112.

30. Chung IH, Park MH, Kim DH, Jeon GS. Endobronchial stent insertion to manage hemoptysis caused by lung cancer. *J Korean Med Sci* 2010;**25**(8):1253–5. Epub 2010 Jul 21. PubMed PMID: 20676346; PubMed Central PMCID: PMC2908804.

31. Saji H, Furukawa K, Tsutsui H, et al. Outcomes of airway stenting for advanced lung cancer with central airway obstruction.

Interact Cardiovasc Thorac Surg 2010;**11**(4):425–8. Epub 2010 Jul 23. PubMed PMID: 20656802.

32. Milisavljevic D, Stankovic M, Tasic-Dimov D, Radovanović Z, Stankovic P. Stridor as initial clinical presentation of tracheal chondroma. *Acta Otorrinolaringol Esp* 2011;**62**(2):164–6. Epub 2010 Mar 25. PubMed PMID: 20346431.

Airway polyps

33. Kalcioglu MT, Can S, Aydin NE. Unusual case of soft palate hairy polyp causing airway obstruction and review of the literature. *J Pediatr Surg* 2010;**45**(12):e5–8. Review. PubMed PMID: 21129531.

34. Becker SS. Surgical management of polyps in the treatment of nasal airway obstruction. *Otolaryngol Clin North Am* 2009;**42**(2):377–85. Review. PubMed PMID: 19328899.

35. Tanguay J, Pollanen M. Sudden death by laryngeal polyp: a case report and review of the literature. *Forensic Sci Med Pathol* 2009;**5** (1):17–21. Epub 2008 Sep 25. Review. PubMed PMID: 19291432.

36. Pawankar R. Nasal polyposis: an update: editorial review. *Curr Opin Allergy Clin Immunol* 2003;**3** (1):1–6. Review. PubMed PMID: 12582307.

37. Probst L, Stoney P, Jeney E, Hawke M. Nasal polyps, bronchial asthma and aspirin sensitivity. *J Otolaryngol* 1992;**21**(1):60–5. Review. PubMed PMID: 1564752.

Laryngeal papillomatosis

38. Bo L, Wang B, Shu SY. Anesthesia management in pediatric patients with laryngeal papillomatosis undergoing suspension laryngoscopic surgery and a review of the literature. *Int J Pediatr Otorhinolaryngol* 2011;**75** (11):1442–5. Epub 2011 Sep 9. PubMed PMID: 21907420.

39. Li SQ, Chen JL, Fu HB, Xu J, Chen LH. Airway management in pediatric patients undergoing suspension laryngoscopic surgery for severe laryngeal obstruction caused by papillomatosis. *Paediatr Anaesth* 2010;**20**(12):1084–91. doi: 10.1111/j.1460–9592.2010.03447.x. PubMed PMID: 21199117.

40. Coope G, Connett G. Juvenile laryngeal papillomatosis. *Prim Care Respir J* 2006;**15**(2):125–7. Epub 2006 Mar 9. PubMed PMID: 16701772.

41. Soldatski IL, Onufrieva EK, Steklov AM, Schepin NV. Tracheal, bronchial, and pulmonary papillomatosis in children. *Laryngoscope* 2005;**115**(10):1848–54. PubMed PMID: 16222208.

42. Kendall KA. Current treatment for laryngeal papillomatosis. *Curr Opin Otolaryngol Head Neck Surg* 2004;**12**(3):157–9. PubMed PMID: 15167022.

Anterior mediastinal mass

43. Bassanezi BS, Oliveira-Filho AG, Miranda ML, Soares L, Aguiar SS. Use of BiPAP for safe anesthesia in a child with a large anterior mediastinal mass. *Paediatr Anaesth* 2011;**21**(9):985–7. doi: 10.1111/j.1460–9592.2011.03607.x. PubMed PMID: 21793982.

44. Blank RS, de Souza DG. Anesthetic management of patients with an anterior mediastinal mass: continuing professional development. *Can J Anaesth* 2011;**58**(9):853–9, 860–7. Epub 2011 Jul 21. English, French. PubMed PMID: 21779948.

45. Garey CL, Laituri CA, Valusek PA, St Peter SD, Snyder CL. Management of Anterior Mediastinal Masses in Children. *Eur J Pediatr Surg*. 2011 Jul 12. [Epub ahead of print] PubMed PMID: 21751123.

46. Gardner JC, Royster RL. Airway collapse with an anterior mediastinal mass despite spontaneous ventilation in an adult. *Anesth Analg* 2011;**113**(2):239–42. Epub 2011 May 19. PubMed PMID: 21596865.

47. Sendasgupta C, Sengupta G, Ghosh K, Munshi A, Goswami A. Femoro-femoral cardiopulmonary bypass for the resection of an anterior mediastinal mass. *Indian J Anaesth* 2010;**54**(6):565–8. PubMed PMID: 21224977; PubMed Central PMCID: PMC3016580.

48. Choi WJ, Kim YH, Mok JM, Choi SI, Kim HS. Patient repositioning and the amelioration of airway obstruction by an anterior mediastinal tumor during general anesthesia - A case report. *Korean J Anesthesiol* 2010;**59**(3):206–9. Epub 2010 Sep 20. PubMed PMID: 20877707; PubMed Central PMCID: PMC2946040.

49. Chiang JC, Irwin MG, Hussain A, Tang YK, Hiong YT. Anaesthesia for emergency caesarean section in a patient with large anterior mediastinal tumour presenting as intrathoracic airway compression and superior vena cava obstruction. *Case Report Med* 2010;**2010**:708481. Epub 2010 Oct 13. PubMed PMID: 20981348; PubMed Central PMCID: PMC2957859.

50. Abdelmalak B, Marcanthony N, Abdelmalak J, *et al.* Dexmedetomidine for anesthetic management of anterior mediastinal mass. *J Anesth* 2010;**24**(4):607–10. Epub 2010 May 8. PubMed PMID: 20454810.

51. Galway U, Doyle DJ, Gildea T. Anesthesia for endoscopic palliative management of a patient with a large anterior mediastinal mass. *J Clin Anesth* 2009;**21**(2):150–1. PubMed PMID: 19329025.

52. Slinger P, Karsli C. Management of the patient with a large anterior mediastinal mass: recurring myths. *Curr Opin Anaesthesiol* 2007;**20**(1):1–3. PubMed PMID: 17211158.

53. Carroll CD, Saunders NC. Respiratory papillomatosis: a rare cause of collapse in a young adult presenting to the emergency department. *Emerg Med J* 2002;**19**(4):362–5. PubMed PMID: 12101164; PubMed Central PMCID: PMC1725930.

10

Use of Heliox in managing stridor: an ENT perspective

D. John Doyle

Introduction

Stridor is noisy inspiration from turbulent gas flow in the upper airway. It is often seen in partial to near complete airway obstruction, and should always command immediate attention. Wherever possible, attempts should be made to establish without delay the cause of the stridor (e.g., foreign body, vocal cord edema, tracheal compression by tumor, functional laryngeal dyskinesia, etc.) Nasopharyngoscopy can be helpful in many such cases. This chapter will discuss in detail the use of Heliox for temporarily treating stridor in the setting of ENT pathology.

Airway obstructing conditions such as epiglottitis or tracheal stenosis may be viewed as breathing through an orifice (defined as involving flow through a tube whose length is smaller than its radius). Gas flow through an orifice is always somewhat turbulent [1]. Under such conditions, the approximate flow across the orifice varies inversely with the square root of the gas density. This is in contrast to laminar flow conditions, where gas flow varies inversely with gas viscosity. Note that while the viscosity values for helium and oxygen are similar, their densities are very different, as shown in Table 10.1.

The usual available mixtures of helium and oxygen are 30% O_2 : 70% He and 20% O_2 : 80% He and are usually administered by a nonrebreathing face mask in patients who face an increased work-of-breathing effort because of the presence of airway pathology (e.g., edema) but in whom endotracheal intubation is preferably withheld at this time. As indicated above, the low density of helium allows it to play a significant clinical role in the management of some forms of airway obstruction associated with gas turbulence.

Treatment with Heliox is not new. For instance, Rudow *et al.* [2] provide the following vignette.

Table 10.1. Density of various gases

Gas	Density at 20°C
Air	1.293 g/l
Nitrogen	1.250 g/l
Nitrous oxide	1.965 g/l
Helium	0.178 g/l
Oxygen	1.429 g/l

A 78-year-old woman developed airway obstruction from a thyroid carcinoma that extended into her mediastinum and compressed her trachea. She had a 2-month history of worsening dyspnea, especially when positioned supine. On examination, inspiratory and expiratory stridor was present. Noted on the chest X-ray were a large superior mediastinal mass and pulmonary metastases. Clinically, the patient was exhausted and in respiratory distress.

Almost instant relief was obtained by giving the patient a mixture of 78% He : 22% O_2, with improvements in measured tidal volume and oxygenation. Later, a thyroidectomy was carried out to relieve the obstruction. Here, anesthesia was conducted by applying topical anesthesia to the airway with awake laryngoscopy and intubation performed in the sitting position. Once the airway was secured using an armored tube, the patient was given a general anesthetic with an intravenous induction. Following the surgery, extubation occurred without complication.

Another interesting clinical vignette has been published by Khanlou and Eiger [3]. They present the case of a 69-year-old woman in whom bilateral vocal cord paralysis developed after radiation therapy and in whom Heliox was successfully used to temporarily manage the resultant upper airway obstruction until she was able to receive a tracheostomy.

A final clinical vignette related to Heliox is from Polaner [4], who reports on the use of the laryngeal mask airway (LMA) and Heliox in a 20:80 mixture for the administration of anesthesia to a 3-yr-old boy with asthma and a large anterior mediastinal mass. Clinical management involved an unusual combination of management strategies: the child was kept in the sitting position, spontaneous ventilation with a halothane-in-heliox inhalation induction was used, and airway stimulation was minimized by use of the LMA. However, the author cautions that cases such as these can readily take a deadly turn, noting that "one must, of course, always be prepared to intervene with either manipulations of patient position in the event of airway compromise (including upright, lateral, and prone) or more aggressive strategies, such as rigid bronchoscopy and even median sternotomy (in the case of intractable cardiovascular collapse), or to allow the patient to awaken if critical airway or cardiovascular compromise becomes evident at any time during the course of the anesthesia".

Management options

The first issue of clinical concern in the setting of stridor is whether or not intubation or a surgical airway is immediately necessary to extricate the patient from death or injury. Obviously, some patients will need immediate intubation to rescue the airway while some patients in whom intubation is close to impossible will probably require a surgical airway. If, however, intubation can be delayed for a period of time, a number of other options can be considered, depending on the severity of the situation and other clinical details.

These potential options include:

- expectant management with full monitoring, oxygen by face mask, and positioning the head of the bed for optimum conditions (e.g., 45–90°);
- use of nebulized racemic epinephrine (0.5 to 0.75 ml of 2.25% racemic epinephrine added to 2.5 to 3 ml of normal saline) in cases where airway edema may be the cause of the stridor (4% cocaine in a dose not exceeding 3 mg/kg may also be used, but not together with racemic epinephrine);
- use of dexamethasone (Decadron®) 4–10 mg IV q 8–12 h or solumedrol 40–60 mg IV q 6–8 h in cases where airway edema may be contributing to the

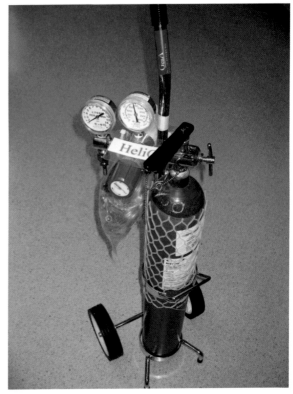

Figure 10.1. An E-size tank of heliox, with a nonrebreathing face mask for gas delivery.

stridor; note that some time (in the range of hours) may be needed for dexamethasone to work fully;
- use of Heliox (70% helium, 30% oxygen); the effect is almost instantaneous (Figure 10.1).

Some causes of stridor

Stridor has many potential causes. It may occur as a result of foreign bodies (e.g., aspirated peanut, aspirated wire), tumor formation (e.g., laryngeal papillomatosis, squamous cell carcinoma), infections (e.g., epiglottitis, retropharyngeal abscess, croup), subglottic stenosis (e.g., following prolonged intubation), airway edema (e.g., following instrumentation of the airway intubation), as well as a result of laryngomalacia (the most common congenital cause of stridor), subglottic hemangioma (rare), and vascular rings compressing the trachea. Abnormalities of vocal cord function can also be responsible. Congenital anomalies of the airway are present in 87% of all cases of stridor in infants and children [1].

Table 10.2 lists some causes of stridor in children.

Table 10.2. Differential diagnosis of pediatric stridor

Infectious

    Croup

    Epigiottitis

    Tracheitis

    Retropharyngeal abscess

Non-infectious

    Symptoms at birth

        Laryngeal web

        Vocal cord paralysis

        Cystic hygroma

        Subglottic stenosis

    Symptoms after neonatal period

        Subglottic hemangioma

        Laryngeal papilloma

        Laryngomalacia

        Tracheomalacia

        Vascular ring/sling

    Acquired

        Foregin body aspiration

        Foreign body ingestion

        Spasmodic croup

        Laryngospasm

        Psychogenic stridor

        Angioedema

        Paratracheal mass (teratoma, lymphoma)

        Vocal cord paralysis (secondary to intubation)

        Subglottic stenosis (secondary to intubation)

From Marin J, Baren J. Pediatric upper airway infectious disease emergencies. EB Medicine November 2007. Volume 4, Number 11. http://www.ebmedicine.net/topics.php?paction=showTopicSeg&topic_id=128&seg_id=2538.

Diagnosis

Stridor is usually diagnosed on the basis of symptoms and physical examination, with a view to revealing the underlying problem or condition. Chest and neck X-rays, CT scans, and/or MRIs may reveal structural pathology. Flexible fiberoptic bronchoscopy can also be very helpful, especially in assessing vocal cord function or in looking for signs of compression or infection.

Case study

A 58-year-old female patient presented for surgery for recurrent head and neck cancer. She had been judged to have a difficult airway at multiple occasions in the past. Her airway difficulties had been largely the result of preexisting glottic pathology related to her cancer; her rather limited mouth opening (about 3 cm) also complicated management. She was intubated utilizing an awake fiberoptic intubation that was rather challenging due to the complexity of her pathology.

Upon extubation while wide awake and with full reversal of neuromuscular blockade, the patient became severely stridorous. This was treated by two doses of 8 mg Decadron (one administered pre extubation), two doses of nebulized racemic epinephrine (0.5 ml of 2.25% epinephrine added to 2.5 ml saline), and assisted mask ventilation with the patient sitting up at $60°$. On standby we had available almost every airway gadget ever manufactured, an experienced ENT surgeon, a number of experienced anesthesiologists, and everything needed for a surgical airway.

Unfortunately, the patient did not improve and was starting to tire out. Reintubation would have been even more difficult than it had been earlier. A surgical airway was starting to look like our only way out.

Administering a mixture of helium (70%) and oxygen (30%) was considered, to be delivered using a nonrebreathing face mask at 10 liters per minute. Within a mere five to 10 breaths the stridor vanished and the patient's work of breathing became much more manageable. The patient was then brought to the recovery room with a large Heliox tank in tow and with full monitoring. She was then weaned off the Heliox over several hours.

In conclusion: Heliox adminstred with a nonrebreathing face mask should be readily available in every operating room suite to assist in the treatment of stridor.

Clinical pearls

- Stridor is usually diagnosed on the basis of symptoms and physical examination.
- The first issue in the setting of stridor is whether or not intubation or a surgical airway is immediately necessary to extricate the patient from death or injury.

- Gas flow through an orifice is always somewhat turbulent. Under such conditions, the approximate flow across the orifice varies inversely with the square root of the gas density. This is in contrast to laminar flow conditions, where gas flow varies inversely with gas viscosity.
- The usual available mixtures of helium and oxygen are 30% O_2 : 70% He and 20% O_2 : 80% He.
- Use of nebulized racemic epinephrine (0.5 to 0.75 ml of 2.25% racemic epinephrine added to 2.5 to 3 ml of normal saline) can be useful in cases where airway edema may be the cause of the stridor.
- Consider also use of dexamethasone (Decadron®) 4–10mg IV q 8–12 h or methylprednisolone (Solumedrol®) 40–60 mg IV Q 6–8 h in cases where airway edema may be contributing to the stridor; note that some time (in the range of hours) may be needed for dexamethasone to work fully.
- Heliox administered with a nonrebreathing face mask should be readily available in every operating room suite to assist in the treatment of stridor.

References

1. Holinger LD. Etiology of stridor. *Ann Otol Rhinol Laryngol* 1980;**89**:397–400.

2. Rudow M, Hill AB, Thompson NW, *et al.* Helium-oxygen mixtures in airway obstruction due to thyroid carcinoma. *Can Anaesth Soc J* 1986;**33**: 498.

3. Khanlou H, Eiger G. Safety and efficacy of heliox as a treatment for upper airway obstruction due to radiation-induced laryngeal dysfunction. *Heart Lung* 2001;**30**:146–7.

4. Polaner DM. The use of heliox and the laryngeal mask airway in a child with an anterior mediastinal mass. *Anesth Analg* 1996;**82**: 208–10.

Prevention and management of airway fires

D. John Doyle

Introduction

An airway fire is potentially deadly complication that may occur during tracheotomy surgery, during laser surgery and with a number of other procedures [1–4]. The objective of this chapter is to introduce readers to the prevention and management of airway fires. The discussion includes the American Society of Anesthesiologists Operating Room Fire Algorithm (Figure 11.1), a checklist-like protocol for dealing with airway fires (Table 11.1) as well as some British recommendations specific to tracheotomy surgery (Table 11.2). Operating room fires are best divided into airway fires and non-airway fires. A recent report by the American Society of Anesthesiologists provides specific guidance for both these scenarios (Figure 11.1).

Some safety principles

Several principles apply to reduce the chance of fires in the settings of ENT surgery.

- Preventive measures do not guarantee that fires will not occur; always be prepared.
- Know the ASA algorithm for operating room fires.
- A simple means to extinguish airway fires (e.g., 50 ml syringe filled with saline) should be immediately on hand. In addition, a CO_2 fire extinguisher is good to have nearby.
- The surgeon should avoid entering the trachea using electrocautery.
- The anesthesiologist must maintain special vigilance at the moment of surgical entry into the trachea.
- The anesthesiologist should keep the administered oxygen levels to the minimum needed when a significant potential for an airway fire is present.

- Nitrous oxide should not be used during airway surgery, since it supports combustion just as does oxygen.

To remove the ETT or not? That is the question

Prevailing conventional wisdom, at least until recently, holds that cases of airway fire call for immediate removal of the endotracheal tube (ETT). While this is a reasonable rule of thumb, it should also be noted that there are some patients where removal of the ETT would in all likelihood result in irreversible loss of the airway. Clinicians in such a setting face a particularly difficult choice: leave the ETT in place and risk fire-related injury to the patient, or remove the ETT and risk deadly loss of the airway.

Both Chee and Benumoff [2] and Ng and Hartigan [5] provide examples where leaving the ETT in place would probably be the best strategy. Chee and Benumoff offer the following commentary: "In certain circumstances, the benefits of leaving the ETT in may outweigh the risks after the airway fire is extinguished. The ETT may still allow acceptable ventilation of the lungs with oxygen, especially when the airway is edematous enough to provide a reasonable seal around the perforated cuff. In addition, the ETT can serve as a conduit for a tube exchanger; this consideration may be extremely important if the airway is difficult to reestablish."

Airway fires in tracheostomy surgery

Airway fires are perhaps most strongly associated with tracheostomy surgery. Table 11.2 provides some recommendations from the British literature in this

Anesthesia for Otolaryngologic Surgery, ed. Basem Abdelmalak and D. John Doyle. Published by Cambridge University Press.
© Cambridge University Press 2013.

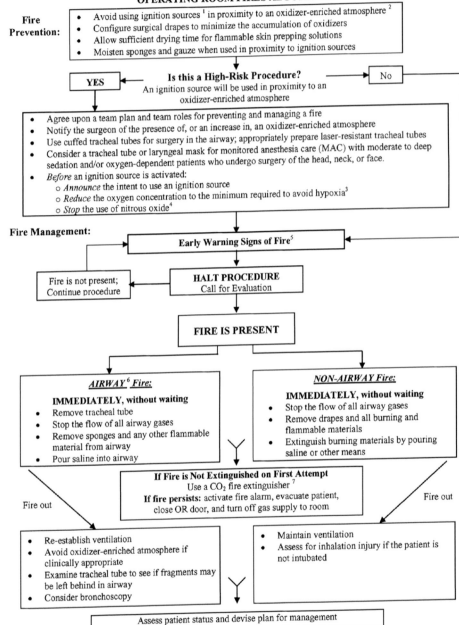

AMERICAN SOCIETY
OF ANESTHESIOLOGISTS

OPERATING ROOM FIRES ALGORITHM

Fire Prevention:
- Avoid using ignition sources [1] in proximity to an oxidizer-enriched atmosphere [2]
- Configure surgical drapes to minimize the accumulation of oxidizers
- Allow sufficient drying time for flammable skin prepping solutions
- Moisten sponges and gauze when used in proximity to ignition sources

Is this a High-Risk Procedure?
An ignition source will be used in proximity to an oxidizer-enriched atmosphere

YES   **No**

- Agree upon a team plan and team roles for preventing and managing a fire
- Notify the surgeon of the presence of, or an increase in, an oxidizer-enriched atmosphere
- Use cuffed tracheal tubes for surgery in the airway; appropriately prepare laser-resistant tracheal tubes
- Consider a tracheal tube or laryngeal mask for monitored anesthesia care (MAC) with moderate to deep sedation and/or oxygen-dependent patients who undergo surgery of the head, neck, or face.
- *Before* an ignition source is activated:
  - o *Announce* the intent to use an ignition source
  - o *Reduce* the oxygen concentration to the minimum required to avoid hypoxia[3]
  - o *Stop* the use of nitrous oxide[4]

Fire Management:

Early Warning Signs of Fire[5]

Fire is not present;
Continue procedure

HALT PROCEDURE
Call for Evaluation

FIRE IS PRESENT

AIRWAY[6] Fire:

IMMEDIATELY, without waiting
- Remove tracheal tube
- Stop the flow of all airway gases
- Remove sponges and any other flammable material from airway
- Pour saline into airway

NON-AIRWAY Fire:

IMMEDIATELY, without waiting
- Stop the flow of all airway gases
- Remove drapes and all burning and flammable materials
- Extinguish burning materials by pouring saline or other means

If Fire is Not Extinguished on First Attempt
Use a CO_2 fire extinguisher [7]
If fire persists: activate fire alarm, evacuate patient, close OR door, and turn off gas supply to room

Fire out   Fire out

- Re-establish ventilation
- Avoid oxidizer-enriched atmosphere if clinically appropriate
- Examine tracheal tube to see if fragments may be left behind in airway
- Consider bronchoscopy

- Maintain ventilation
- Assess for inhalation injury if the patient is not intubated

Assess patient status and devise plan for management

[1] Ignition sources include but are not limited to electrosurgery or electrocautery units and lasers.
[2] An oxidizer-enriched atmosphere occurs when there is any increase in oxygen concentration above room air level, and/or the presence of any concentration of nitrous oxide.
[3] After minimizing delivered oxygen, wait a period of time (*e.g.*, 1–3 min) before using an ignition source. For oxygen dependent patients, *reduce* supplemental oxygen delivery to the minimum required to avoid hypoxia. Monitor oxygenation with pulse oximetry, and if feasible, inspired, exhaled, and/or delivered oxygen concentration.
[4] After stopping the delivery of nitrous oxide, wait a period of time (*e.g.*, 1–3 min) before using an ignition source.
[5] Unexpected flash, flame, smoke or heat, unusual sounds (*e.g.*, a "pop," snap or "foomp") or odors, unexpected movement of drapes, discoloration of drapes or breathing circuit, unexpected patient movement or complaint.
[6] In this algorithm, airway fire refers to a fire in the airway or breathing circuit.
[7] A CO_2 fire extinguisher may be used on the patient if necessary.

Figure 11.1. American Society of Anesthesiologists operating room fire algorithm. From [3].

Table 11.1. Management of airway fires (courtesy Dr. B. Abdelmalak)

Prevention and preparedness:

1. Keep oxygen concentration around 30%, less if possible. Use O_2/air mixture. Avoid N_2O.

2. Use a "laser safe" endotracheal tube.

3. Inflate endotracheal tube cuff with a dyed normal saline to provide an early indicator of cuff rupture.

4. Use a preprepared 50 ml syringe of saline to extinguish any fire and flood the surgical field if a fire occurs.

5. Have an extra endotracheal tube available for re-intubation in case a fire occurs.

6. Inform the surgical team working on the airway of any situation where high concentrations of oxygen are being used.

In the case of an airway fire:

1. Stop lasering. Stop ventilation. Turn O_2 off (as well as N_2O if it was mistakenly in use).

2. Inform the surgical team and assign someone to call control desk for help.

3. Remove the burning ET tube and drop it in a bucket of water if available.

4. Put out the fire with your improvised fire extinguisher (see 4 above).

5. The area should be flushed with saline.

When the fire is extinguished:

1. Ventilate the patient with 100% oxygen via face mask (or supraglottic airway if appropriate).

2. When stable, assess the extent of airway damage. Consider using a ventilating rigid bronchoscope; debris and foreign bodies should be removed.

3. Reintubate the patient if significant airway damage is found.

4. Where appropriate, arrange for admission to an ICU.

5. Supportive therapy, including ventilation, antibiotics, and extubate when appropriate.

6. Tracheotomy may be needed.

Note: removing the endotracheal tube may be inappropriate in some cases (see text).

regard. Table 11.3 from a review by Rogers *et al.* [4] provides a list of airway fire cases that illustrates in detail the variety of clinical outcomes that may occur.

Chicken model

In a study by Roy and Smith [6] the authors used a chicken model consisting of a size 6.0 endotracheal tube inserted into the cranial end of the degutted central cavity. An electrosurgical unit set for 15 W and grounded to the whole raw chicken served as an ignition source. Oxygen was then delivered through the endotracheal tube at varying concentrations and flows. A test was considered negative if no ignition could be obtained after 4 minutes of electrocautery applied to tissue. The authors found the following:

> At an O_2 concentration of 100% and a flow rate of 15 l/min, ignition with a sustained flame was obtained between 15 and 30 s after initiation of electrocautery. At 100% O_2 at 10 l/min, ignition was obtained at 70 s with immediate sustained flame. At an O_2 concentration of 60%, ignition occurred at 25 s and sustained fire after 60 s. At an O_2 concentration of 50% ignition with a sustained flame occurred between 128 and 184 s. At an O_2 concentration of 45%, neither ignition nor sustained flames could be obtained in any trial.

Based on these results, the authors concluded that decreasing oxygen concentrations to under 50% would be expected to decrease the risk of an electro-cautery-ignited airway fire during oropharyngeal surgery. This study provides empirical support to current practices of keeping oxygen concentrations around 30% (or lower where practical), as recommended by the ASA [3].

Flooding the surgical site with carbon dioxide

Ho *et al.* [7] hypothesized that flooding the surgical field with carbon dioxide might be an effective technique in preventing airway fires during open tracheostomy. To study this possibility they cut through the trachea of pigs ventilated with oxygen using cautery while flushing the surgical field with carbon dioxide at 10 l/min. Five times out of five, fire was induced when the cautery cut through the tracheal wall with no carbon dioxide being used. However, five times out of five, fire was not induced when carbon dioxide was used. The authors concluded that flooding the surgical site with carbon dioxide helps prevent airway fires during open tracheostomy using cautery. This practice, however, does not appear to be widespread.

Table 11.2. Airway fire – tracheostomy

Recommendations

All theatre staff should be aware that an airway fire may occur during tracheostomy. Have a bowl of saline and drapes available on the surgical instrument trolley at all times. Have a fire extinguisher immediately available. In practice, a carbon dioxide fire-extinguisher will be the usual choice. Halon fire-extinguishers are significantly better for operating theatre fires but their use is declining owing to environmental concerns.

Have a self-inflating ventilation bag (e.g. Ambu bag) available in case it becomes necessary to ventilate the patient with room air.

Do not use nitrous oxide or any of the flammable/explosive anesthetic agents.

Use a single-lumen endotracheal tube which is long enough to allow the tip to be advanced to the carina (the carina is approximately 24–25 cm from the teeth in an average male.) Change any *in situ* double-lumen endotracheal tube for a single-lumen tube before tracheostomy.

Use saline to inflate the endotracheal cuff. Make sure there is no leak of anaesthetic gases past the endotracheal cuff.

Use the lowest safe FiO_2 in either nitrogen (air/oxygen mixture) or helium.

If the tracheostomy wound is significantly deep (e.g. in an obese patient) use a suction device to clear any build up of diathermy products from within the wound.

Before the trachea is opened, advance the endotracheal tube down the trachea so the tip is close to the carina in order to minimize the likelihood of damage to the cuff when the trachea is incised. Consider using a fibre-optic bronchoscope to position the tip of the endotracheal tube close to the carina. If the tube is too short, consider changing it for a longer one.

Control all bleeding points and obtain a meticulously dry operative field. Incise the trachea using either a scalpel, scissors or a harmonic knife. Never use diathermy to cut through the trachea.

Once the trachea has been opened and the surgeon is ready to insert the tracheostomy tube, stop ventilating, deflate the endotracheal tube cuff and withdraw the endotracheal tube carefully under direct vision until the tip is just above the tracheal hole (do not remove the tube completely at this stage). Be prepared to push the endotracheal tube back down the trachea to secure the airway if there are any difficulties, whether while inserting the tracheostomy, or during the initial ventilation through the tracheostomy.

If bleeding occurs once the trachea has been incised, first ensure that the airway is secured with either a tracheostomy or endotracheal tube with the cuff inflated. If there is cuff leak from the trachea, then temporarily stop ventilation and ligate or suture. If unavoidable, use bipolar diathermy while using suction to clear oxygen and products from the wound. Consider pushing damp swabs into the wound to occlude any air leak.

Once the tracheostomy tube is secure in the trachea, inflate the tracheostomy cuff and suck out the tube using a suction catheter, checking that the suction tube passes easily though the whole length of the tube. If this is satisfactory, then commence ventilation through the tracheostomy.

In the event of fire, immediately disconnect the patient from the anaesthetic machine, switch off the anaesthetic gas flow, disconnect the gas pipelines and ventilate with room air using a self-inflating bag. Use an airway filter if there is smoke in the theatre. Extinguish the fire. Consider flushing saline down the endotracheal tube to extinguish any intraluminal fire. Consider removing or changing the tube to minimize the inhalation of toxic products of combustion and spread of fire into the tracheo-bronchial tree. However, changing the tube may be more risky than leaving it in if the patient was previously difficult to intubate or the airway has become oedematous.

Table 11.3. Case reports of airway fire during tracheostomy

Author	Mechanism	Diathermy	Oxygen source	Oxygen conc.	Action	Burns site	Burns severity
Bowdle *et al.* (1987)	Divided thyroid isthmus	NK	Percutaneous transtracheal	100%	Drapes removed	Right neck Anesthetist	2nd degree 2nd degree
Le Clair *et al.* (1990)	Bleeding tracheal vessel cauterized	NK	ETT	100%	Manual pressure	Trachea	Superficial
Bailey *et al.* (1990)	NK	NK	ETT	100%	Web swabs	Trachea	Superficial
Mandych *et al.* (1990)	Subcutaneous fat cauterized	Coagulation	Face-mask (LA)	5 liters/ min	Drapes removed	Chin, neck	Partial thickness
Aly *et al.* (1991)	Incised trachea	NK	ETT	NK	NK	Trachea	Superficial
Lew *et al.* (1991)	Incised trachea	Cutting	ETT	100%	Manual pressure, Saline down ETT	Hypopharynx, trachea	Death: 13 days
Marsh and Riley (1992)	Incised trachea	Coagulation	DL ETT	100%	Wet swab	Skin	'Charring'
Wilson *et al.* (1994)	Incised trachea	Cutting	ETT	100%	Manual pressure	None	None
Michels *et al.* (1994)	Incised trachea	NK	ETT	100%	NK	None	None
Lim *et al.* (1997)	Bleeding tracheal vessel cauterized	NK	ETT	100%	Saline to wound	None	None
Chee & Benumof (1998)	NK	Coagulation	ETT	100%	Saline down ETT	Skin	Superficial
Thompson *et al.* (1998)	Bleeding tracheal vessel cauterized	Coagulation	Bronchoscope	50%	Manual pressure	Lower neck	2nd degree
Thompson *et al.* (1998)	Bleeding tracheal vessel cauterized	Coagulation	ETT	NK	Manual pressure	None	None
Thompson *et al.* (1998)	Bleeding tracheal vessel cauterized	Blend	ETT	100%	Web swab	None	None
Bauer & Butler (1990)	Incised trachea	NK	ETT	100%	Manual pressure, saline to wound	Larynx, epiglottis, trachea	Death: instant

Reproduced with permission from Rogers ML, Nickalls RW, Brackenbury ET, *et al.* Airway fire during tracheostomy: prevention strategies for surgeons and anaesthetists. *Ann R Coll Surg Engl* 2001;83(6):376–80. Note the use of the British term "diathermy" to denote cautery. Copyright The Royal College of Surgeons of England.
NK, not known; ETT, endotracheal tube; DL ETT, double-lumen endotracheal tube; LA, local anaesthetic.

Two case studies

Case one

Sosis [1] described the following case report of a laser-ignited airway fire.

> The patient was a 56-year-old ASA physical status I man weighing 79 kg who presented with hoarseness. CO_2 laser excision of a vocal cord polyp was planned. Anesthesia was induced with 100 μg of fentanyl, 400 mg of thiopental, and tracheal intubation was facilitated with succinylcholine 100 mg iv. A 6-mm ID Xomed® (Jacksonville, FL) Laser Shield endotracheal tube was placed. Its cuff was inflated with 5 ml of isotonic saline. No leak of anesthetic gases was heard during positive pressure ventilation. The CO_2 laser was set to 20 W in the pulsed mode of operation with a duration of 0.2 s per pulse. Anesthesia was maintained with 4 1/min N_2O and 2 1/min O_2 along with isoflurane up to 1.5% as delivered by a calibrated vaporizer. Intermittent iv boli of atracurium provided paralysis.

> Near the end of the resection, the surgeon noticed bleeding at the edge of one of the vocal cords. Actuation of the laser for hemostasis resulted in smoke emerging from the patient's mouth with flames noted by the surgeon to be coming from the endotracheal tube. The anesthetist also noted flames in the disposable corrugated anesthesia circuit connected to the tracheal tube. The flames were doused with saline. Breath sounds were absent and an obvious leak of anesthetic gas could be heard when the ventilator cycled. The patient's lungs were not being ventilated. The delivery of nitrous oxide and oxygen was terminated and the ventilator turned off. The endotracheal tube was quickly removed, the lungs ventilated via mask, and the trachea was reintubated with a polyvinylchloride (PVC) endotracheal tube. Fiber optic bronchoscopy subsequently revealed extensive burns to the trachea and both bronchi. No fragments of the endotracheal tube were seen in the respiratory tract. The Xomed® tube was later noted to be intact with a ruptured cuff and with evidence of combustion of the cuff and distal shaft. The patient had a long intensive care unit stay requiring positive pressure ventilation, antibiotics, and vigorous pulmonary toilet. He subsequently underwent a permanent tracheostomy and had several dilation procedures.

(Take home message: in such cases avoid nitrous oxide, which supports combustion. Use air instead. Also, it might have been possible to stop the bleeding by other means.)

Case two

Consider the following second case, offered by Chee and Benumof [2].

A 28-yr-old, 100-kg man was scheduled for elective tracheostomy. The patient's lungs had been ventilated in the intensive care unit for 35 days after emergency craniotomy for a closed head injury. During the course of intensive care unit stay the patient remained comatose and adult respiratory distress syndrome developed, which was now resolving. The airway evaluation revealed an in situ 8.0-mm ID polyvinylchloride ETT, swollen lips, an edematous tongue protruding out of the mouth and an oropharynx filled with secretions.

General anesthesia was induced with 300 mg intravenous propofol and maintained with 0.4% inspired isoflurane and a 35% oxygen/air mixture. The vital signs remained stable within 10% of the baseline values. Electrocautery was used for coagulation by the surgeons. The patient was administered 100% oxygen immediately before insertion of the tracheostomy tube. Suddenly, the surgeons reported a blue flame shooting up vertically from the patient's neck. The breathing circuit was disconnected immediately from the ETT; 20 ml saline, 0.9%, was flushed into the ETT. The fire extinguished promptly.

(Take home message: in such cases keep the FiO_2 as low as possible and be careful to enter the trachea using scissors instead of electrocautery.)

Summary

An airway fire is potentially deadly complication that may occur during tracheotomy surgery, during laser surgery and with a number of other procedures. The American Society of Anesthesiologists operating room fire algorithm is a good starting point in the prevention and management of these events. In general, cases of airway fire call for immediate removal of the endotracheal tube (ETT) and flooding of the field with saline. While this is a reasonable rule of thumb, it should also be noted that there are occasional patients where removal of the ETT would in all likelihood result in irreversible loss of the airway. Some authors have suggested that flooding the surgical site with carbon dioxide will help prevent airway fires during open tracheostomy using cautery.

Clinical pearls

- Operating room fires are best divided into airway fires and non-airway fires. A recent report by the American Society of Anesthesiologists provides specific guidance for both scenarios.
- An airway fire is potentially deadly complication that may occur during tracheotomy surgery, during laser surgery and with a number of other procedures.

- Preventive measures do not guarantee that fires will not occur; always be prepared.
- A simple means to extinguish airway fires (e.g., 50 ml syringe filled with saline) should be immediately on hand. In addition, a CO_2 fire extinguisher is good to have nearby.
- The surgeon should avoid entering the trachea using electrocautery; additionally, the anesthesiologist must maintain special vigilance at the moment of surgical entry into the trachea.
- The anesthesiologist should keep the administered oxygen levels (fraction of inspired oxygen, FiO_2) used to the minimum needed when a significant potential for an airway fire is present.

- Nitrous oxide should not be used during airway surgery, since it supports combustion just as does oxygen.
- Prevailing conventional wisdom holds that cases of airway fire call for immediate removal of the endotracheal tube (ETT). While this is a reasonable rule of thumb, it should also be noted that there are some patients where removal of the ETT would in all likelihood result in irreversible loss of the airway.
- Flooding the surgical field with carbon dioxide might be an effective technique in preventing airway fires during open tracheostomy.

References

1. Sosis MB. Airway fire during CO2 laser surgery using a Xomed Laser endotracheal tube. *Anesthesiology* 1990;**72**(4):747–9.

2. Chee WK, Benumof JL. Airway fire during tracheostomy: extubation may be contraindicated. *Anesthesiology* 1998;**89**(6):1576–8.

3. Caplan RA, Barker SJ, Connis RT, *et al.* Practice advisory for the prevention and management of operating room fires.

Anesthesiology 2008;**108**(5): 786–801; quiz 971–2. Available online at http://www.asahq.org/publicationsAndServices/orFiresPA.pdf.

4. Rogers ML, Nickalls RW, Brackenbury ET, *et al.* Airway fire during tracheostomy: prevention strategies for surgeons and anaesthetists. *Ann R Coll Surg Engl* 2001;**83**(6):376–80.

5. Ng JM, Hartigan PM. Airway fire during tracheostomy: should we extubate? *Anesthesiology* 2003; **98**(5):1303.

6. Roy S, Smith LP. What does it take to start an oropharyngeal fire? Oxygen requirements to start fires in the operating room. *Int J Pediatr Otorhinolaryngol* 2011; **75**(2):227–30.

7. Ho AM, Wan S, Karmakar MK. Flooding with carbon dioxide prevents airway fire induced by diathermy during open tracheostomy. *J Trauma* 2007; **63**(1):228–31. PubMed PMID: 17622897.

Chapter

12

Anesthesia for septoplasty and rhinoplasty

Ursula Galway and Daniel Alam

Introduction

Septoplasty and rhinoplasty are both commonly performed surgical procedures. Most of these procedures are performed on an outpatient basis, often in a free-standing surgical facility. Septoplasty surgery can be performed to relieve symptoms of nasal obstruction or as a component of rhinoplasty surgery. Often, it is combined with turbinate reduction surgery. Patients with obstructive sleep apnea (OSA) may undergo septoplasty to facilitate use of continuous positive airway pressure (CPAP). Rhinoplasty surgery is performed for cosmetic or reconstructive purposes to alter the appearance of the nose. The indication for surgery may be purely cosmetic, post trauma, reconstructive after tumor resection or to improve nasal breathing.

Anesthetic management

Preoperative management

A patient presenting for rhinoplasty or septoplasty should have a preoperative workup directed by their preexisting medical conditions. Most patients presenting for septoplasty are young and healthy but some may have OSA. Older patients may present for reconstruction of their nose following basal cell carcinoma resection and may have significant comorbidities owing to their age. Additional testing should be directed by their history and physical exam.

If the surgery is to be performed in an ambulatory surgical center, it is imperative that the patient is a suitable candidate for outpatient surgery in a free-standing surgical center. Patients with uncontrolled chronic disease such as uncontrolled hypertension, unstable angina, symptomatic asthma, or brittle diabetes should not be operated on in this setting [1].

Other potential contraindications include patients with a difficult airway, history of malignant hyperthermia, morbid obesity, severe OSA and chronic pain. These patients should have their operation in a hospital setting.

All patients should have a thorough airway evaluation. Septoplasty patients may have nasal obstruction from a deviated septum and thus may be more difficult to ventilate.

Postoperative bleeding is one of the most common complications after nasal surgery. Patients should cease to use NSAIDs and aspirin for 2 weeks before surgery [2]. Preoperative antibiotics are optional.

Intraoperative management

There are several anesthetic options available for patients undergoing septoplasty or rhinoplasty. Factors to consider include the length of surgery, the number of procedures being performed, the degree of expected bleeding, the invasiveness of the procedure and what the patient is willing to tolerate. Patient preference is another factor in deciding on the anesthetic technique to be used. The main surgical requirements are patient immobility, a clear surgical field and smooth emergence from anesthesia.

Local anesthesia with sedation

Many nasal procedures can successfully be performed under local anesthesia with sedation. The advantages include the avoidance of airway instrumentation and positive-pressure ventilation, less intravenous medication administration and avoidance of inhaled anesthetic agents.

When an endotracheal tube is not in place, there is less coughing, bucking or straining at emergence, all

Anesthesia for Otolaryngologic Surgery, ed. Basem Abdelmalak and D. John Doyle. Published by Cambridge University Press.
© Cambridge University Press 2013.

of which can lead to bleeding from the surgical site. With less intravenous administration of opioids and no inhaled anesthetic administration, there are fewer episodes of nausea and emesis. The disadvantages of local anesthesia with sedation include patient awareness, the possibility of patient movement, pain with inadequate block, oversedation resulting in hypoventilation, and even potential for loss of the airway. Another potential risk of this approach is a probable need for emergency airway management in the setting of unexpected or brisk intraoperative bleeding leading to aspiration or frank obstruction as the airway is not secure and the patient has an altered sense of awareness.

Initially a topical decongestant is applied. Cocaine, phenylephrine or oxymetazoline can be applied to the nasal mucosa to provide vasoconstriction. The nose can be packed with local-anesthetic-soaked gauze and then supplemented with submucosal injection of local anesthetic with epinephrine. Commonly, 1% lidocaine (10 mg/ml) with 1:100 000 or 1:200 000 epinephrine is used. The epinephrine will shrink the nasal mucosa and decrease intraoperative bleeding. The most painful part is the administration of the local anesthetic. At this point the patient can be given a small dose of a short-acting agent such as propofol and then lightened again for the remainder of the procedure. With rhinoplasty, excessive infiltration of local anesthetic will lead to distortion and thus interfere with the assessment of cosmetic results, so care must be taken not to inject too much. Sedation can be administered with any combination of medications; however, patients can become disorientated and uncooperative with sedative medications so care should be taken to avoid oversedation. Surgical procedures performed on the face under sedation pose a risk of a surgical fire. This is due to the proximity of an open oxygen-delivery system with a high oxygen concentration near the face (nasal cannula or face mask) in the presence of electrocautery. As discussed in more detail in the chapter on airway fires (Chapter 11) for a fire to occur the triad of fuel (oxygen tubing, drapes, sponges), oxygen and an ignition source (electrocautery in this case) is needed. Patients having surgery under sedation should be placed on supplemental oxygen, although several precautions should be taken to avoid a fire. In general, surgical drapes should be configured to minimize accumulation of oxygen, flammable skin preparation solution should be allowed to dry before drapes are applied

and gauze and sponges should be moistened before use in proximity to electrocautery. If moderate or deep sedation is required for the procedure or if the patient displays oxygen dependence, it may be advisable to use a sealed oxygen-delivery system such as an endotracheal tube or a supraglottic airway. If neither of these factors is present and an open oxygen-delivery system is to be used (i.e., nasal cannula), several precautions can be taken to avoid the risk of fire. Only the minimum oxygen requirement to avoid hypoxia should be delivered. Prior to the use of electrocautery, oxygen should be stopped or decreased to the minimum required. Then, one should wait a few minutes to allow dispersion of the oxygen before electrocautery is used. Insufflation with medical air or scavenging of the operative field with suction are other ways to decrease the buildup of oxygen near the operating field [3].

Operative and recovery times have been shown to be shorter for patients undergoing surgery with local anesthesia with sedation compared with general anesthesia. There may also be less emesis, epistaxis and nausea as well as earlier discharge times [4].

General anesthesia

General anesthesia may be preferred for more extensive, longer or anticipated large-volume blood-loss procedures. The advantages of general anesthesia include the potential for total patient analgesia and immobility, less patient cooperation requirement and control of the airway by intubation or laryngeal supraglottic airway, reducing risk of aspiration of secretions, blood or irrigation fluids [2]. Disadvantages include the potential for coughing on the endotracheal tube upon emergence, more nausea and vomiting, higher doses of intravenous medications, a longer recovery and postoperative disorientation. A general anesthetic may be performed with either a supraglottic airway or an endotracheal tube. During induction of anesthesia and mask ventilation an oral airway may be needed to alleviate the effects of the nasal obstruction if significant septal deviation is present.

Maintenance of anesthesia can be with volatile inhaled anesthetic, total intravenous anesthesia (TIVA) or a balanced anesthesia technique. A continuous IV opioid-based technique with alfentanil or remifentanil allows for a reduction in the total amount of volatile anesthesia given and significantly blunts the tracheal response to the endotracheal tube. This also allows for improved hemodynamic stability and rapid smooth emergence. Remifentanil may cause a significant opioid-induced vagally mediated bradycardia, especially if given as a bolus, which may lead to decreased cardiac output and hypotension. A propofol infusion provides the advantages of decreasing blood pressure and decreasing the incidence of postoperative nausea and vomiting as well as being rapidly metabolized, resulting in a quicker emergence. Inhalational anesthesia can be used and also provides the advantage of decreasing blood pressure, thus lessening blood loss. During emergence, patients may buck or cough on the endotracheal tube, increasing venous pressure and increasing bleeding and swelling. This should be avoided if possible.

Patients may be disorientated after general anesthesia and may attempt to rub their nose. As this can disrupt the surgical sutures the patient should be watched very carefully until they are back to their baseline mental status.

General anesthesia with supraglottic airway versus general anesthesia with endotracheal tube

A supraglottic airway can be used to secure the airway after administration of general anesthesia. The supraglottic airway will provide a patent airway and allow the patient to breathe spontaneously under deeper levels of anesthesia without airway obstruction. Although it can prevent blood and secretions from entering the airway and stomach [5], it does not protect adequately for aspiration of blood or gastric secretions into the lungs.

Some studies show significantly less sore throat with a supraglottic airway than an endotracheal tube [3]. However, a review of the literature shows a wide variation in the incidence of postoperative sore throat for both supraglottic airways and endotracheal tubes, with the incidence after endotracheal intubation ranging from 14 to 50% and after a supraglottic airway ranging from 6 to 34% [4]. A supraglottic airway causes less cardiovascular response with insertion as compared to an endotracheal tube [5]. The supraglottic airway allows for a less stimulating emergence from anesthesia, thus less coughing and bucking.

The main limiting features of the supraglottic airway are the potential for aspiration and potential difficulties in sealing/placement. Other disadvantages of using a supraglottic airway include the potential for dislodgement, especially with movement of the head by the surgeon during surgery, and the possibility of laryngospasm as the vocal cords are not protected from blood or secretions.

General anesthesia with an endotracheal tube ensures better airway protection from secretions or blood loss from the operative field. A regular endotracheal, reinforced tube (Figure 12.1) or oral Rae tube (Figure 12.2) may be used. The endotracheal tube should be fixed in the midline to avoid any asymmetry of the face.

Throat packs made from saline-soaked gauze can also be used to prevent blood and secretions from entering the stomach. As mentioned previously, the disadvantages to using an endotracheal tube include a more significant cardiovascular response to insertion and more stimulation and airway irritation during emergence, although both can be managed with careful induction, and a well-planned smooth extubation.

Intraoperative considerations
Bleeding

Bleeding is one of the biggest complications of nasal surgery. Minimization of intraoperative blood loss allows the surgeon to have an operative field which he can visualize well. Blood loss can be minimized by applying epinephrine-containing local anesthetic or cocaine to the nasal mucosa, maintaining a slight head-up position, and the use of controlled hypotension in appropriate individuals.

Vasoconstrictors

The use of vasoconstrictors shrinks the nasal mucosa and constricts blood vessels, resulting in less surgical bleeding. Phenylephrine is an α-adrenergic agonist which can be used as a vasoconstrictor. It is supplied as a liquid and is sprayed directly into the nose. Mucosal absorption can lead to hypertension and even cardiovascular decompensation. The initial dose should not exceed 0.5 mg (500 μg). Should it occur, severe hypertension should be either waited out, treated with a short-acting direct vasodilator or an α-antagonist. Avoid β-blockers in this setting, especially long-acting agents like metoprolol and labetalol.

Oxymetazoline is a vasoconstrictor and an imidazoline-derivative sympathomimetic amine. It directly stimulates α-adrenergic receptors and exerts little or no effect on β-adrenergic receptors. Three sprays of

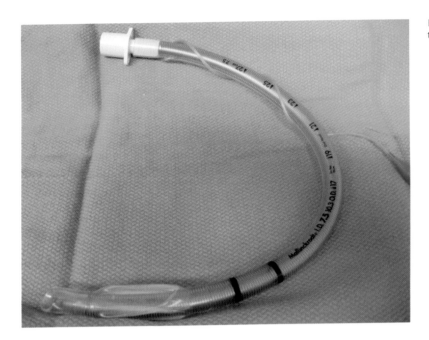

Figure 12.1. Reinforced endotracheal tube.

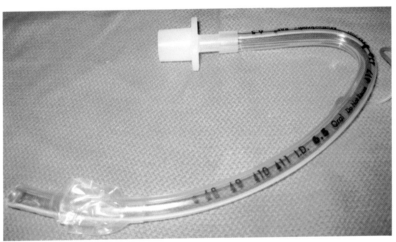

Figure 12.2. Oral Rae endotracheal tube.

0.05% oxymetazoline spray can be used in each nostril [5]. Cocaine is both a local anesthetic and a vasoconstrictor with sympathomimetic effects. Cocaine-soaked pledgets applied to the nasal mucosa provide both local anesthesia and vasoconstriction. Peak plasma levels are reached at 30 minutes and remain elevated for 120 minutes. Cocaine sensitizes the organs to epinephrine and blocks the uptake of released epinephrine at peripheral nerve terminals. Therefore, cocaine should be avoided in hypertensive patients, those on monoamine oxidase inhibitors and those with coronary artery disease or arrhythmias as it may cause detrimental cardiovascular effects. Intranasal doses of 0.5–1 mg/kg increase heart rate and systolic blood pressure, while a dose of 2 mg/kg sensitizes the myocardium to arrhythmogenic effects of epinephrine, and doses in the range of 5–10 mg/kg depress the heart. Cocaine can cause ventricular fibrillation, hypertension, cardiac arrest, tachycardia or respiratory depression in susceptible people. Cocaine is available in both 4% (40 mg/ml) and 10% (100 mg/ml) solutions, although the 4% solution is the most commonly used in medical practice. The recommended intranasal maximum dose of 4% solution of cocaine is 1.5 mg/kg. Each drop of 4% cocaine contains about 3 mg of cocaine. Cocaine is metabolized through ester hydrolysis by plasma pseudocholinesterase. Intranasal cocaine combined with epinephrine lowers plasma cocaine levels due to reduced absorption; however, it may lead to more incidences of arrhythmias and other cardiac events. Epinephrine acts directly on sympathetic neurons, stimulating the postsynaptic norepinephrine receptors.

The combination of reuptake inhibition of the cocaine and the direct synaptic stimulation of epinephrine may lead to excessive hypertension and tachycardia. While cocaine is an effective anesthetic and vasoconstrictor, the long-acting cardiac effects which extend to hours beyond the surgery are an issue that has led to a tendency for surgeons to use cocaine less frequently than in the past. The use of lidocaine with epinephrine and oxymetazoline in combination yields the same effect without the myocardial sensitization.

Controlled hypotension

Surgeons may sometimes request a controlled lowering of blood pressure to allow for less bleeding and improve visualization of the surgical field. Controlled hypotension may be defined as reduction of the systolic blood pressure to 80–90 mmHg and a reduction of the mean arterial pressure (MAP) to 50–65 mmHg or a reduction in MAP by one-third of its baseline value. A slow return to normal pressures postoperatively is ideal as a rapid return to normal pressures may cause reactionary hemorrhage.

Drugs used for controlled hypotension include the following:

• Inhalational anesthetics

Inhalational anesthetics lower MAP and systemic vascular resistance (SVR) via vasodilatation and their negative inotropic effect. They are readily titratable, provide surgical anesthesia and have a rapid onset and offset.

• Sodium nitroprusside

Sodium nitroprusside is a direct vasodilator which acts through nitric oxide release. It has a rapid onset and offset and is easy to titrate. Disadvantages include the potential for cyanide toxicity, rebound hypertension, sympathetic stimulation, increased pulmonary shunt, coronary steal, and tachycardia. An arterial line is ordinarily used whenever sodium nitroprusside is used, as well as a volumetric infusion pump.

• Nitroglycerin

Nitroglycerin is also a direct vasodilator. It also has a rapid onset and offset and is easy to titrate,

and causes limited tachycardia and no coronary steal. It too can increase pulmonary shunt. It may cause methhemoglobinemia and inhibition of platelet aggregation.

• β-Blockers

β-Blockers decrease myocardial contractility, SVR and heart rate. Some, such as esmolol, have a rapid onset and offset and are titratable. Disadvantages include decreased cardiac output, bradycardia, heart block and bronchospasm.

• Calcium channel blockers

Calcium channel blockers cause vasodilatation via decreased transmembrane calcium movement. They work rapidly and have no effect on airway reactivity. However, they can cause cardiac depression, bradycardia and conduction blockade.

Historically drugs such as trimethaphan, pentolinium and phentolamine have been used for controlled hypotension. Recently, dexmedetomidine has been shown also to decrease bleeding and intraoperative fentanyl consumption in septoplasty operations.

Relative contraindications to controlled hypotension include patients with severe cardiovascular disease, cerebrovascular disease, peripheral vascular disease, renal or hepatic impairment [6]. It is important to monitor the electrocardiogram for ST segment depression, which would indicate myocardial ischemia is occurring.

Untreated or poorly controlled hypertension is a relative contraindication as cerebral autoregulation may be shifted to a higher pressure set point. As a result, patients may be prone to cerebral ischemia at higher pressures than in normal individuals.

Care should be taken with patients with preexisting pulmonary disease as decreased arterial oxygen tension and increased alveolar–arterial oxygen gradients have been known to occur with deliberate hypotension, due to ventilation/perfusion mismatch and increase in physiological dead space.

Positioning

ENT patients are usually placed supine, often with the head of the bed elevated 15–30° with the bed turned 90–180° from the anesthesiologist. The elevation of the head 15–30° may cause a decrease in blood pressure due to decreased venous return to

117

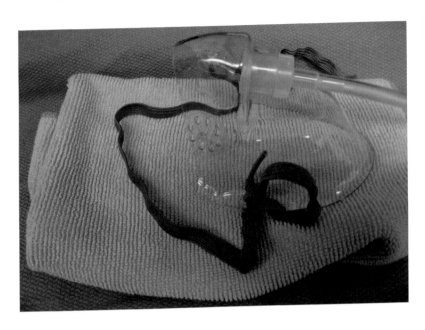

Figure 12.3. Modified simple face mask with upper portion removed using scissors.

the heart, allowing for less bleeding and better visualization of the surgical field. However, as excessive hypotension may occur in dehydrated or susceptible patients, caution should be taken to monitor the blood pressure closely. Eyes should be protected. With rhinoplasty surgery, the eyes should be protected in a way that allows early recognition of orbital injury, i.e., with ointment and minimal tape. The ETT and tubing should be directed toward the foot of the bed. A shoulder roll is placed and the neck extended.

Emergence

After nasal surgery, emergence cough or straining will produce venous engorgement and increase bleeding from the surgical site, so the necessity for a smooth extubation provides a challenge for the anesthesiologists. The stomach can be suctioned at the end of surgery prior to extubation to eliminate blood from the stomach. TIVA with propofol, a remifentanil or alfentanil infusion, IV lidocaine given prior to emergence or lidocaine sprayed directly on the vocal cords can all lessen the chances of coughing. Dexmedetomidine has also been used with success to improve extubation. Deep extubation can be performed to avoid coughing on the endotracheal tube but should be performed only with extreme caution if at all. Deep extubation may be dangerous, as there may be significant blood in the stomach which could

lead to aspiration. Trickling of blood from the surgical site can irritate the vocal cords, leading to laryngospasm. If the airway is lost following deep extubation, reintubation may be difficult due to the accumulation of blood in the airway. Mask ventilation after rhinoplasty may be difficult and undesirable due to the newly reconstructed nose; thus the patient could be difficult to ventilate should any airway issues arise post extubation. After extubation care should be taken not to place excessive pressure on a newly constructed nose with a face mask. Nasal cannulae or a face tent can be used to deliver supplemental oxygen postoperatively. A facemask can be modified by cutting off the top portion, thus avoiding nasal pressure (Figure 12.3). Post septoplasty, the nasal cavities may be packed and septal splints may be placed. During rhinoplasty if nasal bone osteotomies are performed the nose is packed and dorsal nasal splints are placed. The patient will be obliged to breathe through their mouth and if obstruction occurs an oral airway may be needed. Antiemetics should be given to patients to minimize PONV as vomiting and retching can lead to bleeding. The head of the bed should also be kept elevated.

Postoperative considerations

In the recovery area the patient's head should be elevated at 30° and a cold compress applied. A dressing sponge is folded and taped under the nose if there is any evidence of bleeding. Proper postoperative pain control, avoidance of hypertension, vomiting and Valsalva maneuvers can help minimize epistaxis or bleeding under the septal or nasal skin flaps. Short-acting intravenous narcotics, oral narcotics or acetaminophen can be used for pain control. NSAIDs should be avoided because of the potential for platelet inhibition and increased bleeding.

One study showed the majority of readmissions for septoplasty were for bleeding, with a strong association between NSAID use and readmission due to bleeding. If nasal packing is in place, anti-staphylococcal antibiotics [7] are often given. Activity should be kept to a minimum. Home-going postoperative medications include an oral opiate and prophylactic antibiotics. Overnight observation may be needed for patients with severe underlying medical conditions, uncontrolled pain or severe OSA.

Complications

Complications of septoplasty and rhinoplasty include bleeding, infection, traumatic neuromuscular injury and poor esthetic result. However, less common complications such as endocarditis, meningitis, brain abscess, hemorrhage and asphyxiation from nasal packing have been described in the literature.

Summary

The majority of septoplasties and rhinoplasties are performed on healthy patients in the outpatient setting; however, occasionally patients present with medical comorbidities or OSA. These surgeries can be performed with local anesthesia and sedation or general anesthesia with an LMA or endotracheal tube. The main intraoperative concern includes the minimization of bleeding with use of vasoconstrictors and submucosal epinephrine, controlled hypotension and a smooth emergence. Postoperatively patients need to be observed for bleeding but can usually be discharged home on the same day.

Case study – anesthesia for septoplasty and turbinate reduction

Preoperative management

A 25-year-old male presented for septoplasty and turbinate reduction for septal deviation and nasal obstructive symptoms. He had no major medical problems except for severe gastroesophageal reflux disease (GERD), for which he was on a proton pump inhibitor. Despite treatment he continued to have gastric reflux symptoms. He had no cardiac, pulmonary or respiratory problems. He had been NPO for over 8 hours and had not taken any medications on the morning of surgery. An 18-gauge intravenous catheter was inserted and the patient was given intravenous metoclopramide and famotidine as well as oral sodium citrate for aspiration prophylaxis. The plan was to perform the surgery on an outpatient basis.

Intraoperative management

The patient was brought to the operating room and standard monitors were applied. The decision was made by the anesthesiologist to perform a rapid sequence intubation with cricoid pressure because of the history of severe GERD. Anesthesia was induced with propofol, fentanyl and succinylcholine and the airway was easily intubated with a size 7 endotracheal tube. Anesthesia was maintained with an infusion of intravenous propofol and alfentanil with oxygen and nitrous oxide mix. The patient did not receive any further doses of neuromuscular blockade and was breathing spontaneously. The surgeon packed the throat to prevent blood and secretions from entering the stomach. Three sprays of 0.05% oxymetazoline were introduced into each nostril for vasoconstriction and the nasal septum was topicalized with 1% lidocaine with 1:100 000 epinephrine. Surgery proceeded uneventfully. Upon emergence, the patient's mouth was thoroughly suctioned and the throat pack was removed. He was breathing spontaneously with good tidal volumes, a strong head lift and was following commands. He began coughing violently so the endotracheal tube was removed.

Some bleeding was noted coming from his nose so the head of the bed was elevated and gauze was placed under his nose. He was brought to the recovery room on oxygen via simple face mask.

Postoperative management

In the recovery room, the patient's vital signs were stable; however, he continued to have some bleeding from his nose. Shortly after presenting to the recovery room, he began to have multiple episodes of emesis. Intravenous ondansetron was given, which stopped his nausea and vomiting; however, bleeding from his nose had worsened at this point. The surgeon was

119

called to the bedside. He examined the patient, placed pressure on the nose and placed nasal packing. This helped decrease the bleeding from profuse to mild. The decision was made to admit the patient overnight for observation due to epistaxis. Overnight the bleeding resolved and on postoperative day 1 he was discharged home in stable condition.

Complications

As illustrated by this case, this patients' surgical course was complicated by severe epistaxis which required admission to the hospital for further observation. This adds a significant financial and time burden for the patient, surgeon and the hospital. The bleeding may have been caused or aggravated by the coughing on extubation and by the violent bouts of emesis in the recovery room. Although maintenance of anesthesia with a propofol infusion is useful in preventing postoperative nausea and vomiting, the patient could have benefited from receiving intravenous dexamethasone at commencement of surgery and ondansetron prior to emergence. Although coughing on the endotracheal tube is sometimes unavoidable, perhaps the administration of intravenous lidocaine prior to extubation could have prevented or lessened the coughing.

Clinical pearls

- Most patients presenting for septoplasty are young and healthy although some may have OSA; older patients may present for nasal reconstruction following basal cell carcinoma resection and may have significant comorbidities.

- Postoperative bleeding is one of the most common complications after nasal surgery. Patients should cease to use NSAIDs and aspirin for 2 weeks before surgery.
- In septoplasty cases the main anesthetic goals are patient immobility, a clear surgical field and smooth emergence from anesthesia.
- Surgical procedures performed on the face under sedation pose a risk of a surgical fire. This is due to the proximity of an open oxygen-delivery system with a high oxygen concentration near the face (nasal cannula or face mask) in the presence of electrocautery.
- Supraglottic airways have been used successfully during general anesthesia for septoplasty surgeries. They provide a patent airway and allow the patient to breathe spontaneously under deeper levels of anesthesia without airway obstruction. However, while they can prevent blood and secretions from entering the airway and stomach, they do not protect adequately from aspiration of blood or gastric secretions into the lungs. They also offer the potential for dislodgement, especially with movement of the head by the surgeon, and a potential for laryngospasm exists as the vocal cords are not completely protected from blood or secretions.
- After nasal surgery, cough or straining at emergence will produce venous engorgement and increase bleeding from the surgical site – hence the necessity for a smooth extubation.
- After extubation care should be taken not to place excessive pressure on a newly constructed nose (rhinoplasty) with a face mask.

References

1. Duncan PG. Day surgical anaesthesia: Which patients? Which procedures? Can J Anaesth 1991;38(7):881–2.

2. Fedok FG, Ferraro RE, Kingsley CP, Fornadley JA. Operative times, postanesthesia recovery times, and complications during sinonasal surgery using general anesthesia and local anesthesia with sedation. Otolaryngol Head Neck Surg [Clinical Trial Comparative Study] 2000;122(4):560–6.

3. Higgins PP, Chung F, Mezei G. Postoperative sore throat after ambulatory surgery. Br J Anaesth 2002;88(4):582–4.

4. Zuccherelli L. Postoperative upper airway problems. S Afr J Anaesth Analg 2003;9(2)12–6.

5. Webster AC, Morley-Forster PK, Janzen V, et al. Anesthesia for intranasal surgery: a comparison between tracheal intubation and the flexible reinforced laryngeal mask airway. Anesth Analg 1999;88(2): 421–5.

6. Ward CF, Alfery DD, Saidman LJ, Waldman J. Deliberate hypotension in head and neck surgery. Head Neck Surg 1980;2(3): 185–95.

7. Georgalas C, Obholzer R, Martinez-Devesa P, Sandhu G. Day-case septoplasty and unexpected re-admissions at a dedicated day-case unit: a 4-year audit. Ann R Coll of Surg Engl 2006;88(2):202–6.

Chapter

13

Anesthesia for endoscopic sinus surgery

Paul Kempen

Introduction

Historically, the use of optical instruments to examine the nasal passages dates back over 100 years. In 1903, Hirshmann was the first to document the use of a cystoscope in diagnostic and surgical applications for nasal and sinus disorders, known as functional endoscopic sinus surgery (FESS). The early years of nasal endoscopy were primarily dedicated to diagnostic applications. FESS strived to provide for adequate airway drainage and aeration with minimal trauma. Developments over the last few decades have led to an increasingly wide array of surgical procedures. In the 1960s, fiberoptic technology enabled the elimination of significant internal heating. Although in 1965 the first color images of the maxillary antrum were presented, the fiberoptic limitations in field of vision and illumination, as well as the inadequacy to precisely localize surgical biopsy, confined utilization and acceptance in surgical procedures. In the early 1970s, improvements in optics greatly facilitated advances leading to increased utilization of endoscopes in ENT. With the introduction of stereotactic imaging, increasingly, utilization of endoscopic ENT surgery to address complex problems and tumors, beyond those localized to the nasal passage and adjacent sinus structures, followed. As the scope and clinical precision of endoscopic surgery advanced, the importance of anesthetic management in facilitating and ensuring intraoperative homeostasis, hemostasis and absolute immobility facilitated the development of inter-specialty cooperation to include surgical exposure of the ventral central nervous system by ENT surgeons for neurosurgeons [1].

Clinical goals

These collaborations are of particular importance, given the close approximation of the nasal passages to the internal carotid and ethmoidal arteries, the pituitary gland, skull base, superior cervical laminae and the ocular orbit [2]. Anesthesiologists have contributed significantly, using anesthetic techniques to mitigate intraoperative hemorrhage into the surgical field, thus significantly improving visualization of the surgical field. Controlling intraoperative ventilation, arterial and venous blood pressures and eliminating coughing, retching and vomiting during emergence are important anesthetic contributions to improved surgical outcomes [3]. Preventing secondary bleeding and CSF leaks after subarachnoid surgery in the perioperative period is attributed to a smooth emergence and avoidance of manual positive pressure ventilation after extubation. Modern, combined ENT-neurosurgical procedures can result in large defects in bone and limitations in the occlusive closure of the nasocranium. The initial friability of cranial closures presents specific anesthetic challenge at emergence. All of the above perturbations are meticulously avoided specifically to prevent CSF leaks and bleeding. These goals are further complicated by the need to ensure adequate respiration without positive pressure ventilation after extubation and during emergence in pituitary and cranial base surgery. Comorbidities further complicate recognized limitations in the native airway, including obstructive sleep apnea, obesity, and residual anesthetic effects.

While multiple studies have suggested a specific advantage of individual anesthetic techniques during FESS (the most simple, frequently performed, and typically outpatient operations), they nevertheless suffer from significant limitations regarding the influence of specific patient factors. These attempts to standardize anesthetic management for FESS stressed a short, standard and bloodless outpatient procedure, at times performed in a physician's office

Anesthesia for Otolaryngologic Surgery, ed. Basem Abdelmalak and D. John Doyle. Published by Cambridge University Press.
© Cambridge University Press 2013.

or free-standing outpatient surgical center promoting TIVA, local anesthetics, LMA utilization, and moderate induced hypotension to facilitate operative visibility approaching "cadaveric bleeding conditions". This contrasts significantly with the increasing scope and invasiveness of endoscopy in modern ENT surgery, especially in conjunction with multi-specialty cooperative operations, specifically neurosurgical, orbital, and orthopedic cervical spine surgery. These complex surgeries often lead to prolonged and at times staged procedures over multiple days. The increasing frequency of morbid obesity and multiple other comorbidities in the patient population in general significantly reduces the clinical success or practical application of "fast-track" techniques utilizing a supraglottic airway (SGA) without pharmacological neuromuscular blockade in all patients. Increasingly, the application of modern anesthetic techniques in any endoscopic sinus surgery (ESS) must be tailored primarily to the many and variable patient and surgical parameters, while facilitating surgical objectives only secondary to patient safety, as primary anesthetic goals. Thus, the anesthetic management of ESS must consider and formulate anesthetic techniques across a wide spectrum of procedures performed, surgical lesions, patient comorbidities, surgical durations, complications and outpatient vs. intensive care, including surgical staging over multiple days. It is evident that no single anesthetic technique will be optimal for any surgery in every patient, but that anesthetic management for ESS procedures has reached a complexity of sub-specialty anesthesia.

Surgical considerations for functional endoscopic sinus surgery

Hirshmann's early attempt to combat sinus pathology was founded on the appreciation that healthy sinus functional states required normal ventilation and drainage of sinus secretions without obstruction due to mucosal swelling, inflammation or other mechanical impediments. Functional endoscopic sinus surgery (FESS) strives to enable direct examination *in situ* with subsequent correction of encountered chronic changes and barriers which limit sinus drainage and aeration. Reduction of abnormal tissue mass, creation of effective drainage via larger sinus passages or complete obliteration of smaller sinuses as focal problems became operative goals [4]. FESS is a relatively safe surgical procedure, although the limited

evidence available suggests that FESS has not been demonstrated to be superior to medical treatment in chronic rhinosinusitis [5].

Anesthetic management
Preoperative considerations

These should be conducted in the usual fashion as described in Chapter 3. Of particular importance to the surgeries discussed here is the issue with sinusitis and upper respiratory infection (URI). Infection should be controlled with the appropriate antibiotics prior to these (for the most part) elective sinus surgeries. The optimal way to manage uncomplicated URI is controversial; however, most clinicians would proceed with the planned surgery, provided that there is no associated fever, severe wheezing, infected secretions, or any other symptoms or signs of active infection as in bacterial sinusitis, or pneumonia.

Intraoperative management
Anesthetic technique

While many intranasal procedures can be performed with adequate patient selection without general anesthetics, increasingly the availability of anesthetic specialists, minimal adverse effects of newer anesthetic agents, increasing numbers of pediatric and geriatric patients, widespread training of surgeons utilizing fast-track general anesthesia techniques, and increased emphasis on patient satisfaction have all fostered the incorporation of general anesthesia into the daily surgical pattern.

Anesthetic goals
Patient immobility

Early anesthetic management strived to provide patient immobility, enabling FESS within the superficial nasal passages. FESS was typically associated with a small danger of surgical excursion into the surrounding cranial structures. Procedures using topical vasoconstrictors and anesthetic agents, in combination with sedatives or general anesthetics, prevailed [4].

Dry surgical field

As availability of anesthesia services and technological advancement in the specialty proceeded, additional goals included attempts to provide improved surgical operative conditions and outcomes for FESS. With FESS, operating in often very close quarters within the airway, small amounts of intraoperative bleeding significantly obscured visualization and accuracy in surgical resections, soiled optical lenses, and prolonged operative time. Studies directed at a reduction in operative estimated blood loss (EBL) correlated with increased surgical visualization using various anesthetic techniques followed. The minimal amount of blood loss during FESS, even when doubled, may appear to be trivial in most instances, yet can contribute to surgical difficulty, delay and inefficiency.

Smooth, fast emergence

Emergence from general anesthesia can similarly produce untoward problems, when coughing and straining occur, contributing to postoperative bleeding, nausea, and vomiting. With FESS typically presenting as short, outpatient and especially elective procedures, fast-tracking with the use of supraglottic airway (SGA) techniques and total intravenous anesthesia (TIVA) (propofol and short duration narcotics) has become commonplace and was believed to produce optimization of surgical visual fields in selected patients [3,6–8]. The optimization of the operative surgical visual field can be accomplished through joint efforts of both teams by suppressing local hemodynamics in the surgical field: avoiding hypertension or facilitating appropriate, moderate hypotension, maintaining low heart rates by the anesthesiologist and application of combined topical/injected vasoconstrictors with local anesthetic agents, positioning to optimize drainage from the surgical field, and good surgical technique by the surgeon.

Use of supraglottic airways

The use of SGA over endotracheal tubes (ETT) appears additionally advantageous, providing reduced incidence and severity of coughing intraoperatively and during emergence [9]. Contraindications for the use of SGA include an increased risk of aspiration, including patients with a full stomach, significant obesity, and/or lower oesophageal sphincter insufficiency [3]. The SGAs typically enable routine extubation at lighter levels of anesthetic depth secondary to increased LMA tolerance. Once hemostasis is ensured, the smooth emergence reduces secondary hemorrhage. The importance of hemostasis has led to occasional use of intraoperative lasers on rare occasions, further complicating anesthetic management [3,10]. Incorporation of stereotactic and CT-guided imaging as well as robotic procedures to increase operative precision has similarly complicated anesthetic management and prolonged surgical durations [11,12].

SGAs will typically provide an adequate protective seal of the airway intraoperatively while enabling controlled extubation at a minimal level of anesthesia to prevent coughing, hypertension or significant pulmonary aspiration of blood from the field. The SGAs are also designed for use in spontaneously breathing patients where, theoretically, lower intrathoracic pressures reduce venous stasis in the surgical tissues. The larger diameter of the SGAs compared with that of an ETT provides significantly less resistance and pressure fluctuations during air exchange, facilitating larger tidal volumes and lower mean intrathoracic pressures to minimize venous congestion [3,9]. Limitations of SGA spontaneous respiration techniques include possible intraoperative patient movement, which may occur suddenly when surgery progresses from topically anesthetized tissues to normally sensitive structures under lighter depth of anesthesia. Hypercarbia is often commonplace in spontaneously breathing patients when intraoperative narcotics are employed and this is easily corrected at emergence. Positive-pressure ventilation via the LMA is frequently possible if needed to assist or control ventilation, but increased thoracic pressure can contribute to venous distention, facilitating bleeding and leakage of inhaled agents into the environment. Although modern fiberoptics and video projection onto screen monitors allow the surgeon's face to remain significantly distant from any volatile anesthetic leak itself, small amounts of anesthetics escaping from the shared airway and inhalation by surgeon and co-workers remain undesirable. Excessive or increasing LMA gas leak during pressurized ventilation can also indicate decreasing compliance, inadequate depth of anesthesia, or impending patient movements found with dissipation of intended neuromuscular blocking agents [13]. Gas leakage may be eliminated/mitigated by TIVA techniques and appropriate choice of LMA (or use of Proseal®-style LMA) to facilitate occlusive characteristics. Short, corrugated, and flexible airway extensions ("Bennett connectors") or flexible LMA styles are preferred by some surgeons to reduce protrusion and the presence of airway tubing near the operative field.

More on total intravenous anesthesia (TIVA)

Propofol/remifentanil TIVA with spontaneous respiration (PRTSR) is considered by some an optimal strategy to avoid emergence problems and provide flexibility, and minimize nausea, vomiting, and EBL, while ensuring rapid induction and emergence. Multiple studies support PRTSR as advantageous in facilitating hemodynamic conditions, minimizing EBL and thus optimizing surgical conditions, visibility, and efficiency. Although topical and injected local vasoconstrictors are useful to minimize blood loss from the soft tissue, penetration into the ossified structures can be limited and bleeding from resected bone is felt more amenable to hemodynamic measures of suppression. The EBL during FESS typically ranges from 1 to 200 ml of blood and is thus typically of little consequence to patient welfare. However, the presence of increasing amounts of blood in the surgical field is of concern to the surgeons, limiting operative visualization and extending surgical duration [6–8]. The use of EEG monitoring (i.e., bispectral index; BIS) objectifies continuous TIVA drug delivery and control of anesthetic depth, especially when the intravenous infusion site is not readily accessible, as when arms are tucked away from the anesthesia provider to provide optimal access for the surgeon. The various intraoperative and emergence advantages (due to anesthetic technique alone) may be small or negligible over expertly managed endotracheal intubation techniques using TIVA, inhalational anesthetics, endotracheal topical anesthesia and deep extubation [14]. The use of laryngeal tracheal anesthetic kits (LTA) at induction can facilitate smooth extubation in short procedures lasting less than 20–30 minutes. These topical anesthetic effects mitigate reflex responses during positioning, intraoperatively and, when still effective, at extubation [15]. Ultimately the choice of anesthetic technique for FESS will invariably result from an active interaction subject to surgeon, hospital and anesthesia provider assessment, specifically in light of patient-specific considerations.

Endoscopic sinus surgery (ESS): increasingly difficult surgeries and patients

As the patient population increasingly presents with significant cardiovascular and pulmonary comorbidities, gastrointestinal reflux disease, and obesity, anesthetic techniques for simple FESS procedures directed at optimal patient populations increasingly require flexibility to address multiple individual patient issues. Modern ESS in tertiary care settings will include neurosurgical, ophthalmologic, and cervical orthopedic procedures, often leaving the complicated exposure and closure of the surgical site to trained ENT specialists [16–18]. Complicated and repeated ENT ESS entails much longer surgical durations and increased bleeding and requires invasive monitoring. The procedures may occasionally be staged over several days with interval intensive care unit (ICU) management of an intubated patient. While the ETT can allow small amounts of blood to accumulate above the balloon cuff within the trachea and pharynx, it can also drain into the esophagus. This can typically be prevented intraoperatively by surgical packing of the laryngeal outlet or typically is easily removed with suction prior to or during the extubation process itself. In contrast to the dangers of intraoperative aspiration of stomach contents in at-risk patients during LMA techniques with spontaneous respiration, endotracheal intubation and neuromuscular blockade maximize intraoperative safety with respect to aspiration and patient movement. Gastric aspiration remains a danger prior to and after extubation. Passage of a suction catheter by the surgeon under direct vision at the end of surgery is recommended to remove any surgically accumulated secretions and also to protect the surgical site from injury. As the surgical duration increases and the need for neuromuscular blockade presents itself, limitations in the utility of the LMA become apparent. Although many anesthesiologists will utilize LMAs for increasingly longer surgical periods, a danger of gastric content aspiration, poor LMA seal or the need for high ventilation pressures will limit their use in many patients, where endotracheal intubation is not already associated with clear advantages. While TIVA techniques may in many instances be appropriate and possible, the combination with or principle use of inhalational agents may also have advantage in the intubated patient. Ultimately, the type of anesthetic agents utilized will be primarily predicated on team preferences, patient parameters, and cost considerations. Sudden and rapid bleeding can interrupt infusion pump delivery via pressure-sensitive pump alarms, with pressurized infusions/transfusions occurring through common IV sites. Peripheral IV sites may be inaccessible due to surgical positioning and also infiltrate, with interruption of anesthetic delivery. While the use of EEG monitoring may thus be highly desirable in TIVA anesthetics to confirm drug delivery, the presence of the electrodes may interfere with stereotactic markers, as well as cause field interference and interfere with image-guided surgery. As surgery complexity increases, arterial and central catheters become indicated and offer continual pressure measurement, with ensured anesthetic and vasoactive drug delivery. Inhalational anesthetic agents can alternatively be continually monitored along with ventilation, thus ensuring appropriate delivery, anesthetic depth, and ventilation. Although many anesthesiologists may use the EEG monitors to gauge depth of anesthesia as a means to expedite emergence, the use of the BIS to reduce intraoperative awareness has been demonstrated to provide no advantage over monitoring inhaled agent end tidal concentrations [19].

Repeat surgeries and emergencies

Postoperative bleeding, cerebrospinal fluid leaks, infections, recurrent tumors and staged procedures are the primary indications for repeat anesthetics in patients after initial ESS procedures. Especially in emergency procedures, where gastric content aspiration is of significant concern, the need to aspirate gastric contents at the beginning and/or end of the procedure should be deferred to the ENT surgeon. Decompression of the stomach content may be needed prior to surgery to prevent intraoperative reflux of gastric acid into the surgical field. Similarly, blood and gastric contents should be removed prior to emergence and extubation as far as is possible to prevent aspiration, coughing and vomiting postoperatively. It is vitally important to recognize the extent of prior surgery and any cervical and cranial base disruptions. Placement of intraoral and especially intranasal implements of any kind, except under direct visualization, can lead to intracranial insertion and significant morbidity whenever protective ossified barriers have been surgically removed. Knowledge of any retained surgical packing, closure barriers, types and extent will ultimately put the surgeon in the best position to insert any drainage or monitoring equipment that is required under direct endoscopic visualization. Intubation of the trachea is an anesthetic procedure performed typically under direct visualization via the oral cavity, thus obviating these concerns at induction. Transnasal intubation should be strictly avoided. Insertion of gastric tubes, temperature probes, and solid airway devices may occur without the security of direct visual confirmation of placement and can lead to disruption of surgical surfaces and transposition across membranous surgical closures. The minimal degree of barrier protection from such membranous closure will provide inadequate protection from intracranial migration of inserted tubings for the duration of the patient's life, especially after extensive cranial base procedures.

Repeat and staged procedures themselves will typically occur in fasted patients. Emergency procedures require significant concern regarding gastric content reflux and pulmonary aspiration, especially in patients with significant CSF leakage. Symptoms of nausea, vomiting, headache, dehydration, neurological defects, and obtundation secondary to pneumocephalus and intracranial CSF hypotension may be further accentuated by meningitis due to CSF leaks. While small and traumatic CSF leaks are corrected with high rates of success, larger neurosurgical and skull base surgeries require complicated closures and may result in high CSF leak rates approaching 30–58% [16,17,20]. CSF leaks are often believed by surgeons to start in the early postoperative period and specifically at emergence, due to fluctuations of CSF pressure across the closure site. Leaks are attributed specifically to postoperative coughing, gagging, snoring, and snorting [17]. Infection in these patients can further lead to intracranial sinus thrombosis and considerable associated morbidity. Preoperative therapeutic administration of narcotics may also delay gastric motility and increase gastric content. Rapid sequence induction (RSI) may proceed in the usual fashion as indicated, whereby active positive-pressure ventilation is avoided to prevent gastric as well as intracranial air insufflation, as an additional specific concern. Knowledge of the previous intubation conditions and success often facilitates a decision favoring RSI. In the event of a known difficult airway, transoral placement of an airway after induction of anesthesia may favor SGA over ETT, or conversion to ETT after securing the airway with an intubating LMA. Awake intubation is often associated with significant gagging and hemodynamic perturbations. However, the overall patient safety may in some circumstances warrant awake intubation procedures over postinduction measures, particularly as the CSF leak will be subsequently addressed surgically. Vomiting, however, may soil the surgical site and introduce contamination to the CSF and risk–benefit analysis is warranted. The possible and confirmed presence of significant pneumocephalus warrants the omission of nitrous

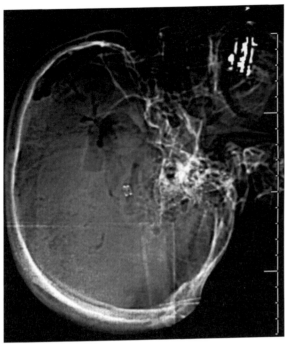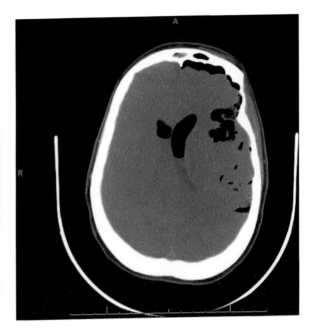

Figures 13.1 and 13.2. The Scout roentgenogram and MRI demonstrate extensive pneumocephalus including intraventricular gas in the preoperative films.

oxide as a component of anesthetic care, as the presence of a CSF leak does not ensure the escape of sudden gas expansion after nitrous oxide administration.

An additional and specific postanesthetic concern arises from postoperative CSF leakage, described as remote cerebellar hemorrhage (RCH). While in the setting of ESS, the connotation of "remote" may be considered a misnomer, RCH had originally been reported after cervical spine surgery and recently has most frequently been associated with frontotemporal craniotomy performed in the supine position [21–23]. RCH has been further associated with surgeries located from the cranial apex to lumbar spinal areas, which produce CSF leaks. The clinical presentation of RCH is typically that of significant headache, possibly initially with characteristics of postdural puncture headache, which subsequently progresses to cerebellar symptomology and may lead to severe neurological compromise from subtentorial compression from hemorrhage. The onset of symptoms typically occurs postoperatively after intervals of hours to days. The role of anesthetic administration itself remains unclear, although anesthetic agents, positive-pressure ventilation and the emergence phenomenon are known to have significant

physical effects on intracranial dynamics. The pathophysiology of this entity is described as one of intracranial hypotension, leading to sagging of cranial structures, subarachnoid vascular compromise and cerebellar hemorrhage. This is supported by the fact that typically bleeding occurs extraaxially, initially located along the tentorium, upper vermis, and cerebellar sulci, where the cerebellar veins provide for outflow. Growing consensus supports the development of secondary intraparenchymal hemorrhage due to a combination of anatomic venous predisposition and mechanical effects, leading to venous parenchyma engorgement. Whether the stretching or interruption of these veins leads to occlusion remains unclear.

While clearly a rare postoperative complication, the importance of RCH becomes significant as a legal liability whenever a Salem sump, temperature probes or other tubes are placed nasally and orally in patients with prior skull-based operations. The patient shown in Figures 13.1 and 13.2 presented postoperatively with an emergency CSF leak after C1–2 anterior resection and an oragastric tube was placed to decompress the stomach. Extensive preoperative pneumocephalus and intraventricular air was noted radiologically. Figure 13.3 demonstrates the complete absence of

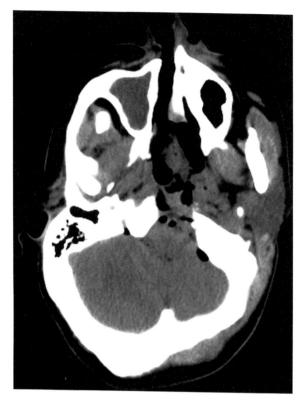

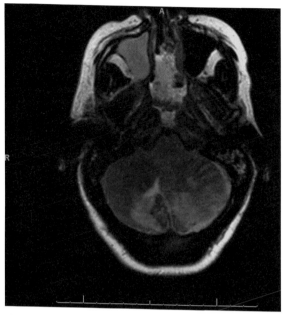

Figure 13.4. Intracerebellar hemorrhage is evident and developed 20 hours postoperatively. Extensive operative site packing is noted and closely approximates and protects the anterior pons separated by Alloderm® graft. The right frontal sinus is filled with fluid.

Figure 13.3. This slightly tilted computer tomograph shows a wide (18 mm diameter) defect in the anterior ossified skull base structures with intracranial air and only limited soft tissue separating the pharynx from the medulla at the lower level of the cerebellum.

nasal packing, leaving only a thin membranous covering of the defect and adjacent intrathecal air. Postoperative control CT demonstrated a new small subarachnoid hemorrhage along the left frontal lobe (not shown) and extraaxial subdural hemorrhage along the tentorium and falx cerebelli. The patient emerged from anesthesia after control CT 4 hours post-induction without neurological deficit, but became obtunded 20 hours postoperatively. Extraaxial pericerebellar hemorrhage was noted on MRI (Figure 13.4) and required neurosurgical intervention. Although neither RCH or transoral intracranial placement of a Salem sump was ever documented in prior literature, the orogastric insertion became implicated as causative in the posterior cerebellar bleeding, especially in conjunction with the caudal extent of surgical resection below the hard palate (Figure 13.5). Placement of all tubes in patients after any endoscopic surgery should be undertaken only in a manner to prevent access to the cranium for life, to prevent access to the residual non-ossified membranes.

Anesthetic emergence techniques for ESS

The goals of emergence and extubation after ESS are particularly challenging. Preoperative discussion of the emergence plan with the surgeon and the patient is useful to optimize emergence [24]. Nasal post-surgical packing will require oral breathing patterns. The surgical use of local anesthetic agents typically causes limited pain upon emergence, including even the most complicated neurosurgical procedures. Both facts should be stressed reassuringly to the patient preoperatively. SGA utilization is effective to facilitate awake removal of the airway without stressful coughing, hypertension or venous congestion at the surgical site. Meticulous control of surgical bleeding and removal of all blood and packing should occur prior to emergence. Intubation of the trachea requires increased attention to detail to optimize emergence. Deep extubation (at surgical planes of anesthesia) necessitates adequate spontaneous respiration and avoidance of tracheal stimulation from oral secretions including surgical bleeding through complete emergence [14]. Deep extubations should only be undertaken in fasted patients without danger of gastric content aspiration, as well as only in patients exhibiting

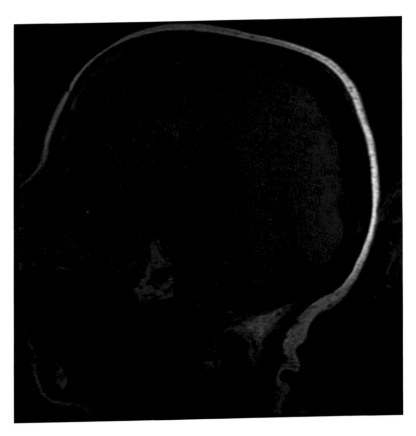

Figure 13.5. This sagittal MRI scan shows extensive posterior nasopharyngeal surgical changes deep to the CSF spaces, including a wide skull base defect and resection of the body of C1 and the Dens axis. The fat packing in the defect appears as the lighter triangular image. The extent of this transnasal surgery clearly extends below the hard palate to the top of the body of C2, hidden from view behind the soft palate but providing direct access to the surgical site from the oropharynx.

adequate probability of spontaneous respiration without significant need of supportive measures. Positioning of the patient in the lateral and head-dependent position is useful to drain secretions from the mouth, but may have limitations if pressure on the nose is a surgical concern. Insertion of an oral airway to ensure ventilation until the patient emerges sufficiently to maintain spontaneous respiration and protective reflexes deserves consideration. This will also prevent clenching on the ETT producing airway obstruction, as well as preventing ETT removal. Frequently, and especially for the shortest procedures requiring intubation, the utilization of laryngotracheal anesthesia (LTA) kits during intubation to distribute 4% lidocaine into the trachea can effectively obtund cough reflexes for periods of 20–30 minutes and allow complete emergence without significant stimulation from the ETT, facilitating awake extubation and maintenance of a spontaneous airway patency. After prolonged surgical procedures, the introduction of topical intratracheal lidocaine prior to emergence can similarly help provide for smooth emergence [14].

Several methods provide for effective intratracheal topical anesthesia at the end of surgery [15]. The instillation of 4–10% lidocaine into the ETT cuff at intubation has been advocated to allow diffusion of lidocaine from within the cuff into the adjacent mucosal. This typically requires a period of up to 60 minutes to become effective. A significant limitation of this technique is that only tissue in contact with the cuff will become anesthetized. Also, the injection and especially the withdrawal of the solution is difficult and requires specific attention to ensure an adequately deflated cuff at extubation. Lidocaine can be topically injected via an endotracheal tube *in situ*. The active administration of topical agents in this fashion may induce coughing, if the patient is not effectively anesthetized and immobilized by neuromuscular blocking agents at the time of injection. Using specifically designed laryngotracheal instillation of topical anesthesia (LITA™) tubes (Sheridan Catheter Corp, Argyle, NY) allows instillation above and beyond the ETT cuff, as they are designed to spray the solution in a circumferential fashion at both sites via an integral port [25,26]. Another endotracheal tube type designed to provide low suction immediately above the cuff to reduce silent aspiration of secretions in long-term intubated patients (TaperGuard EvacTM-Mallenckrodt[TM], Tyco Healthcare[TM], Pleasanton, CA, USA) can effect delivery above the cuff only. Both provide for injectate delivery without manipulation of the ETT or cuff. However, the injection of the solution itself may still stimulate cough reflexes with either ETT, producing movement and intrathoracic pressure changes, unless a significant depth of anesthesia is ensured. The cost of such specialty ETTs is also significantly 3–4-times that of standard ETTs.

Standard ETTs can also be cost-effectively utilized to effect application of topical anesthetics to the tracheal mucosa exterior to the ETT itself. This requires injection of 2–4% lidocaine under deep anesthesia or complete neuromuscular blockade via the 90° elbow connecter, between the ETT and the circle system [15,27]. The local anesthetic is very slowly injected during a large tidal volume breath applied upon deflation of the ETT cuff. Again, as the deflation of any ETT can cause unwanted movement and permit tracheal flow of pharyngeal secretions, adequate anesthesia/paralytic dosing, as well as the slow deflation of the ETT cuff with 5–10 mmHg PEEP, contributes to akinetic patients during the procedure. Typically 5 ml of solution is slowly injected directly down the ETT after the onset of gas egress is heard. The 5 ml injection is timed to correspond to the continual flow of the 3 liter positive-pressure breath emerging around the ETT from the larynx. It is important to ensure the liquid enters the ETT and not the circle circuit. The installation of lidocaine should be distributed across the complete breath volume and the effect will reliably last 20 minutes from the time of instillation. The liquid solution adheres to the ETT surface via surface tension and returns along the outside ETT surface with the airflow. The ETT cuff is now reinflated and the lidocaine is afforded 20–30 seconds to take effect, rapidly anesthetizing the trachea proximal to the ETT tip. It is advantageous to place the ETT only as deep as needed below the cords at intubation, to limit the length of tracheal mucosa needed to be anesthetized or the amount of lidocaine injected. Subsequent to effective topical anesthesia application, the deep anesthesia and/or neuromuscular blockade is reversed, adequate spontaneous respiration is achieved and the effectiveness of the topical agent can be assessed by rapid deflation and immediate reinflation of the cuff ("the Cuff test" – a maneuver which reliably causes

coughing if anesthesia is inadequate). Failure of the patient to adversely respond at sub-MAC concentrations of volatile anesthetic with movement or any change in respiration will now allow ETT removal without concern for laryngospasm or agitation. Should reaction be evident during the cuff test, a repeated installation of an additional 5 ml of lidocaine is typically effective in the rare failure of a single application. Alternately, if the cuff test results in reactions at 30 seconds post installation, ETT cuff reinflation and repeat testing after an additional 30 seconds often either allows complete redistribution of the lidocaine or time for effective anesthesia to develop. Smokers or individuals with thick tracheal secretions will benefit from the higher (i.e., 4% lidocaine) concentration to effectively penetrate to the mucosa. Reversal of neuromuscular blockade, discontinuing the volatile agents with substitution of high-flow nitrous oxide and allowing CO_2 to rise toward 40 torr immediately after the lidocaine instillation will facilitate both subsequent rapid return of respiration and emergence.

Similarly, judicious use of intravenous narcotics titrated to an adequate respiratory pattern at this point will facilitate mitigation of any pain, coughing or retching as long as respirations are ensured. In this manner, patients can completely emerge under spontaneous respiration, while following complex commands, to have the ETT removed in a very safe manner. This method is particularly useful after pituitary and cranial base surgeries where positive-pressure ventilation, coughing, and hemodynamic perturbations are noticeably undesirable. Effective antiemetic administration contributes to minimal retching and vomiting during emergence and postoperatively. Dexamethasone may be requested by some surgeons and should be administered early after induction to avoid the rare syndrome of perineum burning and provide time for this slow-onset drug to become effective [28,29].

Complications

Please see Table 13.1.

Table 13.1. Complications of endoscopic sinus surgery [2–4,30–32]

Minor complications include:

Nasolacrimal duct injury

Synechiae

129

Table 13.1. (*cont.*)

Subcutaneous emphysema

Ostial stenosis or closure

Epiphoria

Anosmia

Minor bleeding

Major complications include:

Airway compromise due to uvula edema, clots, tissue or packing debris

Invasion of the adjacent cortex/pituitary gland

Carotid, ethmoid artery invasion/bleeding

Cranial venous sinus thrombosis

Orbital hematoma and emphysema

Cerebrospinal fluid leak

Penetration into the brain, intracranial infection

Blindness, hemi- or bilateral, resulting from orbital trauma or damage to the optic nerve

Hemorrhage requiring transfusions or surgical control

Death

Summary

Functional endoscopic sinus surgery is among the most challenging of ENT procedures for a variety of reasons, including the need for immobility, hemostasis, and, especially, gentle emergence from anesthesia. The use of total intravenous anesthesia is a frequent anesthetic choice for these surgeries. One particularly important aspect, perhaps more than the kind of anesthetic administered, is the proper use of nasal decongestant agents to reduce the likelihood of intraoperative bleeding that would increase the difficulty of the procedure. Finally, the importance of antiemetic prophylaxis should not be forgotten.

Case Study

A 61 kg, 160 cm tall, 71-year-old female presented for FESS after two previous ENT surgeries, a decade previously, which concerned polyps. She now has progressive airway congestion while using decongestant and steroid therapy. Prior medical history included tracheostomy placement (now healed), right upper lobe resection, PEG tube placement and total esophagectomy performed 1 year previously. She

exhibited an end cervical esophagostomy with neckostomy pouch for secretion control and baseline BP of 170/70. General anesthesia with endotracheal intubation was chosen, as supraglottic airways may have proved ineffective with absence of the upper esophageal recess and potential air leak through the cervical left lateral esophagostomy drainage. Her intrathoracic airway was deviated by mediastinal retraction rightward, but not compromised, as shown in the roentgenogram (Figure 13.6).

Anesthesia was induced with propofol, fentanyl and rocuronium for endotracheal intubation after preoxygenation. Manual mask ventilation led to distention of the esophagostomy appliance prior to intubation, which was then drained. The patient was positioned with the head elevated 10–15°. Topical vasoconstriction and local anesthetics were placed by the surgeon. Propofol and remifentanil were titrated with inhalational 50% N_2O in oxygen. Neuromuscular blockade was maintained throughout. Systolic blood pressure was controlled between 110 and 120 mmHg systolic (under consideration of baseline pressures) with anesthetic agents alone. Peak inspiratory pressures remained below 20 mmHg. The repeat surgical ENT procedure lasted less than 1 hour, incurring no measurable blood loss. As the patient aroused to respond to her name, the endotracheal tube was removed without coughing or agitation. While initially breathing only on command, she then resumed spontaneous respiration as residual remifentanil effects dissipated. She received dexamethasone and ondansetron intraoperatively to prevent nausea and recovered uneventfully.

Clinical pearls

- Functional endoscopic sinus surgery is among the most challenging of ENT procedures for a variety of reasons including the need for immobility, hemostasis, and, especially, gentle emergence from anesthesia. That said, no single anesthetic technique will be optimal for any surgery in every patient.

- The optimization of the operative surgical visual field can be accomplished through joint efforts of both teams by avoiding hypertension or facilitating appropriate moderate hypotension, maintaining low heart rates, using local anesthetic agents combined with topical or injected vasoconstrictors, by positioning to optimize drainage from the surgical field, and by good surgical technique.

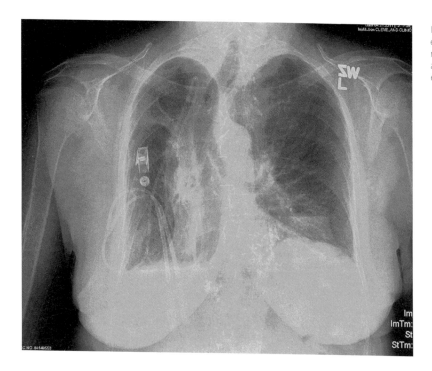

Figure 13.6. Roentgenogram shows extensive postsurgical changes with mediastinal and tracheal shift to right after right upper lobectomy and esophagectomy.

- The use of supraglottic airways (SGA) over endotracheal tubes (ETT) for simple sinus surgeries appears advantageous, providing less coughing intraoperatively and with emergence. Contraindications to SGA use include patients with increased risk of aspiration, or significant obesity that makes ventilation difficult. Another challenge with SGA use is that positive-pressure ventilation via a SGA often results in contamination of the OR with volatile anesthetic. Endotracheal intubation and neuromuscular blockade maximize intraoperative safety with respect to aspiration and patient movement.
- Short corrugated airway extensions ("Bennett connectors") or flexible LMA styles are preferred by some surgeons to reduce protrusion and the presence of airway tubing near the operative field.
- While many believe that TIVA is superior to inhalational anesthetic in sinus surgery, it should be noted that peripheral IV sites may be inaccessible due to surgical positioning and occasionally infiltrate, with interruption of IV anesthetic delivery. While the use of EEG monitoring can help confirm drug delivery, the presence of the electrodes may become undesirable to many surgeons and may interfere with the surgical navigation system. Inhalational anesthetic agents can alternatively be continually monitored along with ventilation, thus ensuring appropriate delivery, anesthetic depth, and ventilation.
- Passage of a suction catheter by the surgeon under direct vision at the end of surgery is recommended to remove any surgically accumulated secretions and also to protect the surgical site from injury.
- In the immediate post-sinus surgery period active positive-pressure ventilation is avoided to prevent gastric as well as intracranial air insufflation.

References

1. Maran AG. Endoscopic sinus surgery. *Eur Arch Otorhinolaryngol.* 1994;**251**(6):309–18.

2. Maniglia AJ. Fatal and other major complications of endoscopic sinus surgery. *Laryngoscope* 1991;**101**:349–54.

3. Danielsen A, Gravningsbråten R, Olofsson J. Anaesthesia in endoscopic sinus surgery. *Eur Arch Otorhinolaryngol* 2003;**260**(9): 481–6.

4. Danielsen A, Olofsson J. Endoscopic endonasal sinus surgery: a review of 18 years of practice and long-term follow-up. *Eur Arch Otorhinolaryngol* 2006;**263**(12):1087–98.

5. Khalil HS, Nunez DA. Functional endoscopic sinus surgery for

chronic rhinosinusitis. *Cochrane Database Syst Rev.* 200619;3: CD004458. PMID:16856048.

6. Eberhart LH, Folz BJ, Wulf H, Geldner G. Intravenous anesthesia provides optimal surgical conditions during microscopic and endoscopic sinus surgery. *Laryngoscope* 2003;**113**(8):1369–73.

7. Beule AG, Wilhelmi F, Kühnel TS, Hansen E, Lackner KJ, Hosemann W. Propofol versus sevoflurane: bleeding in endoscopic sinus surgery. *Otolaryngol Head Neck Surg* 2007;**136**(1):45–50.

8. Wormald PJ, van Renen G, Perks J, Jones JA, Langton-Hewer CD. The effect of the total intravenous anesthesia compared with inhalational anesthesia on the surgical field during endoscopic sinus surgery. *Am J Rhinol* 2005;**19**(5):514–20.

9. Atef A, Fawaz A. Comparison of laryngeal mask with endotracheal tube for anesthesia in endoscopic sinus surgery. *Am J Rhinol* 2008; **22**(6):653–7.

10. Gerlinger I, Lujber L, Jarai T, Pytel J. KTP-532 laser-assisted endoscopic nasal sinus surgery. *Clin Otolaryngol Allied Sci* 2003; **28**(2):67–71.

11. Eichhorn KW, Bootz F. Clinical requirements and possible applications of robot assisted endoscopy in skull base and sinus surgery. *Acta Neurochir Suppl* 2011;**109**:237–40.

12. Parikh SR, Cuellar H, Sadoughi B, Aroniadis O, Fried MP. Indications for image-guidance in pediatric sinonasal surgery. *Int J Pediatr Otorhinolaryngol* 2009;**73**(3):351–6.

13. Gilbey P, Kukuev Y, Samet A, Talmon Y, Ivry S. The quality of the surgical field during functional endoscopic sinus surgery – the effect of the mode of ventilation – a randomized, prospective, double-blind study. *Laryngoscope* 2009; **119**(12):2449–53.

14. Kempen PM. Extubation in adult patients: who, what, when, where, how and why? *J Clin Anesth* 1999;**11**:441–44.

15. Ecklund J, Kempen PM. Consider the use of lidocaine in the cuff of the ETT, but be aware of the risks and alternatives. In Marucci C, Cohen NA, Metro DG, Kirsch JR, eds. *Avoiding Common Anesthesia Errors*. Philadelphia: Wolters Kluwer. pp. 43–8.

16. Rutka JT. Craniopharyngioma. *J Neurosurg* 2002;**97**(1):1–2.

17. Snyderman CH, Kassam AB, Carrau R, Mintz A. Endoscopic reconstruction of cranial base defects following endonasal skull base surgery. *Skull Base* 2007; **17**(1):73–8.

18. Nayak JV, Gardner PA, Vescan AD, Carrau RL, Kassam AB, Snyderman CH. Experience with the expanded endonasal approach for resection of the odontoid process in rheumatoid disease. *Am J Rhinol*. 2007 Sep-Oct;**21**(5): 601–6.

19. Avidan MS, Jacobsohn E, Glick D, *et al.*; BAG-RECALL Research Group. Prevention of intraoperative awareness in a high-risk surgical population. *N Engl J Med* 2011;**365**(7):591–600.

20. Basu D, Haughey BH, Hartman JM. Determinants of success in endoscopic cerebrospinal fluid leak repair. *Otolaryngol Head Neck Surg* 2006;**135**(5):769–73.

21. Brockmann MA, Nowak G, Reusche E, Russlies M, Petersen D. Zebra sign: cerebellar bleeding pattern characteristic of cerebrospinal fluid loss. Case report. *J Neurosurg* 2005; **102**(6):1159–62.

22. Farag E, Abdou A, Riad I, Borsellino SR, Schubert A. Cerebellar hemorrhage caused by cerebrospinal fluid leak after spine surgery. *Anesth Analg* 2005; **100**(2):545–6.

23. Friedman JA, Ecker RD, Piepgras DG, Duke DA. Cerebellar hemorrhage after spinal surgery: report of two cases and literature review. *Neurosurgery* 2002;**50** (6):1361–3; discussion 1363–4.

24. Mehta U, Huber TC, Sindwani R. Patient expectations and recovery following endoscopic sinus surgery. *Otolaryngol Head Neck Surg* 2006;**134**(3):483–7.

25. Gonzalez RM, Bjerke RJ, Drobycki T, *et al.* Prevention of endotracheal tube-induced coughing during emergence from general anesthesia. *Anesth Analg* 1994;**79**:792–5.

26. Diachun CA, Tunink BP, Brock-Utne JG. Suppression of cough during emergence from general anesthesia: laryngotracheal lidocaine through a modified endotracheal tube. *J Clin Anesth* 2001;**13**(6):447–51.

27. Burton AW, Zornow MH. Laryngotracheal lidocaine administration. *Anesthesiology* 1997;**87**(1):185–6. Kempen PM:Reply

28. Neff SP, Stapelberg F, Warmington A. Excruciating perineal pain after intravenous dexamethasone. *Anaesth Intensive Care* 2002; **30**(3):370–1.

29. Steward DL, Grisel J, Meinzen-Derr J. Steroids for improving recovery following tonsillectomy in children. *Cochrane Database Syst Rev.* 2011 Aug 10;(8):CD003997.

30. Holden JP, Vaughan WC, Brock-Utne JG. Airway complication following functional endoscopic sinus surgery. *J Clin Anesth* 2002;**14**(2):154–7.

31. Pepper JP, Wadhwa AK, Tsai F, Shibuya T, Wong BJ. Cavernous carotid injury during functional endoscopic sinus surgery: case presentations and guidelines for optimal management. *Am J Rhinol* 2007;**21**(1):105–9.

32. Bhatti MT, Schmalfuss IM, Mancuso AA. Orbital complications of functional endoscopic sinus surgery: MR and CT findings. *Clin Radiol* 2005; **60**(8):894–904.

Chapter

14

Anesthesia for transsphenoidal pituitary surgery

Gazanfar Rahmathulla, Robert Weil and David E. Traul

Introduction

The transsphenoidal approach is a common surgical technique utilized to perform resection of lesions found in the sella turcica. In the early 1900s, the transsphenoidal technique was promoted as a less invasive and safer alternative to the transcranial approach to pituitary tumors [1]. While the popularity of the transsphenoidal approach fluctuated over the next century, the modern advent of microsurgical and endoscopic techniques has facilitated its present-day acceptance as an attractive option for the resection of lesions in the sella region, including chordomas, craniopharyngiomas, and pituitary tumors.

Surgical procedure

Transsphenoidal pituitary resection allows total, or near-total, tumor removal with the goals of achieving neuroendocrine remission as well as providing pituitary fossa decompression. Generally, the transsphenoidal approach to the sella region can be divided into two techniques: (1) the sublabial approach involves an incision made beneath the upper lip into the gum and subsequently through the septum and (2) the transnasal approach involves dissection through the nasal cavity wall using microsurgical or endoscopic instruments inserted through the nostrils. With either approach, insertion of a CSF drain in the lumbar region may be used to manipulate CSF levels in order to optimize surgical conditions. Injection of saline or air through the drain and into the spinal column may help the lesion descend into the surgical field. Additionally, opening of the lumbar drain may help alleviate any CSF leakage present postoperatively. After tumor removal, the integrity of the sella is then reconstructed. Often a Valsalva maneuver is performed to detect a CSF leak and, if present, the sella is packed with an autologous fat graft

from the abdominal region. At our institution, the endonasal technique is typically favored, with the sublabial approach reserved for patients in whom the transnasal approach would be difficult or contraindicated (e.g., a child with small nostrils).

Anesthetic management

The anesthetic management of patients undergoing transsphenoidal resection of pituitary tumors requires the anesthesiologist to not only consider the surgical aspects of the procedure, but to also have a firm understanding of the unique implications that the underlying neuroendocrine pathology may have in terms of their secondary effect on various body systems. The majority of patients presenting for transsphenoidal pituitary tumor resection will have a non-functioning endocrine tumor producing symptoms of mass effect such as headache, nausea/vomiting, or visual disturbances. Alternatively, some patients will have some pituitary abnormality of hypo- or hypersecretion warranting a thorough evaluation by an endocrinologist prior to surgery. At our institution roughly 60% of patients undergoing surgery have a nonfunctional tumor (or express gonadotropins on immunohistochemical staining only). Fifteen percent have acromegaly, 15% Cushing's disease, 5% have prolactin-secreting tumors, and 5% have a craniopharyngioma or Rathke's cleft cyst.

Preoperative evaluation

As with any patient undergoing a neurosurgical procedure, a routine preoperative workup for transsphenoidal pituitary resection patients would include a history and physical examination with emphasis on the neurologic system. A full neurologic evaluation that includes mental status, cranial nerve function,

Anesthesia for Otolaryngologic Surgery, ed. Basem Abdelmalak and D. John Doyle. Published by Cambridge University Press.
© Cambridge University Press 2013.

motor and sensory testing, reflexes, and coordination testing should be documented prior to surgery in order to properly assess any postoperative deviations. Additionally, any comorbidity such as cardiovascular disease, respiratory disease, or renal disease should be adequately evaluated, with further testing completed as warranted by the specific patient requirements. Previous surgeries and anesthetic experiences are important data prior to proceeding with surgery. Laboratory work should include a complete blood count, basic chemistry panel, and, if indicated, coagulation studies.

Neuroimaging with computerized tomography (CT) and magnetic resonance imaging (MRI) is essential for a differential diagnosis, to plan the surgical approach, and to assess the configuration of the sphenoid sinus. MRI T_1-weighted images, with and without intravenous contrast, define the anatomy of the sella and the relationship of the lesion to the parasellar structures, including the cavernous sinus and the carotid arteries, and the optic chiasm. T_2-weighted images help visualize cystic lesions within the sella. Coronal images help define the location of the internal carotid arteries, the distance between them, and the presence of ectatic loops which to a substantial degree the surgeon should be aware of prior to a transsphenoidal approach. CT scans are preferred to MR imaging to define the three types of sphenoid sinus, namely, presellar (partially), sellar (completely), and conchal (solid) sinus, based on the degree of pneumatization. It also helps define the location of the intersphenoid septum to the sella and the location of its insertion in relation to the carotid arteries, enabling the surgeon to utilize knowledge of this anatomy to maintain midline orientation during surgery.

Prior to surgery, a complete neuroendocrine evaluation is required and should include a thyroid panel, as well as serum levels of cortisol, adrenocorticotropic hormone (ACTH), testosterone, follicle stimulating hormone, luteinizing hormone, and prolactin. A pregnancy test should be obtained in women of childbearing age. Pre- and perioperative hormone replacement may be indicated to medically optimize the patient prior to undergoing transsphenoidal pituitary resection [2].

Nonfunctioning pituitary tumors

Patients with nonfunctioning pituitary tumors will often present later in the course of the disease with tumors larger than 1 cm (pituitary macroadenoma). Patients with macroadenomas typically present with headaches or signs of local cranial nerve compression

(visual disturbances). Rarely, these patients may have signs of elevated intracranial pressure (ICP) that must be taken into consideration during anesthetic management. The conditions of hypopituitarism, hypothyroidism and adrenal insufficiency must also be ruled out or managed with perioperative hormone replacement in this subset of patients.

Functioning pituitary tumors

When the pituitary tumor is functional in nature, the neuroendocrine workup will be essential in guiding the evaluation of comorbidities secondary to the associated endocrine dysfunction. Typically, a functioning pituitary tumor is a single-cell-type tumor that presents with signs and symptoms associated with overproduction of the associated hormone. The clinical condition associated with each type of functional pituitary tumor requires special consideration.

Patients with acromegaly have overproduction of growth hormone from the pituitary, and the secondary effects of this hormone excess present a wide range of challenges to the anesthesiologist. Acromegalic patients express a characteristic phenotype, including soft tissue and bony hypertrophy of the oral, pharyngeal, and laryngeal structures, which may narrow the airway [3]. Obstructive sleep apnea (OSA) is common in acromegalic patients as well. Predictably, these characteristics are a frequent cause of difficult tracheal intubation [4], and require the immediate availability of alternative ventilation and intubation tools prior to the start of anesthesia induction. Cardiovascular disturbances such as hypertension, conduction disorders, cardiomegaly, and valvular disease are a major cause of mortality and morbidity in acromegalic patients [5] and appropriate cardiovascular workup, which must include echocardiography, is essential. Diabetes mellitus is also associated with acromegaly and perioperative blood glucose monitoring should be performed.

Cushing's disease is caused by the overproduction of ACTH and has secondary effects on organ systems important to the anesthesiologist. Ischemic heart disease, left ventricular hypertrophy, and systemic hypertension are common [6] and represent a significant cause of perioperative morbidity. Diabetes mellitus, osteoporosis, skin fragility, and possible exophthalmos are other common conditions associated with Cushing's disease that demand attention in the operating room. Cushingoid patients also have a higher body mass index, with concomitant OSA, which may make tracheal intubation unpredictable.

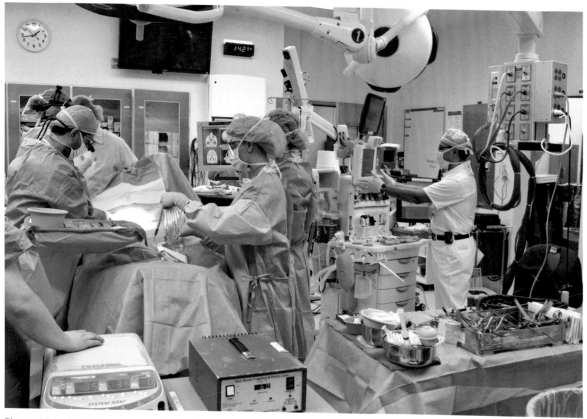

Figure 14.1. Operating room organization. The patient is supine and the head is positioned slightly away from the center of the operating room. The primary surgeon should stand to the right of the patient. Anesthesia team and equipment are placed on the left side of the patient near the head. Neuronavigation is optimally placed to adequately visualize the localizing device, at the same time allowing easy visualization for the main operator and assistant.

Prolactinomas are encountered more frequently in woman than in men, and constitute the most frequently encountered hyperfunctioning pituitary adenoma in patients, although most do not undergo transsphenoidal resection of the lesion. While hyperprolactinemia causes endocrine-related conditions in both men and woman, the effects of these disorders typically are not associated with specific concerns to the anesthesiologist. Of note, medical therapy for hyperprolactinemia may consist of the use of bromocriptine, a dopamine agonist, therefore warranting careful use or avoidance of butyrophenone antiemetics (i.e., droperidol).

Operative room setup and procedural planning

The use of the fluoroscope (C-arm) to help localize and direct the approach to the sphenoid sinus has

been gradually taken over by neuronavigation in most modern operative neurosurgical units [7]. At the authors' institution, the setup is such that the patient's head is positioned slightly away from the center of the room, away from the anesthesia team. Neuronavigation is placed in front of the operating surgeon to be more convenient to visualize the approach at any point of time during surgery. The surgical team usually stands to the right of the patient, with the nurse and equipment at the foot end of the operating table (Figure 14.1).

Intraoperative management

Tracheal intubation can be performed with a standard endotracheal tube; however, some neurosurgeons may prefer a reinforced tube or an oral RAE tube. Nasal intubation should be avoided due to the nature of the surgical approach. As mentioned previously, patients

135

with acromegaly or Cushing's disease may be difficult to ventilate and intubate, and alternative intubating techniques such as awake fiberoptic intubation may be indicated. Once intubated, securing the endotracheal tube to the left side of the mouth, avoiding tape over the upper lip, maximizes operating conditions for the surgeon. The surgeon, to minimize drainage into the oropharynx, often places a throat pack.

A second peripheral intravenous line is placed and invasive blood pressure monitoring, typically via radial artery catheterization, should be considered in patients with coexisting heart disease, or with poorly controlled hypertension. A central venous line is not necessary in most patients with adequate peripheral access unless indicated by the presence of cardiovascular comorbidity in the patient.

After intubation, in order to decrease the amount of bleeding and to optimize surgical conditions, the surgeon preps the nasal mucosa using a combination of local anesthetic and a vasoconstrictive agent such as phenylephrine or epinephrine. Although systemic absorption of these agents is usually minimal, inadvertent intravascular injection of these agents may result in cardiac arrhythmias or severe hypertension [8,9]. Therefore, vigilant monitoring of EKG and blood pressure is important during this phase of the procedure. The use of non-selective β-blockers to treat the hypertension may result in unopposed alpha activity of epinephrine, thereby worsening the hypertension. In such cases, phentolamine or a direct-acting vasodilator may be required.

Positioning of the patient supine with the upper torso elevated helps facilitate venous return from the head. While this semi-seated position may increase the risk of venous air embolism (VAE), the angle of head elevation is usually not severe enough to warrant placement of intracardiac air detection devices such as transesophageal echo or precordial Doppler. At our institution, Mayfield pins position the patient's head with the neck slightly extended and turned to the right, allowing adequate space for midline approach by a right-handed surgeon. The anesthesia circuit is then secured down the left side of the patient, anticipating access to the right abdominal area for fat graft harvesting. Careful arrangement of peripheral intravenous lines, monitoring wires and the anesthesia breathing circuit prior to draping is required to allow unhindered access to the patient's head.

The goals of anesthetic management for transsphenoidal pituitary resection include the maintenance of hemodynamic stability, optimization of surgical conditions, sustaining cerebral perfusion and oxygenation, and rapid emergence. Specific challenges to these goals inherent to the transsphenoidal approach include increased stimulation as compared to the transcranial approach and the critical nature of immobility of the patient due to the proximity of the brain tissue and neurovasculature to the surgical field. An inhaled volatile-agent-based maintenance plan with muscle paralysis and intravenous titration of short-acting opioids will often provide adequate surgical conditions. However, in some patients the associated increase in CSF pressure from inhaled agents may be undesirable [10,11]. Total intravenous anesthesia regimens consisting of propofol and opioid infusions with muscle paralysis avoid the increase in CSF pressure seen with inhaled gas-based techniques while providing acceptable surgical conditions [12]. Frequently, we use an inhaled gas with low solubility (sevoflurane) combined with an opioid infusion such as remifentanil. The use of remifentanil allows rapid emergence while providing hemodynamic stability during the operation [13]. Alternative narcotic infusions used include fentanyl infusion 2 μg/kg/h or sufentanil infusion 0.4 μg/kg/h, which have provided clinically apparent smooth emergence from anesthesia

At the end of the procedure, insertion of nasal packing by the surgeon aids in hemostasis and helps prevent oozing of fluids into the oropharynx. Prior to extubation, meticulous suctioning of the oropharynx is performed. If a sublabial approach is necessary, the surgeon may perform suctioning of the oropharynx under direct visualization. Extubation should proceed once the patient meets extubation criteria. To prevent coughing that might lead to dislodgement of the packing material, low-dose remifentanil infusion or lidocaine bolus (0.5 mg/kg) intravenously may be used immediately before extubation. Once extubated, the patient receives supplemental oxygen via a simple mask. Due to the nasal packing, positive-pressure ventilation through a mask should be avoided. The use of an oral airway may be required for patients with OSA. In patients who do not require preoperative glucocorticoid replacement therapy, strict avoidance of perioperative corticosteroids is practiced in order to preserve the validity of postoperative hypothalamic–pituitary–adrenal (HPA) axis testing. Pre-emergence administration of a 5HT-3 receptor antagonist or butyrophenones is used to prevent nausea/vomiting and is based on patient risk factors.

Table 14.1. Potential complications of the transsphenoidal approach

Anesthetic/perioperative (2.8%)	
Local nasal/sinus complications [19]	Septal perforations [20] (6.7%), epistaxis (3.4%), sinusitis (8.5%)
Intrasellar/parasellar	CSF leak (3.9%), meningitis (1.5%), carotid artery injury (1.1%)
Neurological	Vision loss (1.8%), ophthalmoplegia (1.4%), CNS injury (1.3%)
Endocrinological	Pituitary insufficiency (19.4%), diabetes insipidus (17.8%)

Postoperative/recovery

Patients undergoing transsphenoidal pituitary resection should be observed in the post-anesthesia care unit by personnel trained to perform an accurate screening of the patient's neurologic system, including careful assessment of cranial nerve function. Due to the proximity of the cranial nerves II–VI to the pituitary region, any postoperative visual field deficits or extraocular motility dysfunction should be reported to the surgical team for consideration of immediate postoperative brain imaging or possible re-exploration under general anesthesia. Excessive rhinorrhea should prompt investigation of a possible CSF leak, especially when accompanied by headache. Opioids or nonsteroidal drugs are used to treat incision pain associated with transsphenoidal resections, but narcotics should be titrated carefully in a patient with OSA.

After transsphenoidal pituitary resection, most patients remain in the hospital for 24–48 hours for continued monitoring of neurologic status and for the required postoperative testing of endocrine function. Although nearly all patients with normal HPA axis function preoperatively do not require postoperative hormone replacement [14], all patients should be screened for hypopituitarism after tumor removal. At our institution, a morning total serum cortisol level above 15 μg/dl postoperatively is used as a predictor of normal HPA axis function [15,16]. In addition to pituitary function studies, all patients are monitored for disorders of water imbalance. Diabetes insipidus (DI) can occur after transsphenoidal pituitary resection and, although usually transient, may require administration of desmopressin (DDAVP). Alternatively, the syndrome of inappropriate antidiuretic hormone secretion (SIADH) may develop spontaneously after surgery or by excessive use of exogenous DDAVP. Hyponatremia associated with SIADH may require treatment with free-water restriction or, if severe, hypertonic saline can be used for treatment.

Complications

Potential complications of the transsphenoidal approach to pituitary tumors can be classified as shown in Table 14.1 [17,18]. With an experienced surgeon, transsphenoidal pituitary resection is a safe and effective treatment for pituitary tumors and major complications are uncommon. While the potential risk of a VAE is increased with a semi-sitting patient, reports of VAE during transsphenoidal surgery are rare [21]. Minimal blood loss is expected during most transsphenoidal pituitary resections; however, the proximity of the lesion to the internal carotid artery (ICA) in some patients can facilitate inadvertent puncture of the vessel, leading to significant blood loss [22]. Hemorrhage due to rupture of the ICA can usually be controlled by direct compression or with a muscle graft. Deliberate hypotension may be needed for suturing of the neurovasculature. Persistent CSF leaks following surgery are uncommon but have the potential to cause severe headaches, meningitis [23], symptomatic pneumocephalus [24] and death.

Summary

Transsphenoidal pituitary resection is a common surgical procedure that offers unique challenges to the anesthesiologist. The heterogeneity of the patient population and their medical condition requires a fundamental knowledge of the nature of pituitary disease and management. Understanding the specific demands of the surgical technique allows the anesthesia provider to facilitate the procedure and increase the efficacy of the intervention. Additionally, predicting and managing the peri- and postoperative complications allows the anesthesiologist to maximize the safety of the patient.

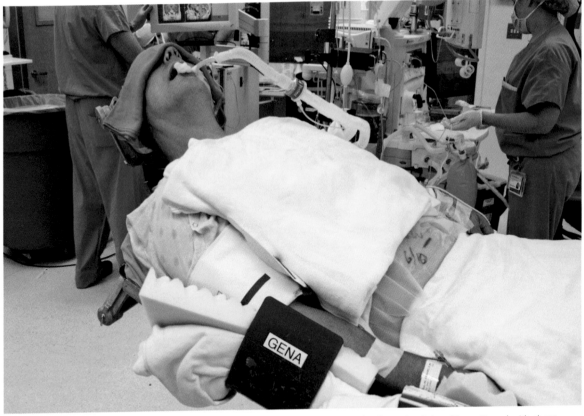

Figure 14.2. Patient positioning. View of the patient from the right (surgical team) side. The patient's head is positioned with about 15° rotation to the right and slight extension, being fixed in a Mayfield head holder. This facilitates access to the surgical site by the right-handed surgeon.

Case study

A 46-year-old man complaining of difficulty sleeping was diagnosed with a pituitary lesion found incidentally on brain MRI performed during workup of suspected central sleep apnea. Further questioning revealed intermittent visual disturbances described as partial loss of visual fields but the patient was unsure whether the symptom was bilateral or unilateral. His past medical history was otherwise normal except for borderline hypertension. He had arthroscopic surgery on both knees and on his left shoulder without any general anesthesia complications. Family history was notable for Huntington's disease in his paternal grandmother and aunt. Physical exam revealed blood pressure of 138/97; pulse 58; weight 106 kg; and height 1.87 m. The rest of the physical exam was unremarkable. Laboratory workup including complete blood count and chemistry panel was normal except for elevated serum glucose of 158 mg/dl. Serum levels of TSH, GH, LH, FSH, and ACTH were all within normal range. A 24-hour urinary cortisol level was elevated at 78 µg. Visual field testing performed 1 month previously revealed superior bitemporal hemianopsia. A brain MRI showed a $27 \times 22 \times 20$ mm^3 sellar and suprasellar lesion with optic nerve compression consistent with pituitary adenoma. It was believed a transnasal transsphenoidal resection of pituitary adenoma was his best option.

On the day of surgery, the patient was brought to the operating room with an 18-gauge peripheral IV. The patient was positioned supine on the operating table and standard ASA monitors were placed. Induction of anesthesia was performed with lidocaine 50 mg, propofol 200 mg, rocuronium 80 mg, and fentanyl 100 µg intravenously. A 7.5 mm cuffed endotracheal tube was positioned under direct laryngoscopy without difficulty. The nasal mucosa was infiltrated with 2% lidocaine and epinephrine (1:100 000) for local anesthesia and hemostasis.

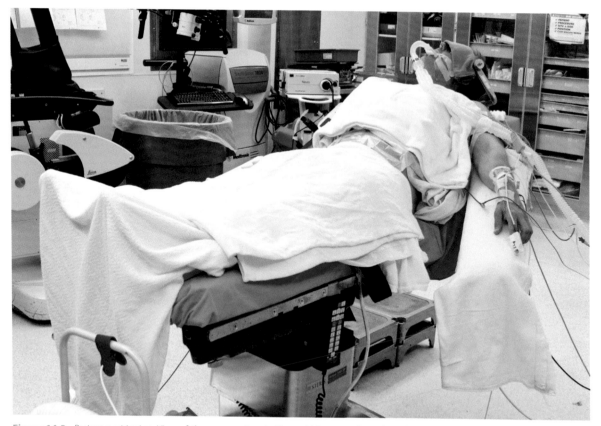

Figure 14.3. Patient positioning. View of the same patient in Figure 14.1 as seen from the left (anesthesia) side. The anesthesia circuit is secured to the left side of the patient to allow access for possible abdominal fat graft harvesting on the side of the surgical team.

A left radial arterial line was placed as was an additional 18-gauge peripheral IV. The patient's head was secured in a Mayfield clamp, and then placed in a semi-seated position with the neck slightly extended and rotated to the right (Figures 14.2 and 14.3). The patient's arms were tucked and a warm air blanket was positioned over the patient's lower torso, allowing room for a possible abdominal fat graft. The chest was covered with blankets, and a skin temperature probe was placed in the left axilla. The anesthesia machine was positioned to the patient's left, allowing the surgeon full access to the head. Surgical instruments were located towards the patient's feet to ensure adequate access to the patient by the operating microscope, frameless stereotaxic equipment, and, if needed, a fluoroscopy machine (Figure 14.4).

Anesthesia maintenance with 0.5 MAC sevoflurane and remifentanil infusion (0.05–0.2 µg/kg/min) was used and adjusted to maintain adequate cerebral perfusion pressure in accordance with the patient's blood pressure. Muscle paralysis was maintained with periodic boluses of rocuronium. An ABG was analyzed 1 hour after surgical start time to monitor the patient's blood count and chemistry values including serum glucose, which was 130 mg/dl. The surgery proceeded uneventfully, and 30 min prior to the end of surgery 4 mg of ondansetron was administered IV. After closure of the surgical site, the sevoflurane was discontinued and remifentanil continued at 0.05 µg/kg/min. Neostigmine 4 mg and glycopyrrolate 0.8 mg were administered for reversal of neuromuscular blockade and the patient was extubated after following commands of hand squeezing and demonstrating protective airway reflexes. The remifentanil infusion was discontinued. The patient was admitted to the recovery room and frequent neurological checks revealed no abnormalities in cranial nerve function. Postoperative serum studies including complete blood count and comprehensive metabolic panel were normal. He was discharged to the neurosurgical floor after 2 hours of recovery room monitoring. On the first postoperative day, his morning serum

139

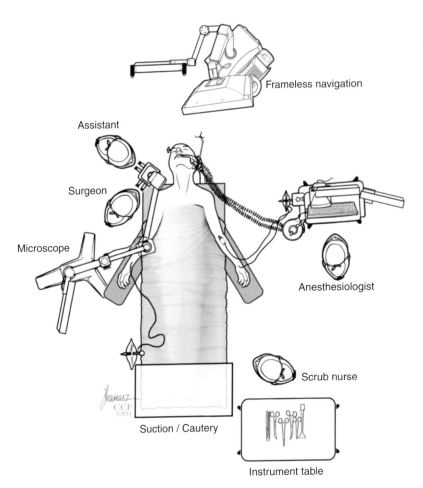

Figure 14.4. Operating room organization. With the patient properly positioned, the nursing team and instrument table are placed near the patient's feet to provide the ability for the microscope, frameless navigation system and possibly fluoroscopy to access the head. Reprinted with permission, Cleveland Clinic Center for Medical Art & Photography © 2012. All rights reserved.

cortisol level was 46.6 μg/dl; having passed his pre-operative ACTH stimulation test and with adequate level > 15 μg/dl on postoperative day one, supplemental adrenal steroids were not indicated [16]. The patient complained of mild head pain, which was improved with oral pain medication. There was no evidence of diabetes insipidus (DI). He was discharged home on the evening of postoperative day one with scheduled follow-up in an outpatient neurosurgery clinic, where repeat endocrinological studies, including an ACTH stimulation test, were normal.

Clinical pearls

- Two transsphenoidal approaches to the sella region exist: (1) a sublabial approach that involves an incision made beneath the upper lip into the gum and subsequently through the septum and (2) a transnasal approach involving dissection

through the nasal cavity wall using instruments inserted through the nostrils.

- Insertion of a CSF drain in the lumbar region may be used to manipulate CSF levels in order to optimize surgical conditions. Injection of saline or air through the drain and into the spinal column may help the lesion descend into the surgical field.
- The majority of patients presenting for transsphenoidal pituitary tumor resection will have a nonfunctioning endocrine tumor producing mass effect symptoms such as headache, nausea/vomiting, or visual disturbances. Alternatively, some patients will have some pituitary abnormality of hypo- or hypersecretion warranting an evaluation by an endocrinologist.
- A neurologic evaluation that includes mental status, cranial nerve function, motor and sensory testing, reflexes, and coordination testing should

be documented prior to surgery in order to properly assess any postoperative deviations.

- Acromegalic patients have soft tissue and bony hypertrophy of the oral, pharyngeal, and laryngeal structures, which may narrow the airway. OSA is common in acromegalic patients as well. Predictably, these characteristics are a frequent cause of difficult tracheal intubation.

- The goals of anesthetic management for transsphenoidal pituitary resection include the maintenance of hemodynamic stability, optimization of surgical conditions, sustaining cerebral perfusion and oxygenation, and smooth emergence.

- In patients who do not require preoperative glucocorticoid replacement therapy, strict avoidance of perioperative corticosteroids is practiced in order to preserve the validity of

postoperative hypothalamic–pituitary–adrenal (HPA) axis testing.

- Due to the proximity of the cranial nerves II–VI to the pituitary region, any postoperative visual field deficits or extraocular motility dysfunction should be reported to the surgical team for consideration of immediate postoperative brain imaging or possible re-exploration under general anesthesia. Excessive rhinorrhea should prompt investigation of a possible CSF leak.

- Diabetes insipidus (DI) can occur after transsphenoidal pituitary resection and, although usually transient, may require administration of desmopressin (DDAVP). Alternatively, the syndrome of inappropriate antidiuretic hormone secretion (SIADH) may develop spontaneously after surgery or by excessive use of exogenous DDAVP.

References

1. Lanzino G. Transsphenoidal approach to lesions of the sella turcica: historical overview. *Barrow Q* 2002;**18**(3).

2. Inder WJ, Hunt PJ. Glucocorticoid replacement in pituitary surgery: guidelines for perioperative assessment and management. *J Clin Endocrinol Metab* 2002;**87**(6):2745–50.

3. Seidman PA, Kofke WA, Policare R, Young M. Anaesthetic complications of acromegaly. *Br J Anaesth* 2000;**84**(2):179–82.

4. Schmitt H, Buchfelder M, Radespiel-Troger M, Fahlbusch R. Difficult intubation in acromegalic patients: incidence and predictability. *Anesthesiology* 2000;**93**(1):110–4.

5. Rajasoorya C, Holdaway IM, Wrightson P, Scott DJ, Ibbertson HK. Determinants of clinical outcome and survival in acromegaly. *Clin Endocrinol (Oxf)* 1994;**41**(1):95–102.

6. Arnaldi G, Angeli A, Atkinson AB, *et al.* Diagnosis and complications of Cushing's syndrome: a consensus statement.

J Clin Endocrinol Metab 2003; **88**(12):5593–602.

7. Kaye AH, Black PML. *Operative Neurosurgery*. London: Churchill Livingstone; 2000.

8. Pasternak JJ, Atkinson JL, Kasperbauer JL, Lanier WL. Hemodynamic responses to epinephrine-containing local anesthetic injection and to emergence from general anesthesia in transsphenoidal hypophysectomy patients. *J Neurosurg Anesthesiol* 2004; **16**(3):189–95.

9. Chelliah YR, Manninen PH. Hazards of epinephrine in transsphenoidal pituitary surgery. *J Neurosurg Anesthesiol* 2002; **14**(1):43–6.

10. Talke P, Caldwell J, Dodsont B, Richardson CA. Desflurane and isoflurane increase lumbar cerebrospinal fluid pressure in normocapnic patients undergoing transsphenoidal hypophysectomy. *Anesthesiology* 1996;**85**(5): 999–1004.

11. Talke P, Caldwell JE, Richardson CA. Sevoflurane increases lumbar cerebrospinal fluid pressure in normocapnic patients undergoing

transsphenoidal hypophysectomy. *Anesthesiology* 1999;**91**(1):127–30.

12. Cafiero T, Cavallo LM, Frangiosa A, *et al.* Clinical comparison of remifentanil-sevoflurane vs. remifentanil-propofol for endoscopic endonasal transphenoidal surgery. *Eur J Anaesthesiol* 2007;**24**(5):441–6.

13. Gemma M, Tommasino C, Cozzi S, *et al.* Remifentanil provides hemodynamic stability and faster awakening time in transsphenoidal surgery. *Anesth Analg* 2002;**94**(1):163–8.

14. Jane JA Jr, Laws ER Jr. The surgical management of pituitary adenomas in a series of 3,093 patients. *J Am Coll Surg* 2001; **193**(6):651–9.

15. Marko NF, Gonugunta VA, Hamrahian AH, *et al.* Use of morning serum cortisol level after transsphenoidal resection of pituitary adenoma to predict the need for long-term glucocorticoid supplementation. *J Neurosurg* 2009;**111**(3):540–4.

16. Marko NF, Hamrahian AH, Weil RJ. Immediate postoperative cortisol levels accurately predict postoperative

hypothalamic-pituitary-adrenal axis function after transsphenoidal surgery for pituitary tumors. *Pituitary [Research Support, Non-U.S. Gov't]* 2010;**13**(3):249–55.

17. Ciric I, Ragin A, Baumgartner C, Pierce D. Complications of transsphenoidal surgery: results of a national survey, review of the literature, and personal experience. *Neurosurgery [Research Support, Non-U.S. Gov't Review]* 1997;**40** (2):225–36; discussion 236–7.

18. Black PM, Zervas NT, Candia GL. Incidence and management of complications of transsphenoidal operation for pituitary adenomas. *Neurosurgery* 1987;**20**(6): 920–4.

19. Nabe-Nielsen J. Nasal complication after transsphenoidal surgery for pituitary pathologies. *Acta Neurochir (Wien) [Research Support, Non-U.S. Gov't]* 1989; **96**(3–4):122–5.

20. Sherwen PJ, Patterson WJ, Griesdale DE. Transseptal, transsphenoidal surgery: a subjective and objective analysis of results. *J Otolaryngol* 1986;**15**(3):155–60.

21. Arora R, Chablani D, Rath GP, Prabhakar H. Pulmonary oedema following venous air embolism during transsphenoidal pituitary surgery. *Acta Neurochir (Wien)* 2007;**149**(11):1177–8.

22. Fukushima T, Maroon JC. Repair of carotid artery perforations during transsphenoidal surgery. *Surg Neurol* 1998;**50**(2): 174–7.

23. Kaptain GJ, Kanter AS, Hamilton DK, Laws ER. Management and implications of intraoperative cerebrospinal fluid leak in transnasoseptal transsphenoidal microsurgery. *Neurosurgery* 2011;**68**(1 Suppl Operative): 144–50; discussion 150–1.

24. Rao G, Apfelbaum RI. Symptomatic pneumocephalus occurring years after transphenoidal surgery and radiation therapy for an invasive pituitary tumor: a case report and review of the literature. *Pituitary [Case Reports Review]* 2003;**6**(1):49–52.

Chapter

15

Anesthesia for neck dissection and laryngectomy

David W. Healy and Carol R. Bradford

Introduction/background

Cancers of the aerodigestive system are rare. Each year they account for 2.5% of the new cases of cancer in North America [1]. Of these, there are approximately 3560 new cases of laryngeal cancer. Squamous cell carcinoma is the most common type. The major risk factors for the development of laryngeal cancers are tobacco and alcohol use, acting synergistically to increase the risk of cancer [2]. The 5 year survival rate for laryngeal squamous cell carcinoma is 64% [3].

Mortality has remained largely unchanged over the past 20 years [1], with some authorities reporting a decline in survival [3], occurring despite improvement in surgical techniques, supplemented by perioperative chemotherapy and radiotherapy. Recent research has focused on molecular biology to provide new treatment options and target therapy.

The terms neck dissection and laryngectomy describe a wide variety of surgical procedures that attempt to remove a cancer and its main route of spread. The extent of a given procedure is dictated by the extent of the cancer. Neck dissection is commonly performed in the treatment of different cancers of the head and neck to remove metastatic tumor deposits and the route of spread. Balancing anesthesia for the surgical requirements of these procedures can be a significant challenge.

Surgical procedures

The treatment of laryngeal cancer has three primary goals:

1. Tumor removal.
2. Prevention of spread and recurrence
3. Preservation of organ function (phonation and swallowing) if possible.

Partial laryngectomy

Partial laryngectomy is performed in an attempt to remove the tumor but preserve the organ or its function [4]. Limited disease may also be treated by laser and microsurgery.

Total laryngectomy

Total laryngectomy is the removal of the larynx in its entirety. A tracheal stoma is formed by bringing the cut end of the trachea to the neck surface. The trachea is therefore independent of the esophagus, which remains in continuity with the oral cavity and pharynx. During the procedure a perforation is made between the trachea and esophagus (tracheoesophageal puncture – TEP) to allow later placement of a voice prosthesis. The prosthesis allows air to pass into the pharynx and oral cavity when the tracheal stoma is occluded, thereby allowing the maintenance of voice. It consists of a one-way valve, preventing secretions and food soiling the trachea and respiratory tract (Figure 15.1). Occasionally the procedure is supplemented with microvascular free tissue transfer (see Chapter 14), which may be required for pharyngeal reconstruction after laryngo-pharyngectomy or in an attempt to prevent cutaneous fistula formation due to poor tissue quality after chemo-radiation.

Neck dissection

Neck dissection is commonly performed during laryngectomy for cancer to prevent and treat any local spread of the primary disease.

The lymph nodes of the neck are divided into six main levels [5], which are further subdivided according to the degree of metastatic spread (Figure 15.2). The extent of a neck dissection can be described

Anesthesia for Otolaryngologic Surgery, ed. Basem Abdelmalak and D. John Doyle. Published by Cambridge University Press.
© Cambridge University Press 2013.

(a)

(b)

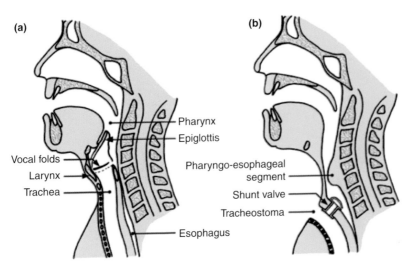

Pharynx
Epiglottis
Vocal folds
Larynx
Trachea
Pharyngo-esophageal segment
Shunt valve
Tracheostoma
Esophagus

Figure 15.1. Sagittal section of the head and neck region (a) before laryngectomy, and (b) after laryngectomy with a shunt valve placed in the wall between the trachea and esophagus. Reproduced with kind permission from Springer Science and Business Media: *Annals of Biomedical Engineering* 2006;**34**: 1897, Tack, J.W. Figure 15.1. All rights reserved.

according to the number of lymph node levels dissected and removed, and the degree of removal of additional structures. The procedure is termed selective when the contents of a limited lymph level or levels are removed, or radical when all lymph nodes and some additional structures (spinal accessory nerve, internal jugular vein, and sternocleidomastoid muscle) are removed. The procedure is said to be modified when something less than the radical neck dissection is performed, but more extensive than the purely selective neck dissection.

Anesthetic management

Preoperative evaluation

A careful airway evaluation is an essential part of preparation for a patient undergoing laryngectomy with neck dissection. A history of previous difficult direct laryngoscopy and intubation should be sought, and must be considered in light of more recent changes to the airway due to pathology or treatment. For example, preoperative radiation may have been used to shrink the tumor and reduce metastatic spread. Neck radiation changes can make airway management difficult as its presence is an independent predictor of failure for both bag-mask ventilation and Glidescope intubation [6,7]. The assessment should be supplemented by nasendoscopy, performed in clinic by the otolaryngologist, as well as neck computerized tomography (CT) findings where available.

If the airway findings are unfavorable a method of intubation maintaining spontaneous ventilation is recommended [8]. During assessment, consideration of an awake tracheostomy should always be given. The performance of an awake tracheostomy decision should be made during discussion between the otolaryngologist and the anesthesiologist with consideration given to any symptoms of airway obstruction, tumor location, and appearance on nasendoscopy. For example, a friable, invasive tumor, located above or within the glottis, with symptoms of airway obstruction will usually be managed with awake tracheostomy. If intubation from above is considered, one method is to perform awake fiberoptic intubation; however, other methods such as awake videolaryngoscopy (Glidescope™, Airtraq™, Pentax AWS™) have been described in this setting [9–11]. Deep inhalation anesthesia with standard direct laryngoscopy is yet another option.

Patients with head and neck cancer are frequently elderly and often have comorbidites associated with tobacco and alcohol ingestion. All patients should have a cardiac workup guided by symptomatology and functional capacity. Regarding overall cardiovascular assessment, major head and neck surgery is classified as intermediate-risk surgery (1–5% risk of preoperative myocardial infarction or death) according to the American College of Cardiology/American Heart Association (ACC/AHA) guidelines [12]. The presence of active cardiac conditions, cardiac risk factors, and level of functional capacity should guide further preoperative cardiac investigations. A baseline electrocardiogram is often performed. In general it is advisable for patients to continue their daily β-blocker and withhold ACE inhibitors and angiotensin receptor blockers (ARBs) on the day of surgery [13].

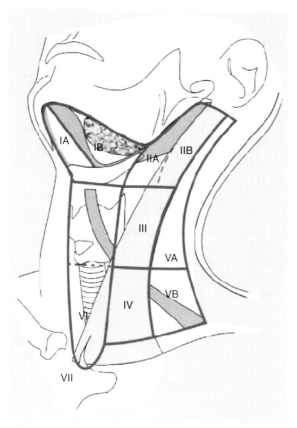

Figure 15.2. Anatomic diagram of the neck depicting the boundaries of the six neck levels and three neck sub-levels. Reproduced with permission from the *Archives of Otolaryngology Head and Neck Surgery* 134(5); 536–8, 2008. Copyright © 2008 American Medical Association. All rights reserved.

Chronic obstructive pulmonary disease is associated with smoking. A complete history should be taken looking for any recent breathing difficulty, precipitating factors of dyspnea, β-agonist reversibility, and recent episodes of infection (increasing symptoms with sputum). The goal is optimization of their current respiratory condition and avoidance of complications (worsening symptoms, infection, or respiratory failure).

Nutritional status is extremely important as the patient's intake may be limited in the period before surgery. This should be optimized by dietician advice before surgery and may require supplementation by enteral feed (via a small-bore feeding tube) in the perioperative period.

Patients should be instructed in the use of a patient-controlled analgesia device (PCA) before surgery. Methods of communication (especially regarding pain, nausea, and comfort) should be discussed and practiced before surgery as the patient may be without a voice for a variable period of time.

A blood sample for a blood type and antibody screen should be sent from the preoperative area, for instance during initial IV access. If antibodies are detected two units of blood should be cross-matched immediately. If blood can be made available and delivered to the operating room within 30 minutes, a cross-match is not required if significant antibody interactions are absent from the initial screen.

Intraoperative management

Access and monitoring

Intravenous access should occur in the preoperative area and a blood sample sent for a CBC and cross-match. Other blood tests should be guided by patient morbidity and drug history.

Standard monitoring is commenced with an additional five-lead electrocardiogram.

The decision to place an arterial line, before induction of anesthesia, should be guided by the patient's comorbidities. Surgical requirements do not necessitate it to be placed before induction.

Anesthesia is induced through a small IV (18 gauge) then a large bore IV is placed after induction. The practice preference of the author for the second IV access line is to place a 14-gauge IV in the lower limb saphenous vein; however, others place a large IV in the upper limb.

For deep vein thrombosis prophylaxis a pneumatic intermittent calf compression is commenced before induction and a subcutaneous dose of heparin is often given.

Induction and maintenance

For an asleep intubation technique we induce with propofol and fentanyl, and give an intermediate-acting neuromuscular blocking agent (vecuronium). Nerve function monitoring is required later in the case during neck dissection; however, neuromuscular blockade is useful at the beginning of the procedure. We check neuromuscular function with a neuromuscular twitch monitor before dosing vecuronium to ensure correct lead placement.

Anesthesia is maintained with inhaled isoflurane (or any other inhalational anesthetic). Intense analgesia or deep inhalational anesthesia is required to allow the return of neuromuscular function as the surgeons start

145

the neck dissection phase of the procedure. Potent opioid infusions (e.g., remifentanil or sufentanil) are beneficial to maintain a constant depth of adequate analgesia with a standard depth of inhaled anesthesia. Another method to allow the return of neuromuscular function is the "single agent technique" where deep sedation using high concentrations of inhalational anesthesia is used. Intravenous anesthesia with propofol is another option but can accumulate during long surgeries. A balanced anesthetic technique is preferable to deep inhalational anesthetic or total intravenous anesthetic (propofol) techniques; to avoid the hypotension associated with the latter two techniques.

An estimate of filling pressure to guide fluid balance is important. At The University of Michigan we use the systolic pressure variation of the arterial line tracing to help guide fluid replacement [14]. Alternatively a central line, at a different location from the neck dissection, may be placed after a consideration of risk–benefit. We use crystalloid to replace the preoperative fasting deficit, followed by a combination of colloid (starch) and crystalloid to replace losses. The hematocrit is monitored with intermittent arterial blood gas measurements. Of note, excessive crystalloid administration should be avoided as it may lead to swelling of the operative site.

A tracheostomy is performed by the surgeons at the beginning of the case; an appropriately sized armored endotracheal tube should be available in the surgical field.

The patient is then often turned 180° from the anesthesia machine. Care must be taken to ensure that all monitors and infusion lines make the turn intact. There are many methods to ensure success, and these are best taught under instruction in the operating room.

Emergence

The prime goals at emergence from anesthesia in any head and neck case should be the provision of adequate analgesia, cardiovascular stability, and the prevention of coughing. If using a short-acting opioid infusion for the case, such as remifentanil, extra longer-acting opioid (e.g., morphine) should be given in good time to be active at extubation and continued as required through the immediate recovery period. Alternatively the patient may emerge on a low-dose opioid infusion (e.g., remifentanil) allowing a gradual return of spontaneous ventilation. Supplemental opioid

analgesia is then provided in the post-anesthesia care unit (PACU).

Extubation is relatively simple, removing the endotracheal tube from the tracheal stoma (the end of the trachea brought out to the anterior neck) once spontaneous ventilation is well established with an adequate minute volume. This should occur after the patient has been turned back 180° with the head near the anesthesia machine. An oxygen face mask is placed around the neck to deliver supplemental oxygen during emergence.

Postoperative/recovery

The patient should be transferred to the PACU with supplemental oxygen and portable pulse oximetry. Full monitoring should be quickly resumed, and attention paid to adequacy of ventilation and oxygenation.

Humidified oxygen should be supplied via a tracheostomy mask. A PCA should be provided. Communication via a pick board or writing paper should be focused on eliciting any evidence of pain or distress to allow expeditious treatment.

Care is then transferred to either the ICU or step-down unit as the patient will generally not require ventilatory support, but will require care of the fresh tracheal stoma.

Complications

Major:

- respiratory failure
- myocardial ischemia
- pulmonary embolus secondary to deep vein thrombosis
- nerve injury (dependent upon extent of neck dissection); most commonly accessory nerve to trapezius
- hematoma formation; may be precipitated by coughing or hypertension at emergence

Summary

The terms neck dissection and laryngectomy describe a wide variety of surgical procedures that attempt to remove a cancer and its main route of spread. The extent of procedures is dictated by the extent of the cancer. Similarly, the anesthetic care of patients undergoing such procedures can involve a wide variety of techniques, the key features of which should be: careful assessment and management of the airway; management of co-morbidities associated with smoking, alcohol and aging; and a technique that facilitates the return of neuromuscular function during the neck dissection with the goal being the prevention of surgical nerve injury.

Case study
Description

The patient is a 52-year-old male, 5′11″ (180 cm) in height, weighing 258 lbs (117 kg), with a history of coronary artery disease (drug-eluting stent placed in LAD artery 2 years prior to the scheduled surgery), hypertension, and multiple sclerosis. He has a remote history of pancreatitis secondary to alcohol 10 years previously; 20 pack year smoking history.

Current medications: aspirin, alprazolam (Xanax), doxazosin (Cardura), glatiramer acetate (Copaxone), rosuvastatin (Crestor), duloxetine (Cymbalta), fentanyl patch, oral morphine, Roxicodone (Oxycodone), metoprolol (Lopressor), spironolactone (Aldactone).

He is obese, BMI 36; HR 62; BP 140/75.

Airway examination reveals poor dentition, good neck extension, with mouth opening > 30 mm, Mallampati 3, a thyromental distance of > 6 cm.

No evidence of tracheal deviation.

Chest clear. Heart sounds heard and normal.

Upper motor neuron signs on examination of the left lower limb.

Contrast CT of the neck revealed an irregular mass involving the epiglottis, vallecula, bilateral aryepiglottic folds and extending to the true vocal cords and anterior commissure (Figure 15.3). Several borderline lymph nodes are present on the left side at levels II and III. These were correlated with increased uptake on PET.

The surgical clinic note revealed nasendoscopy findings of a supraglottic mass involving the vallecula and bilateral aryepiglottic fold, extending to the true vocal cord. He was graded as a T4 N2 M0 squamous cell carcinoma after direct laryngoscopy and biopsy. He had a cycle of induction chemotherapy that resulted in only minimal reduction in size. He was scheduled for total laryngectomy with bilateral selective neck dissection and transesophageal puncture.

Preoperative
Evaluation

This involved an assessment of the severity and extent of comorbidities with consideration of optimization before surgery.

Cardiovascular

Following his drug-eluting stent placement, dual therapy consisting of aspirin and clopidogrel was continued for 1 year after the procedure. Aspirin was continued to protect the stent according to the ACC/AHA guidelines [15]. Given the benefit in terms of preventing cardiac stent occlusion

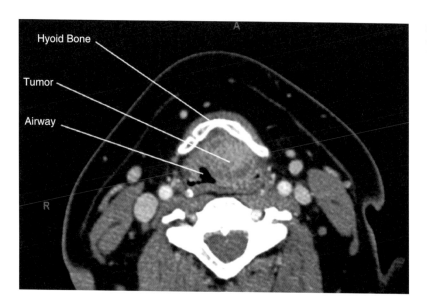

Figure 15.3. Contrast CT scan of neck at level of the hyoid demonstrating the supraglottic carcinoma.

compared with the risk of increased surgical bleeding, aspirin was continued throughout the perioperative period.

Regarding the need for cardiology workup before surgery, major head and neck surgery is classified as intermediate-risk surgery according to the the ACC/AHA guidelines [12]. The patient's functional capacity was low due to obesity, and mild right-sided weakness secondary to multiple sclerosis. If ACC/AHA guidelines are strictly applied the case could continue without further workup and simply with heart rate control. However, the patient saw his cardiologist, who requested a stress echo before surgery. The stress echo demonstrated an ejection fraction of 55% with no evidence of reversible ischemia. The patient's hypertension was well controlled on current medication.

Pain

The patient is on a significant amount of opioid analgesia, which must be considered in the postoperative plan for pain control.

Preparation

IV access in preop with an 18G catheter (dorsum of left hand).

Standard monitors placed + 5 lead EKG.

Preparation for an awake fiberoptic intubation (see Chapter 6: Awake intubation).

Arterial line placed in left radial artery under local anesthesia.

Type and cross blood sample sent to transfusion laboratory

Intraoperative

Remifentanil infusion commenced at 0.02 µg/kg/min for awake intubation.

Awake fiberoptic intubation performed; a size 6.5 plain endotracheal tube (ETT) placed.

Propofol induction 140 mg.

Vecuronium 4 mg.

Remifentanil increased to 0.05 µg/kg/min.

Isoflurane inhalational anesthesia commenced.

Eyes taped.

Sufentanil bolus of 5 µg given, infusion commenced at 0.25 µg/kg/h, remifentanil discontinued.

Patient turned 180° to the anesthesia machine.

Temperature-sensing urinary catheter placed.

Forced-air warmer placed on lower body.

14G catheter IVI placed in left lower limb (saphenous vein); connected to fluid warmer.

Lactated Ringer's (1 liter) given via IVI.

Antibiotics given (ampicillin/sulbactam 1.5 g).

Baseline ABG sent; starting hematocrit (HCT) checked.

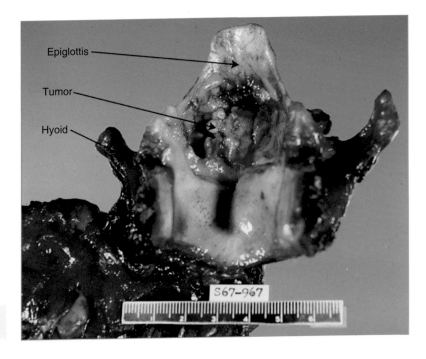

Epiglottis

Tumor

Hyoid

S67-967

Figure 15.4. Specimen post laryngectomy with neck dissection removed "en-bloc". Image courtesy of the Department of Otolaryngology, University of Michigan Health System.

Hetastarch (1 liter) given slowly; guided by blood pressure, heart rate, urine output and systolic pressure variability.

Surgeons perform a tracheostomy; place a 6.5 armored ETT sutured to chest.

Surgeons make sure blue cuff can just be seen at the tracheal site (to avoid endobronchial intubation), end-tidal carbon dioxide returned, and adequate tidal volume with airway pressures $< 30\,cmH_2O$.

Surgeons continue with laryngeal resection and neck dissection.

The tissue sample is removed and sent to pathology (Figure 15.4).

Surgeons form the tracheal stoma.

Emergence

Sufentanil infusion stopped in sufficient time to allow return of spontaneous ventilation, but with residual analgesic efficacy.

Isoflurane anesthetic stopped.

Patient turned back to 0° (head near anesthesia machine).

Gentle suction (via a small endobronchial suction tube) to tracheal stoma.

Spontaneous ventilation returns, augmented by pressure-supported ventilation.

Reduction of pressure support, patient maintains an adequate tidal volume. Patient follows command. Endotracheal tube is removed.

Transport to PACU with supplemental oxygen and pulse oximetry

Postoperative

Patient monitored closely in PACU:

- recovery from anesthesia
- maintain cardiorespiratory stability, fluid balance, temperature control

References

1. R. Siegel, E. Ward, Brawley O, Jemal A. Cancer statistics, 2011: the impact of eliminating socioeconomic and racial disparities on premature cancer deaths. *CA Cancer J Clin* 2011;**61**:212–36.

2. Elwood JM, Pearson JC, Skippen DH, Jackson SM. Alcohol, smoking, social and occupational factors in the aetiology of cancer of the oral cavity, pharynx and larynx. *Int J Cancer* 1984;**34**: 603–12.

3. Hoffman HT, Porter K, Karnell LH, *et al.* Laryngeal cancer in the United States: changes in demographics, patterns of care, and survival. *Laryngoscope* 2006;**116**(Suppl 111): 1–13.

4. Pfister DG, Laurie SA, Weinstein GS, *et al.* American Society of Clinical Oncology clinical practice guideline for the use of larynx-preservation strategies in the treatment of laryngeal cancer. *J Clin Oncol* 2006;**24**:3693–704.

5. Robbins KT, Shaha AR, Medina JE, *et al.* Consensus statement on the classification and terminology of neck dissection. *Arch*

- provide timely and appropriate administration of analgesia and anti-emesis
- commence opioid PCA
- observe surgical site integrity and function of bulb drains then transfer to step-down unit once recovery complete.

Clinical pearls

- The terms neck dissection and laryngectomy describe a wide variety of surgical procedures that attempt to remove a cancer and its main route of spread. The extent of a given procedure is dictated by the extent of the cancer.
- The treatment of laryngeal cancer has three primary goals: tumor removal, prevention of spread and recurrence, and preservation of organ function (phonation and swallowing) where possible.
- A partial laryngectomy is performed in an attempt to remove the tumor but preserve the organ or its function
- During a total laryngectomy a perforation is often made between the trachea and esophagus (tracheoesophageal puncture – TEP) to allow subsequent placement of a voice prosthesis.

  This prosthesis allows air to pass into the pharynx and oral cavity when the tracheal stoma is occluded, thereby allowing the maintenance of voice
- Neck radiation changes can make airway management difficult as its presence is an independent predictor of failure for both bag-mask ventilation and GlideScope intubation.
- Systolic blood pressure variation of the arterial line tracing can help guide fluid replacement. Alternatively a central line, at a different location from the neck dissection, can be used.

Otolaryngol Head Neck Surg 2008;**134**:536–8.

6. Kheterpal S, Martin L, Shanks AM, Tremper KK. Prediction and outcomes of impossible mask ventilation: a review of 50,000 anesthetics. *Anesthesiology* 2009;**110**:891–7.

7. Aziz MF, Healy D, Kheterpal S, *et al.* Routine clinical practice effectiveness of the Glidescope in difficult airway management: an analysis of 2,004 Glidescope intubations, complications, and failures from two institutions. *Anesthesiology* 2011;**114**:34–41.

8. American Society of Anesthesiologists Task Force on Management of the Difficult Airway. Practice guidelines for management of the difficult airway: an updated report by the American Society of Anesthesiologists Task Force on Management of the Difficult Airway. *Anesthesiology* 2003;**98**:1269–77.

9. Doyle DJ. Awake intubation using the GlideScope video laryngoscope: initial experience in four cases. *Can J Anaesth* 2004;**51**:520–1.

10. Dimitriou VK, Zogogiannis ID, Liotiri DG. Awake tracheal intubation using the Airtraq® laryngoscope: a case series. *Acta Anaesthesiol Scand* 2009;**53**:964–7.

11. Suzuki A, Kunisawa T, Takahata O, *et al.* Pentax-AWS (Airway Scope®) for awake tracheal intubation. *J Clin Anesth* 2007;**19**:642–3.

12. Fleisher LA, Beckman JA, Brown KA, *et al.* ACC/AHA 2007 Guidelines on perioperative cardiovascular evaluation and care for noncardiac surgery. *J Am Coll Cardiol* 2007;**50**: 159–242.

13. Coriat P, Richer C, Douraki T, *et al.* Influence of chronic angiotensin-converting enzyme inhibition on anesthetic induction. *Anesthesiology* 1994;**81**:299–307.

14. Rooke GA, Schwid HA, Shapira Y. The effect of graded hemorrhage and intravascular volume replacement on systolic pressure variation in humans during mechanical and spontaneous ventilation. *Anesth Analg* 1995;**80**:925–32.

15. Fleisher LA, Beckman JA, Brown KA, *et al.* 2009 ACCF/AHA focused update on perioperative beta blockade incorporated into the ACC/AHA 2007 guidelines on perioperative cardiovascular evaluation and care for noncardiac surgery: a report of the American College of Cardiology Foundation/ American Heart Association task force on practice guidelines. *Circulation* 2009;**120**:169–276.

Chapter

16

Anesthesia for head and neck flap reconstructive surgery

Edward Noguera, Brian Burkey and Basem Abdelmalak

Introduction

A tissue transfer in the form of a free or a pedicle flap is a surgical technique by which autologous tissue(s) composed of fascia, skin, fat, functioning muscle, nerve or composites is rotated or transferred on a supporting vascular supply. The graft is transferred to a new location of the body by using microvascular surgical techniques (in the free flap) or rotated (in the pedicle flap) to reconstruct anatomical defects in a permanent fashion. Some of the advantages to the use of free flaps in head and neck surgery patients include highly successful reconstruction of complex defects [1], repair of contaminated defects with vascularized flaps leading to improvement of wound healing, better cosmetic results, separation of compartments such as intracranial structures from the digestive tract, improved functionality of critical structures (e.g., the tongue in swallowing), and high tolerance of radiation therapy postoperatively. Thus, such procedures became somewhat routine procedures especially in tertiary and quaternary medical care facilities. For appropriate safe anesthetic care, the anesthesiologists need to have a clear understanding of these surgical procedures, and their implications that affect anesthetic management such as: careful planning for difficult airway management including tracheostomy if airway is compromised, positioning and careful understanding of graft donor and recipient sites considerations, choice of intraoperative monitoring, considerations related to the length of surgery and thermoregulation, flap perfusion considerations, planning postoperative care and level of care. This is in addition to considerations related to coexisting morbidities in this elderly population who commonly present with tobacco and alcohol abuse.

Surgical background/considerations

Flaps can be categorized based on their blood supply. If the flap vessels are transferred intact with the rotated flap, then the tissue is termed a pedicle flap. If the flap is moved from a distant site and the flap vessels are re-anastomosed to the recipient site vessels, then the tissue is termed a microvascular free tissue transfer or "free" flap. In general, pedicle flaps are used when they are adequate to reconstruct an adjacent defect safely and there is no loss of function. Pedicled flaps are highly reliable and can be completed in less time compared to the more labor intensive free flaps. Over the last 20 years, the field of microvascular free tissue transfer has advanced [2] and today the vast majority of complex reconstructions are performed with free flap transfer because of the high success rates, the capacity for replacing head and neck tissue with similar tissue from other areas of the body, and the capacity for complex three-dimensional reconstructions not possible with pedicle flaps secondary to inherent tethering and other anatomic issues [3]. In the majority of patients, the harvest vs. recipient sites of the flap are apart in such a way that it allows for the simultaneous harvest of the flap while the resection is progressing at the recipient site, thus providing for a reduced operative time. This so-called "two-team" approach also allows the individual surgeons to focus all their efforts on only one aspect of the procedure, which has resulted in shorter procedure duration and thus fewer after hours surgery, less surgeon burnout and higher professional satisfaction.

The most common pedicle flaps used are the myocutaneous flaps, such as the pectoralis major myocutaneous flap and the latissimus myocutaneous flap. The former is still popular for reconstruction of lateral pharyngeal wall defects, pharyngeal defects after total laryngectomy, and neck cutaneous defects. Muscle flaps are used to cover the carotid artery after radical neck dissections where the carotid artery is sacrificed and reconstructed with a saphenous vein graft. All the pedicled flaps add little complexity to the surgical or anesthetic management of the head and neck tumor patient, as they can be accomplished quickly and the tissue is fairly close to the primary resection site. As well, vascular issues are less critical since the flap vessels remain intact.

Free tissue transfer reconstruction has provided the reconstructive surgeon with vastly more options for donor sites. The quality, quantity, and availability of each tissue and supporting vascular structures along with donor site characteristics play a major role in flap selection. Factors such as skin and soft tissue volume and color, vessel length and caliber, innervation capacity, bone quality and availability, donor site location, and potential morbidity are all taken into account for final selection. Donor site morbidities include functional losses and cosmetic deformities.

For head and neck surgery patients, a group of patients have been well characterized as gaining the most benefit from free flap reconstructions. These patients typically tend to have poor healing (chemo and radiation therapy exposure, recurrent cancer, prior surgical repairs), defects of the anterior mandibular arch and pharyngoesophageal defects. The most common "free flaps" used in head and neck surgery involve the following.

Fasciocutaneous flaps

These are used to repair small and moderate soft tissue defects. The radial forearm fasciocutaneous flap and anterolateral thigh flap are very reliable and have become the most utilized flaps in the field. Both flaps allow for a two-team approach due to their distant anatomical location from the primary resection site.

Muscle and myocutaneous flaps

These flaps are used to cover large-volume defects. There are two main donors: the rectus abdominis and the latissimus myocutaneous flaps. Both have large-

caliber vessels with adequate pedicles. The skin of the myocutaneous flap provides coverage of relatively large head and neck defects, such as scalp defects, and the muscle provides for good sealing potential of problematic defects, such as CSF leaks. The latissimus muscle is harvested in lateral decubitus position and is therefore less commonly utilized.

Vascularized bone flaps

These are used primarily to reconstruct oromandibular defects. Several options are available: the fibula osteocutaneous flap, the radial forearm osteocutaneous flap, the scapula osteocutaneous flap and the iliac crest-internal oblique osteocutaneous flap. The scapular free flap requires several changes in patient positioning during the procedure and does not allow for a two-team approach, which lengthens the procedure duration [4]. The radial forearm donor site provides high-quality bone and so is used primarily for maxillary reconstructions. The iliac crest flap was highly popular in the early 1990s due to its abundant bone and reliable nature, but its bulk has made it a less popular choice in the USA more recently. The fibula osteocutaneous flap is clearly the workhorse flap for oromandibular reconstruction and constitutes 50–80% of bone flaps in large series [5].

Better understanding of blood supply to different anatomic regions of the body, improvement of techniques and technologies, along with formal training has led to the development and creation of a wide variety of flaps that can potentially be used by reconstructive surgeons. Flap survival rates now average 95% or greater in most series of reconstructions performed by dedicated microvascular surgeons. Moreover, microvascular techniques are now considered the standard of care for the repair of many defects and it is, therefore, expected that anesthesiologists become more familiar with the dominant flaps in use for head and neck surgery and the proper anesthetic management of such cases.

The prognosis of patients requiring such extensive head and neck resections and reconstructions depends on many patient, tumor and other treatment factors; however, it is not unusual to do large combined resections and flap reconstructions that take 8–14 hours on patients with only a 30–60% chance of long-term cure. This is due to several factors. First, patients many times want a reasonable chance of cure no matter the effort and surgery is often a central part of the best treatment, frequently with postoperative radiation therapy. Second, untreated head and neck cancers create horrible local problems during the 6–18 months that will transpire before death, including fistulas, ulcers, severe otalgia and local pain, and tissue necrosis. All this makes surgery a much better option even if cure is unlikely, as it may change the method of death and allow the patient to have quality time with family and to pursue lifelong goals of travel, etc. Finally, the maturation of free flap reconstruction has allowed extensive surgery with a minimal impact on cosmesis and function, with a high success rate, and with quick healing that permits the patient to return to active life without prolonged rehabilitation.

Anesthetic considerations
Preoperative assessment and preparation
Patients who benefit from free flaps in ENT surgery are usually patients with cancer. Microvascular surgery techniques can also be used for traumatic injuries, congenital defects, prior infections or secondary reconstructions. In general, trauma patients tend to be younger and, thus, there is a trend towards lower incidence of chronic medical conditions. Acute medical problems such as intoxication syndromes, intracranial hypertension or multisystem organ dysfunction from multiple trauma will delineate clinical management. For example, trauma patients may have acute airway issues with unstable spine or possible pneumothorax that may become clinically relevant during the middle of a surgical procedure. These repairs are likely to be scheduled on an elective basis but within a period of time post-trauma that might coincide with acute or chronic medical complications common in trauma patients (e.g., healthcare-associated pneumonia, DVT, acute malnutrition, pulmonary embolism, nosocomial infections, prolonged ICU stay, prolonged hospital stay, etc.). In contrast, patients with upper aerodigestive tract cancers tend to be elderly and chronically exposed to tobacco, alcohol, other recreational substances and chronic opioid therapy for chronic pain management. Other common comorbidities include: atherosclerosis, coronary artery disease, cardiac arrhythmias, hypertension, COPD, diabetes, chronic renal insufficiency, chronic malnutrition and cachexia syndrome, and tendency to thrombotic complications associated with cancer. Some of these patients have also been exposed to radiation

therapy and/or chemotherapeutic agents before reconstruction with free flap is planned [6]. Other patients, instead, are awaiting free flap reconstruction to have radiation therapy.

A through preoperative assessment is warranted. The topic of preoperative assessment is discussed in detail in Chapter 3. Following clinical algorithms and guidelines established by the American Society of Anesthesiologists (ASA) is recommended. It is also recommended to review the potential toxicity of chemotherapeutic agents used in ENT cancer patients (hematologic, cardiac, pulmonary and renal toxicity) before anesthesia is planned.

There are several implications of radiation therapy before free flap reconstruction. Radiation therapy to the neck structures leads to scarring and difficulties establishing the airway (decreased extension or flexion of the neck). Radiation therapy to the mediastinum can also induce dose-dependent pericarditis, pericardial effusion, and/or rapid progression of coronary artery disease and heart failure. Thus, it is advised that patients with a history of radiation therapy to the mediastinum are carefully evaluated for ischemic heart disease regardless of age. Radiation therapy also leads to higher risk of fistulas due to poor tissue healing. Poor healing might lead to different infectious complications, further malnutrition, use of total parenteral nutrition and overall increased morbidity.

Anesthesiologists can face free flap repairs in two main scenarios: elective and emergency. Free-flap-related emergencies are routinely related to flap ischemia secondary to: hematoma formation, arterial or venous thrombosis.

Aside from the general anesthetic implications for coexisting comorbidities, perhaps the most important anesthetic implications of tissue transfers are:

(a) careful planning for difficult airway management including tracheostomy if the airway is compromised
(b) positioning and careful understanding of graft donor and recipient site considerations
(c) choice of intraoperative monitoring
(d) considerations related to the length of surgery and thermoregulation
(e) flap perfusion considerations
(f) planning postoperative care and level of care.

Communication with the surgical team is the key. It will greatly help delineate many of the following considerations.

Airway management

Free flap reconstruction requires general anesthesia. The airway is secured via tracheal intubation (orotracheal or nasotracheal or tracheostomy). Often the very tumors that indicated the extensive resection and flap reconstruction and/or the effects of radiation render the airway extremely difficult, and awake intubation technique is required to safely establish the airway. While many airway devices can be employed with the awake technique, the flexible fiberoptic scope is very helpful as it offers the option of navigating around the tumor, to visualize the glottis.

Tracheostomy is carried out as the initial part of the resection in those cases where there is an expectation of significant swelling of the tissues of the upper aerodigestive tract either during the procedure or in the first 48 hours of the postoperative period, e.g., resection of oral tongue or tongue base cancers. In these cases, accidental displacement of an endotracheal tube postoperatively would create a life-threatening situation since subsequent reintubation would be extremely difficult, if not impossible. Additionally, tracheostomy may be carried out initially in those cases where the oro/nasotracheal tube itself interferes with the resection of the tumor, e.g., supraglottic laryngeal tumors. Frequently, patients present to the operating room with *in situ* tracheostomy which are placed due to obstruction of the upper airway by the tumor (e.g., advanced supraglottic tumors).

It is important to anticipate acute and chronic complications of tracheostomy be familiar with the different appliances used to manage patients with tracheostomy. It is always possible to face an emergency tracheostomy-related complication during anesthesia for free flap reconstructions.

Tracheostomy tubes can be removed when the patient has a stable airway without significant edema, which generally is seen within 7–21 days after the procedure. The tract heals primarily within 1 week, with a minimal secondary scarring.

Positioning

Position of the patient for head and neck surgery is usually supine but some variations in positioning might be required to harvest tissue from the donor site. Ultimate positioning must allow for necessary monitoring and adequate exposure of the head and neck and flap donor sites. Often two nursing teams and sterile sites are used to allow for simultaneous harvesting of the flap during the resection, and room must be provided to allow the teams to work without interrupting each other or contaminating sterile fields. Positioning of the anesthesia machine can be done at the foot of the patient or off to one side, depending on local preference and patient safety-related issues (Figures 16.1–16.3).

Patients need to be adequately padded to prevent pressure ulcers and leg compression devices used for thromboprophylaxis.

Monitoring

Surgical field avoidance can constitute a challenge in terms of applying appropriate monitors to the patient, including but not limited to electrocardiogram leads placement away from donor and recipient sites, and positioning and securing the breathing circuit.

Knowledge of surgical sites and proposed surgical intervention is important in planning placement of venous or arterial catheters. Thoughtful planning and communication with the surgical team are paramount.

Electrocardiogram pads

EKG pads should be placed away from the donor site without compromising ischemia or arrhythmia detection. Obtaining a baseline tracing with the current arrangement of leads is advised to compare and delineate trends as the case proceeds.

Central venous pressure monitoring

The use of an internal jugular vein catheter is discouraged as this might compromise the venous return of pedicle flaps. Subclavian vein central catheters are likely to be appropriate for most procedures; however, femoral vein catheters or peripherally inserted central catheters (PICCs) are likely to be better options if central access is necessary. One must bear in mind the risk/benefit ratio of central lines (i.e., central access, central venous pressure monitoring) to optimize hemodynamic management along with prevention of potential complications such as deep vein thrombosis for PICC lines or infectious complications of femoral lines. At the authors' institution peripheral venous pressure monitoring and trending is sometimes used in lieu of central venous pressure monitoring [7]. Such values and trends are interpreted in the context of other parameters

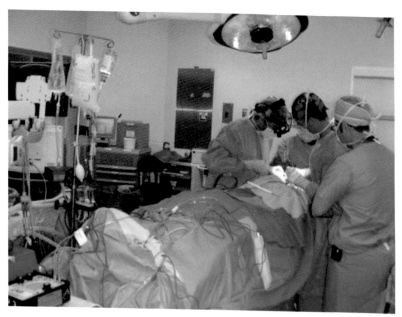

Figure 16.1. The two images show an example of operating room arrangement in a lengthy otolaryngologic flap surgery. The anesthesia and surgical equipment are arranged in such a way to provide the surgical team free access not only to the head of the patient but also to the flap harvest site. The anesthesia machine is rotated in a way to allow simultaneous continuous monitoring of the surgical field, ventilator, as well as the patient's monitor.

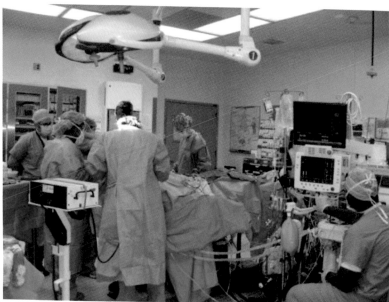

such as blood pressure, heart rate, fluid intake and urine output as well as systolic blood pressure variability to ascertain the blood volume status of these patients.

Breathing circuit

As in any other general anesthesia all alarms that help diagnose accidental disconnection of breathing circuits or large leaks along with oxygen sensors should be checked for proper functioning. The breathing circuit should be long enough to allow the anesthesia machine to be safely stationed away from the surgical field to allow room for surgeons, instruments and microscopes. All connections of the breathing circuits should be tightened to make sure disconnections do not occur when the circuit is covered by surgical drapes.

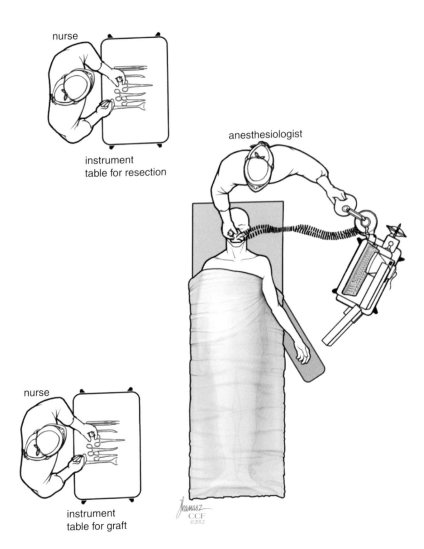

nurse

instrument
table for resection

anesthesiologist

nurse

instrument
table for graft

Thermoregulation

Esophageal temperature monitors are used in most other surgical procedures, yet might not be the best option for free flaps in head and neck surgery patients. The goal is to minimize lines and monitors around the face and neck area; therefore an axillary temperature probe is often used. Skin temperature probes carry the risk of being inaccurate. Thus, clinicians have used bladder or rectal temperature monitors instead. Significant hypothermia can develop during anesthesia for free flap surgeries [8]. Hypothermia can lead to vasoconstriction and development of flap ischemia. Intraoperative hypothermia is also associated with increased blood loss, higher wound infection rates, and pharmacokinetic changes that prolong anesthetic and other medication effects and further increase in morbidity [9]. Prevention of hypothermia is especially important during the anesthetic management for microvascular surgeries. Forced-air warming devices such as the Bair Hugger™ can lack efficacy in these surgeries due to the large skin surface area involved in the surgical fields. Thus, a small body surface area is available for forced-air warming devices to be applied to. Therefore, it is recommended that other clinical measures are taken to prevent hypothermia. A combination of underbody and surface forced-air warming blankets, warming of intravenous fluids or blood products, increased room temperature and radiant heat facilitate hypothermia prevention.

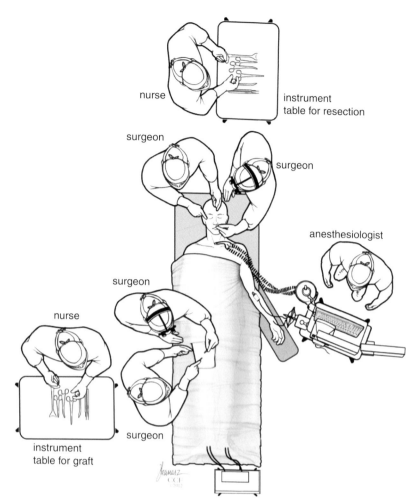

nurse

instrument
table for resection

surgeon

surgeon

anesthesiologist

surgeon

nurse

surgeon

instrument
table for graft

Figure 16.3. A cartoon showing the operating room organization during the phase of simultaneous graft harvest, and completion of tumor resection of a free flap otolaryngologic surgery; please note the orientation and location of the anesthesia machine and the anesthesiologist, allowing for simultaneous monitoring of the patient's monitor, IV fluids, and both surgical fields. Reprinted with permission, Cleveland Clinic Center for Medical Art & Photography © 2012. All rights reserved.

Anesthetic management

Induction of general anesthesia

Intravenous anesthetic induction can be used safely in patients who are judged not to have a difficult airway, or after awake intubation in those with difficult airway. Inhalational induction can also be safely done in patients with *in situ* or freshly placed (under local anesthesia) tracheostomies.

Anesthesia maintenance

A balanced anesthesia technique is preferred; there is little role for regional anesthesia techniques in free flap surgery for head and neck cancer patients. Inhalational maintenance or total intravenous anesthesia (TIVA) are appropriate. There is a paucity of data indicating what techniques are most appropriate. However,

anesthetic goals such as amnesia and analgesia must be accomplished throughout.

A motionless surgical field is important, especially during the anastomosis of vascular structures when microvascular techniques are in use. Muscle relaxants can be used during this time; however, if the surgical team utilizes a nerve monitoring technique, muscle relaxants will need to be avoided. Another option to achieve motionless surgical fields is to increase the anesthetic depth. Continuous infusions of opioids such as fentanyl, remifentanil or sufentanil can also be used to achieve a motionless surgical field and provide analgesia.

Remifentanil has been prospectively studied for the prevention of movement during balanced anesthesia without muscle relaxation during craniotomy [10]. Immobility can be reached between doses of 0.1 and 0.21 µg/kg/min. Chances of movement at

157

0.13 µg/kg/min are about 50%. Probability of movement at a dose 0.21 µg/kg/min is about 20%; however, side effects such as bradycardia and hypotension can be seen between doses of 0.13 and 0.17 µg/kg/min.

Remifentanil's potency and half-life make it ideal for easy clinical titration during very stimulating surgical procedures; however, the hemodynamic profile provided by it (bradycardia and hypotension) and lack of prolonged clinical analgesic effect make it less desirable during free flap surgery. Postoperative analgesia is nearly nonexistent after infusion is stopped. Therefore, opioid infusions of fentanyl or sufentanil are recommended as they provide a smooth analgesic effect that extends into the postoperative period and can also provide motionless surgical fields when muscle relaxants are not desirable.

The authors' choice is the use of fentanyl infusion titrated around 2 µg/kg/h. At this dose, fentanyl provides a motionless field with very stable hemodynamics (no observed bradycardia or hypotension) as well as easy titration according to time constraints (i.e., unplanned prolongation of surgery or unexpected termination of surgery). At this dose, fentanyl allows recovery of spontaneous ventilation promptly after stopping the infusion in short cases without delay in extubation. For more prolonged cases – as is usually the case with free flap reconstruction – if fentanyl infusion is stopped about 30 minutes before emergence from anesthesia, patients usually recover from anesthesia smoothly with appropriate analgesia and full recovery of spontaneous ventilation without delay of extubation when feasible. Of note, fentanyl infusions are less costly than remifentanil or sufentanil infusions.

Due to the length of the flap reconstructions, re-dosing prophylactic antibiotics every 4 to 6 hours is needed in addition to routine pre-incision intravenous antibiotic administration.

Fluid management

Judicious use of intravenous fluids (crystalloids or colloids) and avoidance of hypovolemia and hypotension are important to maintain homeostasis and help avoid ischemia to the flap. On the other hand, too much fluid, once redistributed, can increase tissue edema formation within the flap with detrimental consequences in flap perfusion and survival. Some surgical teams advocate the use of dextran as a rheologic agent to prevent thrombosis. Dextran can be initiated intraoperatively and continued postoperatively for up to 48 hours.

There is paucity of data regarding the choice of intravenous fluids for flap reconstruction surgery. Neither crystalloids nor colloids have been studied prospectively in flap reconstruction surgery patients. Fluids that maintain the intravascular volume are preferred. Colloids are more effective for plasma volume expansion as their contents diffuse poorly into the interstitial space and create oncotic pressures that keep water in the intravascular space. Crsytalloids are used as maintenance fluids and hypotonic solutions should be avoided. The use of vasoactive drugs (i.e., phenylephrine, norepinephrine or vasopressin) is discouraged during microvascular reconstructions. Vasopressors can worsen or induce ischemia of the graft by intense vasoconstriction of the microvasculature. A thorough hemodynamic assessment with invasive monitoring might be necessary when sustained hypotension (i.e., circulatory shock) and use of vasopressors are needed. While a retrospective study that compared flap patients who received intraoperative vasopressors with those who did not reported no difference in graft outcomes, the authors cautioned against the use of vasopressors for these surgeries [11].

Blood transfusions

There is usually no brisk and sudden blood loss in microvascular surgery cases due to the meticulous and extreme attention on the head and neck surgeons' part regarding hemostasis and careful dissection; however, continuous oozing over a long period of time may result in anemia. Some patients may present at a well-compensated anemic state (of chronic nature) so red blood cell transfusion is sometimes required. The goal is to maintain adequate perfusion to end organs and ascertain adequate perfusion of the grafts. A reasonable target is a hematocrit of 25–30 secondary to the commonly associated comorbidities, and physiological considerations regarding oxygen-carrying capacity in and to the graft. A higher hematocrit may not prove to be superior as it might affect blood rheology.

Avoidance of hyperviscosity of the blood is thought to help decrease the potential for vessel thrombosis; thus, blood transfusions for hematocrits above 30 are considered unnecessary.

Flap perfusion considerations

For a comprehensive review on the impact of anesthetics, vasopressors and blood transfusion on graft perfusion, the reader is directed to Chapter 23 of this volume.

Emergence

Smooth emergence from general anesthesia is desirable. Avoidance of extreme fluctuations in blood pressure, especially hypertension, is advised to minimize risks of bleeding, disruption of new anastomoses, and potential flap failure from hematoma formation. Agitation upon emergence should also be avoided due to its potential to cause accidental dislodgement of drains and tracheostomy appliances or even disruption of flaps.

As during maintenance of anesthesia, avoidance of hypertension, tachycardia or sustained hypotension during emergence from anesthesia will help protect the viability of the graft(s).

In general, most patients can be separated from mechanical ventilation at the end of the procedure if weaning parameters are met. The decision to extubate patients after free flap reconstruction should be made jointly with the surgical team. Even if the patient is clinically fit for liberation from ventilatory support there are several other clinical factors that help to make the decision:

(a) feasibility of reintubation and anticipated difficult airway even after repair
(b) possibility of severe airway edema from new graft placement
(c) individual patient monitoring needs
(d) anticipated surgical complications due to technical difficulties and potential need for reexploration
(e) medical intraoperative complications that require admission to intensive care units with need for postoperative mechanical ventilation.

In general, lengthy procedures, prolonged emergence and lack of adequate spontaneous respiratory efforts or questionable protection of the airway usually call for a delayed extubation or liberation from mechanical ventilation in the recovery area. If extubation is decided in the operating room, this should be accomplished smoothly to minimize extreme hemodynamic variations, extreme cough, straining or any clinical situation (such as hypoxemia) that can jeopardize the safety of the patients and ultimately the viability of the grafts.

Postoperative care planning

Individualized care plans might help make a decision for postoperative ventilatory support. Some patients will benefit from mechanical ventilation and sedation postoperatively even if extubation is deemed to be safe at the end of the procedure. For example, patients with a history of schizophrenia, severe anxiety disorders, or claustrophobia who can potentially progress to postoperative delirium and agitation may pose a clinical challenge to adequately monitor the viability and survival of the grafts. The need for graft surveillance and diligent vigilance of the graft postoperatively has led to the creation of specialized units in medical centers in order to avoid delayed recognition of graft complications. Some of these specialized units have mechanical ventilation capabilities and enhanced nurse:patient ratios to accomplish postoperative care.

Postoperative monitoring

The goal of postoperative monitoring of the patient with flap reconstruction is similar to that seen in all major head and neck procedures. General homeostasis and adequate organ function secure the basis of a healthy, viable graft. Monitoring of the flap is of paramount importance postoperatively. Flap monitoring is generally achieved with visual checks (general inspection of color, turgor, edema, and capillary refill) and Doppler ultrasound assessment of the exposed cutaneous portions of the flap, if available. These are carried out hourly for the first 24–48 hours, then checked every 4 hours or so over the next 3–5 days. The critical period for vessel thrombosis is the initial 24–48 hours after the procedure, and early detection of vessel/flap problems requires rapid return to the operating room for exploration and vessel revision if necessary. Flap exploration may be necessary in up to 10% of flaps, and generally successful resuscitation occurs in 50% of these explorations. More invasive monitoring such as laser-Doppler flowmetry, transcutaneous pulsoximetry, duplex ultrasound, pH monitoring and others is available, but has potential complications, including disruption of the flap vessel anastomoses and false-positive results creating unnecessary postoperative explorations. With flap success rates above 95%, the use of more invasive monitoring seems ill-advised. Tracheostomy tubes can be removed when the patient has a stable airway without significant edema, which generally is seen within 7–21 days after the procedure. The tract heals primarily within 1 week, with a minimal secondary scar.

Anticoagulation of the free flap patient postoperatively is a highly debated topic. No controlled studies show a benefit of any particular anticoagulation regimen in this cohort of patients. Antiplatelet drugs have been shown effective in increasing flap survival in traumatic reimplantations, e.g., finger and arm, but no data exist in the more controlled setting of microvascular free tissue transfer. Some institutions advocate infusions of dextran-40 at 25 ml/h for up to 48 hours postoperatively, and give 81 mg aspirin for 21 days postoperatively starting on the morning of postoperative day 1. However, if there is a contraindication to anticoagulation, e.g., intracranial cases, then anticoagulation is avoided.

Complications

Several potential complications can arise during the care of free flap reconstruction surgery patients and are related to increased morbidity postoperatively. The following are considered the most common complications during anesthesia for microvascular surgery.

Intraoperative

Complications that commonly occur during anesthesia for free flap reconstruction are:

Hypotension: hypotension usually ensues after induction of general anesthesia and is often related to hypovolemia. A thorough evaluation of the patient's hemodynamics and possible causes of hypotension should be carried out. Common causes of hypotension include cardiac dysrhythmias, myocardial ischemia, hypovolemia, anaphylactic reactions, and medication side effects. Bleeding is a general cause of hypotension during free flap reconstruction and it is usually not brisk but continuous and difficult to quantify.

Hypothermia: anticipation and prevention of hypothermia is a key element of the anesthetic management for flap reconstructive surgery. Prolonged surgical times and heat loss from the surgical field (donor and recipient sites) seem to be the main reasons associated with hypothermia during free flap surgery. Lack of warming strategies during these cases can lead to severe hypothermia and intense vasoconstriction, which increases the risk of flap ischemia.

A combination of underbody and surface forced-air warming blankets, warming of intravenous fluids or blood products, increased room temperature and radiant heat facilitates hypothermia prevention.

Breathing circuit failure: during anesthesia for free flap surgery, the breathing circuit is usually hidden under the surgical drapes to maintain optimal sterile conditions of both donor and transplant sites. The breathing circuit should be long enough to maintain the anesthesia machine safely away from the surgical sites but close enough to the patient's airway. The breathing circuit should also be compliant enough to allow titration of tidal volumes and flexible enough to allow easy repositioning of the patient without causing disconnections. Breathing circuit leaks and failure to effectively ventilate the patient thereby are potential complications that might be lethal if unrecognized. All connections from the anesthesia machine to the patient's airway should be tightened to ascertain appropriate seals before final position and preparation of surgical sites.

Dislodgement of vascular catheters: intravenous and arterial catheters and their tubing connections can potentially be dislodged during turning or positioning of the patient. It is recommended that all catheters are secured to the skin to prevent kinking, dislodgement, obstruction or extravasation of medications that are injected. Regardless of the anesthesia technique, patency of the intravenous line must be ascertained before infusion of anesthetics starts. All IV sites should be easily accessible for patency assessment or for blood sampling.

Postoperative

Multiple complications may arise during the recovery phase after general anesthesia. Most common postoperative complications in this phase include hypoxemia, hypercarbia, cardiac dysrhythmias, acidosis, prolonged sedation, uncontrolled pain, hypo- or hypertension, anxiety, emergence delirium, hypothermia, shivering, nausea, and vomiting. Some of these problems can be explained by the pharmacodynamics and kinetics of anesthetic agents. Symptoms and signs of postoperative complications in the recovery area should be addressed promptly and aggressively as many of these complications tend to have a "snowball" effect if not immediately addressed (e.g., upper airway obstruction and respiratory insufficiency are not resolved until obstruction is addressed).

Specific postoperative complications for free flap patients include hypothermia, and flap failure due to ischemia or hematoma. Hypothermia is a potential complication that, as mentioned above, can lead to graft ischemia by intense vasoconstriction. Active rewarming appears to be an effective intervention to treat hyperthermia in the recovery phase of anesthesia but certainly prevention of hypothermia is the best clinical approach. The most feared complication in free flap surgery is the development of flap ischemia due to hematoma formation or thrombosis of the vascular grafts [12]. To prevent thrombosis, many surgical centers advocate the use of low-dose heparin infusions or dextran-40. There is a scarcity of data indicating the most effective prophylactic measure to prevent thrombosis of vascular pedicles. Early identification of flaps at risk of ischemia leads to prompt interventions and possible salvage of the flaps.

Summary

Otolaryngologic flap reconstructive surgery, while lengthy, risky and complex, can be performed with a high degree of safety. The anesthetic management includes careful planning of difficult airway issues such as tracheostomy if the airway is compromised, considerations to positioning, understanding of surgical sites (donor and recipient), choice of intraoperative monitoring, considerations related to the length of surgery and thermoregulation, flap perfusion considerations, planning postoperative care and level of care. This is in addition to considerations related to coexisting morbidities in this elderly population, who commonly present with tobacco and alcohol abuse. Clear communication with otolaryngology colleagues will help greatly for proper planning and execution of these considerations, helping to ensure a favorable outcome.

Case study

A 62-year-male with a history of tongue cancer presents for glossectomy, neck dissection and free latissimus myocutaneous flap reconstruction. Past medical history includes chronic atrial fibrillation for which he is on warfarin therapy, hypertension treated with lisinopril, COPD – emphysema type, active smoker, history of alcohol abuse, type 2 diabetes mellitus on oral hypoglycemics and SQ glargine insulin. He had radiation therapy 5 weeks prior to his surgery and has

not been able to eat solids for the past month due to tongue mass. He continues to smoke cigarettes and drink vodka daily.

Patient states he was admitted to an emergency room 7 weeks ago with difficulty breathing and swallowing. He states that he can no longer swallow solids and liquids are becoming more difficult to swallow in the past week. He denies any fever, chest pain or dyspnea on exertion.

Due to anticipated difficult airway resulting from his large tongue mass, the patient was intubated awake using a flexible fiberoptic bronchoscope. Sedation for awake intubation was accomplished with 3 mg of midazolam IV in increments of 1 mg, and 50 μg of fentanyl IV. Topicalization was achieved with atomized 4% lidocaine, using a standard atomizer, and 2% lidocaine jelly applied to the dorsum of a size 10 Williams airway. In addition, 4% lidocaine was sprayed to the hypopharynx and supraglottic area using a syringe attached to a MADgic® catheter.

Induction of anesthesia was then achieved with 70 mg of propofol, 100 μg of fentanyl and 40 mg of rocuronium. After induction, an arterial catheter and an 18G IV catheter were inserted. This catheter was connected to a pressure transducer to intermittently measure the peripheral venous pressure, as a surrogate to the volume status. A Foley catheter was inserted as well as a rectal temperature probe. Antithrombotic stockings were then applied to the legs and a forced-air warming blanket applied to the skin except for the two operative fields (graft recipient and harvest sites). A fentanyl infusion was started at 2 μg/kg/h. After induction of anesthesia, no additional muscle relaxant was given. Anesthesia was maintained with sevoflurane in an air/oxygen mixture and the fentanyl infusion.

A tracheostomy was performed, and the orally inserted ETT replaced by a cross-field sterile reinforced tube.

Lactated Ringer's solution was used as the maintenance fluid, while Hextend® and albumin 5% were used for colloid replacement of intraoperative blood loss. The use of colloid is justified on the basis of decreasing the amount of total crystalloid administered, with the goal of decreasing the amount of tissue edema globally and locally at the graft site. Arterial blood gas analysis was followed throughout the surgery; a unit of red blood cells was given in response to a hematocrit of 26%.

The fentanyl infusion was discontinued 30 minutes from the anticipated emergence time, followed by the discontinuation of the sevoflurane, after which the patient emerged from anesthesia. The ETT was then replaced with a #6 Shiley tracheostomy tube, which was secured with sutures and ties, and a Trach Collar mask was used to provide supplemental oxygen. The patient was then discharged to the recovery room, followed by admission to a step-down unit three hours later for graft monitoring.

Clinical pearls

- A clear understanding of proposed donor sites and the planned surgical intervention is important to avoid placement of internal jugular vein catheters in the middle of the surgical field or the placement of a radial artery line or a peripheral IV at the donor site.
- Careful positioning and careful pressure points padding is very important in these lengthy surgeries, together with surgical field avoidance while allowing for easy monitoring of both patient monitor and surgical field(s).

- Maintenance of normothermia in these procedures is essential to avoid hypothermia and its associated complications.
- Maintaining normovolemia, together with an adequate hematocrit ($\approx 30\%$) to ensure appropriate oxygen-carrying capacity will help ensure adequate graft perfusion.
- The use of colloids is justified on the basis of decreasing the amount of total crystalloid administered, with the goal of decreasing the amount of tissue edema both globally and at the graft site.
- The use of vasoactive drugs (i.e., phenylephrine, norepinephrine or vasopressin) is discouraged during microvascular reconstructions. Vasopressors can worsen or induce ischemia of the graft by intense vasoconstriction of the microvasculature.
- Careful postoperative care planning is necessary to ensure proper matching of patient and graft monitoring needs and the capabilities of the specialized unit and its nursing staff.

References

1. Wehage IC, Fansa H. Complex reconstructions in head and neck cancer surgery: decision making. *Head Neck Oncol* 2011;3:14.

2. Clymer MA, Burkey BB. Other flaps for head and neck use: temporoparietal fascial free flap, lateral arm free flap, omental free flap. *Facial Plastic Surg* 1996;12(1):81–9.

3. Girod DA TT, Shnayder Y. Free tissue transfer. In Flint P HB, Lund V, Niparko J, Richardson M, Robbins KT, Thomas J, eds. *Cummings Otolaryngology Head & Neck Surgery*, Vol. 2, 5th edn. Philadelphia: Mosby Elsevier; 2010. pp. 1080–99.

4. Coleman SC, Burkey BB, Day TA, *et al.* Increasing use of the scapula osteocutaneous free flap. *Laryngoscope* 2000;110(9): 1419–24.

5. Burkey BB, Coleman JR Jr. Current concepts in oromandibular reconstruction. *Otolaryngol Clin North Am* 1997;30(4):607–30.

6. Correa AJ, Burkey BB. Current options in management of head and neck cancer patients. *Med Clin North Am* 1999;83(1): 235–46, xi.

7. Munis JR, Bhatia S, Lozada LJ. Peripheral venous pressure as a hemodynamic variable in neurosurgical patients. *Anesth Analg* 2001;92(1):172–9.

8. Robins DW. The anaesthetic management of patients undergoing free flap transfer. *Br J Plastic Surg* 1983;36(2): 231–4.

9. Sessler DI. Mild perioperative hypothermia. *N Engl J Med* 1997;336(24):1730–7.

10. Maurtua MA, Deogaonkar A, Bakri MH, *et al.* Dosing of remifentanil to prevent movement during craniotomy in the absence of neuromuscular blockade. *J Neurosurg Anesthesiol* 2008;20(4):221–5.

11. Chen C, Nguyen MD, Bar-Meir E, *et al.* Effects of vasopressor administration on the outcomes of microsurgical breast reconstruction. *Ann Plastic Surg* 2010;65(1):28–31.

12. Esclamado RM, Carroll WR. The pathogenesis of vascular thrombosis and its impact in microvascular surgery. *Head Neck* 1999;21(4): 355–62.

Chapter

17

Anesthesia for thyroid and parathyroid surgery

Twain Russell and Richard M. Cooper

Introduction

Most patients undergoing thyroid surgery have thyroid cancer, a symptomatic thyroid goiter, or a contraindication to or failure of medical management of their hyperthyroidism. The National Cancer Institute estimates that 37 000 women and 11 000 men were diagnosed with primary thyroid cancer in the USA in 2011. It is the fifth most common cancer among women yet accounts for less than 2% of cancer deaths. Papillary and follicular thyroid cancers account for approximately 80% and 15% of cases respectively and are generally cured by early recognition and surgical excision. Medullary thyroid cancer may produce calcitonin or be associated with other endocrine adenopathies or familial medullary cancer. The least common form of primary thyroid cancer is anaplastic and is associated with a very unfavourable prognosis with or without surgery (http://www.cancer.gov/cancertopicswyntk/thyroid; accessed Oct. 28, 2011).

Preoperative assessment for thyroid surgery

There are several specific issues that significantly affect the anesthetic management for patients undergoing thyroid surgery. In addition to the general considerations pertaining to anesthesia, specific attention should be directed to the assessment of thyroid function, the size and location of the thyroid gland, its relationship to the trachea and adjacent vascular structures, and the co-existence of a multiple endocrine neoplasia (MEN1 or 2).

Thyroid function

With very few exceptions, thyroid surgery is elective. The signs and symptoms of thyrotoxicosis are nonspecific but include nervousness, heat intolerance and perspiration, tachycardia, fatigue, insomnia, weakness and tremulousness, diarrhea and weight loss. Patients may have anemia, leukopenia or thrombocytopenia and coagulopathy. Patients with Graves' disease may have exophthalmos. Patients should be medically optimized preoperatively with the goal to achieve a euthyroid state to reduce the risk of a thyroid storm. Radioactive iodine ablation or an anti-thyroid drug (propylthiouracil or methimazole) may be administered for several weeks preoperatively. In addition, Lugol's solution may help reduce iodine uptake and the vascularity of the gland. Readiness for surgery may be judged by symptom resolution and normalization of weight and heart rate. Anti-thyroid drugs can cause agranulocytosis, hepatitis, aplastic anemia, and lupus-like syndromes.

Patients with uncontrolled hyperthyroidism who require urgent surgery may have atrial fibrillation, congestive heart failure and/or myocardial ischemia. These patients should be treated with anti-thyroid medications, steroids and β-blockers. The anesthesiologist must be prepared to deal with thyroid storm, a condition that may resemble malignant hyperthermia. In such cases, care must be taken to control heart rate with a titratable β-blocker such as esmolol, especially in the setting of acute heart failure. Sympathetic nervous system activation should be minimized with adequate anesthesia and the avoidance of sympathomimetic drugs. Volatile anesthesia requirements are unchanged but the clearance and distribution volume of propofol are increased, resulting in increased drug infusion requirements. Intra-arterial blood pressure monitoring and high-dependency care are recommended, especially in patients with uncontrolled hypertension, patients with poor cardiovascular status, or cases expected to last a long time. Removal

Anesthesia for Otolaryngologic Surgery, ed. Basem Abdelmalak and D. John Doyle. Published by Cambridge University Press.
© Cambridge University Press 2013.

of the thyroid does not result in the immediate resolution of the thyrotoxic state since the half-life of T_4 is 7 days. Anti-thyroid medication can be ceased but β-blocker therapy may need to be continued in the postoperative period.

Hypothyroidism may also be a problem in some patients. However, it is extremely rare for an untreated hypothyroid patient to present requiring urgent thyroid surgery. It should also be borne in mind that hypothyroid patients with unstable coronary disease may not tolerate full thyroid supplementation without producing cardiac ischemia.

Airway difficulty

Patients presenting with complaints of hoarseness, vocal changes, or previous mediastinal, neck or re-operative thyroid surgery are likely to have had diagnostic laryngoscopy (or videostroboscopy) performed by the surgeon and the findings should be reviewed along with any relevant diagnostic imaging. The majority of patients presenting for thyroid surgery pose little additional risk of difficult ventilation and intubation [1,2]. Routine airway assessment should be performed. In a small proportion of patients with enlarged thyroids it may be difficult to ventilate via mask or supraglottic airway, to intubate or even to create an emergency surgical airway. Thyroid enlargement can be associated with laryngeal deviation, laryngeal edema, tracheal compression, and an anterior vascular neck mass. Consideration should be made as to the location or multiple locations of any potential obstruction as the management options vary.

Symptoms of dysphagia, recumbent dyspnea, or a change in voice or stridor should alert the anesthesiologist to airway compromise and possible difficulties with airway management following induction.

For patients with a retrosternal goiter and tracheal compression or superior vena cava syndrome, several induction strategies have been advocated, including intravenous induction with neuromuscular blockade and direct laryngoscopy, inhalational induction, and awake flexible bronchoscopic intubation [3]. The management depends on the unique features of the individual case and the skills of the anesthesia and surgical staff [3,4].

Deviation of the larynx and compression of the trachea may occur from a large cervical or retrosternal goiter. Stridor in adults implies an airway narrowing of greater than 50% reduction in diameter or a diameter less than 4–5 mm. The absence of stridor is reassuring but does not exclude significant airway narrowing.

Preoperative airway evaluation using multi-slice 3D CT and high-resolution virtual laryngoscopy based on spiral CT data for patients with severe tracheal stenosis may be useful. In the setting of a benign goiter a compressed tracheal segment opens with endotracheal tube placement.

Retrosternal goiter

There is no universal agreement regarding a definition of a retrosternal goiter (RSG) although generally more than 50% of its mass must be below the thoracic inlet to qualify. Most are outgrowths of the cervical thyroid but rarely a primary intrathoracic goiter arises from thyroid tissue located in the mediastinum. Surgery is usually required since medical therapy rarely arrests growth and malignancy surveillance is difficult.

The most common presenting symptoms are respiratory (dyspnea, choking, inability to sleep comfortably), hoarseness and dysphagia. Less common features include impending airway obstruction, superior vena cava obstruction and Horner's syndrome. Symptoms of supine presyncope are very rare but suggest vascular compression. Clinical symptoms correlate well with the preoperative CT measurements of tracheal and esophageal displacement, retrotracheal extension and the degree of tracheal compression [5].

A preoperative neck and chest CT scan is generally performed in patients suspected of having RSG to assess trachea deviation or compression, goiter size, and mediastinal extension. The cervical route is successful in removing the majority of RSG but in high-risk patients the resources to perform a sternotomy should be available. Factors favoring the need for a sternotomy include the presence of an ectopic goiter, adherence to the surrounding mediastinal tissues, previous thyroid surgery, malignancy, thyroid gland volume, and extension of the goiter to or below the aortic arch or tracheal carina or into the posterior mediastinum [6].

SVC compression

Superior vena cava syndrome results from venous hypertension causing facial, neck, and mucosal membrane engorgement, and increased intracranial pressure including headache and altered mental status. Elevation of both upper limbs may produce facial plethora as a consequence of jugular venous compression (Permberton's sign). SVC obstruction may result in airway edema, dependence on spontaneous ventilation for venous return, and hemodynamic instability. Dyspnea and hoarseness may reflect edema of the vocal cords.

Surgical bleeding is often increased due to increased central venous pressure. Intravenous access in the legs rather than in the arms and invasive blood pressure monitoring should be considered.

Multiple endocrine neoplasia syndromes

Hyperparathyroidism due to an adenoma or hyperplasia is the most common presenting symptom of multiple endocrine neoplasia 1 syndrome (MEN1). The most common tumors associated with MEN1 are parathyroid adenoma, pituitary adenoma, pancreatic tumours (gastrinomas and insulinomas), and skin tumors (angiofibromas, collagenomas, and lipomas).

Medullary thyroid cancer is associated with MEN2 syndrome, of which there are three subtypes: Type 2A is associated with pheochomocytoma and hyperparathyroidism; Type 2B is associated with pheochromocytoma, mucosal neuromas, intestinal ganglioneuromas, and Marfanoid body habitus; and a third subtype, FMTC or familial medullary thyroid carcinoma.

Anesthesia technique for thyroid surgery

Patients are commonly positioned supine with both arms by the side, a sandbag between the scapulae and the head resting on a padded cushion to enhance head extension. Reverse Trendelenburg positioning of 15–25° will assist with venous drainage and surgical access. Eye protection is of particular importance in patients with exophthalmos. As with most head and neck cases, access to the airway will be limited during the procedure so the endotracheal tube should be taped securely and padded to prevent pressure areas.

General anesthesia with tracheal intubation and muscle relaxation is usually employed although Laryngeal Mask Airway (LMA®) and other supraglottic airways have been used with both spontaneous respiration and intermittent positive-pressure ventilation in thyroid surgery. This allows flexible bronchoscopic assessment of recurrent laryngeal nerve function and may reduce coughing and straining on emergence, potentially reducing the risk of a neck hematoma. A plan should be made in advance with the surgical team to manage laryngospasm and LMA displacement during the surgery. Local anesthesia with sedation has been used successfully [7].

The surgeon will often infiltrate local anesthetic and epinephrine 1:200 000 subcutaneously prior to incision to reduce bleeding and to confer some postoperative analgesic effect. Acetaminophen, nonsteroidal anti-inflammatory drugs, or weak opioids are usually adequate to ensure most patients are comfortable. Bilateral superficial cervical plexus blocks reduce opiate requirements but are rarely required. These patients are at high risk of postoperative nausea and vomiting, which can increase the risk of postoperative neck hematoma. A suitable combination is a serotonin 5-HT_3 receptor antagonist with dexamethasone 4–8 mg, which may also help reduce postoperative airway edema. Before wound closure a Valsalva maneuver for 15–20 s is often requested to assess hemostasis and lymphatic integrity.

Smooth emergence and recovery from anesthesia are important. Airway manipulation and head and neck movement should be minimized during emergence to avoid straining. Suctioning of saliva from the pharynx should be performed during deep anesthesia. Patients can be extubated, ideally in the semi-sitting position either fully awake or (in special circumstances) in a deep plane of anesthesia. The authors favor a "no touch" emergence technique with the ETT removed when the patient responds to commands. Deep extubation reduces the incidence of coughing, bucking, and straining but at an increased risk of airway obstruction and aspiration [8,9]. Alternatively, a Bailey maneuver may be employed (see Case study) wherein a supraglottic airway is substituted for the ETT while the patient is still under neuromuscular blockade and deep anesthesia [8]. The depth of anesthesia, oxygen concentration, ventilatory support, and sequestration of secretions are all potentially under control. (Although this technique has several advantages, it should be regarded as "a high-risk maneuver in high-risk patients" and is best practiced in low-risk patients to ensure the requisite skills.)

There are several pharmacological interventions to suppress cough and smooth emergence. These can be used routinely or in the patient at increased

165

risk of emergence coughing, such as smokers or patients at increased risk of neck hematomas. Total intravenous anesthesia has been shown to lower the incidence of coughing on emergence for non-thyroid surgery [10–12]. Lidocaine topically applied to the ETT cuff prior to intubation [13], given intravenously 5 minutes before extubation and intra-cuff alkalinized lidocaine have also been shown to reduce cough on extubation [12]. A low-dose remifentanil infusion (0.01 to 0.05 µg/kg/min) throughout the extubation period reduces cough without prolonging wake-up [14].

Complications of thyroid surgery

Postoperative respiratory distress

Postoperative respiratory distress or compromise in the setting of neck surgery can be life-threatening, requiring immediate expert management. While providing supportive care, early consideration of the differential is required as the definite therapy depends on the etiology. Immediate and early complications of thyroid surgery include neck hematoma, vocal cord paralysis from recurrent laryngeal nerve injury, tracheomalacia, pneumothorax, airway edema, and thyroid crisis. Subsequently, seroma, chyle fistula, tracheal or esophageal injury and hypocalcemia are additional concerns. A broader differential diagnosis, unrelated specifically to thyroid surgery, must also be kept in mind.

Neck hematoma

The incidence of hematoma post thyroidectomy is reported in the literature as 0% to 1.6%, with the majority developing within 4 hours of surgery and almost all within 24 hours [15–17]. The risk of hematoma formation increases with bilateral surgery, Graves' disease, associated neck dissection, malignancy, and antiplatelet or anticoagulant therapy. A neck hematoma can produce life-threatening airway compromise by direct pressure on the laryngeal structures.

Neck hematomas may present with neck pain or pressure, swelling, excessive drain volumes, voice changes, dysphagia, stridor, dyspnea, and agitation. Symptom progression to airway obstruction is variable and requires very careful vigilance and early intervention. Progression to obstruction, hypoxia, and agitation unquestionably compromises outcome.

The order, timing, and location of life-saving interventions depend on the patient's location, severity of symptoms, and availability of resources. Temporizing management strategies such as elevation of the head of the bed, helium/O_2, nebulized adrenaline, and steroids may be useful but must not delay definite management. Removal of sutures and hematoma evacuation should be performed immediately if the patient is in extremis or if immediate airway management is not available. Hematoma evacuation may assist some patients by relieving direct hematoma compression but it will not resolve airway obstruction from perilaryngeal edema.

If time permits, an awake endoscopic evaluation with topical anesthesia but very judicious sedation should be performed. It is generally well tolerated, has minimal risks and provides useful information on laryngeal position and swelling to help plan the most appropriate airway strategy. There are many induction and intubation options in the patient with a neck hematoma, including inhalation induction, awake bronchoscopic or videolaryngoscopic intubation and tracheostomy under local anesthesia. Each technique has limitations and the surgical team should be fully prepared to proceed with a surgical airway if complete airway obstruction occurs or intubation and ventilation attempts fail.

The choice of intubation techniques will depend upon the clinical circumstances, available resources and local expertise. It is unlikely that an adequately controlled trial will ever establish the preferred technique. The authors believe that in the face of life-threatening obstruction or oxygen desaturation, the quickest technique is likely to be direct or videolaryngoscopy. An inhalation induction in the face of partial airway obstruction is unlikely to provide sufficient depth of anesthesia to permit airway instrumentation. An awake technique in a struggling, hypoxic, and uncooperative patient is an extreme test of the laryngoscopist's technical skill but at some centers flexible bronchoscopy-assisted intubation would be the technique of choice. In any case, it is prudent to be prepared for an emergency (and potentially difficult) surgical airway.

Thyroid crisis

Thyroid storm is a rare but life-threatening exacerbation of uncontrolled hyperthyroidism precipitated by medication withdrawal, trauma, infection, medical illness, intravenous radio-contrast, amiodarone or surgery, with a mortality of 20–30% [18]. Presentation usually occurs in the postoperative period with symptoms including extreme anxiety, fever, vomiting, tachypnea, tachycardia, cardiovascular instability, cardiac failure, dehydration, electrolyte derangements (hypokalemia, hypercalcemia, hyponatremia, hypomagnesemia), respiratory and metabolic acidosis, altered consciousness, and hepatic dysfunction. It is a clinical diagnosis with several important differentials including malignant hyperthermia, sepsis, pheochromocytoma, metastatic carcinoid, malignant neuroleptic and serotonergic syndromes. This condition probably results from thyrotropin receptor antibodies stimulating excess thyroidal synthesis and secretion of T_4 and T_3 [18].

The management of thyroid storm includes: [18]

(i) blocking of the sympathetic response (β-blockers)

(ii) blocking thyroid hormone synthesis (PTU or methimazole)

(iii) blocking thyroid home release (dexamethasone, lopanoic acid or Lugol's solution)

(iv) blocking T_4 to T_3 conversion (β-blocker, PTU, lopanoic acid, steroids)

(v) supportive measures (restoring electrolyte and fluid status, anti-pyretics and active cooling, treatment of heart failure, supplemental oxygen, and ventilation). Dantrolene and magnesium sulfate have also been used effectively.

Post-thyroidectomy tracheomalacia

Post-thyroidectomy tracheomalacia (PTTM), defined as dynamic airway collapse of at least 50% of tracheal diameter, results from longstanding extrinsic tracheal compression and subsequent removal of the compressive goiter. The true incidence of tracheomalacia is difficult to determine due to a lack of a universal definition, the heterogeneity of thyroid disease and variability in patients' access to healthcare [19]. In a review of 12 studies, Bennett *et al.* found five patients of 1969 patients (0.3%) suffering PTTM and Lacoste *et al.* found none among over 3000 thyroidectomies [20]. Bennett *et al.* concluded that CT imaging overestimated the severity of intubation difficulty and that the risk of PTTM has been exaggerated [21]. There is a diversity of "opinions" regarding this problem [3] but bronchoscopic identification of dynamic airway collapse has recently been provided [22]. Identification of this entity by surgical palpation or post-extubation obstructive symptoms probably under-diagnoses the disorder but may accurately reflect those patients who are likely to require intervention. The risk factors for PTTM are believed to be longstanding goiter, trachea compression, and retrosternal extension. Bronchoscopic examination through a supraglottic airway following extubation can reveal intrathoracic expiratory collapse with spontaneous ventilation. If the supraglottic airway is successfully placed, this technique allows for control of the anesthetic depth and oxygen concentration, sequesters the secretions, and enables the clinician to assess the severity of respiratory embarrassment, at least during quiet respiration [22].

Recurrent laryngeal nerve (RLN) palsy

The RLN innervates the intrinsic laryngeal musculature and gives sensory innervation to the larynx. Unilateral RLN palsy is usually well tolerated but may result in hoarseness, breathlessness, and an ineffective cough. Delayed aspiration may also occur. Bilateral RLN palsy is generally more dramatic, presenting with early stridor and breathlessness requiring urgent re-intubation.

Some surgeons advocate preoperative evaluation of the vocal cords since vocal cord dysfunction may be asymptomatic. Routine intraoperative identification of the recurrent laryngeal nerve and good surgical technique minimizes the risk of nerve injury. RLN palsy most commonly occurs with an intact RLN rather than a transsected nerve: 3.45% vs. 0.45% [20,23]. There are numerous mechanisms of nerve injury including ischemia, contusion, stretching resulting from traction, entrapment, thermal, and transection [23]. The incidence of permanent nerve injury is < 1% [20] and temporary nerve injury 3–4% [23,24], which usually recovers within 2 weeks to 6 months. The risk of injury is increased with malignancy [25], anatomical variability [26], secondary surgery [24], and inexperienced operators. Although bilateral RLN palsy is rare, thyroidectomy is the leading cause of this injury.

Intraoperative nerve monitoring is safe and simple but whether it is effective in reducing RLN damage remains to be established [27,28]. The benefits may be greatest in patients at high risk of nerve injury (e.g., secondary cancer surgery) or patients with known RLN palsy on the contralateral side. A 2006 survey found 13.8% of American endocrine surgeons routinely used intraoperative electrophysiological monitoring while 23.9% used it selectively [28].

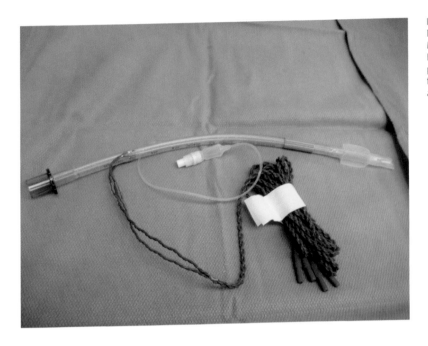

The RLN can be stimulated directly or via the vagus. The response can be assessed by inspection or palpation of the cricoarytenoid or vocal cord movement. Alternatively, a silicone, wire-reinforced endotracheal tube with surface or embedded electrodes can be accurately placed just above the vocal cords, to provide an intralaryngeal surface EMG recording [29] (e.g., Medtronic Xomed NIM™ EMG Endotracheal Tube, Minneapolis, MN; see Figures 17.1 and 17.2). False-negative responses – failure to locate the nerve – may occur with poor vocal cord contact (incorrect ETT positioning, electrode/ETT migration, small ETT or head and neck movement), deep anesthesia, muscle paralysis, local anesthesia lubricants or neuromuscular fatigue from prolonged or repeated exposure to electrical stimuli. The outer diameter of these ETTs is approximately 1 mm larger than standard ETTs of the same internal diameter. Correct placement of the exposed electrodes can be easily verified with videolaryngoscopy. These endotracheal tubes increase cost, require a stylet, cannot be used in the presence of neuromuscular blockade, and may suffer from cuff herniation with over inflation.

Postoperative assessment of RLN integrity can be determined by visualizing vocal fold mobility during spontaneous ventilation using direct or video- or flexible laryngoscopy, the latter with [25] or without a supraglottic airway. The management of unilateral RLN palsy is supportive but some surgeons favor immediate re-exploration.

Hypocalcemia

Transient hypocalcemia, the most common complication following total thyroidectomy, occurs in approximately 5.4–20% [30,31] of cases depending on the type of surgery performed, although permanent hypocalcemia is rare. The cause of hypocalcaemia may be direct trauma to the parathyroid glands, devascularization of the glands, or removal of the glands during surgery. In patients at high risk of postoperative hypocalcemia, such as total thyroidectomy with central neck dissection, parathyroid autotransplantation may be considered.

Patients at risk of iatrogenic hypoparathyroidism should have ionized calcium (or albumin-adjusted total calcium) levels monitored postoperatively until calcium levels demonstrate that parathyroid function is intact. Alternatively, a normal postoperative PTH level can predict normocalcemia after thyroid surgery.

Hypocalcemia usually presents after 24 hours with perioral tingling, twitching or tetany and can progress to seizures or ventricular arrhythmias if left untreated. Clinical signs include carpopedal spasm during blood pressure cuff inflation (Trousseau's sign), facial twitching by tapping over the facial nerve at the

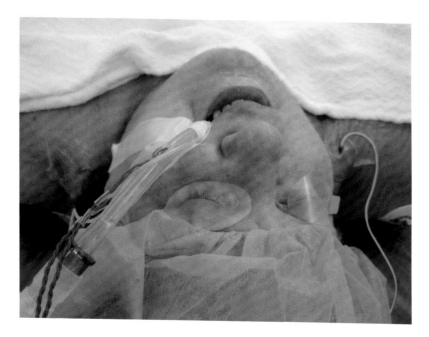

parotid gland (Chvostek's sign) and the ECG may show a prolonged QT interval. Patients who have symptomatic hypocalcemia in the early postoperative period or whose calcium levels continue to fall require rapid treatment. Patients with symptoms and serum calcium lower than 7.0 mg/dl (1.75 mmol/l) or ionized calcium level lower than 3.6 mg/dl (0.9 mmol/l) can be treated with 1 g calcium gluconate (10%) by slow intravenous infusion followed by oral replacement.

Parathyroid surgery

Primary hyperparathyroidism may result from benign parathyroid adenoma (85%), multiple gland hyperplasia (15%) and carcinoma of the parathyroid glands (< 1%). Most of the clinical manifestations of primary hyperparathyroidism are due to hypercalcemia but the classic description of "moans, groans, and abdominal pain" is rare. Most patients have mild or nonspecific signs and symptoms including skeletal muscle weakness, nephrolithiasis, polyuria and polydipsia, renal failure, anemia, peptic ulcer disease, vomiting, pancreatitis, hypertension, prolonged PR interval, short QT interval, generalized osteopenia, bone pain, decline in mental function, personality changes, and mood disturbances [32]. Other conditions can cause hypercalcemia, such as bone metastases, vitamin D intoxication, milk-alkali syndrome, sarcoidosis, and prolonged immobilization. An

elevated ionized Ca and urinary Ca in association with increased parathyroid hormone confirms the diagnosis of hyperparathyroidism.

Operative intervention remains the only curative therapy for patients with primary hyperparathyroidism. Surgery is effective with minimal risk so is commonly recommended even in asymptomatic patients. Symptomatic patients with significant hypercalcemia require medical control with hydration, furosemide and bisphosphonates (palmidronate or etidronate) before undergoing surgery. Plicamycin, glucocorticoids, calcitonin or dialysis may be required for refractory or severe hypercalcemia. Avoidance of hypoventilation (which increases ionized Ca) and maintenance of hydration and urine output is important during the perioperative period. Hypercalcemia may result in cardiac arrhythmias and alter the sensitivity to neuromuscular blockers.

Secondary hyperparathyroidism is caused by parathyroid gland hyperplasia as a compensatory response to hypocalcemia from a primary disease process, commonly chronic renal failure. The initial treatment is directed at controlling the underlying primary disease. Parathyroidectomy is indicated when medical therapy or dialysis fails to relieve the symptoms of bone pain, pruritus, and malaise or to control calcium and phosphate levels [32]. Patients with secondary hyperparathyroidism are more medically challenging. They require preoperative assessment of the underlying cause and are at risk of postoperative "hungry bone" syndrome, which causes acute-onset severe hypocalcaemia, usually with hypomagnesemia and hypophosphatemia.

Traditionally parathyroidectomy was performed with a midline incision and bilateral neck dissection, although minimally invasive parathyroidectomy (MIP) is growing in acceptance. With traditional surgery, if an adenoma is detected, the presence of a normal gland makes further exploration unnecessary, though some surgeons will attempt to identify and remove virtually all of the parathyroid glands with autotransplantation of a small amount of parathyroid tissue.

MIP can be performed with regional anesthesia, a smaller skin incision, shorter lengths of stay, a lower incidence of transient hypocalcemia, low complication rates and comparable success. Preoperative localization of abnormal parathyroid glands is achieved with sestamibi ^{99m}Tc scans while interoperatively use is made of focused parathyroid resection and in conjunction with PTH sampling at 5-minute intervals. Resection is considered curative if there is a greater than 50% decrease in venous or arterial intraoperative parathyroid hormone (iPTH) levels at 5, 10, or 15 minutes post resection compared to the baseline sample. If the iPTH level fails to decrease by 50% the surgeon can re-explore the neck for a second adenoma or additional hyperplastic tissue before waking the patient [33,34].

There are several possible operative adjuncts for the MIP operation, including radio-guided gamma probes, the video-assisted approach, and laparoscopic techniques. Very small adenomas and those located in aberrant locations, such as the mediastinum or posterior to the trachea, are not amenable to ultrasound examination. MIP may not be suitable if the patient has concomitant thyroid surgery, multi-glandular parathyroid disease, inadequate preoperative localization, or previous parathyroid surgery [34].

Case study
Preoperative evaluation

A 42-year-old female presented for elective total thyroidectomy. She complained of increasing neck enlargement over 6 months and recent recumbent dyspnea but no voice changes, dysphagia, odynophagia or symptoms suggestive of hyper- or hypothyroidism. On examination, she was 155 cm, 100 kg (BMI 40 kg/m^2). Elevation of her arms over her head produced facial plethora and jugular venous distension (Pemberton's sign). Her oropharyngeal view was a Mallampati 3, the thyromental distance was 7 cm, interincisor gap was 4 cm and neck circumference was 38 cm. Preoperative endoscopy revealed laryngeal deviation to the right with diminished right vocal cord mobility. Thyroid function tests and hematology labs were within normal limits. A CT scan of the neck with contrast showed a large heterogeneous thyroid gland, extending 20 cm from above the hyoid to the level of the aortic valve in the anterior mediastinum. There was right-ward tracheal deviation and compression to a minimum of 5 mm, 6 cm inferior to the glottis. The brachiocephalic veins and superior vena cava were compressed (Figure 17.3).

Induction of anesthesia

An induction and intubation plan was made after consultation with the ENT and thoracic surgeons. Plan A was a bronchoscopy-assisted intubation under topical anesthesia with sedation. Plan B was intravenous induction with tracheal intubation using a videolaryngoscope or rigid bronchoscope.

A femoral venous catheter and left radial arterial line were inserted in the semi-recumbent position and standard anesthesia monitoring was applied. A rigid bronchoscope, 2 units of red pack cells and the surgical teams were immediately available.

With the patient in the seated position and the anesthesia team to the patient's right, oxygen was administered by nasal cannulae and sedation with remifentanil (0.05 μg/kg/min), and midazolam (1 mg IV) was commenced, monitoring for cardiovascular or respiratory stability. A mixture of equal parts of lidocaine jelly (2%) and lidocaine (2%) sweetened with added sweetener ("Pacey's Paste", Figure 17.4) was applied to the oropharynx. The adequacy of topical anesthesia was assessed and reinforced by applying lidocaine ointment (5%) to a laryngoscope blade and slowly advancing this along the patient's tongue until the gag was suppressed. A pre-warmed 6.5-mm wire-reinforced endotracheal tube was advanced over an adult bronchoscope and easily passed beyond the tracheal narrowing. The cuff was inflated with alkalinized lidocaine (40 mg) [12]. Sevoflurane was slowly increased while maintaining spontaneous ventilation. Then the bed was adjusted to a supine position and after establishing that manual

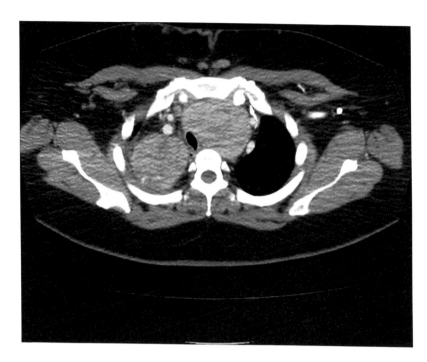

Figure 17.3. The CT scan shows a large retrosternal thyroid compressing the intrathoracic trachea and causing rightward deviation. This image with contrast shows compression of the left brachiocephalic vein and a collateral vessel in the anterior chest wall.

positive-pressure ventilation was tolerated, rocuronium and mechanical ventilation were instituted.

Maintenance of anesthesia

General anesthesia was maintained with sevoflurane and fentanyl. Prior to emergence, granisetron and dexamethasone were administered for PONV prophylaxis and to decrease postoperative airway edema. The retrosternal cervical goiter and ectopic mediastinal goiter were removed via a neck incision and sternotomy with minimal blood loss and recurrent laryngeal nerves identification and protection. Before wound closure a Valsalva maneuver was performed to assess venous hemostasis and lymphatic integrity.

Emergence and recovery from anesthesia

At the completion of the case a Bailey's maneuver was performed [9]. The oropharynx was suctioned to remove secretions. A nasogastric tube was advanced through the drainage tube of a Proseal LMA®. Under deep anesthesia with muscle relaxation, a videolaryngoscope was used to position the gastric tube behind the endotracheal tube and into the esophagus. The Proseal LMA was advanced over the gastric tube and once proper positioning was established, the cuff of

the ETT was deflated and the latter was removed. A bronchoscopic adapter was affixed to the LMA and bronchoscopy confirmed the laryngeal view. The muscle relaxant was reversed and the absence of tracheomalacia and laryngeal movement were assessed as spontaneous ventilation resumed. Emergence with the PLMA was well tolerated and the patient removed the airway with minimal coughing after recovering consciousness. She was transferred to PACU, where a chest X-ray was performed. After an uneventful 60 minutes in PACU she was transferred to the high-dependency unit. Her preoperative total corrected calcium fell from 2.45 mmol/l (normal = 2.2–2.6 mmol/l) to its lowest level of 1.96 mmol/l 6 hours postoperatively before normalizing prior to discharge on day 5 with supplements. Levothyroxine 0.15 mg daily was commenced.

Clinical pearls

- With very few exceptions, thyroid surgery is elective. Readiness for surgery may be judged by symptom resolution and normalization of weight and heart rate.
- A small proportion of patients with enlarged thyroids may be difficult to ventilate via mask or supraglottic airway.

171

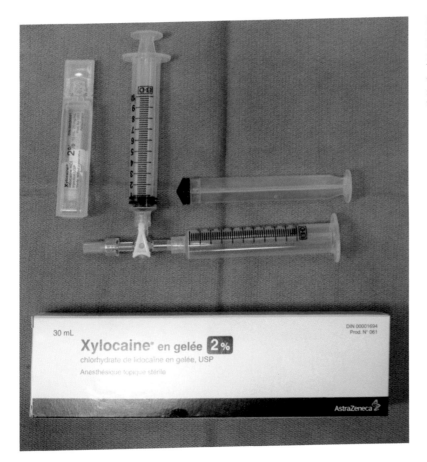

Figure 17.4. Pacey's paste (described by Dr. John A. Pacey) consists of 5 ml 2% lidocaine and 5 ml of lidocaine jelly, mixed by way of a three-way stopcock. The sticky suspension can be sweetened with sugar or a small amount of artificial sweetener and is applied by catheter to the posterior oropharynx.

- Symptoms of dysphagia, recumbent dyspnea, a change in voice or stridor should alert the anesthesiologist to possible compromised airway and possible difficulties with airway management following induction of anesthesia.
- For patients with a retrosternal goiter with tracheal compression or superior vena cava syndrome, several induction strategies have been advocated, including intravenous induction with neuromuscular blockade and direct laryngoscopy, inhalational induction, and awake flexible bronchoscopic intubation; specific management will depend on the unique features of the individual case and the skills of the clinical staff.
- Superior vena cava syndrome may result in airway edema, dependence on spontaneous ventilation for venous return, and hemodynamic instability. Dyspnea and hoarseness in such patients may reflect edema of the vocal cords. Surgical bleeding is often increased due to increased central venous pressure. Intravenous access in the legs rather than in the arms and invasive blood pressure monitoring should be considered.
- Deep extubation reduces the incidence of coughing, bucking, and straining but at an increased risk of airway obstruction and aspiration.
- A Bailey maneuver, wherein a supraglottic airway is substituted for the ETT while the patient is still under neuromuscular blockade and deep anesthesia, may be helpful. The depth of anesthesia, oxygen concentration, ventilatory support, and sequestration of secretions are all potentially under control. Although this technique has several advantages, it should be regarded as "a high-risk maneuver in high-risk patients" and is best practiced in low-risk patients to ensure the requisite skills.
- For post-thyroidectomy neck hematoma, removal of sutures and hematoma evacuation should be performed immediately if the patient is in extremis or if immediate airway management is

not available. Hematoma evacuation may assist some patients by relieving direct hematoma compression but it will not resolve airway obstruction from perilaryngeal edema.

- The management of thyroid storm includes:

  - blocking of the sympathetic response (β-blockers)
  - the blocking of thyroid hormone synthesis (PTU or methimazole)
  - the blocking of thyroid hormone release (dexamethasone, lopanoic acid or Lugol's solution)
  - the blocking of T_4 to T_3 conversion (β-blocker, PTU, lopanoic acid, steroids)
  - supportive measures (restoring electrolyte and fluid status, anti-pyretics and active cooling, treatment of heart failure, supplemental oxygen

and ventilation). Dantrolene and magnesium sulfate have also been used effectively.

- A silicone, wire-reinforced endotracheal tube with surface or embedded electrodes can be accurately placed at the level of the vocal cords, to provide an intralaryngeal surface EMG recording (e.g., Medtronic Xomed NIM™ EMG Endotracheal Tube, Minneapolis, MN).

- Postoperative hypocalcemia, should it occur, usually presents after 24 hours with perioral tingling, twitching or tetany and can progress to seizures or ventricular arrhythmias if left untreated. Clinical signs include carpopedal spasm during cuff inflation (Trousseau's sign), facial twitching by tapping over the facial nerve at the parotid gland (Chvostek's sign), and a prolonged QT interval on the ECG.

References

1. Amathieu R, Smail N, Catineau J, et al. Difficult intubation in thyroid surgery: myth or reality? Anesth Analg 2006;103(4):965–8.

2. Farling PA. Thyroid disease. Br J Anaesth 2000;85(1):15–28.

3. Cook TM, Morgan PJ, Hersch PE. Equal and opposite expert opinion. Airway obstruction caused by a retrosternal thyroid mass: management and prospective international expert opinion. Anaesthesia 2011; 66(9):828–36.

4. Radauceanu DS, Dunn JOC, Lagattolla N, Farquhar-Thomson D. Temporary extracorporeal jugulosaphenous bypass for the peri-operative management of patients with superior vena caval obstruction: a report of three cases. Anaesthesia 2009;64 (11):1246–9.

5. Mackle T, Meaney J, Timon C. Tracheoesophageal compression associated with substernal goitre. Correlation of symptoms with cross-sectional imaging findings. J Laryngol Otol 2007;121(4):358–61.

6. White M, Doherty G, Gauger P. Evidence-based surgical management of substernal goiter. World J Surg 2008;32(7): 1285–300.

7. Spanknebel K, Chabot JA, DiGiorgi M, et al. Thyroidectomy using local anesthesia: a report of 1,025 cases over 16 years. J Am Coll Surg 2005;201(3): 375–85.

8. Koga K, Asai T, Vaughan RS, Latto IP. Respiratory complications associated with tracheal extubation. Timing of tracheal extubation and use of the laryngeal mask during emergence from anaesthesia. Anaesthesia 1998;53(6):540–4.

9. Nair I, Bailey PM. Use of the laryngeal mask for airway maintenance following tracheal extubation. Anaesthesia 1995; 50(2):174–5.

10. Hans P, Marechal H, Bonhomme V. Effect of propofol and sevoflurane on coughing in smokers and non-smokers awakening from general anaesthesia at the end of a cervical spine surgery. Br J Anaesth 2008;101(5):731–7.

11. Hohlrieder M, Tiefenthaler W, Klaus H, et al. Effect of total intravenous anaesthesia and balanced anaesthesia on the frequency of coughing during emergence from the anaesthesia. Br J Anaesth 2007;99(4): 587–91.

12. Estebe JP, Gentili M, Le CP, Dollo G, Chevanne F, Ecoffey C. Alkalinization of intracuff lidocaine: efficacy and safety. Anesth Analg 2005;101(5): 1536–41.

13. Minogue SC, Ralph J, Lampa MJ. Laryngotracheal topicalization with lidocaine before intubation decreases the incidence of coughing on emergence from general anesthesia. Anesth Analg 2004;99(4):1253–7.

14. Aouad MT, Al-Alami AA, Nasr VG, et al. The effect of low-dose remifentanil on responses to the endotracheal tube during emergence from general anesthesia. Anesth Analg 2009;108(4):1157–60.

15. Rosato L, Avenia N, Bernante P, et al. Complications of thyroid surgery: analysis of a multicentric study on 14,934 patients operated on in Italy over 5 years. World J Surg 2004;28(3): 271–6.

16. Bononi M, Bonapasta SA, Scarpini M, et al. Incidence and circumstances of cervical hematoma complicating thyroidectomy and its relationship to postoperative vomiting. *Head Neck* 2010;**32**(9):1173–7.

17. Rosenbaum MA, Haridas M, McHenry CR. Life-threatening neck hematoma complicating thyroid and parathyroid surgery. *Am J Surg* 2008;**195**(3):339–43; discussion 43.

18. Nayak B, Burman K. Thyrotoxicosis and thyroid storm. *Endocrinol Metab Clin North Am* [Review] 2006;**35**(4):663–86, vii.

19. Abdel Rahim A, Ahmed M, Hassan M. Respiratory complications after thyroidectomy and the need for tracheostomy in patients with a large goitre. *Br J Surg* 1999;**86**(1):88–90.

20. Lacoste L, Gineste D, Karayan J, et al. Airway complications in thyroid surgery. *Ann Otol Rhinol Laryngol* 1993;**102**(6):441–6.

21. Bennett A, Hashmi S, Premachandra D, Wright M. The myth of tracheomalacia and difficult intubation in cases of retrosternal goitre. *J Laryngol Otol* 2004;**118**(10):778–80.

22. Lee C, Cooper RM, Goldstein D. Management of a patient with tracheomalacia and supraglottic obstruction after thyroid surgery. *Canadian J Anaesth* 2011;**58**(11):1029–33.

23. Snyder SK, Lairmore TC, Hendricks JC, Roberts JW. Elucidating mechanisms of recurrent laryngeal nerve injury during thyroidectomy and parathyroidectomy. *J Am Coll Surg* 2008;**206**(1):123–30.

24. Chan W-F, Lang BH-H, Lo C-Y. The role of intraoperative neuromonitoring of recurrent laryngeal nerve during thyroidectomy: a comparative study on 1000 nerves at risk. *Surgery* 2006;**140**(6):866–73.

25. Maroof M, Siddique M, Khan RM. Post-thyroidectomy vocal cord examination by fibreoscopy aided by the laryngeal mask airway. *Anaesthesia* 1992;**47**(5):445.

26. Nemiroff PM, Katz AD. Extralaryngeal divisions of the recurrent laryngeal nerve: surgical and clinical significance. *Am J Surg* 1982;**144**(4):466–9.

27. Angelos P. Recurrent laryngeal nerve monitoring: state of the art, ethical and legal issues. *Surg Clin North Am* 2009;**89**(5):1157–69.

28. Sturgeon C, Sturgeon T, Angelos P. Neuromonitoring in thyroid surgery: attitudes, usage patterns, and predictors of use among endocrine surgeons. *World J Surg* 2009;**33**(3):417–25.

29. Johnson S, Goldenberg D. Intraoperative monitoring of the recurrent laryngeal nerve during revision thyroid surgery. *Otolaryngol Clin North Am* 2008;**41**(6):1147–54.

30. Pattou F, Combemale F, Fabra S, et al. Hypocalcemia following thyroid surgery: incidence and prediction of outcomes. *World J Surg* 1998;**22**(7):718–24.

31. Bacuzzi A, Dionigi G, Del Bosco A, et al. Anaesthesia for thyroid surgery: perioperative management. *Int J Surg* 2008;**6** Suppl 1:S82–5.

32. Mihai R, Farndon JR. Parathyroid disease and calcium metabolism. *Br J Anaesth* 2000;**85**(1):29–43.

33. Chen H, Pruhs Z, Starling JR, Mack E. Intraoperative parathyroid hormone testing improves cure rates in patients undergoing minimally invasive parathyroidectomy. *Surgery* 2005;**138**(4):583–7; discussion 7–90.

34. Monchik JM, Barellini L, Langer P, Kahya A. Minimally invasive parathyroid surgery in 103 patients with local/regional anesthesia, without exclusion criteria. *Surgery* 2002;**131**(5):502–8.

Chapter

18

Anesthesia for obstructive sleep apnea surgery

Ursula Galway and Alan Kominsky

Introduction

Obstructive sleep apnea (OSA) is a sleep-related breathing disorder that involves periodic, partial or complete upper airway obstruction despite an ongoing effort to breathe. It is caused by the repetitive collapse or partial collapse of the pharyngeal airway during sleep. This leads to apneas (complete obstruction of the airway), hypopneas (partial obstruction leading to desaturation) and respiratory effort-related arousals (RERAs – partial obstruction leading to arousal but no significant desaturation). The prevalence of OSA is estimated to be 2% in women and 4% in men [1].

Typically the OSA patient suffers obstruction of the airway in the presence of continued movement of the diaphragm. Attempted inspiration continues and arterial oxygen saturation may fall. This hypoxia leads to partial arousal from sleep, with a sudden reopening of the airway and an intake of breath. This may be followed by brief hyperventilation and the cycle begins again. These events may cause episodic sleep-associated oxygen desaturation and hypercarbia. The severity of the disease is determined by the number of these respiratory events per hour, known as the RDI or respiratory disturbance index [2]. Central sleep apnea is a condition in which the brain's respiratory control center is imbalanced during sleep. The brain does not respond to changing levels of carbon dioxide. During periods of apnea there is no effort to breathe, no chest wall movement and no obstruction during pauses. Hyperpnea may follow these apneic spells. Central sleep apnea may be caused by conditions such as heart failure and stroke.

OSA leads to disturbed sleep and possible daytime sleepiness. Consequently, patients can be a danger to themselves and others, particularly if driving. More serious long-term consequences include a rise in sympathetic tone, ischemic heart disease, hypertension, tachyarrhythmias, deterioration in cognitive function, pulmonary hypertension, cor pulmonale, congestive heart failure, cardiovascular accident/stroke and sudden death. These sequelae are the result of the physiologic consequences of the respiratory events. In severe cases, pulmonary hypertension and polycythemia occur due to prolonged hypoxemia. Systemic hypertension occurs due to increased levels of catecholamines. According to the National Commission on Sleep Disorders Research, there are 38 000 cardiovascular deaths per year in the United States secondary to OSA [3]. Untreated, the 15-year mortality for adults with severe OSA is 30% [4]. OSA in itself is associated with an increase in postoperative complications and is an independent risk factor for increased morbidity and mortality [5,6].

Clinical features that suggest the presence of OSA include increased neck circumference (> 17 inches in men > 16 inches in women), body mass index ≥ 30 kg/m^2, Mallampati score of 3 or 4, retrognathia, macroglossia, tonsillar hypertrophy, enlarged uvula, high narrow hard palate, and/or nasal abnormalities [7].

Continuous positive airway pressure (CPAP) is considered the first line of treatment for patients with OSA; however, surgery may be considered if this treatment is not tolerated.

Diagnosis

OSA is diagnosed by clinical history and an overnight sleep study or polysomnography (PSG). OSA is suspected by the occurrence of daytime sleepiness, loud snoring, witnessed breathing interruptions or awakenings due to gasping or choking. The severity of OSA cannot be predicted clinically, therefore

Anesthesia for Otolaryngologic Surgery, ed. Basem Abdelmalak and D. John Doyle. Published by Cambridge University Press.
© Cambridge University Press 2013.

objective testing is required. Polysomnography includes monitoring of chest wall movement, airflow dynamics, heart rate, blood pressure, arterial oxygen saturation, electroencephalogram, electrooculogram, and chin electromyogram during sleep. Obstructive events are recorded as apnea hypopnea index (AHI) or respiratory disturbance index (RDI). The American Academy of Sleep Medicine currently recommends the use of RDI in the determination of sleep apnea severity. RDI is defined as the total number of apneas, hypopneas, and respiratory effort-related arousals during sleep divided by the number of hours of recorded sleep. In contrast the AHI is defined as the total number of apneas and hypopneas during the study divided by the number of hours of recorded sleep. OSA is confirmed if the number of RDIs is >15 events per hour or greater than five events per hour in a patient who also reports unintentional sleep episodes during waking hours, daytime sleepiness, un-refreshing sleep, fatigue, insomnia, waking up, breath-holding, gasping, choking, or bed-partner description of snoring and breathing interruptions. OSA is classified as mild, moderate or severe based on the respiratory disturbance index [7].

   Mild: RDI 5–14
   Moderate: RDI 15–29
   Severe: RDI>30

Medical treatment

Positive airway pressure (PAP) is considered the first line of treatment for patients with OSA. PAP treatment attempts to maintain a competent airway through the application of continuous positive airway pressure (CPAP), bi-level positive pressure (BiPAP) or auto-titrating positive pressure (APAP). It can be applied via the oral, nasal or oronasal route. PAP is the treatment of choice for all severities of OSA. PAP has the potential to reduce cardiac dysrhythmias, stabilize blood pressure, and improve hemodynamics. PAP has been found to be protective against cardiovascular death and improves survival [8].

   Oral appliances (OA) may also be used. Oral appliances may improve airway patency by enlarging the upper airway and improving upper airway muscle tone. They may be used by those intolerant of CPAP who have mild to moderate OSA.

   Behavioral treatment used in the treatment of OSA includes weight loss, positional therapy, and avoidance of sedatives and alcohol at bedtime.

Surgical treatment

Despite being the first line of treatment, CPAP is often poorly tolerated by patients. More than 50% of patients with OSA are intolerant of CPAP. Patients turn to surgical correction in an attempt to find a cure. Surgery may be considered in patients who have obstructing anatomy that is surgically correctable or when PAP or OA are inadequate or poorly tolerated. It may also be considered as an adjunct when obstructive anatomy compromises other therapies [4].

   Patients who fail medical management or desire surgical therapy should initially be evaluated for eligibility for surgery. The presence and severity of OSA must be confirmed before undergoing surgery. Thus, a preoperative PSG is warranted. Desired outcomes include resolution of clinical signs and symptoms, normalization of sleep, AHI, and oxygen saturation [9]. Indications for surgery depend on the severity of the sleep apnea, symptoms, and comorbid conditions, and the anatomical location of the obstruction. Patients should be counseled on the surgical options, goals, risk, benefits, and possible complications. Surgeries can be performed singly or in a staged manner [4].

   Surgical treatment has a variable success rate, with patients seldom receiving a total cure. Surgical success has been defined as an AHI less than 20/h and a reduction of the AHI by 50% or more after surgery. Surgical cure is defined as AHI <5/h [4]. After any surgical procedure for OSA, patients should undergo follow-up evaluation including objective testing as well as clinical assessment for residual symptoms [9].

   Anatomically, resistance can occur anywhere from one to four places; intranasal, at the level of the palate (type 1), at the palate and the base of tongue (type 2) or at the base of the tongue alone (type 3) [10]. The palate of patients with OSA has increased muscle and fat content compared with control patients [11]. Any of these locations may be targeted during surgery in an attempt to reduce obstruction. Surgical treatment involves either modification of the obstructing upper airway or, rarely, total bypass of the upper airway (tracheostomy) (Table 18.1).

Nasal procedures

The three anatomic areas that can contribute to OSA as a result of increased nasal resistance include the alar cartilage/nasal valve area, the septum and the

Table 18.1. Surgical procedures and anesthetic choices for OSA

Anatomical location	Surgical procedure	Anesthesia
Nasal	Septoplasty, Functional rhinoplasty, Turbinate reduction, Nasal polypectomy	Local ± sedation or general anesthesia with supraglottic airway or endotracheal tube
Oral/ oropharyngeal/ nasopharyngeal	UPPP, UPF, Tonsillectomy/adenoidectomy	General anesthesia with endotracheal tube
Hypopharyngeal	GA, Tongue reduction surgery	General anesthesia with endotracheal tube
Laryngeal	Epiglottoplasty, Hyoid suspension	General anesthesia with endotracheal tube
Global airway	MMA, Maxillomandibular expansion	General anesthesia with nasotracheal tube
Trachea	Tracheostomy	Local ± sedation or general anesthesia with supraglottic airway or endotracheal tube

turbinates [12]. Nasal surgeries aimed at reducing OSA symptoms include septoplasty, functional rhinoplasty, turbinate reduction, and nasal polypectomy. Septoplasty and turbinate reduction are the most common nasal surgeries. Improvements in OSA post nasal surgery may only be minimal but can improve AHI scores and may decrease CPAP pressure requirements [13,14].

Oral, oropharyngeal and nasopharyngeal procedures

Uvulopalatopharyngoplasty

Uvulopalatopharyngoplasty (UPPP) involves removal of the redundant soft palate, pharyngeal tissues and as the uvula. This attempts to widen the oropharyngeal inlet. The tonsils are also removed. Early complications such as wound dehiscence, bleeding and infection are rare. Late complications can include velopharyngeal insufficiency, postnasal secretions, pharyngeal discomfort, odynophagia, tongue numbness, stenosis, and dysphagia [12]. The success rate is reported to be between 40% and 60%, with a cure rate of 16% as it only addresses oropharyngeal obstruction and not hypopharyngeal obstruction [4]. Newer techniques have been developed that are tissue-sparing with similar results.

Uvulopalatal flap (UPF)

This procedure is a modification of the UPPP involving superior suspension of a limitedly resected uvula toward the hard–soft palate junction. There is no difference in

the outcome between the UFP and UPPP groups; however, there is less pain in the UFP group [12].

Laser-assisted uvuloplasty

This is an office-based procedure in which the soft palate is reshaped using a CO_2 laser. This is not approved as a treatment option for OSA [9].

Radiofrequency ablation of the tongue

Radiofrequency energy is used to reduce the size of the base of tongue. This procedure is an adjunct to other treatments and not a primary treatment for OSA [4].

Tonsillectomy/adenoidectomy

Please refer to Chapter 32 for more on tonsillectomy and adenoidectomy.

Hypopharyngeal procedures

Tongue advancement/stabilization surgeries

Genioglossus advancement (GA)

This surgery involves the pulling forward of the base of tongue in an attempt to reduce obstruction caused by the tongue. It is often paired with UPPP and hyoid suspension. A rectangular osteotomy is performed intraorally on the mandibular symphyseal bone, which also contains the geniotubercle. This bone is advanced anteriorly, rotated to allow bony overlap, and immobilized with a titanium screw. Thus, the geniotubercle with the genioglossus insertion is moved forward without moving the mandible. This results in the tongue

177

being moved forward. Complications may include infection, hematoma, injury to the genioglossus muscle, and paresthesia of the lower teeth [12].

Tongue-reduction surgeries

The tongue size can be reduced via partial glossctomy, tongue ablation or lingual tonsillectomy.

Laryngeal procedures
Epiglottoplasty

Hyoid suspension

The hyoid bone, located just below the mandible, is involved in maintaining upper airway patency. The hyoid bone is identified via an external neck incision and then surgically repositioned anteriorly by attaching it to the thyroid cartilage or suspending it from the mandible. Complications may include infection, seroma, and dysphagia. The procedure is often combined with UPPP or GA [12].

Global airway procedures
Maxillomandibular advancement (MMA)

When abnormalities of the maxillofacial skeleton are the main contributor to OSA, MMA can be considered. MMA achieves enlargement of the entire upper airway. Anatomic abnormalities which may benefit from MMA include hypopharyngeal and/or velo-oropharyngeal narrowing. The surgery is designed to enlarge the velo-orohypopharyngeal airway without direct exploitation of the pharyngeal tissue [15]. Intraoral osteotomy of the maxilla and mandible is performed. A Le Fort 1 is created with bilateral sagittal split osteotomies of the mandible. The maxilla and mandible are advanced anteriorly and are stabilized with titanium plates, screws, or bone grafts. Advancement of the mandible results in advancement the tongue and suprahyoid muscles. Advancement of the maxilla results in advancement of the velum and velopharyngeal muscles. Transient vagally mediated bradycardia can occur secondary to maxillary or mandibular advancement [16]. It is the most effective OSA surgery available. The surgical success rate is 86%, with a cure rate of 43% [4]. Intraoperative blood loss can be between 100 and 500 ml. Complications may include infection, bleeding, malocclusion, and permanent numbness [12].

Maxillomandibular expansion

Osteotomies are performed above the roots of the maxillary teeth, between the roots of the maxillary central incisors and between the mandibular central incisor teeth. Distractors are placed and left in place for 3 months.

They provide stability to the maxilla and mandible, allowing for slow expansion until the new bone has ossified. It is less invasive than MMA; however, treatment time is lengthened [12].

Tracheostomy

Tracheostomy is the first reported treatment for OSA; however, it is rarely done these days for OSA. Tracheostomy totally bypasses the upper airway. It is the most effective treatment; however, patient acceptance is low. It is now used as a temporary measure for airway protection in the perioperative period (in morbidly obese patients) or as a long-term treatment option in severely obese patients or patients with craniofacial anomalies in whom all other forms of treatment have failed [12]. Complications can include infection, tissue necrosis, bleeding, recurrent bronchitis, granulation tissue, stoma stenosis, and tracheo-innominate fistula formation [4].

Multimodal procedures

Any of the above-mentioned surgical procedures can be performed singly, multiply or as staged procedures. Often a patient will undergo UPPP/UPF and GA/HA/radiofrequency tongue base reduction first. After a 4–6 month healing period a PSG can be obtained to assess outcome. If OSA persists, a MMA can be considered as a phase 2 operation. The surgical success rate of multimodal procedures is 66% [4].

Anesthetic management of a patient undergoing OSA surgery
Preoperative management

Optimal care begins with a tailored preoperative assessment to aid patient risk stratification and optimization [1].

Preoperative history and physical exam

A thorough history and physical exam should be obtained evaluating all of the patients' disease processes and co-morbidities. Patients with OSA are

Table 18.2. Comorbidities associated with OSA [8]

Cardiac	Respiratory	Metabolic	Neurologic	Others
Treatment-resistant hypertension	Asthma	Type 2 diabetes	Stroke	Alcoholism
Congestive heart failure, cor pulmonale	Pulmonary hypertension	Metabolic syndrome		GERD
Ischemic heart disease		Hypothyroidism		
Atrial fibrillation, dysrhythmias		Morbid obesity		

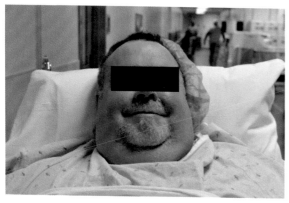

Figure 18.1. Classic appearance of a patient with obstructive sleep apnea. Image courtesy of Dr. B. Abdelmalak. Reprinted with permission, Cleveland Clinic Center for Medical Art & Photography © 2012. All rights reserved.

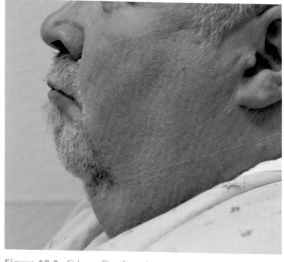

Figure 18.2. Side profile of an obstructive sleep apnea patient showing a short thyromental distance. Image courtesy of Dr. B. Abdelmalak. Reprinted with permission, Cleveland Clinic Center for Medical Art & Photography © 2012. All rights reserved.

more likely to have the comorbidities listed in Table 18.2. These disease conditions need to be optimized as well as possible prior to undergoing anesthesia and surgery. Some comorbidities may be the direct sequelae of the chronic hypoxia and hypercarbia caused by the OSA. Consultation with specialists such as cardiology and pulmonology may be warranted, especially if significant comorbidities exist.

Preoperative testing should be directed by the pre-existing comorbidities. A preoperative EKG may show signs of heart strain, ventricular hypertrophy, arrhymia or hypertension. A chest X-ray may show cardiomegaly or chronic preexisting respiratory conditions.

A preoperative echocardiogram may be warranted if suspicion of right heart failure or pulmonary hypertension exists. Complete blood count may show signs of polycythemia if the patient is chronically hypoxemic. A basic metabolic panel should be obtained to assess any electrolyte abnormalities, particularly if the patient is on any diuretics for hypertension. A coagulation panel is not necessary unless the patient is on chronic anticoagulation or has a history of bleeding abnormalities.

Airway assessment

A thorough airway exam is of the utmost importance. Patients with OSA may be difficult to intubate or ventilate. The upper airway abnormalities which lead to OSA can be the same abnormalities which lead to a difficult airway. Snoring and OSA were found to be independent risk factors for difficult mask ventilation [17]. Difficult intubation was found to occur eight times more often in OSA patients than in control patients [18]. An OSA patient (Figure 18.1) is likely to have tonsil or uvula hypertrophy, anterior positioning of the larynx, retro-or micrognathia, nasal obstruction, thick neck, high Mallampati score (Figure 18.2) and a decreased thyromental distance (Figure 18.3) [2]. Old anesthesia records if available should be reviewed, looking in particular for ventilation or intubation difficulties and whether there has been any interval changes in weight and its impact on the airway. The patient should be educated regarding the possibility of an awake intubation.

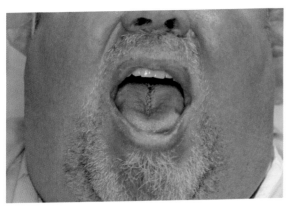

Figure 18.3. Mallampati grade 4 oropharyngeal view in an obstructive sleep apnea patient. Image courtesy of Dr. B. Abdelmalak. Reprinted with permission, Cleveland Clinic Center for Medical Art & Photography © 2012. All rights reserved.

Surgical evaluation

The preoperative ENT evaluation will include a direct visual exam and a fiberoptic nasopharyngoscopy to assess anatomic abnormalities that may be contributing to OSA [12]. Fiberoptic nasopharyngoscopy allows the surgeon to assess the entire airway from nose to larynx.

The Muller maneuver (maximal inspiratory effort against closed nose and mouth) can give some insight into the level at which the obstruction occurs and the dimensions of the obstruction.

A CT scan can provide good airway and bony resolution and an MRI allows evaluation of the palate, tongue base, and posterior pharyngeal wall. These tests may sometimes be ordered preoperatively [10].

Aspiration prophylaxis

Obese patients, due to their high intraabdominal pressure, larger gastric fluid volume and lower gastric pH, may be at risk of aspiration. Consideration should be given to aspiration prophylaxis with antacid, proton pump inhibitor, and esophageal motility stimulant prior to induction.

Preoperative sedation

Unsupervised preoperative sedation should be avoided. OSA patients are at higher risk of obstruction and apnea after the administration of sedatives. If sedatives are to be given, it should only be done in a monitored environment.

Intraoperative management

Special consideration should be given to the OSA patient with regard to anesthetic technique, choice of pain medication, airway management, and prevention of airway edema.

Choice of anesthetic technique

General anesthesia with a secured, intubated airway is preferable because of the risk of aspiration of blood from the surgical site and the patient's likelihood of obstruction when sedated. There is also the risk of laryngospasm if blood or secretions touch the vocal cords in an unsecured airway. OSA patients have a propensity towards airway collapse, sleep deprivation, and blunting of physiological response to hypoxia and hypercarbia. This makes them especially susceptible to the respiratory depressant effects of sedatives, opioids, and inhaled anesthetics. These drugs reduce the brain's arousal response and may worsen the number of respiratory events, leading to hypoxemia and hypercarbia [2]. Patients with OSA receiving oral or parenteral opioids are 12–14 times more likely to have postoperative oxygen desaturations than those receiving nonopioid analgesic agents [19]. One study showed that patients receiving 2.9 µg/kg fentanyl versus 1.7 µg/kg fentanyl intraoperatively had more obstruction after extubation and other extubation problems [20]. However, these procedures may be quite painful and if only short-acting narcotics are used, additional doses of narcotics may be needed in PACU, delaying discharge. It may be prudent to judiciously dose longer-acting narcotics at the beginning of the surgery so that they do not delay extubation at the conclusion of this relatively short procedure, and at the same time remain effective while in the recovery room. With that in mind, careful thought should be given when selecting intraoperative medications. Consideration should also be given to the use of non-narcotic analgesics or short-acting narcotic analgesics. Anesthesia can be maintained using total IV anesthesia such as a propofol infusion, due to its quick onset and offset. A short-acting narcotic infusion such as remifentanil or alfentanil may also be used. Insoluble anesthetic agents such as desflurane, which are more quickly eliminated when discontinued, should be considered for maintenance of anesthesia. However, all other inhalational anesthetics may be safely used as long as they are discontinued at the appropriate time towards the end of surgery based on their solubility.

Airway management

As mentioned, patients with OSA may have a difficult airway and should be managed accordingly. Patients may have excess oro- and hypopharyngeal soft tissue leading to significant obstruction during induction of anesthesia. They may also have mandibular or maxillary deficiencies, macroglossia, lingual tonsil hypertrophy, enlarged uvula, redundant pharyngeal tissue, large neck circumference, an anterior larynx, and a long airway, making direct laryngoscopy difficult. Patients ramping from scapulae to head and utilizing the sniffing position may help improve visualization of the glottis. The patient should breathe 100% oxygen for 3 minutes with a tightly fitting mask to ensure adequate pre-oxygenation. Two-person mask ventilation with the aid of oral or nasal airways may be needed. An awake intubation should be considered if there is any question of difficulty of ventilation or intubation. Video-assisted laryngoscopy may be useful in helping visualize the larynx if unable to do so with direct laryngoscopy [21]. The ASA difficult airway algorithm should always be followed [22]. Patients undergoing MMA need to be nasally intubated for the surgery. Procedures such as radiofrequency ablation of the tongue and laser-assisted uvuloplasty are often done as an adjunct to other treatments; however, if performed alone, anesthesia is not required. After surgery has been completed, patients should be extubated fully awake with full reversal of neuromuscular blockade. They should demonstrate purposeful movement and adequate strength and tidal volume. If bleeding is a concern the surgeon may request a deep extubation, as coughing during emergence may worsen bleeding. A deep extubation should be performed with extreme caution. Although the decrease in coughing achieved with a deep extubation is beneficial, there is a serious risk of loss of airway or laryngospasm with a deep extubation. Even if the patient was previously easy to intubate and ventilate, the postoperative airway has now been traumatized and may be edematous, bloody, and very different from the airway that was there to begin with. Extubation over a tube exchanger may be appropriate. The stomach can be suctioned prior to emergence as blood from the surgical site may have gathered in the stomach, causing stomach irritation with the resultant nausea and emesis, which can be a potential aspiration risk. Nasal packing worsens sleep apnea, and should be avoided after nasal surgery by using quilting septal sutures, septal splints, nasal tubes or nasaopharyngeal airways sewn in place [2].

Preventing airway edema

Postoperative airway edema after upper airway surgery is a concern. Although rare, airway obstruction leading to reintubation or tracheostomy most commonly occurs within hours after surgery. Airway edema may occur due to the airway surgery itself or during intubation attempts. Although controversial, systemic steroids may reduce airway edema and can be given prior to surgery and several times postoperatively. Dexamethasone, 10–15 mg, is given every 6–12 hours. Antibiotics prevent infection-induced edema and may be administered perioperatively. Application of ice packs postoperatively reduces edema [2].

Postoperative management

Postoperative complications after OSA surgery include respiratory events, infection, cardiovascular events, and bleeding. A prospective cohort study utilized the Department of Veterans Affairs National Surgical Quality Improvement Program (NSQIP) database for the years 1991–2001 to look at postoperative complications of 3130 patients undergoing inpatient UPPP with or without other concurrent procedures. They found the incidence of 30-day serious complications including death was 1.6%. Incidence of death was 0.2%, respiratory complications 1.1%, cardiovascular complications 0.3% and hemorrhage 0.3% [23].

Special consideration should be given to the following.

Analgesia

As mentioned previously, it is best to minimize opioids and sedatives, which may suppress respiratory drive and lead to life-threatening hypoxia. Patients should be warned of postoperative discomfort. Mild pain can be treated with oral opioids, acetaminophen or tramadol, best given in the liquid form. Small intravenous doses of short-acting opioids such as fentanyl can be given. Non-steroidal anti-inflammatory agents should be used with caution due to their potential to cause platelet dysfunction and bleeding. Sedating antiemetics such as prochlorpromazine should be avoided as they may cause the patient to obstruct postoperatively.

181

Oxygenation and disposition

Postoperatively, OSA patients may have a rebound of delta or rapid eye movement sleep and may be prone to more severe sleep apnea. This is likely for the first 24–48 hours [24,25]. Patients with OSA have a greater increase in AHI after surgery, peaking on postoperative day 3 and returning to preoperative level on night 7 [26]. Most serious complications occur in the first 24 hours. The ASA guidelines state that monitoring of patients with OSA postoperatively should be for a median of 3 hours longer than for those without OSA.

Patients with OSA should be monitored for a median of 7 hours after the last episode of airway obstruction or hypoxemia while breathing room air in an un-stimulating environment [1]. These guidelines, however, may really not be reasonable as most patients will continue to have apnea after surgery as surgery is not initially curative [2]. Airway complication rate for UPPP ranges from 1.4–10.3%. [20,27]. Although patients post OSA surgery may have a higher incidence of respiratory complications, ICU care may only be appropriate for the sickest of OSA patients [20,28]. One study suggests that postoperative ICU monitoring is not needed for most OSA patients and the decision should be made on an individualized basis taking into consideration the patient's other medical comorbidities, the degree of airway crowding, and the number of simultaneous surgical procedures being performed as well as the potential for postoperative edema. Complications tend to be higher in patients undergoing UPPP along with other procedures particularly concurrent nasal procedures [27].

Supplemental oxygen should be given to the patients until they are able to maintain baseline oxygen saturation on room air, bearing in mind that supplemental oxygen may increase the duration of apneic episodes and may delay the detection of atelectasis, transient apnea and hypoventilation by pulse oximetry. During hospitalization, patients should have continuous pulse oximetry until they are at least back to their baseline. This does not necessarily need to be done in an ICU but can be done in a step-down unit or by telemetry. Pulse oximetry should be applied until the room air saturation is at least above 90%. Intermittent oximetry monitoring has minimal benefit and is not recommended. Positive airway pressure devices can be used after most upper airway surgeries, except for maxillary or mandibular advancement due to the potential for subcutaneous emphysema [2].

According to the ASA practice guidelines for the perioperative management of patients with OSA, those undergoing airway surgery such as UPPP are not candidates for this surgery on an outpatient basis [1]. As far as discharge plans go, a reasonable goal should be that patients' walking oxygen saturation, respiratory event frequency, and degree of hypoxemia should be no worse at discharge than at baseline [2].

Patient positioning

Patients with OSA who sleep in the lateral, prone or sitting position usually have less apnea/hypopnea episodes than in the supine position. Although there is insufficient literature to guide us on optimal positioning in the postoperative setting, most agree on the avoidance of the supine position. In recovery, patients should be placed in the off-supine position.

Postoperative hemorrhage

Patients may be prone to postoperative bleeding, especially after tonsillectomy. Good blood pressure control and perhaps the avoidance of NSAIDS pre- and postoperatively may help reduce bleeding events.

Summary

The OSA patient presenting for OSA surgery presents a number of challenges to the anesthesiologist. These patients may have a number of cardiac and respiratory comorbidities as well as very challenging airways. Consideration should be given to optimization of medical comorbidities preoperatively, careful airway management, and minimization of sedating pain medications intraoperatively. Postoperatively airway edema, hemorrhage, and respiratory complications are a concern and the patient should be recovered in a monitored setting until they return to their baseline.

Case study – anesthesia for OSA surgery

Preoperative management

A 40-year-old male presented to an ENT surgeon for evaluation for UPPP for OSA. He had a known history of severe OSA diagnosed by polysomnography. He was placed on CPAP therapy but does not tolerate it, and thus wants to explore a surgical option.

He had a BMI of 50 and weighed 160 kg. His vital signs included blood pressure of 140/75, heart rate 63 and oxygen saturation of 96% on room air. He had a history of type 2 diabetes on oral hypoglycemic agents and a history of hypertension, well controlled on an ACE inhibitor and β-blocker. He is a current smoker. Fiberoptic nasopharyngoscopy was performed by his ENT surgeon and showed excessive redundant oropharyngeal tissue with collapsibility.

Physical exam revealed a morbidly obese gentleman with normal cardiovascular, respiratory, and neurological examinations. Preoperative workup included a complete blood count (CBC) and basic metabolic panel (BMP), which were both normal. EKG showed normal sinus rhythm. An airway examination revealed normal mouth opening with a Mallampati score of 4, macroglossia, and excessive soft tissue in the pharyngeal area. He had a normal thyromental distance but an excessively thick neck. The patient reported no previous anesthetic complications, except for a broken tooth and sore throat after undergoing gallbladder surgery 2 years previously. He was instructed to discontinue smoking and also instructed to withhold his ACE inhibitor and oral hypoglycemic agents on the morning of surgery but to take his β-blocker.

Intraoperative management

The patient was seen and examined by the anesthesiologist on the morning of surgery, who decided to proceed with an awake fiberoptic intubation based on the airway exam and history of dental trauma with intubation in the past, indicating a difficult airway. The patient was given 1 mg of midazolam only after he was brought into the operating room and monitors were applied. Glycopyrrolate 0.2 mg was given as an antisialagogue. He was sedated with a dexmedetomidine infusion with a 1 μg/kg bolus over 20 minutes followed by an infusion of 0.5 μg/kg/h. His airway was topicalized with aerosolized 4% lidocaine.

He was successfully intubated with a 7.5 mm ID endotracheal tube via a flexible fiberoptic intubating bronchoscope. Anesthesia was then induced with propofol, fentanyl, and rocuronium. Anesthesia was maintained with air, oxygen, and desflurane with intermittent small boluses of fentanyl. Intravenous antibiotics were given. Dexamethasone 8 mg IV was given for PONV prophylaxis and to decrease postoperative airway edema. Surgery proceeded uneventfully. Prior to emergence intravenous lidocaine was given to help prevent coughing and ondansetron was given as an antiemetic. His neuromuscular blockade was fully reversed. Only after the patient had been shown to be breathing spontaneously, with adequate tidal volume and respiratory rate, strong head lift, and responding to commands, was he extubated. He was brought to the recovery room on 10 liters of oxygen per minute delivered via simple face mask in the sitting position.

Postoperative management

In the recovery room the patient complained of 6/10 pain. He was treated with small boluses of intravenous fentanyl and an elixir of oxycodone/acetaminophen with some relief. He was noted to be somnolent with episodes of apnea, airway obstruction, and oxygen desaturation of around 80%. He was placed on his CPAP mask with some improvement of the apneic and hypoxic episodes. He was then sent to an ENT step-down unit with telemetry and continuous pulse oximetry monitoring on CPAP therapy. On postoperative day 1 he experienced less pain and was noted to be more awake, with no daytime apneic or hypoxic episodes. He was weaned off the CPAP mask but kept on 2 l/min of oxygen via nasal cannula. The oxygen was weaned later in the day as he maintained a room air saturation of 96%. At night the CPAP mask was placed and no hypoxic episodes were noted. On postoperative day 2 he was discharged home on oral pain medications.

Complications

As this case study describes, although patients undergo surgical procedures in an attempt to cure their OSA symptoms, these apneic and hypoxic episodes may continue or possibly worsen in the early postoperative period. Postoperatively, OSA patients may have a rebound of delta or rapid eye movement sleep and may be prone to more severe sleep apnea with a greater increase in AHI after surgery compared with preoperative AHI, peaking on postoperative day 3. Thus, it is imperative to monitor the patients' oxygen saturation continuously, to be cautious with intravenous narcotics, and to possibly consider the use of CPAP therapy in the first few postoperative days.

Clinical pearls

- Serious long-term consequences of OSA include a rise in sympathetic tone, ischemic heart disease, hypertension, tachyarrhythmias, deterioration in cognitive function, pulmonary hypertension, cor

183

pulmonale, congestive heart failure, cardiovascular accident/stroke and sudden death.

- Clinical features that increase the likelihood that OSA is present include increased neck circumference (>17 inches in men > 16 inches in women), body mass index 30 kg/m^2 or more, Mallampati score of 3 or 4, retrognathia, macroglossia, tonsillar hypertrophy, an enlarged uvula, a high narrow hard palate, and/or nasal abnormalities.

- OSA is classified according to the respiratory disturbance index (RDI):

  o Mild: RDI 5 to 14
  o Moderate: RDI 15 to 29
  o Severe: RDI 30 or more

- The upper airway abnormalities which lead to OSA can be the same abnormalities which lead to a difficult airway; difficult intubation is eight times more frequent in OSA patients than in control patients. Snoring and OSA are independent risk factors for difficult mask ventilation.

- Consideration should be given to aspiration prophylaxis. Unsupervised preoperative sedation should be avoided.

- General anesthesia with a secured, intubated airway is preferable because of the risk of aspiration of blood from the surgical site and the patient's likelihood of obstruction when sedated.

There is also a risk of laryngospasm if blood or secretions touch the vocal cords in an unsecured airway.

- Systemic steroids may reduce surgery- and/or intubation-induced airway edema and can be given prior to surgery as well as postoperatively.

- Postoperatively, it is best to minimize opioids and sedatives, which may suppress respiratory drive; acetaminophen or tramadol are commonly used in such a setting. Non-steroidal anti-inflammatory agents should be used with caution due to their potential to cause platelet dysfunction and bleeding. Sedating antiemetic agents such as prochlorperazine should be avoided as well.

- Patients with OSA have a greater increase in AHI after surgery compared with preoperative AHI, peaking on postoperative day 3 and returning to preoperative level on night 7. Most serious complications occur in the first 24 hours. ASA guidelines state that monitoring of patients with OSA postoperatively should be for approximately 3 hours longer than for those without OSA.

- During hospitalization, patients should have continuous pulse oximetry (with supplemental oxygen when needed) until they are at least back to their baseline.

- Postoperatively, patients with OSA should be monitored until they reach baseline status. ICU care may be needed for the sickest of OSA patients.

References

1. Gross JB, Bachenberg KL, Benumof JL, et al. Practice guidelines for the perioperative management of patients with obstructive sleep apnea: a report by the American Society of Anesthesiologists Task Force on Perioperative Management of patients with obstructive sleep apnea. Anesthesiology 2006;**104** (5):1081–93; quiz 117–8.

2. Mickelson SA. Anesthetic and postoperative management of the obstructive sleep apnea patient. Oral Maxillofac Surg Clin North Am 2009;**21**(4):425–34.

3. Office GP. National Commission on Sleep Disorders Research. Wake up America; A National Sleep Alert. Government Printing Office; 1993.

4. Holty JE, Guilleminault C. Surgical options for the treatment of obstructive sleep apnea. Med Clin North Am 2010;**94**(3):479–515.

5. Liao P, Yegneswaran B, Vairavanathan S, Zilberman P, Chung F. Postoperative complications in patients with obstructive sleep apnea: a retrospective matched cohort study. Can J Anaesth 2009;**56**(11): 819–28.

6. Marshall NS, Wong KK, Liu PY, et al. Sleep apnea as an independent risk factor for all-cause mortality: the Busselton Health Study. Sleep 2008;**31**(8):1079–85.

7. Epstein LJ, Kristo D, Strollo PJ Jr, et al. Clinical guideline for the evaluation, management and long-term care of obstructive sleep apnea in adults. J Clin Sleep Med 2009; **5**(3):263–76.

8. Seet E, Chung F. Obstructive sleep apnea: preoperative assessment. Anesthesiol Clin 2010;**28**(2):199–215.

9. Aurora RN, Casey KR, Kristo D, et al. Practice parameters for the surgical modifications of the upper airway for obstructive sleep apnea in adults. Sleep (Rochester) 2010; **33**(10):1408–13.

10. McMains KC, Terris DJ. Evidence-based medicine in sleep apnea surgery. Otolaryngol Clin North Am 2003;**36**(3):539–61.

11. Stauffer JL, Buick MK, Bixler EO, *et al.* Morphology of the uvula in obstructive sleep apnea. *Am Rev Respir Dis* 1989;**140**(3):724–8.

12. Li KK. Surgical therapy for adult obstructive sleep apnea. *Sleep Med Rev* 2005;**9**(3):201–9.

13. Friedman M, Tanyeri H, Lim JW, *et al.* Effect of improved nasal breathing on obstructive sleep apnea. *Otolaryngol Head Neck Surg* 2000;**122**(1):71–4.

14. Verse T, Maurer JT, Pirsig W. Effect of nasal surgery on sleep-related breathing disorders. *Laryngoscope* 2002;**112**(1):64–8.

15. Caples SM, Rowley JA, Prinsell JR, *et al.* Surgical modifications of the upper airway for obstructive sleep apnea in adults: a systematic review and meta-analysis. *Sleep (Rochester)* 2010;**33**(10):1396–407.

16. Jaffe R, Samuels S. *Anesthesiologist's Manual of Surgical Procedures*, 4th edn. Philadelphia: Lippincott Williams & Wilkins; 2009.

17. Kheterpal S, Han R, Tremper KK, *et al.* Incidence and predictors of difficult and impossible mask ventilation. *Anesthesiology* 2006;**105**(5):885–91.

18. Siyam MA, Benhamou D. Difficult endotracheal intubation in patients with sleep apnea syndrome. *Anesth Analg* 2002;**95**(4):1098–102.

19. Bolden N, Smith CE, Auckley D, Makarski J, Avula R. Perioperative complications during use of an obstructive sleep apnea protocol following surgery and anesthesia. *Anesth Analg* 2007; **105**(6):1869–70.

20. Esclamado RM, Glenn MG, McCulloch TM, Cummings CW. Perioperative complications and risk factors in the surgical treatment of obstructive sleep apnea syndrome. *Laryngoscope* 1989;**99**(11):1125–9.

21. Marrel J, Blanc C, Frascarolo P, Magnusson L. Vidoelaryngoscope improves intubating conditions in morbidly obese patients. *Eur J Anesthesiol* 2007;**24**(12): 1405–9.

22. ASA Task Force on Management of the Difficult Airway: Practice guidelines for management of the difficult airway, an updated report. *Anesthesiology* 2003;**98**:1269–77.

23. Kezirian EJ, Weaver EM, Yueh B, *et al.* Incidence of serious complications after

uvulopalatopharyngoplasty. *Laryngoscope* 2004;**114**(3):450–3.

24. Johnson JT, Sanders MH. Breathing during sleep immediately after uvulopalatopharyngoplasty. *Laryngoscope* 1986;**96**(11):1236–8.

25. Troell RJ, Powell NB, Riley RW, Li KK, Guilleminault C. Comparison of postoperative pain between laser-assisted uvulopalatoplasty, uvulopalatopharyngoplasty, and radiofrequency volumetric tissue reduction of the palate. *Otolaryngol Head Neck Surg* 2000;**122**(3):402–9.

26. Chung F, Liao P, Fazel H, *et al.* Evolution of sleep pattern and sleep breathing disorders during first seven nights after surgery – a pilot study. *Sleep (Rochester)* 2009; **32**(Suppl. S):A217–8.

27. Mickelson SA, Hakim I. Is postoperative intensive care monitoring necessary after uvulopalatopharyngoplasty? *Otolaryngol Head Neck Surg* 1998;**119**(4):352–6.

28. Haavisto L, Suonpaa J. Complications of uvulopalatopharyngoplasty. *Clin Otolaryngol Allied Sci* 1994; **19**(3):243–7.

Chapter

19

Anesthesia for carotid body tumor resction

Maged Argalious and Sivan Wexler

Introduction

The normal carotid body is a small cluster of chemo-receptors located on the posterior aspect of the bifurcation of the common carotid artery (Figures 19.1 and 19.2) monitors changes in arterial oxygen tension and pH of the blood and, in turn, influences the rate and depth of respiration, and to a lesser extent heart rate. It was first anatomically described in 1743 by Albrecht von Haller [1].

The carotid body receives its blood supply from the common or external carotid artery and its innervation primarily from sensory (afferent) fibers of the glossopharyngeal (IX) nerve, with lesser contributions from the vagus (X) nerve and superior cervical ganglion of the sympathetic nervous system.

Carotid body tumors (CBTs), also called paragangliomas, are highly vascular tumors (Figure 19.1) arising from these chemoreceptors cells, which develop from the neural crest region during embryogenesis.

While carotid body tumors are rare, diagnosed with an incidence of about 1:30 000 in the general population, they account for 60% of head and neck paragangliomas [2].

There are three distinct types: familial, sporadic and hyperplastic forms.

The hyperplastic type generally develops in response to chronic hypoxemia, and thus is common in patients with a history of COPD, congenital cyanotic heart disease and living in high-altitude (> 5000 feet) areas.

A family history of paraganglioma syndrome should be considered in all cases particularly if bilateral tumors exist.

CBTs commonly present clinically as a painless cervical mass. On physical examination, this non-

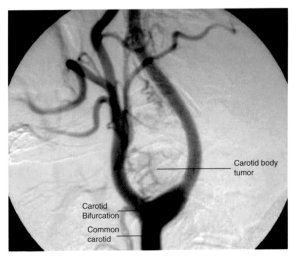

Figure 19.1. Carotid angiogram showing a carotid body tumor causing splay of internal and external carotid arteries (image courtesy of Dr. Robert Lorenz, Head and Neck Institute, Cleveland Clinic).

tender, rubbery, pulsatile lesion is more easily displaced laterally than vertically (Fontaine's sign). Although CBTs are usually benign, they can be malignant, with a metastatic rate of 2% to 9%. Malignant CBTs typically occur in patients between 30 and 60 years of age and are more commonly of the familial type [3]. Large carotid body tumors (> 5 cm) can cause transient or permanent cranial nerve deficits, most commonly involving the vagus nerve [1]. Most CBTs are nonfunctioning tumors but norepinephrine-, epinephrine-, serotonin- and histamine-secreting tumors have been described.

Shamblin et al. introduced a system to classify these tumors according to tumor size and the degree of involvement of the internal carotid artery. Tumors that do not compress or involve both carotid vessels

Anesthesia for Otolaryngologic Surgery, ed. Basem Abdelmalak and D. John Doyle. Published by Cambridge University Press.
© Cambridge University Press 2013.

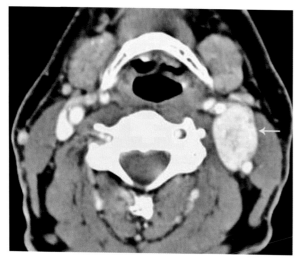

Figure 19.2. CT scan demonstrating a carotid body tumor at the carotid bifurcation (arrow) (image courtesy of Dr. Robert Lorenz, Head and Neck Institute, Cleveland Clinic).

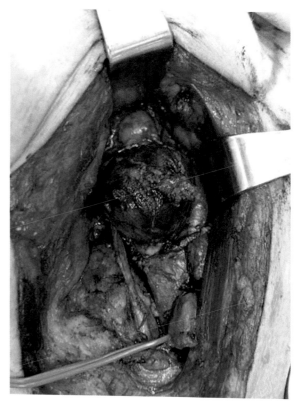

Figure 19.3. Carotid body tumor resection (image courtesy of Dr. Joseph Scharpf, Head and Neck Institute, Cleveland Clinic).

are classified as Shamblin I, tumors that compress the carotid vessels are Shamblin II, and those that involve the carotid vessels are Shamblin III [4].

Carotid body tumor surgery

Surgery for resection of carotid body tumors (Figure 19.3) is the only curative treatment; radiotherapy may be indicated in cases of giant or recurrent carotid body tumors or in malignant tumors with metastases to the regional lymph nodes. Surgical treatment is always associated with the risk of damage to major vascular structures and to cranial nerves. Preoperative embolization appears to reduce blood loss, facilitate surgical resection, and reduce operating time and morbidity [5].

Preoperative preparation

Preoperative cardiac evaluation for this procedure should be conducted in the usual fashion, keeping in mind that carotid body tumor excision is considered to be an intermediate-risk surgery. The classification of cardiac risk in noncardiac surgery is based on the incidence of cardiac death and nonfatal myocardial infarction (1–5% in intermediate risk surgeries) and the ACC/AHA guidelines [6] for preoperative evaluation.

Airway management

Preoperative airway assessment should focus on any radiation history to the neck which can reduce tissue compliance, increase tissue friability as well as increase intubation difficulty. Large CBTs may cause marked compression of the pharyngeal wall, making conventional laryngoscopy as well as endoscopy difficult. This is especially true when large bilateral CBTs are present [3].

It is important to note that carotid body tumors have a tendency to grow longitudinally and have even been reported to reach the skull base (cephalad extension), causing a reduction in submandibular space compliance. In such cases where there is concern regarding the cranial extent of the tumor, mandibular subluxation may be necessary for adequate exposure and nasoendotracheal intubation should be considered [7].

Consideration should be given to securing the airway before anesthetic induction when airway assessment points to a difficult intubation and/or ventilation.

Documentation of baseline cranial nerve deficits and assessment of vocal cord mobility (vagal nerve involvement) is of paramount importance. Preoperative imaging modalities including CT scan, 3D CT scan, MRI and MRA are invaluable in assessing the extent of tumor involvement of major vessels (internal jugular vein patency) and intracranial tumor extension, whether extradurally to the posterior fossa or less commonly to the middle fossa. Rarely, signs of intracranial hypertension can occur, either as a result of obstruction of venous sinuses and the occurrence of hydrocephalus, or due to mass effect from the tumor.

While most carotid body tumors are non-secreting, a proper history-taking is important to identify patients with a tumor secreting catecholamine (hypertension, sweating) or serotonin (diarrhea, flushing, headaches) and initiate lab tests (normetanephrine, 5 HIAA, serotonin). A "type and screen" of the patient's blood is essential in ensuring the availability of blood products intraoperatively [7].

Preoperative assessment helps in optimization of patients' comorbidities and in formulating an anesthetic plan with the goal of reducing perioperative morbidity.

Intraoperative management goals

The operative field of carotid body surgery is a highly reflexogenic and vascular one, and thus the provision of adequate intraoperative analgesia, blood pressure control and a motionless patient are paramount. As cranial nerve injury or stroke is a potential complication of this surgery, anesthetic management should also aim to achieve a rapid awakening for neurologic examination. Techniques aimed at preventing coughing or straining on emergence are equally important in limiting the risk of hematoma formation, which, in light of the anatomical location, carries significant morbidity and mortality in the postoperative period. When carotid artery clamping, reconstruction or repair is required, optimization of cerebral perfusion and brain protection are additional anesthetic considerations.

Monitoring

In addition to standard monitoring, invasive arterial monitoring and large-bore IV access are essential. The tumor's rich vascular blood supply (Figure 19.1), its contact with the carotid arterial system and its proximity to the jugular venous system can result in acute massive blood loss, especially in larger CBTs and those with cephalad intracranial extension. Use of central venous access should be guided by patient comorbidities. Femoral or antecubital access sites are preferable as extensive neck dissection and ipsilateral swelling may render head and neck venous drainage dependent on the contralateral internal jugular vein. Before placement of a central line, tumor involvement of both the internal jugular vein and the superior vena cava should be assessed (imaging). If the internal jugular vein, but not the superior vena cava, has been invaded by tumor, the contralateral basilic, external or internal jugular vein can be used to gain central access. If both have been invaded, the femoral vein should be used.

A urinary catheter is inserted and a forced-air warming blanket is placed over the lower extremities to maintain normothermia.

If the carotid artery is to be occluded intraoperatively, monitoring the adequacy of cerebral perfusion can be done either by periodic neurologic evaluation in patients undergoing resection under regional anesthesia or by the use of electroencephalogram, somatosensory evoked potentials, arterial stump pressure measurement or transcranial Doppler measurement of middle cerebral artery flow velocities in patients under general anesthesia. However, at present, none of the aforementioned neuromonitoring modalities has been shown to improve neurologic outcome [8].

Hemodynamic considerations

The goals of intraoperative hemodynamic management are to maintain normal "baseline" hemodynamics, avoiding extreme swings in blood pressure and heart rate. This can prove challenging especially during periods of lack of surgical stimulation (post-induction hypotension) and periods of intense surgical stimulation (hypertension during surgical manipulation) and may require the use of short-acting antihypertensives (nitroglycerin, nicardipine, clevidipine, esmolol) and vasopressors (phenylephrine, ephedrine, atropine) until a steady state of surgical stimulation is achieved. Patients with depleted intravascular volume, especially with concomitant left ventricular hypertrophy and diastolic dysfunction, are more prone to hemodynamic swings in blood pressure, and judicious fluid loading to achieve euvolemia should be considered. While mild hypotensive anesthesia has been advocated to reduce blood loss, the hemodynamic focus should be on maintaining end-organ perfusion (heart, brain, kidney, liver) by maintaining a normal intraoperative heart rate, blood pressure and cardiac output. Hypotensive techniques risk cerebral hypoperfusion especially in the setting of carotid artery clamping and are contraindicated in patients with end organ injury. When clamping of the carotid artery is contemplated, maintenance of a high normal blood pressure may be more appropriate to maintain distal ipsilateral cerebral perfusion pressure through collaterals from the contralateral side.

Surgical manipulation of the carotid sinus may cause reflex bradycardia, hypotension or even asystole. When this occurs, surgical stimulation should be discontinued. Atropine is effective when bradycardia is persistent. Conversely, marked hypertension and tachycardia on induction or during tumor manipulation should raise the suspicion of a previously undiagnosed functioning CBT [9] or coexisting extra-cervical pheochromocytoma [3]. The anesthetic management of a functional CBT is similar to the management of a pheochromocytoma from a physiological and pharmacological standpoint and may include preoperative alpha and beta sympathetic blockade.

Positioning the head and neck above the level of the heart helps limit blood loss but vigilance is necessary for the increased risk of venous air embolism in this position, should the integrity of a large neck vein be violated inadvertently. Maintaining adequate intravascular volume and positive-pressure ventilation may decrease the risk of this complication.

In the majority of patients transfusion requirements are minimal to none. Still, blood loss can be rapid and substantial and at least 2 units of cross-matched blood should be available. In large tumors ($>$ 6 cm) or in those with extensive carotid artery involvement, consideration should be given to cell-salvage techniques.

Maintenance of anesthesia
General anesthesia

A balanced technique using a combination of intravenous and inhalation anesthetics is commonly used. As the anatomical location of the tumor is a highly reflexogenic one, adequate intraoperative analgesia is an essential component of anesthetic management. This, coupled with the need to avoid neuromuscular blocking agents to facilitate intraoperative nerve identification, makes an opiate-based

technique advantageous. Highly potent synthetic opioids such as fentanyl or sufentanil, given as a loading dose and followed by a continuous infusion, can aid in maintaining stable hemodynamics, facilitate tolerance of the endotracheal tube, and will allow for a smooth emergence. A continuous infusion of the synthetic ultra-short-acting remifentanil can also be used and has the advantage of high potency, easy titratability and rapid offset, thus allowing for a smooth and rapid emergence. Regardless of anesthetic technique chosen, every effort should be made to prevent coughing or straining on emergence, since this may provoke bleeding, contribute to hematoma formation, or disrupt suture lines.

In cases when carotid artery shunting is employed, avoidance of nitrous oxide prevents the potential expansion of micro-air emboli in the distal cerebral circulation.

Particularly in cases where carotid artery cross-clamping is required, physiological and pharmacological management may also be important in improving neurological outcome, as is the case in carotid artery surgery [10]. A normal-to-high arterial pressure should be maintained during carotid cross-clamping to increase collateral cerebral perfusion. Normocarbia should be maintained, since hypocarbia can cause vasoconstriction of cerebral artery blood flow, while hypercarbia can contribute to the occurrence of "steal phenomenon" where blood flow is diverted from maximally dilated ischemic areas to other normal cerebral regions. Since hyperglycemia and hyperthermia are known to worsen neurologic insults, they should be avoided. Most general anesthetics (with the exception of etomidate and possibly ketamine) have been shown to be protective against focal cerebral ischemia. Barbiturate therapy before carotid occlusion has been shown to be protective against focal ischemic injury but this potential advantage must be weighed against significant cardiovascular depression and delayed awakening. Among the volatile anesthetics, isoflurane and sevoflurane have been shown to reduce the critical cerebral blood flow below which ischemic EEG changes appear [11,12].

Regional anesthesia

Carotid body tumor resection can be performed under regional anesthesia. A careful and thorough explanation to the patient (informed consent) is essential to ensure that patients understand the steps involved in both anesthetic and surgical management, since patient cooperation is essential. The decision to use regional anesthesia should be guided by patients' preferences and comorbidities as well as by skills and familiarity of the surgeon and the anesthesiologist with regional techniques.

A regional technique for open carotid surgery requires anesthesia of cervical nerves 2–4, and has been performed successfully with a superficial or deep cervical plexus block, and less commonly under cervical epidural anesthesia or local anesthetic infiltration (or a combination of these methods). Superficial cervical plexus block is the preferred technique since it is easy to perform and has a lower risk of serious complications compared to deep cervical plexus or cervical epidural blocks [13], which can cause subarachnoid or intravascular injections, Horner's syndrome and blockade of the recurrent laryngeal and vagus nerves [14]. When superficial and deep cervical plexus blocks are performed together, the incidence of temporary ipsilateral phrenic nerve paralysis is 55% [15]. In the absence of severe baseline respiratory compromise or contralateral diaphragmatic paresis, unilateral temporary phrenic nerve paralysis is well tolerated.

Inadequate intraoperative anesthesia is common after regional techniques [16] and necessitates additional local anesthetic infiltration or sedation. Vigilance for intravascular injection is of paramount importance in light of the high vascularity of carotid body tumors [17]. Finally, a high incision or a short neck may call for mandibular retraction for adequate surgical exposure. However, none of the above techniques provides anesthetic coverage for this area, which is innervated by the trigeminal nerve.

The principal advantage of regional anesthesia for carotid body surgery is that it allows continuous sensitive monitoring of neurological function when cross-clamping of the internal carotid artery is necessary [18] (see below). An additional advantage is its utility in high-risk cardiac patients where avoidance of general anesthesia is preferred [19]. Other reported advantages of regional anesthesia include a decrease in shunting requirements, decreased cost, avoidance of potential postoperative cognitive decline and fewer blood pressure swings compared with general anesthesia. Disadvantages include poor access to the airway and potential for patient movement. Additionally, acute neurological changes (e.g., stroke or seizure) during cross-clamping or unpredictable patient agitation or distress may necessitate emergency airway management and conversion to GA in non-ideal conditions. Furthermore, pharmacological cerebral protection is not feasible when regional techniques are employed [20].

Carotid artery occlusion and cerebral protection

Internal carotid artery clamping, reconstruction or sacrifice may be required for large grade III tumors or when the internal carotid artery is inadvertently injured.

During carotid artery clamping, the use of internal carotid artery shunting aims to prevent ischemic stroke by maintaining cerebral blood flow. There is wide variation in the use of carotid artery shunting [21]. While some surgeons do not use carotid shunts, based on the rationale that shunting has a small but significant risks of embolic stroke or intimal dissection of the carotid artery [22] and is prone to technical complications such as kinking or occlusion, other surgeons use carotid artery shunting routinely when carotid artery clamping is required [21]. Most surgeons use carotid artery shunting selectively.

In cases done under regional anesthesia, the decision to shunt is based on changes in neurologic examination (gold standard in awake patients) after carotid clamping, indicating the occurrence of cerebral ischemia.

In cases done under general anesthesia, selective shunting is based on the occurrence of EEG or somatosensory evoked potential (SSEP) changes, a reduction in cerebral artery flow velocity or a low distal arterial stump pressure in response to carotid clamping.

Intraoperative EEG is the most commonly used modality in cases done under general anesthesia [23]. High-frequency attenuation or development of low-frequency activity on cross-clamping indicates inadequate cerebral perfusion but may be limited by the inability to detect subcortical ischemic changes [24] and the need for personnel experienced in its use and interpretation. Additionally, changes in anesthetic depth and temperature may mimic ischemia, leading to unnecessary shunting.

SSEPs, on the other hand, have the advantage of examining deeper subcortical structures and may be advantageous in patients with baseline EEG changes. Unfortunately, studies have not shown a clear benefit for SSEP use as a tool to identify cerebral ischemia on cross-clamping. Additionally, SSEPs are also influenced by anesthetic technique and depth as well as temperature.

Distal carotid artery stump pressure (the pressure in the distal internal carotid artery) has been used to assess collateral flow and cerebral tolerance during temporary carotid occlusion, with the assumption that perfusion pressure is an important determinant of cerebral flow. Studies have shown this to be specific but not sensitive in identifying those patients who develop ischemic EEG changes with carotid artery cross-clamping. A carotid stump pressure of < 45 mmHg has been used as a threshold for shunting [25].

Transcranial doppler is used to measure flow velocity in the middle cerebral artery and is followed as an indicator of cerebral blood flow during carotid cross-clamping. Like stump pressure monitoring, sensitivity is poor for identifying patients who could benefit from shunting. Furthermore, it is operator-dependent and an acoustic window may not be found in up to 20% of patients. It is, however, advantageous in detecting emboli and may alert the surgeon to avoid further manipulation which may cause stroke. Despite the large number of methods available for intraoperative neurologic monitoring, no single method has been shown to improve neurologic outcome.

Complications

Postoperative complications after resection of carotid body tumor are listed in Table 19.1. It is important to note that cranial nerve involvement predisposing to postoperative airway obstruction can occur through several mechanisms, including tumor invasion preoperatively, nerve injury or sacrifice intraoperatively or tissue edema causing nerve palsy postoperatively. In addition, postoperative bleeding can result in a rapidly expanding neck hematoma and airway compromise.

Patients undergoing resection of bilateral carotid body tumors and patients with a history of contralateral carotid surgery should have continuous monitoring of oxygenation, ventilation, and hemodynamics postoperatively, since bilateral carotid surgery has been shown to result in the abolition of the normocapnic ventilatory response to progressive hypoxia and can result in apneic episodes [26].

Table 19.1. Postoperative complications after carotid body tumor resection

Cerebrovascular
  Stroke (ischemic or embolic)
  Cranial nerve deficits: glossopharyngeal (IX), vagus (X), hypoglossal (XII) predisposing to airway compromise, either by causing airway obstruction or leading to aspiration

Airway obstruction
  Vocal cord paralysis (vagus nerve)
  Airway edema from neck manipulation during surgery
  Postoperative bleeding leading to expanding neck hematoma

Pulmonary (especially after bilateral carotid surgery)
  Abolition of the normocapnic ventilatory response to hypoxia
  Apneic episodes
  Aspiration pneumonitis (slow gastric emptying)

Cardiovascular (especially after bilateral carotid surgery)
  Decreased baroreceptor sensitivity
  Temporary baroreceptor failure
  Increased blood pressure variability
  Orthostatic hypotension
  Hypertension
  Sick sinus syndrome

Gastrointestinal
  Delayed gastric emptying
  Postoperative ileus

Summary

The perioperative anesthetic management of carotid body tumor resection includes a comprehensive preoperative airway assessment, optimization of patient comorbidities, and identification of symptoms pointing to secreting tumors. Whether regional or general anesthesia is used, the goals of perioperative management are to preserve stable hemodynamics and maintain end-organ perfusion, to prepare for resuscitation of acute major blood loss, to utilize monitoring modalities to identify, avoid, and manage cerebral ischemia, and to provide a smooth controlled emergence. In the postoperative period, complications should be anticipated, diagnosed, and promptly managed. Patients undergoing bilateral carotid tumor surgery should be continuously monitored in an intensive care environment postoperatively

Case study

A 61-year-old male arrived in the PACU after a right carotid body tumor resection. His medical history included stable coronary artery disease, hypertension, and chronic obstructive pulmonary disease. His surgical history included a remote appendectomy and a cervical spine fusion. His medications included aspirin, atorvastatin, and amlodipine.

In the operating room, an arterial catheter was placed in the left radial artery following a smooth induction of anesthesia using propofol, fentanyl, and rocuronium, He was intubated with an 8.0 mm endotracheal tube and maintained on oxygen/air in sevoflurane with a continuous infusion of remifentanil. During temporary occlusion of his right carotid artery, the distal carotid stump pressure was measured at 55 mmHg and carotid cross-clamping proceeded without carotid shunting; the total carotid cross-clamp time was 8 minutes and the patient's intraoperative hemodynamics remained close to his preoperative baseline.

On emergence from anesthesia, and after discontinuation of remifentanil, the patient developed severe hypertension (190/115) requiring intravenous nitroglycerin boluses as well as IV labetalol. His blood pressure on arrival in the PACU was 150/80 mmHg.

Thirty minutes after arrival in the PACU, the PACU nurse noticed a swelling at the incision site. Immediately thereafter, the patient started to complain of shortness of breath despite increased supplemental oxygen. The staff surgeon and anesthesiologist were called to the bedside.

Discussion

While the postoperative dyspnea can be multifactorial in this patient, the presence of a swelling at the incision site should alert the perioperative care team to the possibility of an expanding neck hematoma. Other causes of dyspnea in this patient may be cardiac (myocardial ischemia or acute pulmonary edema secondary to the acute hypertension on emergence), pulmonary (atelectasis, or exacerbation of COPD) or nerve injury related (recurrent laryngeal nerve injury).

A preformulated plan for management of a postoperative neck hematoma is outlined in Table 19.2.

In this patient, a continuous expansion of the neck hematoma despite tight blood pressure control prompted awake fiberoptic intubation after

Table 19.2. Management of postoperative neck hematoma

1. Apply pressure to bleeding site
2. Notify surgery and anesthesia team (call for help)
3. Consider reversal of any residual anticoagulation
4. Tight blood pressure control

Possible outcomes:

A – No further hematoma expansion
Communication with surgical team
Mark the boundaries of the hematoma for early identification of further expansion
Close observation and extended (8–12 hours) monitoring in a critical care environment

B – Continuous expansion of hematoma with no airway compromise
Awake (fiberoptic) intubation either in the PACU or after immediate transfer to the operating room after topical anesthesia to the airway followed by general anesthesia for exploration of wound and drainage of neck hematoma
Assess neurologic status at the end of the case
Consider maintaining the patient intubated postoperatively until resolution of reactionary airway edema

C – Expansion of neck hematoma with rapidly progressive airway compromise (dyspnea, stridor, airway obstruction)
Emergency intubation (ASA algorithm)
Cannot intubate/can ventilate: using face mask, oral or nasal airways, laryngeal mask airway: consider immediate surgical drainage of the neck hematoma followed by further attempts to secure the airway
Cannot intubate/cannot ventilate: surgical airway
Evacuation of hematoma and wound exploration
Neurologic assessment
Maintain airway secured postoperatively

Adapted from Maged Argalious, Postoperative hematoma and airway compromise after carotid endarterectomy Table 29.2. In *Case Studies in Neuroanesthesia and Neurocritical Care*, edited by George A. Mashour and Ehab Farag, Cambridge University Press, 2011.

topicalization of the airway followed by transfer to the operating room for surgical exploration. A small bleeding vessel was secured, and a wake-up test to assess neurologic status was performed in the operating room before patient transfer to the intensive care unit, where he was extubated a few hours later. The rest of his hospital stay was uneventful.

Clinical pearls

- The hyperplastic type of carotid body tumor (CBT) generally develops in response to chronic hypoxemia, and thus it is more common in patients with a history of COPD, congenital cyanotic heart disease and/or living at high altitude.

- Most CBTs are nonfunctioning but norepinephrine-, epinephrine-, serotonin- and histamine-secreting tumors have been described.

- Radiation history to the neck can reduce tissue compliance, increase tissue friability, as well as increase the difficulty of intubation. Large CBTs may make conventional laryngoscopy as well as endoscopy difficult, especially when large bilateral CBTs are present.

- The operative field of CBT surgery is a highly reflexogenic and vascular one, and thus the provision of adequate intraoperative analgesia, blood pressure control, and a motionless patient are paramount.

- Surgical manipulation of the carotid sinus may cause reflex bradycardia, hypotension or even asystole. When this occurs, surgical stimulation should be discontinued. Atropine is effective when bradycardia is persistent. Conversely, marked hypertension and tachycardia on induction or during tumor manipulation should raise the suspicion of a previously undiagnosed functioning CBT.

- As cranial nerve injuries or strokes are potential complications of this surgery, anesthetic management should also aim to achieve a rapid awakening to allow early neurological examination. Techniques aimed at preventing coughing or straining on emergence are important to limit the risk of hematoma formation.

- In addition to standard monitoring, invasive arterial monitoring and large-bore IV access are crucial. Use of central venous access should be guided by patient comorbidities.

- Monitoring the adequacy of cerebral perfusion can be done by periodic neurologic evaluation in patients undergoing resection under regional anesthesia. Patients under general anesthesia may benefit from the use of EEG, SSEP, arterial stump pressure measurement or transcranial Doppler measurement of middle cerebral artery flow velocities. However, at present, none of the aforementioned neuromonitoring techniques has been shown to improve neurologic outcome.

References

1. Kruger AJ, Walker PJ, Foster WJ, *et al.* Important observations made managing carotid body tumors during a 25-year experience. *J Vasc Surg* 2010;**52**:1518–24.

2. Mitchell RO, Richardson JD, Lambert GE. Characteristics, surgical management, and outcome in 17 carotid body tumors. *Am Surg* 1996;**62**:1034–7.

3. Connolly RAJ, Baker AB. Excision of bilateral carotid body tumours. *Anaesth Intens Care* 1995;**23**:342–5.

4. Luna-Ortiz K, Rascon-Ortiz M, Villavicencio-Valencia V, Herrera-Gomez A. Does Shamblin's classification predict postoperative morbidity in carotid body tumors? A proposal to modify Shamblin's classification? *Eur Arch Otorhinolaryngol* 2006;**263**:171–5.

5. Sajid MS, Hamilton G, Baker DM on behalf of Joint Vascular Research Group. A multicenter review of carotid body tumour management. *Eur J Vasc Endovasc Surg* 2007;**34**:127e130.

6. Fleisher L, *et al.* ACC/AHA 2007 guidelines on perioperative cardiovascular evaluation and care for noncardiac surgery: executive summary: a report of the American College of Cardiology/American Heart Association Task Force on practice guidelines (writing committee to revise the 2002 guidelines on perioperative cardiovascular evaluation for noncardiac surgery). *Circulation* 2007;**116**:1971–96.

7. Jensen NF. Glomus tumors of the head and neck: anesthetic considerations. *Anesth Analg* 1994;**78**:112–9.

8. Rerkasem K, Rothwell PM. Routine or selective carotid artery shunting for carotid endarterectomy (and different methods of monitoring in selective shunting). *Cochrane Database Syst Rev* 2009 Oct 7;(4): CD000190.

9. Newland MC, Hurlbert BJ. Chemodectoma diagnosed by hypertension and tachycardia during anesthesia. *Anesth Analg* 1980;**59**:388–90.

10. Stoneham MD, O Warner. Blood pressure manipulation during awake carotid surgery to reverse neurological deficit after carotid cross-clamping. *Br J Anaesth* 2001;**87**(4):641–4.

11. Messick JM Jr, Casement B, Sharbrough FW, *et al.* Correlation of regional cereberal blood flow (rCBF) with EEG changes during isoflurane anesthesia for carotid

endarterectomy: critical rCBF. *Anesthesiology* 1987;**66**:344–9.

12. Grady RE, Weglinski MR, Sharbrough FW, *et al.* Correlation of regional cerebral blood flow with ischemic electroencephalographic changes during sevoflurane-nitrous oxide anesthesia for carotid endarterectomy. *Anesthesiology* 1998;**88**:892–7.

13. Guay J. Regional anesthesia for carotid surgery. *Curr Opin Anaesthesiol* 2008;**21**:638–44.

14. Pandit JJ, Satya-Krishna R, Gration P. Superficial or deep cervical plexus block for carotid endarterectomy: a systematic review of complications. *Br J Anaesth* 2007;**2**:159–69

15. Emery G, Handley G, Davis MJ, *et al.* Incidence of phrenic nerve block and hypercapnia in patients undergoing carotid endarterectomy under cervical plexus block. *Anaesth Intensive Care* 1998;**26**:377–81.

16. Davies MJ, Silbert BS, Scott DA. Superficial and deep cervical plexus block for carotid artery surgery: a prospective study of 1000 blocks. *Reg Anesth* 1997;**26**:377–81.

17. Brooker CD, Lawson AD. Convulsions following bupivacaine infiltration for excision of carotid body tumour. *Anaesth Intensive Care* 1993;**21**:877–8.

18. Lawrence PF, Alves JC, Jicha D, *et al.* Incidence, timing, and causes of cerebral ischemia during carotid endarterectomy with regional anesthesia. *J Vasc Surg* 1998;**27**:329–37.

19. Jones HG, Stoneham MD. Continuous cervical plexus block for carotid body tumour excision in a patient with Eisenmenger's syndrome. *Anaesthesia* 2006;**61**:1214–8.

20. Erickson KM, Cole DJ. Carotid artery disease: stenting vs endarterectomy. *Br J Anaesth* 2010;**S1**: i34–i49.

21. AbuRahma AF, Mousa AY, Stone PA. Shunting during carotid endarterectomy. *J Vasc Surg* 2011;**54**:1502–10.

22. Salvian AJ, Taylor DC, Hsiang YN, *et al.* Selective shunting with EEG monitoring is safer than routine shunting for carotid endarterectomy. *Cardiovasc Surg* 1997;**5**:481–5.

23. Isley MR, Edmonds HL Jr, Stecker M. Guidelines for intraoperative neuromonitoring using raw (analog or digital waveforms) and quantitative electroencephalography: a position statement by the American Society of Neurophysiological Monitoring. *J Clin Monit Comput* 2009; **23**(6):369–90. Epub 2009 Sep 16.

24. Rowed DW, Houlden DA, Burkholder LM, *et al.* Comparison of monitoring techniques for intraoperative cerebral ischemia. *Can J Neurol Sci* 2004;**31**: 347–56.

25. Jacob T, Hingorani A, Ascher E. Carotid Artery Stump Pressure (CASP) in 1135 consecutive endarterectomies under general anesthesia: an old method that survived the test of times. *J Cardiovasc Surg (Torino)* 2007;**48**(6):677–81.

26. Timmers HJLM, Karemaker JM, Wieling W, *et al.* Baroreflex and chemoreflex function after bilateral carotid body tumor resection. *J Hypertens* 2003;**21**:591–9.

Anesthesia for Zenker's diverticulectomy

Ashish Khanna, Benjamin Wood and Basem Abdelmalak

Introduction

First described by Zenker and Von Ziemssen in 1874 as a herniation of pharyngeal mucosa through the posterior wall of the hypopharynx, Zenker's diverticulum, is an acquired disorder typically seen in the sixth to ninth decades of life [1]. Reported incidence is approximately 1 in 800 upper gastrointestinal barium studies [2].

The location of Zenker's diverticulum along with the inherent risks of aspiration at any given stage of surgery (pre-, intra- or postoperative periods) adds an element of unique difficulty in the anesthetic approach to these patients. In this chapter we explore the anesthetic considerations for this unique procedure.

The patient age group involved is also one that carries increased perioperative cardiovascular risk which may translate into increased hemodynamic fluctuations and the need for invasive monitoring.

Surgical anatomy

Anatomically, the outpouching occurs through what has been named "Killian's dehiscence", which is located below the inferior constrictor and above the cricopharyngeus muscle on the posterior hypopharyngeal wall. Precisely speaking, the area of weakness is between the oblique and horizontal components of the cricopharyngeus muscles. This is believed to be a consequence of spasm or dysfunction of the cricopharyngeus muscle [3].

Clinical presentation

The usual Zenker's diverticulum patient presents with dysphagia, globus, halitosis, coughing and regurgitation of undigested food (more when lying down), the latter being a very characteristic and almost diagnostic feature. Chest roentgenogram may show a widening of the upper mediastinum [4]. X-rays of the neck may disclose a collection of air anterior to the fifth and sixth cervical vertebrae.

Confirmatory diagnosis is with a barium swallow (Figure 20.1), which reveals a pouch in the proximal posterior esophagus, with a neck usually located slightly above the level of the cricoid ring, and an endoscopy which visualizes the pouch in the location described above, often filled with undigested food [4,5].

Surgical approaches

Surgical treatment aims at dividing the cricopharyngeus muscle and removing the pouch causing the symptoms. The surgical procedure is generally curative and a majority of the patients live symptom-free for the rest of their lifetime.

The basic surgical approaches may be either open or endoscopic.

Open surgery

- Transcervical surgical approach: the diverticulum is exposed through a lateral neck incision. The sac may be resected (diverticulectomy) or tacked superiorly to the prevertebral fascia (diverticulopexy). These procedures are usually done in conjunction with a cricopharyngeal myotomy (a procedure to surgically weaken the cricopharyngeus muscle and prevent a recurrence of the pathology).

Endoscopic

This approach differs from the open surgery in that no skin incision is required, and the patient is usually

Anesthesia for Otolaryngologic Surgery, ed. Basem Abdelmalak and D. John Doyle. Published by Cambridge University Press.
© Cambridge University Press 2013.

(A)

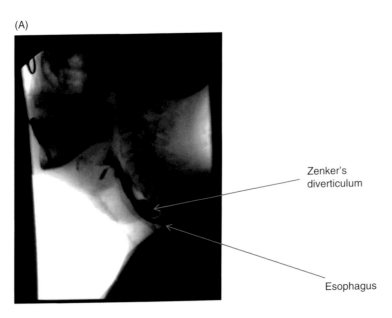

Zenker's
diverticulum

Esophagus

Figure 20.1. (A) A lateral view of a modified barium swallow study showing Zenker's diverticulum. (B) Anteroposterior view of a modified barium swallow study showing Zenker's diverticulum. Reprinted with permission, Cleveland Clinic Center for Medical Art & Photography © 2012. All rights reserved.

(B)

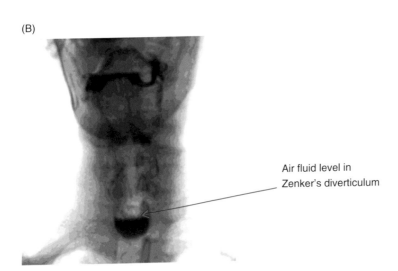

Air fluid level in
Zenker's diverticulum

discharged home the same day or the following morning.

- Dohlman procedure: the diverticulum is exposed with a bivalved (two-blade) endoscope with one blade in the pouch and the other blade in the cervical esophagus. Under direct visualization, the common wall between the pouch and the esophagus is ablated (usually with a carbon dioxide laser) [6].
- Endoscopic staple diverticulotomy: the redundant hypopharyngeal mucosa is not removed and the cricopharyngeus muscle is partially divided. A bivalved endoscope is placed through the mouth to expose the cricopharyngeus. Similar to the Dohlman procedure, one blade is placed in the ZD and the other in the cervical esophagus. The common wall separating the diverticulum from the esophagus is reduced with an endoscopic stapler, which prevents food material from collecting within the diverticulum [7].
- Endoscopic harmonic scalpel technique: [8].

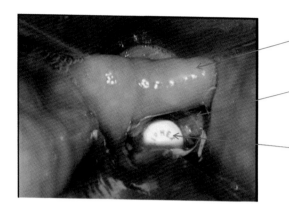

Hypertrophic
cricopharyngeal bar

Zenker's diverticulum

Aciphex tablet

Figure 20.2. An intact pill lodged in a Zenker's diverticulum, intraoperative endoscopic view (Weerda diverticuloscope). Image is courtesy of Dr. Joseph Scharpf of the Head and Neck Institute, Cleveland Clinic, Cleveland, OH.

Anesthetic management
Preoperative considerations

The main preoperative considerations for these patients are:

(1) The diverticulum tends to occur in elderly patients, the age at which coronary artery disease is common, the degree of which needs to be assessed preoperatively.

(2) The pouch contents are alkaline, so aspiration of such content does not result in acid-related aspiration pneumonia [4]. Nonetheless, the condition is not uncommonly associated with recurrent aspiration pneumonitis or even lung abscess [9]. A likely explanation is that aspirated material from the ZD may contain oral pathogens that may lead to infectious complications.

(3) Malnutrition is a common finding in these patients as well.

A thorough evaluation in the outpatient setting is warranted, keeping in mind the elective nature of this procedure. In addition to the routine preoperative evaluation, discussion of which is beyond the scope of this chapter, special emphasis should be given to the above three considerations [9,10].

The day of surgery

Fasting is always important before induction of any general anesthetic. It is even more important in patients with Zenker's, though a fasting period more than the usual 6 hours prior to initiation of induction does not guarantee an empty pouch. Oral premedication should be avoided because premedicants may lodge in the pouch (Figure 20.2) and may be aspirated

to the lung. The use of antacids or H_2 blockers is of no value because the contents of the pouch have an alkaline pH [4,5,11].

Preparation of the operating room

Preparing the operating room prior to surgery revolves around the nature of the procedure (open vs. endoscopic) and whether or not laser is being used. If the surgery is a laserization it would mean adoption of the universal protocol for anesthesia safety during laser procedures, including the use of laser-safe tubes and other necessary precautions for the prevention of airway fires. More discussion on management of lasers is in Chapter 25.

Induction of anesthesia

A main concern during the induction period is to safely secure the airway without increasing the risk of aspiration. It has been suggested that decrease the risk of regurgitation of pouch contents:

(1) the pouch should be emptied preoperatively via external pressure [5]; however, this is not commonly performed in clinical practice for fear of causing iatrogenic regurgitation and subsequent aspiration as well as its unproven benefit [5];

(2) position the patient in a head-up tilt at the time of induction of anesthesia [4].

The different options for the induction of anesthesia and intubation for this procedure are listed below along with a discussion of the pros and cons of each technique.

Awake intubation

Awake intubation is a very reasonable option [9], as maintaining the airway reflexes provides a natural

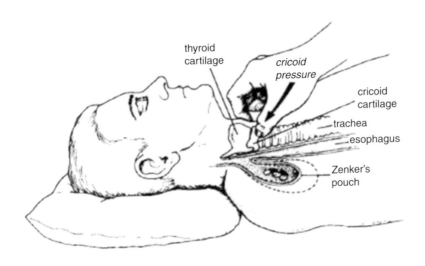

Figure 20.3. Anatomical relationships of the diverticulum to the cricoid cartilage during application of cricoid pressure. (Reproduced from Thiagarajah S, Lear E, Keh M. Anesthetic implications of Zenker's diverticulum. *Anesth Analg* 1990;**70**:109–11, with permission from Wolters Kluwer Health.)

protection against the risk of aspiration of regurgtated pouch contents. This is especially helpful when managing a patient with a large diverticulum extending to the mediastinum and/or an orifice above the cricoid ring as seen on a barium swallow. There are several caveats to be considered though.

Firstly, ensure adequate topicalization of the airway; however, an effort should be made to focus topicalization to the supraglottic region and minimize local anesthetic application to the trachea (i.e. avoid transtracheal block) to maintain protective airway reflexes. It should be noted that this is only a theoretical concern. Many clinicians believe that it takes multiples of the usual local anesthetic dose used to topicalize the trachea to abolish such protective reflexes. Moreover, another concern is that transtracheal injection is known to trigger coughing, which along with straining could theoretically induce regurgitation of pouch contents and potential aspiration [12].

Awake intubation can be accomplished using a variety of airway devices and scopes; however, a flexible fiberoptic scope seems to be the gentlest and least traumatic.

Rapid sequence induction with or without cricoid pressure

The use of cricoid pressure has been debated for many years now in the prevention of aspiration with a possible full stomach while administering a general anesthetic. The size of the pouch and the anatomical position of the orifice of the pouch are some of the factors to be considered while considering applying cricoid pressure. Careful preoperative examination of the barium-swallow results and conferring with the surgeon are helpful steps in determining whether cricoid pressure will be effective or harmful. *Application of cricoid pressure has only been recommended if the neck of the pouch is below the cricoid cartilage* (Figure 20.3).

In most circumstances, though, the neck of the pouch is above the cricopharyngeus muscle, and thus the cricoid ring is always below the neck of the diverticulum [4]. This obviously makes cricoid pressure more harmful than helpful by squeezing the sac, which would result in increasing pressure within the pouch and inducing regurgitation of its contents into the hypopharynx and increasing the likelihood of aspiration.

If the sac is large, extending down into the mediastinum with its orifice at the level of the cricoid cartilage and neck below the cricoid, it is likely that cricoid pressure will obliterate the opening and protect against regurgitation.

Therefore, the application of cricoid pressure in the majority of cases where the sac is small may increase rather than decrease the risk of regurgitation in patients with Zenker's diverticulum [4,13].

Smooth induction with upward head tilt

A smooth induction with a 30° upward head tilt would probably be a safer alternative [4,12]. The avoidance of coughing and straining is critical. After adequate pre-oxygenation, an intravenous hypnotic supplemented with opioids and/or lidocaine with or without mask ventilation with O_2 usually results in a smooth induction.

A non-depolarizing muscle relaxant is administered and endotracheal intubation performed after complete relaxation has been achieved. The cuff of a single-lumen endotracheal tube must be promptly inflated to provide adequate sealing of the airway. The use of succinylcholine is the basis for a traditional rapid sequence, but it has been questioned here because if used alone, and not preceded by a small dose of a non-depolarizing muscle relaxant, it could induce muscle fasciculation, which may cause compression of the pouch and deleterious consequences [12].

Intraoperative

While regurgitation and aspiration may occur during induction of anesthesia and during intubation, they might still happen even after successful uneventful intubation [5]. This is thought to be due to the seepage of fluid around the single-lumen tube cuff during surgical manipulations. Intraoperatively, it has been suggested that a moist gauze pack placed to surround the endotracheal tube will prevent aspiration during surgery [5]. Postoperatively, nursing the patient in a semi-sitting position and avoiding excessive sedation may decrease the risk.

Perforation of the diverticulum

While this may occur during a difficult intubation, with blind attempts at intubation of the trachea, it could also occur during blind placement of a nasogastric tube. A recommended technique is to insert the nasogastric tube under surgical guidance once adequate access to the pouch has been established. Blood loss and air embolism may occur if major vessels are inadvertently severed and retraction of the carotid sheath may cause baroreceptor stimulation that may initiate tachyarrhythmias or bradyarrhythmias [5].

Alternative approaches

Alternatively, the procedure can be performed under regional anesthesia using deep and superficial cervical plexus blocks [14]. Decreasing the risk of aspiration, by preserving protective airway reflexes, is one advantage of regional anesthesia. An awake, alert patient is able to cooperate with the surgeon and to swallow on command, allowing the surgeon to view the pathology in action. After repair of the diverticulum with the incision still open, the patient is fed small spoonfuls of gelatin so the surgeon can ensure the adequacy of correction under direct vision [15]. That said, the majority of Zenker's diverticulum surgery continues to be done today under general endotracheal anesthesia.

Another approach that is now increasing in common practice is that of flexible endoscopic cricopharyngeal myotomy using an endoscopic needle knife and electrocautery without diverticulectomy, performed by the endoscopist/gastroenterologist without the use of general anesthesia. The procedure is usually performed with moderate sedation using midazolam/meperidine and/or fentanyl, after careful preprocedure patient selection. Potential advantages include avoiding general endotracheal anesthesia. In addition, it is performed in an outpatient setting, and resumption of oral intake is faster. Local injection of 1:10 000 epineherine controls bleeding and if a perforation in the wall of the posterior esophagus results from the cricopharyngeal myotomy an endoclip is placed over it. It is a relatively recent procedure, first reported in 1995, as an alternative to open surgical and rigid endoscopically guided cricopharyngeal myotomy with or without myotomy. Outcome data are limited at this stage. However, preliminary data suggest that this is a relatively safe procedure with similar success rates to the standard open surgical and rigid endoscopic procedures in addition to low recurrence rates, and minimal complications [16,17].

Postoperative issues

Desirable as always in neck surgery is a smooth extubation with an awake patient adequately reversed from muscle paralysis, to avoid the risks of neck hematoma compromising the airway. While different approaches to accomplish this goal are described in other chapters, the authors of this chapter utilize a narcotic technique in which a full dose of long-acting narcotic, hydromorphone for example, is given with the incision (0.01–0.02 mg/kg) in 0.4 mg increments 5 minutes apart as blood pressure allows. This approach allows for a smooth wake up, without much cough or strain. Care in the post anesthesia care unit (PACU) should include nursing in the semi-upright position, more so in patients with Zenker's undergoing another surgery in which the sac has not been excised. Most of the surgeons will have the nasogastric tube on gravity drainage for a prolonged period of time and oral feeding will be initiated only after the closure of the surgical anastomoses has been confirmed.

Complications

Fistula
Perforation
Recurrent laryngeal nerve injury
Neck hematoma
Infection
Aspiration pneumonia
Mortality (very rare)

Patients with Zenker's diverticulum for other surgical procedures

The presence of a Zenker's diverticulum in a patient having other elective surgery should not be overlooked because this will increase the risk of regurgitation and pulmonary aspiration during the intraoperative and the postoperative periods. It might be wise to consider excising the pouch before any other elective procedure if possible to prevent silent aspiration.

Summary
Zenker's diverticulum – a story of dos, don'ts, and maybes

In conclusion, a Zenker's diverticulum is very much an enigma, a story of dos, don'ts, and maybes which confronts the anesthesiologist prior to every induction. Some things which stand out as the clear do's are preoperative fasting, smooth induction in a 10–30° head-up tilt or awake intubation. Pertinent perioperative evaluation should include detailed cardiovascular and nutritional status evaluation and optimization. The things not to do would be use of particulate antacid premedication, application of cricoid pressure if the neck of the pouch is above the cricoid ring and blind insertion of a nasogastric tube. Maybes include regional anesthesia techniques utilizing superficial and deep cervical plexus blockade, which have the advantages of an awake and responsive patient with preserved reflexes. However, there are technical difficulties with a variable failure rate and patients acceptability.

All in all, anesthesia for a patient with a Zenker's diverticulum is a fascinating interplay of several surgical and non-surgical issues and is testament to the fact that a relatively simple surgical procedure can never be equated to a straightforward anesthetic course.

Case study

A 70-year-old male presented with a symptomatic Zenker's diverticulum for an open surgical diverticulectomy along with cricopharyngeal myotomy.

Preoperative evaluation

- Comorbidities: COPD on home nocturnal oxygen 2 l/min, baseline oxygen saturation on room air 93–95%, diabetes mellitus well controlled on oral medication, hypertension well controlled.
- Airway: Mallampatti classification III, thyromental distance 2.5 fingers, adequate neck range of motion, circumference 18 inches, dentition intact.
- Vitals: BP 150/78 mmHg; HR 85/min; weight 150 kg; height 180 cm; BMI 46.29 kg/m^2.

Intraoperatively

On the morning of surgery, the patient was NPO >8 hours. Upon arrival to the operating room he was premedicated with midazolam 1 mg IV. Standard ASA monitors were applied. He was positioned with head up at about 10–20° and 4 l/ml of oxygen was applied via a nasal cannula. Awake intubation was elected for an airway exam consistent with a potentially difficult airway, and as a precaution against aspiration as well as utilizing the patient's own airway protective reflexes.

Another 1 mg of midazolam IV was given followed by 50 µg of fentanyl IV. Airway topicalization was started by applying atomized 4% lidocaine to the oropharyngeal mucosa, after which an Ovasappian airway was introduced. At this point another 1 mg of midazolam was given IV to augment his sedation for awake intubation. Then 2 ml of 4% lidocaine were sprayed through a MADgic® catheter introduced through the Ovassapian airway after being formed into the shape of the airway (almost a hockey stick shape). This last spray induced a limited and expected cough as the local anesthetic reached the upper surface of the vocal cords and upper endotracheal mucosa.

A flexible fiberoptic bronchoscope (FFB) pre-loaded with a size 7.5 Parker® flextip tube (the FFB had been pre-warmed through immersion in a warm bottle of saline to avoid lens fogging) was introduced into the airway through the Ovassapian airway. Once the vocal cords were visualized, the FFB was introduced through them, and was advanced for approximately 2.5 inches (6.5 cm), then the ETT was railroaded over it into the trachea. The FFB was then withdrawn, and the anesthetic circuit was connected to the ETT, after inflating its cuff. After confirmation of $ETCO_2$, general anesthesia was induced with 120 mg of propofol and 150 µg of fentanyl. Sevoflurane inhalational anesthetic vaporizer was dialed to 2.5%. Muscle relaxation was then induced with 80 mg of rocuronium. The Ovassapian airway was peeled off the ETT and removed from the airway, and the tube was secured with tape.

Had the patient not had an airway exam consistent with a diffficult airway, general anesthesia could have been induced with 150 µg of fentanyl, 40 mg of lidocaine (to lessen the burning sensation associated with propofol injection), and 250 mg of propofol IV in gradual titrated doses, followed by IV rocuronium 100 mg and gentle positive-pressure ventilation, and intubation. A rapid sequence approach with cricoid pressure would not have been an option because pre-operative imaging had visualized the neck of the diverticulum above the cricoid ring. In such a case cricoid pressure would have squeezed the contents of the bag and actually increased the chances of regurgitation and aspiration. Cricoid pressure may be useful when the neck of the sack is below the cricoid ring and the size of the diverticulum is not very large.

Anesthesia was maintained with sevoflurane in a mixture of air and oxygen. Muscle relaxation was maintained with intermittent boluses of IV rocuronium and analgesia was maintained with IV fentanyl. An orogastric tube was placed in the esophagus under direct vision to help in identification of the diverticulum. The resection was carried out through an incision in the neck. After excising the diverticular sac, the suture lines on the pharyngeal wall were tested for air leaks.

At the end of surgery, with the patient awake, responsive and demonstrating adequate reversal of neuromuscular blockade, the trachea was extubated.

Postoperative care

The patient was then admitted to PACU, where a chest X-ray was found to be negative for any acute changes. In the PACU he was nursed in the semi-upright position and was kept NPO. He spent an uneventful 120 minutes during which his oxygenation was stable and vitals remained unremarkable in the PACU and was then discharged to the floor, once he met the PACU discharge criteria.

Clinical pearls

- Fasting prior to the induction of anesthesia does not guarantee an empty pouch. Oral premedication should be avoided because premedicants may lodge in the pouch.
- Options for induction of general anesthesia include: awake intubation, rapid sequence with cricoid pressure and smooth induction with upward head tilt. However, the application of cricoid pressure during induction of anesthesia for Zenker's diverticulum patients is only recommended if the neck of the pouch is at or below the cricoid cartilage.
- Perforation of Zenker's diverticulum may occur during a difficult intubation, or during blind placement of a nasogastric tube.
- It might be wise to excise a Zenker's diverticulum before proceeding with any other elective surgery as its presence may increase the risk of regurgitation and pulmonary aspiration perioperatively.

References

1. Zenker F, Von Ziemssen H, Krankheiten O. Handbuch der speciellen Pathologie und Therapie. *Supplement Leipzig: Vogel* 1874;7, Part 1:50–87.

2. Dorsey JM, Randolph DA. Long-term evaluation of pharyngo-esophageal diverticulectomy. *Ann Surg* 1971;**173**(5):680–5. Epub 1971/05/01.

3. Last R. *The Pharynx, Anatomy, Regional and Applied*. Edinburgh: Churchill Livingstone; 1973. pp. 643–9.

4. Aouad MT, Berzina CE, Baraka AS. Aspiration pneumonia after anesthesia in a patient with a Zenker diverticulum. *Anesthesiology* 2000;**92**(6): 1837–9.

5. Thiagarajah S, Lear E, Keh M. Anesthetic implications of Zenker's diverticulum. *Anesth Analg* 1990;**70**(1): 109–11.

6. Verhaegen VJ, Feuth T, van den Hoogen FJ, Marres HA, Takes RP. Endoscopic carbon dioxide laser diverticulostomy versus endoscopic staple-assisted diverticulostomy to treat Zenker's diverticulum. *Head Neck* 2011;**33**(2):154–9. Epub 2010/09/18.

7. The UC Davis Health System CfVaS. Available from: http://www.ucdvoice.org/zenkers.html.

8. May JT, Padhya TA, McCaffrey TV. Endoscopic repair of Zenker's diverticulum by harmonic scalpel. *Am J Otolaryngol* 2011. Epub 2011/02/11.

9. Payne WS, King RM. Pharyngoesophageal (Zenker's) diverticulum. *Surg Clin North Am* 1983;**63**(4):815–24.

10. White IL. Severe complication of a Zenker's diverticulum with endoscopic diverticulotomy rescue. *Laryngoscope* 1981;**91**(5):708–19. Epub 1981/05/01.

11. Baron SH. Zenker's diverticulum as a cause for loss of drug availability: a "new" complication. *Am J Gastroenterol* 1982;77(3):152–3.

12. Cope R, Spargo P. Anesthesia for Zenker's diverticulum. *Anesth Analg* 1990;**71**(3):312.

13. Estafanous F. *Anesthesia for Pulmonary and Mediastinal Surgery*, 2nd edn. Philadelphia: Lippincott Williams & Wilkins; 2001.

14. Naja ZM, Al-Tannir MA, Zeidan A, *et al.* Bilateral guided cervical block for Zenker diverticulum excision in a patient with ankylosing spondylitis. *J Anesth* 2009;**23**(1):143–6. Epub 2009/02/24.

15. Adams CF. Regional anesthesia for repair of Zenker's diverticulum. *Anesth Analg* 1990;**70**(6):676.

16. Case DJ, Baron TH. Flexible endoscopic management of Zenker diverticulum: the Mayo Clinic experience. *Mayo Clinic Proc* 2010;**85**(8):719–22. Epub 2010/08/03.

17. Tang SJ, Jazrawi SF, Chen E, Tang L, Myers LL. Flexible endoscopic clip-assisted Zenker's diverticulotomy: the first case series (with videos). *Laryngoscope* 2008;**118**(7):1199–205. Epub 2008/04/11.

Chapter

21

Anesthesia for parotid surgery

Mauricio Perilla, Biao Lei and Daniel Alam

Introduction

The paired parotid glands are the largest among the three major salivary glands in the human body (the other two are the submandibular and subglottic glands). They are located on the side of the cheeks, anterior and inferior to the external ear, resembling an inverted pyramid in shape, with their base extending from the zygomatic arch and their apex overlying and wrapping around the mandibular angle. Because of their superficial localization, they can be palpated. The saliva secretion drains through the Stensen's duct into the parotid papilla, which is located on the buccal mucosa opposite the upper second molar.

The parotid gland is encapsulated between the superficial and deep layers of the parotid gland fascia (PGF). The superficial PGF is thick and covers the parotid gland, extends over the masseter muscle and attaches to the zygomatic arch. There is a lax space between the superficial PGF and the gland, which allows for easy separation. The deep layer of the PGF is thin and underlies the deep lobe of the parotid gland [1].

The facial nerve (extratemporal segment) crosses lateral to the styloid process and approaches the parotid gland posteriorly. It penetrates the parotid gland, and runs in the body of the gland separating the deep and superficial lobes. Here the nerve divides into two major divisions, the superiorly directed temporal-facial and the inferiorly directed cervico-facial branches [2]. Because of the important function of the facial nerve, its preservation is always an important goal of parotid surgery, and will be discussed in detail later.

The great auricular nerve (GAN) is also an important neighboring structure. After emerging from the posterior margin of the sternocleidomastoid muscle, the GAN runs under the platysma towards the mandibular angle, where it divides into three branches. These branches mostly run within the superficial PGF; however, some bundles may penetrate the fascia and run deeply into the gland parenchyma [3–5]. Sacrifice of the GAN branches during parotid surgery is thought to be responsible for the common complication of postoperative ear lobe dysesthesia.

Pathology of the parotid gland

Neoplasm is the most common parotid pathology that warrants surgery. Fortunately, the majority of parotid gland tumors are benign. The most common type is pleomorphic adenoma (also known as benign mixed tumor, 60–70%), followed by Warthin's tumor (also known as papillary cystadenoma lymphomatosum, 14–20%) [6]. Pleomorphic adenoma has a high rate of cure with surgery; however, if left untreated for a prolonged time there is a small but certain rate of degeneration into malignancy [6]. Pleomorphic adenoma most often derives from the superficial lobe, whereas the deeper lobe is involved only 10% of the time [7]. Histologically, pleomorphic adenoma is circumscribed, with either a complete or partial capsule. The capsule itself may contain lesions such as satellite nodules or pseudopodia (fingerlike formations) [7]. Before the 1950s, tumor enucleation was the prototype of surgery for pleomorphic adenoma, with the purpose of minimizing injury to the facial nerve. However, the recurrence rate was reported as high as 23–31%, sometimes even long after the initial surgery [1]. Although controversies still exist, factors such as tumor non-encapsulation, incomplete excision and implantation are currently viewed as responsible for recurrence. For these reasons, currently the

Anesthesia for Otolaryngologic Surgery, ed. Basem Abdelmalak and D. John Doyle. Published by Cambridge University Press.
© Cambridge University Press 2013.

most commonly performed procedure is superficial parotidectomy [7].

Warthin tumor is the second most common benign neoplasm of the parotid gland, accounting for 14–30% of all parotid tumors. It is encapsulated, has a slow growth rate and a low rate (0.3%) of degeneration into malignancy. For that reason, conservative management is often the chosen line of treatment. However, surgery is still the most commonly chosen option (either superficial parotidectomy or enucleation) [8].

Malignant tumors of the parotid gland include mucoepidermoid carcinoma and carcinoma ex pleomorphic adenoma, etc. Surgery, usually parotidectomy, is the most commonly used treatment. Adjuvant therapies include radiotherapy and chemotherapy.

Sialolithiasis is a common obstructive disease of the major salivary glands, which can cause superimposed infection and sialoadenitis. The surgical treatment and anesthesia of sialolithiasis will be briefly discussed below.

Surgical considerations

Brief description of superficial parotidectomy

Complete or limited superficial parotidectomy with facial nerve dissection is still the most commonly performed procedure for benign parotid neoplasm. It gives the surgeon the opportunity to completely remove the parotid tumor with a safe margin of normal gland tissue. The operating procedure is primarily the identification of the facial nerve and its dissection anteriorly along the branches. The "cuff" of the normal parotid tissue surrounding the tumor is thereby preserved. After anesthesia, the patient is placed in a supine position with the head hyperextended and laterally rotated to expose the lesion side upwards. Classically, an S-shaped incision, called the Blair incision, is used, extending from the preauricular to the submandibular region. A skin flap is raised to the anterior parotid border to expose the parotid gland. The facial nerve and its branches are identified and are preserved carefully. The portion of the parotid lateral to the facial nerve is removed [1]. There have been various modifications of surgical techniques, which are beyond the scope of this chapter.

Facial nerve monitoring

Because of its intimate anatomical location and important function, facial nerve injury has always

been a common but dreaded complication of parotid surgery. The incidence of postoperative transient facial nerve paresis was reported to be between 20% and 40%, whereas that of permanent paralysis was about 0–4% [9]. Intraoperative facial nerve monitoring thus became an important technique. The earliest technique in the 1970s relied on mechanical detection of actual facial movements. It was soon abandoned because of the requirement for large supra-threshold stimuli. A more sensitive technique based on electrophysiology stimuli and electromyography (EMG) recording was first developed by Delgado in 1979 [10]. Since then, it has been modified into a sophisticated technique and applied in various surgery fields as well, such as neurosurgeries and otological surgeries. Rea et al. first developed the technique during parotidectomy in 1990 [11]. There are various types of monitors commercially available, usually with multi-channel monitoring. The electrodes are typically placed in the four areas innervated by the facial nerve (frontal, zygomatic, buccal, and marginal mandibular) to monitor two of the muscles groups innervated by the facial nerve, i.e. orbicularis oculi and orbicularis oris [9]. EMG activity in response to continuous neurotonic discharges is monitored, while direct electrical stimuli are intermittently applied through monopolar or bipolar stimulating probes. Both visual and audio signals are generated. To eliminate the nonspecific signals (background noises), additional recording electrodes are also placed in the contralateral side orbicularis oculi/oris. Of note, the nonspecific signals decrease in amplitude as the depth of anesthesia increases [12]. Surgeons use this technique to identify the facial nerve and its branches, to map its contour, and to evaluate nerve integrity and function. The electrodes are inserted near the facial midline and the connections are kept to the side contralateral to surgery to minimize interference with the surgical field. Although these techniques are precise and accurate, most surgeons use neurostimulators with direct observation of facial movement.

Anesthesia for parotidectomy

Preoperative considerations

Preoperative evaluation of patients for parotid surgery should be conducted in the usual fashion. Special attention should be paid to the patient's past medical history. Head and neck cancer has been associated with alcohol and tobacco abuse. Patient interrogation should focus on the patient's history of previous head, neck or facial surgery and history of radiation therapy. Past intubations should be investigated and studies and images such as office-based airway fibrolaryngoscopies and CT or MRI images of head and neck should be reviewed and discussed with the surgical team in order to establish an airway access plan.

The patient's physical exam will focus on tumor displacement of the airway as well as temporomandibular joint mobility; other factors such as mouth opening, sub-mandibular space compliance, thyromental distance, neck diameter, and neck range of motion should be evaluated. Previous radiation has been considered as an independent factor for difficult mask ventilation [13]. Interestingly parotid enlargement has been reported secondary to general anesthesia: "anesthesia mumps" [14].

Intraoperative

During parotidectomy the anesthesiologist has little access to the patient's head, whereas the surgical field is close to the patient's airway. Absolute immobility of the patient is highly desirable during delicate parts of the surgery such as microsurgical manipulation. For these reasons, general anesthesia with endotracheal intubation is usually required. The patient's comfort is another factor to consider, although cases done with local anesthesia have been reported.

The use of muscle relaxants is an important issue in parotidectomy anesthesia. The basis of the EMG recording requires that neurological signals are able to cross the functional neuromuscular junctions, therefore demanding that neuromuscular junctions be least affected by muscle relaxants. On the other hand muscle relaxants are commonly used for general anesthesia, especially for induction to facilitate endotracheal intubation to reduce laryngeal and tracheal damage. Therefore in practice the long-acting muscle relaxants are generally avoided for intubation.

Succinylcholine is a commonly used short-acting depolarizing muscle relaxant. It has rapid onset (30–60 s), quick metabolism by plasma pseudocholinesterase and thus short duration (typically less than 10 min) in the normal population. However, in a few patients with a genetic background of atypical pseudocholinesterase (either heterozygous, 1/50 incidence; or homozygous, 1/3000 incidence), neuromuscular blockade

can be prolonged from 20–30 min up to 4–8 hours. In those situations, blockade cannot be reversed because cholinesterase inhibitors further inhibit pseudocholinesterase and paradoxically prolong the blockade. Other side effects of succinylcholine, such as bradycardia (particularly in children), muscle fasciculation and muscle pain, hyperkalemia (usually increases by 0.5–1 mEq/l in normal population, but can reach life-threatening levels in burn, crush injury, paraplegia, or renal failure patients), increase of intraocular and intracranial pressure, etc., have to be considered carefully before administration. Routine use of succinylcholine is contraindicated in children and adolescents because there are reports of cardiac arrest due to undiagnosed myopathies.

Mivacurium is a non-depolarizing muscle relaxant with short duration of action (reported 95% recovery time is about 14 min). Similar to succinylcholine, mivacurium is also metabolized by pseudocholinesterase; its duration can be prolonged in patients with atypical pseudocholinesterase. However, cholinesterase inhibitors can reverse blockade from mivacurium once muscle contraction to neural stimulation is partially recovered. Thiede et al. studied the use of mivacurium in a small group of 21 patients undergoing parotidectomy [15]. A single dose (0.2 mg/kg IV) of mivacurium was used for intubation. Train-of-four (TOF) of peripheral muscle (adductor pollicis) recovered to 4/4 after the mean time of 19.7 min, whereas the mean time to incision and identification of facial nerve was 31.6 and 61.2 min, respectively. Although none of their patients developed transient facial paresis postoperatively, at the recorded earliest time to incision (21 min), still 14.3% of their patients would have TOF less than 2/4 and thus would be at risk. Considering that the recovery of orbicularis oculi might be sooner than that of adductor pollicis, as reported before [16], there might be fewer patients at risk. In the so-called worst-case scenario, earliest incision on a patient with slowest mivacurium recovery, false-negative responses from the EMG recording cannot be ruled out and must be taken into consideration. Mivacurium is no longer available in North America but is still used in other parts of the world.

We have to keep in mind that light anesthesia and patient arousal can be dangerous and cause serious complications, especially in the absence of neuromuscular blockade. Sufficient anesthesia depth and patient immobility are usually achieved by a balanced anesthetic technique employing a relatively large dose of opioid and inhalational agents. Maintenance with remifentanil, sufentanil or fentanyl combined with isoflurane or desflurane inhalation is also a reasonable option. In certain patients with poor hemodynamic stability, deep anesthesia by opioids and inhalational agents may excessively depress the cardiovascular system. Kizilay et al. thus probed the role of reported partial neuromuscular blockade in the situation of facial nerve monitoring [17]. In their small study of otological surgery, they found that by using atracurium as high as 50% of full neuromuscular blockade would still allow for successful facial nerve monitoring. Whether their result can be applied to parotid surgery has not been proven. It has been reported that the distal segment of the facial nerve is different from the central (cerebellopontine angle and labyrinthine) segment in histology, that the distal segment is surrounded by denser epineurium and therefore has a higher stimulation threshold.

Interestingly, because the nonspecific facial nerve EMG signal decreases in amplitude as anesthesia deepens, it could be used as a means of monitoring the anesthesia depth. Jellish et al. compared the facial nerve EMG vs. BIS in the setting of craniofacial and skull-base surgeries under either TIVA (using propofol and remifentanil) or inhalational general anesthesia (using desflurane). They found that in terms of predicting patient stillness during surgery, the facial nerve EMG has a better negative predictive value than BIS. They also found that TIVA provides more hemodynamic stability compared to desflurane inhalational anesthesia [12].

The introduction of sugammadex seems to provide another interesting strategy for brief muscle relaxation. Sugammadex is a specially designed cyclodextrin compound with a ring-shaped molecular structure. The lipophilic cavity inside the ring binds to aminosteroid compounds such as rocuronium or vecuronium, which are two commonly used nondepolarizing muscle relaxants of intermediate duration. The encapsulation of rocuronium/vecuronium makes them unavailable to diffuse through the neuromuscular junction, creates a reversed concentration gradient to pull out bound rocuronium/vecuronium molecules, and therefore effectively terminates their paralytic effect [18]. In a case report of parotid surgery by Sasakawa et al. [19], rocuronium 0.6 mg/kg was used for intubation for general anesthesia, followed immediately by sugammadex 2 mg/kg to allow for effective facial nerve stimulation. The FDA does not yet approve sugammadex due to concerns about hypersensitivity/allergic reactions.

For parotidectomy in patients with a family history of malignant hyperthermia [20] or affected by myotonic dystrophy [21], total intravenous anesthesia (TIVA) has been reported using awake intubation with 0.2% tetracaine topicalization followed by ketamine bolus, or carefully administered propofol-ketamine boluses maintained with ketamine infusion, or combined propofol-ketamine infusion supplemented with fentanyl.

Complications of parotidectomy

Airway management after parotidectomy with radical neck dissection can be a challenging situation due to aggravating factors like previous neck interventions, radiation therapy, large fluid shift, intraoperative airway manipulation, swollen tissue and residual anesthetic effect. Extubation might be deferred until the airway patency can be guaranteed. Expanding hematoma in the immediate postoperative period is a complication that should be suspected in patients who present with postoperative respiratory failure after this surgical procedure.

As mentioned above, other common complications of parotidectomy include transient facial paresis or permanent facial paralysis due to unintentional iatrogenic facial nerve injury, and ear lobe dysesthesia due to injury to GAN branches. Frey's syndrome is another common complication manifested as "gustatory sweating" on the affected side in response to food intake. It is thought to be secondary to erroneous regeneration of parotid sympathetic nerves into the sweat glands [22]. Different surgical techniques have been attempted to minimize or treat these complications.

Obstructive salivary diseases of parotid glands

Ductal stone formation (sialolithiasis) and ductal stenosis are common causes of obstructive salivary diseases of the parotid glands. Traditionally, sialolithiasis was managed by duct dilatation or papillotomy, which can be performed under local anesthesia. Distal stones may need ductal dissection; resistant cases or intraparenchymal stones may even require sialoadenectomy (e.g., total parotidectomy). Ductal abnormalities are usually treated with bypass or ductal sialodochoplasty [23]. These surgeries are usually performed under general anesthesia, where nasal intubation may be required.

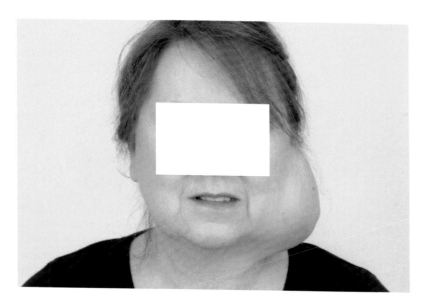

Figure 21.1. Left large parotid tumor extending into the neck. Please note the additional signs of potential difficult airway, including retracted mandible and short thyromental distance. Reprinted with permission, Cleveland Clinic Center for Medical Art & Photography © 2012. All rights reserved.

In recent years, with the advance of modern technologies and availability of specially designed small-caliber endoscopes, procedures such as extra-corporeal shock-wave lithotripsy, sialoendoscopy, laser intra-corporeal lithotripsy, and video-assisted conservative removal of calculi have all been applied in practice with high success rates. These minimally invasive surgeries have shaped the modern management of obstructive salivary diseases of the parotid gland. These procedures can usually be performed on outpatients, under local anesthesia, or supplemented with sedatives and analgesics if necessary [23].

Case study

A 51-year-old woman presented for left parotidectomy and radical neck dissection. Her medical history included morbid obesity, diabetes, hypertension, asthma, obstructive sleep apnea (OSA) and severe cervical myelopathy. Her past surgical history is consistent with cervical fusion (C5–C6).

Preoperative evaluation

The patient had no apparent distress, body mass index (BMI) 38, BP 160/85, HR 88, respiratory rate 22, oxygen saturation (SpO_2) 92% at room air. Airway exam: Mallampati score of 3, short thyromental distance (less than 6 cm), limited neck range of motion, neck circumference 40 cm and a left parotid mass

compromised an extensive area of face and neck (Figure 21.1). An MRI of the neck is presented in Figure 21.2.

Comorbidities

Diabetes mellitus type 2
Obstructive sleep apnea (OSA)
Asthma
Cervical myelopathy

Anesthesia technique

The patient was positioned in supine position on the OR table. ASA standard monitors were applied. Noninvasive blood pressure measurements, heart rate, SpO_2, capnography, respiratory rate, temperature and sedation score were recorded. A preoperative dose of glycopyrrolate 0.2 mg IV was given in order to reduce secretions and improve local anesthetics effect, midazolam 1 mg IV for sedation was given followed by an infusion of remifentanyl (0.05 μg/kg/min). Topicalization of the airway was performed initially, using a small-volume nebulizer (VixOne TM Westmed, AZ) with 4% lidocaine for 8 min followed by oxygen administration and additional oral airway transport topicalization using a multiport system (MADgic Airway, Wolfe Tory Medical Inc., Salt Lake City, UT). The flexible bronchoscope (FOB) was used in order to achieve

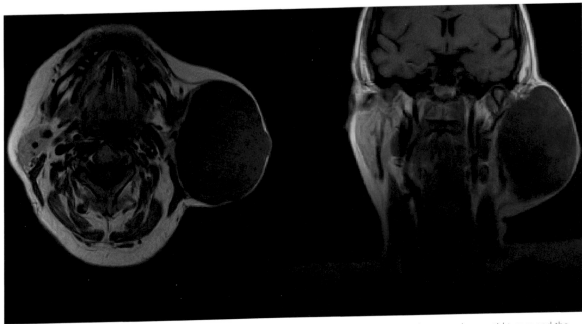

Figure 21.2. MRI of the patient's neck. Axial view (left). Coronal view (right). Note the relationship between the parotid tumor and the parapharyngeal structures compromising the left temporomandibular joint. Reprinted with permission, Cleveland Clinic Center for Medical Art & Photography © 2012. All rights reserved.

additional trans-vocal cord anesthesia with additional lidocaine 1% injected through the work channel. The patient was intubated orally with a Parker tube (Parker Flex-Tip PFHV, Parker Medical), 7.0 mm ID, via the flexible fiberoptic scope. Oral intubation was confirmed clinically and endoscopically. After intubation the patient was able to place her head in the most confortable neck position for surgery. An initial dose of propofol was administered for induction and anesthesia was maintained with sevoflurane, supplemented with remifentanil infusion (0.1–0.2 μg/kg/min). During the procedure no muscle relaxation was given in order to facilitate facial nerve monitoring. After 6 hours of surgery and before the emergence from anesthesia, the clinical assessment of the airway showed no cuff leak. The oral fiberoptic exam confirmed the airway to be severely swollen. The patient was transported intubated to the post-anesthesia care unit. A few hours later, a positive airway leak and a decrease of airway swelling were confirmed. Due to prominent risk factors, extubation was planned using a tube exchanger as a temporary bridge. These factors were obesity, short thyromental distance, previous spine fusion and extensive neck surgery. The patient was successfully extubated and the tube exchanger removed in the post-anesthesia care unit.

Clinical pearls

- For parotidectomy procedures, general anesthesia with endotracheal intubation is usually required, although cases done with local anesthesia have been reported.
- While mildly to moderately enlarged parotid glands rarely impact the airway, very large glands can extend into the neck, displacing the trachea and causing airway distortion and making airway management difficult.
- Because of the importance of the facial nerve, its preservation is a central goal of parotid surgery. This usually requires EMG monitoring and muscle relaxant avoidance.
- Sufficient anesthetic depth and patient immobility are usually achieved by a balanced anesthetic technique employing relatively large doses of opioid and inhalational agents. Light anesthesia and patient movement lead to serious complications, especially in the absence of neuromuscular blockade.

References

1. Hegazy MA, El NW, Roshdy S. Surgical outcome of modified versus conventional parotidectomy in treatment of benign parotid tumors. *J Surg Oncol* 2011;**103**:163–8.

2. Laing MR, McKerrow WS. Intraparotid anatomy of the facial nerve and retromandibular vein. *Br J Surg* 1988;**75**:310–2.

3. Colella G, Rauso R, Tartaro G, Biondi P. Skin injury and great auricular nerve sacrifice after parotidectomy. *J Craniofac Surg* 2009;**20**:1078–81.

4. Zumeng Y, Zhi G, Gang Z, Jianhua W, Yinghui T. Modified superficial parotidectomy: preserving both the great auricular nerve and the parotid gland fascia. *Otolaryngol Head Neck Surg* 2006;**135**:458–62.

5. Porter MJ, Wood SJ. Preservation of the great auricular nerve during parotidectomy. *Clin Otolaryngol Allied Sci* 1997;**22**:251–3.

6. Biorklund A, Eneroth CM. Management of parotid gland neoplasms. *Am J Otolaryngol* 1980;**1**:155–67.

7. Emodi O, El-Naaj IA, Gordin A, Akrish S, Peled M. Superficial parotidectomy versus retrograde partial superficial parotidectomy in treating benign salivary gland tumor (pleomorphic adenoma). *J Oral Maxillofac Surg* 2010;**68**:2092–8.

8. Yoo GH, Eisele DW, Askin FB, Driben JS, Johns ME. Warthin's tumor: a 40-year experience at The Johns Hopkins Hospital. *Laryngoscope* 1994;**104**:799–803.

9. Eisele DW, Wang SJ, Orloff LA. Electrophysiologic facial nerve monitoring during parotidectomy. *Head Neck* 2010;**32**:399–405.

10. Delgado TE, Bucheit WA, Rosenholtz HR, Chrissian S. Intraoperative monitoring of facial muscle evoked responses obtained by intracranial stimulation of the facial nerve: a more accurate technique for facial nerve dissection. *Neurosurgery* 1979;**4**:418–21.

11. Rea JL. Use of a hemostat/stimulator probe and dedicated nerve locator/monitor for parotid surgery. *Ear Nose Throat J* 1990;**69**:566, 570, 573.

12. Jellish WS, Leonetti JP, Buoy CM, *et al*. Facial nerve electromyographic monitoring to predict movement in patients titrated to a standard anesthetic depth. *Anesth Analg* 2009;**109**:551–8.

13. Kheterpal S, Martin L, Shanks AM, Tremper KK. Prediction and outcomes of impossible mask ventilation. A review of 50,000 anesthetics. *Anesthesiology* 2009;**110**:891–7

14. Reilly DJ. Benign transient swelling of the parotid glands following general anesthesia: "anesthesia mumps". *Anesth Analg* 1970;**49**:560–3.

15. Thiede O, Klusener T, Sielenkamper A, *et al*. Interference between muscle relaxation and facial nerve monitoring during parotidectomy. *Acta Otolaryngol* 2006;**126**:422–8.

16. Caffrey RR, Warren ML, Becker KE Jr. Neuromuscular blockade monitoring comparing the orbicularis oculi and adductor pollicis muscles. *Anesthesiology* 1986;**65**:95–7.

17. Kizilay A, Aladag I, Cokkeser Y, *et al*. Effects of partial neuromuscular blockade on facial nerve monitorization in otologic surgery. *Acta Otolaryngol* 2003;**123**:321–4.

18. Baldo BA, McDonnell NJ, Pham NH. Drug-specific cyclodextrins with emphasis on sugammadex, the neuromuscular blocker rocuronium and perioperative anaphylaxis: implications for drug allergy. *Clin Exp Allergy* 2011.

19. Sasakawa T, Iwasaki H, Kurosawa A, *et al*. A case report: a normal dose of rocuronium achieved the desired effect in a short time after the administration of sugammadex during reoperation. *Masui* 2011;**60**:621–4.

20. Wadhwa RK, Tantisira B. Parotidectomy in a patient with a family history of hyperthermia. *Anesthesiology* 1974;**40**:191–4.

21. Yasuda T, Otomo N, Matsuki A, *et al*. Total intravenous anesthesia for two patients complicated with myotonic dystrophy. *Masui* 1999;**48**: 181–4.

22. Sood S, Quraishi MS, Bradley PJ. Frey's syndrome and parotid surgery. *Clin Otolaryngol Allied Sci* 1998;**23**:291–301.

23. Nahlieli O, Baruchin AM. Endoscopic technique for the diagnosis and treatment of obstructive salivary gland diseases. *J Oral Maxillofac Surg* 1999;**57**:1394–401.

Anesthesia for maxillary, salivary gland, mandibular and temporomandibular joint surgery

Gail I. Randel and Tracey Straker

The maxilla

Introduction

Surgery of the maxilla straddles the expertise of oto-rhinolaryngology and oromaxillofacial surgeons. This section of the chapter will focus on non-traumatic maxillary procedures and endoscopic maxillary sinus surgery. The maxilla is composed of two fused bones along the palatal fissure that form the upper jaw. The body of the maxilla is a component of three cavities – the roof of the mouth, the wall of the orbit and the floor and lateral wall of the nasal antrum. The maxillary sinus is housed in the body of the maxilla and is the largest of the paranasal sinuses [1].

Surgical procedure

Maxillectomy surgery may encompass many variations – total maxillectomy with and without orbital exenteration, partial (subtotal) maxillectomy and limited maxillectomy. Limited maxillectomy is defined as surgery that removes one wall of the antrum. An example of a limited maxillectomy is a medial maxillectomy. Subtotal maxillectomy is defined as removal of two walls of the antrum. Total maxillectomy is defined as removal of the total maxilla [2]. Indications for maxillectomy include tumors of the palate, nasal cavity and sinus pathology, salivary gland pathology, fungal infection (mucormycosis), papilloma, angiofibroma and granulomatous disease. A maxillectomy may also be performed for skull base pathology [3]. Benefits of endoscopic maxillectomy include access to ethmoid and sphenoid sinuses, no external scarring, and no loss of bony nasal or anterior maxillary support structures [4].

Anesthetic management

Preoperative evaluation

In addition to the general principles discussed in Chapter 3 a thorough hemostatic assessment should be taken from the patient. Questions regarding liver disease, bleeding from previous surgeries, antiplatelet and anticoagulant medications, herbal medications and a family history of blood dyscrasias should be asked. Baseline screening lab work should include hematocrit and type and screen. Imaging studies such as MRI and CT scan can be of immense help in planning airway management.

Discussions regarding airway management should occur with the patient if an awake technique is to be utilized. Likewise, if there is a strong possibility of postoperative ventilation or tracheostomy, these issues should be discussed. If you will be placing an arterial line, explain the reason for its use.

Jehovah's Witness patients should have a detailed discussion regarding preoperative anemia, possible hemorrhage, and options for cardiovascular resuscitation.

Intraoperative management

These surgeries are performed under general anesthesia. An arterial line is generally needed to facilitate deliberate hypotensive technique and for measuring serial hematocrits. A short-acting muscle relaxant should be used if cranial nerves or SSEPs are monitored.

Airway management usually consists of oral intubation and is not usually an issue. Occasionally, depending on the extent of the tumor, oral intubation may not be possible. Securing the airway nasally or by tracheostomy may be viable alternatives.

Anesthesia for Otolaryngologic Surgery, ed. Basem Abdelmalak and D. John Doyle. Published by Cambridge University Press.
© Cambridge University Press 2013.

The endotracheal tube should be taped to the lower lip and on the opposite side of the incision site. If the airway is difficult, consider an awake technique to secure the airway.

Stomach decompression of swallowed blood should be considered at the end of the surgery. Two large-gauge intravenous lines, blood warmer, warming device and Foley catheter may be necessary in lengthy maxillectomy procedures.

Consider transporting the intubated patient with a propofol infusion to prevent hypertensive episodes and the formation of hematoma, particularly in patients who have had a flap reconstruction.

Postoperative care

Maintaining a normal blood pressure to prevent excessive bleeding or hematoma formation is prudent. Depending on the extent of the surgery, edema formation and possible flap reconstruction, postoperative spontaneous/controlled ventilation through the ETT or tracheostomy tube may be safer options than immediate extubation.

Bridge to extubation techniques may be considered if there are concerns regarding successful extubation. Maintaining continuous access to the difficult airway post extubation is a significant consideration in an algorithm. Extubation over an airway exchange catheter may be considered. The airway exchange catheter is passed down the endotracheal tube. The endotracheal tube is removed over the exchange catheter and the catheter is left *in situ* in the airway. The airway exchange catheter has been left in place as long as 72 hours post extubation [5]. That said, airway management post maxillectomy is usually not a challenge [6].

Cranial nerves V, VI, VII, IX, X and cervical components of the spinomesencephalic tract are responsible for acute and chronic pain of the head, face and neck [7]. Pain can be characterized as either nociceptive (somatic or visceral) or neuropathic (paroxysmal, lancinating pain). Pain management consists of many modalities – pharmacological, herbal, physiotherapy and interventional pain techniques. Cancer pain responds well to opioids, while neuropathic pain responds more readily to tricyclic antidepressants and anticonvulsants. Pain management should be guided by the World Health Organization (WHO) and the American Pain Society guidelines. A three-step ladder approach composed of non-steroidal anti-inflammatory drugs, opioids, and adjuvant medications encompasses the framework of the WHO pain treatment regimen. Adjuvant drugs enhance the effects of analgesics or lessen other symptoms that exacerbate pain. Examples of adjuvant drugs include tricyclics, antidepressants, anticonvulsants, cannabinoids, antispasmodics, biphosphonates, α-adrenergics, steroids, and calcitonin [8,9].

Chronic pain management in head and neck pathology yields variable results. Many of the neurolytic and neuroablative procedures damage pain signals, but can result in motor loss. It should be noted that chronic pain and accompanying changes may manifest as reflex sympathetic dystrophy. Repeated stellate ganglion blocks supplemented by trigeminal nerve blocks have shown some efficacy in chronic pain relief. Rhizotomy of cranial nerves V, IX, X and gamma knife treatment also yield variable results. Favorable results have been reported for spinal cord stimulators in head and face procedures [10,11].

Complications

Maxillectomy procedures have the following associated complications:

1. Hemorrhage – significant blood loss can occur in maxillectomy. The blood loss increases as the dissection goes in an anteroposterior direction. The pterygoid plexus is usually the cause of significant blood loss.
2. Reconstruction may be necessary if the orbital floor is violated in maxillectomy surgery. Orbital exenteration may be needed when the intraorbital contents are violated by tumor. Other ocular complications include enophthalmos, diplopia, ectropion, blepharitis, conjunctivitis, exposure keratopathy, epiphora, and optic atrophy.
3. Swallowing may be compromised, though it is acceptable in most patients.
4. Speech changes are common in maxillectomy as a result of loss of palatal competence and increased speech resonance.
5. Infection and multiple cranial nerve palsies are possible. The optic nerve, maxillary branch of the trigeminal nerve and the sphenopalatine nerve are at risk during maxillectomy resection.
6. Radiation-induced cataracts, blindness, hearing loss, pituitary insufficiency, brain necrosis, nasal crusting, and frontal sinus mucocele formation are also seen following maxillectomy.

211

7. Airway management post maxillectomy is usually not a challenge and cerebrospinal fluid leaks are not common. It has been reported that only 7.7% of patients required a tracheostomy after free flap reconstruction [12].

8. Chronic facial pain syndromes as discussed above.

Conclusion

Maxillectomy procedures provide challenges for anesthesiologists. Among these challenges are blood loss management, cranial nerve monitoring, and at times airway management. Successful surgery involves open dialog between the anesthesiologist, ENT surgeon, and at times the plastic surgeon. The principles set forth above for the perioperative management of the maxillectomy patient aid in a collaborative and successful treatment plan for these patients.

Salivary glands

Introduction

Salivary glands consist of two parotid glands, two submandibular glands, two principal sublingual glands and a large amount of minor salivary glands. The function of the salivary glands is to produce serous secretions, mucous secretions, digestive enzymes, lubrication, and hygienic and bacteriostatic functions [13]. Approximately 80% of salivary gland tumors are found in the parotid gland and are usually benign. Fifty to sixty percent of submandibular tumors are benign [14].

Pleomorphic adenomas constitute about two-thirds of all salivary gland tumors. Malignant tumors include mucoepidermoid carcinomas and adenocystic carcinoma. These tumors cause ulceration and nerve invasion resulting in numbness and facial paralysis [15].

The reader is directed to Chapter 21 on anesthesia for parotid surgery; scant information regarding parotid glands will be included in this chapter. The following sections will deal with submandibular glands.

Surgical procedures

Surgical procedures of the salivary glands are technically challenging procedures. Close proximity to vascular vessels and nerves, anatomic variability, previous surgeries, infection and radiation all contribute to the challenge. Indications for submandibular gland surgery include neoplasm, chronic sialadenitis refractory to medical management, and impacted stones in the hilum of the gland. Benign tumors are usually embedded in the gland and require gland excision, while malignant tumors extend into surrounding tissues. Gland excision and the resection of the contents of the submandibular triangle are usually the appropriate treatment for malignant tumors [16].

Anesthetic management
Preoperative assessment

A thorough assessment of the physical examination and corresponding laboratory values should be done. All comorbidities should be elicited from the patient and optimization established. Discussion between the anesthesiologist and surgeon should include the plans for using neuromuscular blockade and the possibility of hemorrhage. The operating room table is sometimes turned away from the anesthesiologists, and appropriate circuit connections and intravenous extensions should be considered. Submandibular gland surgery is usually a "clean" procedure. In the case of an infection, the need for antibiotics should be discussed.

Intraoperative management

The neoplasm is usually well localized and lateralized from the midline. Impingement on airway structures is usually not a factor. Antibiotics, if needed, should be given 30 minutes to 1 hour prior to incision. Muscle relaxant is usually withheld to facilitate intraoperative monitoring of nerves. There is a possibility of hemorrhage from the facial artery and the anterior fascial vein. While an arterial line is usually not needed for this surgery, a large-bore intravenous line should be considered. Emergence from anesthesia should be planned to be smooth and free from "bucking" to prevent potential neck hematoma.

Postoperative care

Appropriate pain management medication should be ordered. Unless there is an intraoperative complication, disposition to a regular floor bed after the post-anesthesia care unit is appropriate.

Complications

Submandibular gland resection has the following associated complications:

1. Hemorrhage from the facial artery and the anterior facial vein may occur.
2. Infection can occur postoperatively in 2–9% of the patient population.
3. Nerve injury – injury to the marginal mandibular branch of the facial nerve. Injury to this nerve results in lower lip depression. Injury to the lingual nerve results in sensory loss of the anterior two-thirds of the ipsilateral tongue. This injury occurs in 3–6% of cases. Hypoglossal nerve injury causes ipsilateral tongue paralysis.
4. Other complications are xerostomia, gustatory sweating, toxic shock syndrome, and mylohyoid nerve injury [16].

Conclusions

Salivary gland resection poses technical challenges to both the surgeon and the anesthesiologist. The anesthetic management of these procedures mainly involves preservation of motor function of the face. This will allow the surgeon to continuously test and monitor neural integrity. Knowledge of the needs of the surgeon and the safety of the patient chart the clinical pathway of the anesthesiologist. Salivary gland resection is an example of the integrated efforts of both surgeon and anesthesiologist.

Mandible

Introduction

Surgery of the mandible and temporomandibular joint (TMJ) may involve the expertise of several surgical specialties – otorhinolaryngologists and oromaxillaryfacial and plastic surgeons depending on the extent of surgery. This section of the chapter involves surgery of the mandible and temporomandibular joint.

The mandible is composed of the body and two rami that form the lower jaw. The lower teeth are located in the alveolar ridge in the upper part of the body. The quadrangular-shaped ramus continues laterally and upward from the body. The superior aspect of the ramus has two protuberances: anteriorly known as the coronoid process, and posteriorly known as the condylar process.

Table 22.1. Indications for various kinds of mandibular surgery

Mandibular surgery	Indication
Bilateral sagittal split osteotomy (BSSO)	Mandibular deficiency Malocclusion of teeth
BSSO and lower border osteotomy	Facial asymmetry
Mandibular set back with bimaxillary surgery	Mandibular prognathism Mandibular excess Mandibular asymmetry
Maxillo-mandibular advancement	Obstructive sleep apnea
Radical mandibulectomy with reconstruction	Advanced tumor (squamous cell carcinoma with boney invasion), odontogenic tumors, osteosarcoma, chondrosarcoma

The temporomandibular joint is a synovial joint divided into two compartments by a disc that articulates with the temporal bone superiorly and inferiorly with the condylar process of the mandible [1].

Surgical procedure

Surgery for the mandible can range from biopsy to radical mandibular resection (Table 22.1). Often, reconstruction of a major mandibular defect is performed during the initial removal of the lesion. The options for repair of mandibular defects may include screw and plating, pedicled flaps with the osseous component originating from ribs, scapulae, clavicles, or calvarium or free osteocutaneous flaps from the fibula, iliac crest, scapula, radial forearm or clavicle [17]. The associated soft tissue defect requires soft tissue replacement for the resultant defect with a myocutaneous flap (pectoralis major or trapezius flap) or free microvascular composite tissue transfer. Stabilization for the resection defects may include maxillo-mandibular fixation, bone transfer, or external fixator applied to the facial bones [18].

Anesthetic management
Preoperative evaluation

For the preoperative assessment, routine history and physical examination are sufficient in patients without comorbidities. Detailed questioning of patients with head and neck cancer or prior exposure to radiation therapy may aid in choices of airway management. On the other hand, existing comorbidities and decreased exercise tolerance may aid in deciding on the need for invasive monitoring. It is critical to review anesthesiology records from prior surgeries, laboratory values, and imaging studies to delineate the extent of the lesion. Discussion with the surgeon, patient and family regarding airway management, complications and disposition post procedure is essential. Many practitioners utilize an antisialogogue to be administered 30 minutes prior to the procedure, particularly if a difficult airway is anticipated. Usually, nasal intubation is a part of the airway management. A vasoconstrictor is used to prepare the nares by shrinking the nasal mucosa to minimize bleeding with nasal intubation. Midazolam sedation may be provided to achieve a much-needed anxiolysis in these commonly very anxious patients.

Intraoperative management

The introduction of "time out" finalizes the communication regarding surgical requirements during different phases of the procedures (patient position, use of muscle relaxants, order of surgical procedures, antibiotic redosing, temperature of the room and potential requirement for red cell, and blood components transfusion). The nasal intubation may be performed under general anesthesia by direct laryngoscopy or videolaryngoscopy with Magill forceps when an adequate mouth opening is apparent. Nasal fiberoptic intubation with an assistant providing jaw thrust and tongue pull is an alternative airway management technique. If a difficult airway is anticipated, then it is prudent to perform an awake intubation.

When a mature tracheostomy exists, the tracheotomy tube is removed and an armoured (anode) tube is inserted into the tracheostoma. The tube is secured by being sutured in place to provide an uninterrupted access to the operative field and minimized contamination with the use of adhesive tape. A minimum of two large-bore intravenous lines with extensions are used. An arterial line is indicated when rapid response to hemodynamic changes is essential, for close monitoring of patients with multiple comorbidities.

Anesthetic management usually incorporates inhaled agents. Deliberate hypotensive anesthesia is used to maintain the mean blood pressure around 60 mmHg for orthognathic procedures to minimize blood in the operative field. For cases longer than 3 hours, Foley catheters, fluid warmers and warming devices are used. Antiemetics are administered to minimize postoperative nausea and vomiting.

Extubation may occur in the operating room if the patient meets extubation criteria and bleeding and airway swelling are not concerns [5]. Extubation may be delayed due to patient comorbidities. If extubation fails and reintubation is required, then tracheostomy may be warranted for failure to extubate and prolonged intubation greater than 7 days.

Postoperative care

Postoperative management of major reconstruction surgeries may involve care in a monitored setting for postoperative ventilation and monitoring of flap viability. In the postoperative period, humidified oxygen is provided. The patient's head is elevated and ice packs are placed at the surgical area to decrease swelling for orthognathic procedures. Analgesia is provided for pain relief.

Complications

BSSO has the following associated complications:

1. Hemorrhage from the retromandibular vein, inferior alveolar vessels and rarely facial vessels can be managed intraoperatively. If blood enters the stomach, it may cause postoperative nausea and vomiting. A nasogastric tube is placed at induction to facilitate removal of blood prior to extubation and may remain in place in the postoperative phase.
2. Facial edema may occur and can be managed with ice packs, corticosteroids and head elevation.
3. Neurosensory deficits may be associated with the inferior alveolar nerve, lingual nerve and rarely the facial nerves from direct trauma or indirect compression during surgery. Patients temporarily present with numbness of the lower lip and chin.
4. TMJ dysfunction may cause limited mouth opening lasting up to 6 months post-surgery.
5. Difficult reintubation may be caused by bleeding, TMJ dysfunction and facial edema. This can be minimized by preparing for extubation using extubation catheters [5].

Conclusions

Orthognathic procedures pose several potential challenges, tight management of blood pressure to facilitate a bloodless surgical field, extubation in the face of edema and hematoma formation, and preemptive management of nausea and vomiting. An example of an anesthetic management for reconstructive mandibular cancer surgery is discussed in the case presentation at the end of this chapter.

Temporomandibular joint

Introduction

The prevalence of temporomandibular joint dysfunction (TMJ) ranges from 20% to 25% in the general population. Surgery is indicated for TMJ intra-articular pathology such as osteoarthritis, synovitis, fibrosis, ankylosis, recalcitrant pain and reduced interincisor distance. Temporomandibular arthroscopy is preferred over arthrotomy for its less invasive nature and quicker recovery. Significant dysfunction of the TMJ presents as pain and decreased interincisor distance. TMJ dysfunction may be recognized for the first time during laryngoscopy, when the patient's mouth cannot be opened [19,20].

Surgical procedure

Surgical intervention for the TMJ may involve arthrocentesis, arthroscopy, arthroplasty or an open joint procedure. If joint space is adequate then arthroscopy is performed, otherwise arthrotomy is reserved for presence of a tumor or lack of joint space.

Anesthetic management

TMJ surgery is often performed in patients between 20 and 40 years old as an outpatient procedure. The arthroscopy procedure can be performed with an auriculotemporal nerve block and sedation. Most procedures are performed under general anesthesia with nasal intubation to enable the surgeon to evaluate all mandibular positions without interference from the airway [21]. A single 18-gauge intravenous line is appropriate. The patient is positioned supine. The operating room table may be turned away from the anesthesiologist to allow the surgeon access to the surgical field.

Preoperative evaluation

Evaluation of the airway is essential, with additional focus on the patency of the nares. Tip: when a deviated septum is present, the nares with the smallest opening is associated with the larger opening into the nasopharynx. Ideally, one should examine the internal aspect of the nares with a nasoscope to ensure patency from nasal polyps. In a busy practice, this may not be feasible. Instead, check clinically for nasal patency by asking the patient which nostril allows easier breathing. Instruct the patient to compare and contrast patency of the nasal passageways by occluding one nostril with his/her finger pressing the nasal ala against the nasal septum. This exam is performed while exhaling and then repeated for the other nostril.

The patient's nares are further prepared with a nasal vasoconstrictor. Several options exist: 0.05% neosynephrine nasal spray, 0.05% oxymetazoline nasal spray, 4% cocaine. Oxymetazoline has the longest half-life, up to 12 hours, and aids in maintaining patient nares for extubation. If the patient requires an awake nasal intubation, then an antisialogogue (glycopyrrolate or atropine) to be administered 30 minutes prior to surgery is considered.

Intraoperative management

Nasal intubation is further prepared by local anesthetic and a vasoconstricter by cotton-tipped applicators soaked with either cocaine 4% or lidocaine 4% with neosynephrine 0.25% inserted nasally 3–5 minutes prior to intubation. Tip: when four cotton-tipped applicators fit in the nares, it indicates that a 7.5 endotracheal tube will also fit in the nares. This step can be done with the patient awake or after general anesthesia is induced. The following endotracheal tubes have been used: nasal RAE tube, standard endotracheal tube with a curved metal adaptor or reinforced armored tube with tube extension. At our institution, we ascribe to a particular way to protect the eyes and nose and secure the nasoendotracheal tube, as shown in Figure 22.1. Minimal opioids are required since the surgeon often performs auriculotemporal blocks as well as local infiltration of the surgical site. At the end of the procedure, the surgeon may elect to inject 2 mg of dexamethasone and or sodium hyaluronate into the joint space [21,22].

Postoperative care

Recovery requires continued reduction of joint overloading, inflammation, pain, and maximizing joint mobility [23]. Postoperative pain has been significantly reduced by injection of botulin A (Botox) [21].

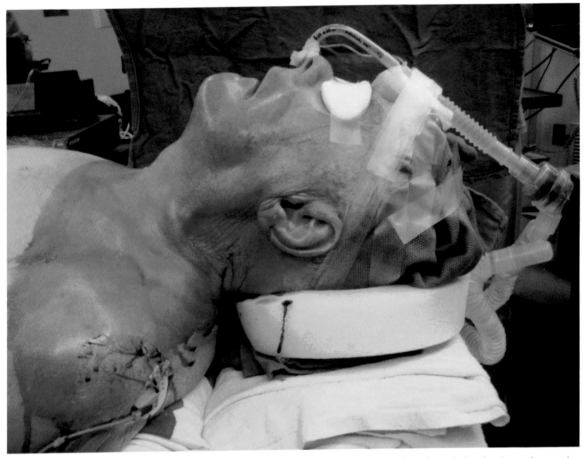

Figure 22.1. Nasal intubation. Safety concerns addressed with lubricant placed in the eyes with ocular occlusive dressing and eye pads. Nasal RAE tube softened in warm water prior to placement. Vaseline gauze is placed around endotracheal tube near the nares to minimize nasal necrosis from ETT pressure. Head wrap and surgical sponge is in place prior to securing the ETT with tape that is secured circumferentially around the head. The head is placed on a foam donut to pad the head.

Complications

TMJ surgery has the following associated complications [21,24]:

(1) otologic injuries (8.6%) involve blood clot, perforation of tympanic membrane;

(2) laceration of external auditory canal, partial hearing loss, vertigo;

(3) neurologic injury (1.7%) may involve cranial nerves V and VII;

(4) arrhythmia, reflex bradycardia;

(5) pulmonary edema.

Conclusions

TMJ arthroscopy is an effective minimally invasive technique to reduce pain and improve the mandibular

range of motion that can be done safely on an outpatient basis.

Case study: anesthesia for mandibular cancer

The patient is an 82-year-old male, 5'9" (175 cm) in height and weighing 85 kg, ASA III physical status, with a verrucous cancer of the oral cavity. He is scheduled for resection of a left mandibular cancer with free flap reconstruction and plating.

Preoperative evaluation

- Comorbidities: oral cancer, obesity, hypertension, paroxysmal supraventricular tachycardia, a few years previously (chemically converted and resolved with toprol and verapamil), hyperlipidemia, gastroesophageal reflux (asymptomatic with medication), anemia, arthritis, cervical spine disease, restless leg syndrome and benign prostatic hypertrophy.

- Past surgical history included wide local excision of an oral soft tissue lesion, debridement of left mandible, radical alveolarectomy, hernia with mesh repair, and TURP.
- Past intubation history: general anesthesia, oral intubation with 7.5 oral RAE ETT with MacIntosh #4 blade, one attempt with Cormach–Lehane view 2, Glidescope large blade 7.5 oral ETT with good view. Mask ventilation not attempted.
- Airway examination: MP III airway, intercisor distance 5 cm, thyromental distance 5 cm, six teeth remaining on left lower mandible, neck extension greatly limited.

Induction of anesthesia

On the day of the procedure, the NPO status was verified. In the preoperative area, the patient was premedicated with intravenous (IV) glycopyrrolate 0.2 mg, 30 minutes prior to induction, and received midazolam 2 mg IV en route to the operating room suite. The anesthesiologist and the surgeons discussed the airway management plan, procedure order and post-surgical recovery location.

After applying standard monitors, the patient was pre-oxygenated with 100% oxygen by face mask. General anesthesia was then induced with 150 µg of fentanyl, 150 mg of propofol followed by rocuronium 10 mg IV for a defasiculating dose prior to 120 mg of succhinylcholine. Easy face-mask ventilation was verified by chest rise and capnography. The patient was intubated using a Glidescope™ (Verathon, Canada) with a 7.5 mm ID nasal RAE endotracheal tube (ETT) through the right nares. The intubation was confirmed by observing the tube passing through the vocal cords, chest rise, the presence of bilateral breath sounds, and capnography. Special notes: the nares were topicalized with cotton tip application of neosynephrine 0.25% and lidocaine 4% mixtures for several minutes after induction was initiated. Using the Glidescope stylet was not an option for nasal intubation. The following steps were taken for preparing for the intubation:

(1) the ETT was prewarmed in warm water and lubricated with jelly;
(2) the cuff was flattened by inflating once to test cuff integrity and deflating the cuff completely.

During intubation and while the Glidescope and ETT were in the oropharynx, the pilot balloon was inflated to raise the bevel of the ETT to the glottic opening. The cuff was deflated as the tube passed through the vocal cords. As an alternative Magill forceps could have been used to assist with directing the tube into the glottis. A 20-gauge right radial arterial line, a second large-bore intravenous line with additonal extensions, was placed while the surgeons placed a Foley catheter. During the time the patient was prepped, the room was warmed, and the patient was padded meticulously. In particular, the surgeon packed a petrolatum gauze around the endotracheal tube at the nares to avoid potential nasal pressure-induced ischemic necrosis (Figure 22.1). The head was wrapped with a blue towel like a turban and a surgical scrub sponge was placed in the center with the ETT resting on the sponge. The ETT is secured by placing tape circumferentially around the head. This step avoids tension of the ETT on the nares during the case.

Maintenance of anesthesia

General anesthesia was maintained with sevoflurane approximately 1.7–2.2%, continued muscle relaxation and opioid analgesia. The case proceeded uneventfully for 12 hours with a total blood loss of 600 ml. Dexamethasone 10 mg IV was given for postoperative nausea and vomiting prophylaxis and to decrease postoperative airway edema.

Emergence and recovery from anesthesia

By the end of the case, the patient was given a total of 700 µg of fentanyl and 4 mg of dilaudid, and a propofol infusion was started at 50 µg/kg/min for planned postoperative continued intubation and mechanical ventilation in the intensive care unit. Postoperative intubation and sedation were maintained in order to support the airway until edema subsided and the flap viability was ensured.

On postoperative day 7, the patient received a tracheostomy since he failed extubation twice due to upper airway obstruction.

Potential complications

- Shared airway surgeries require meticulous attention to securing the airway and using long extensions to allow surgeons room to work and allow the anesthesiologist access to the patient for administration of medications. In addition, the eyes were lubricated with ointment, and taped with ocular adhesive and padded eye pads. This was precautionary since surgical instruments were near the face area.

Other complications

- Bleeding is a potential challenge. Reassessing intravenous access during the case is essential. An arterial line should be used for timely detection of cardiovascular changes and to access metabolic status.
- Nasal necrosis from prolonged nasal intubation. Care was taken to prevent pressure on the nares by placement of the vaseline gauze and taping the tube without tension.
- Nasal epistaxis with the nasal intubation is minimized with a softened, warmed ETT and application of vasoconstrictor to the nares.
- Skin breakdown: padding was placed on all prominent boney parts since this was anticipated to be a long procedure in an elderly patient. In this case, the adhesive pulse oximeter probe was used instead of the clip-on since both of the patient's arms were not available. Since the patient's arms were not readily available during the procedure, the intravenous line was draped over his arm and easy access to the line was maintained when tucking the arm.

Clinical pearls

- Occasionally, depending on the extent of the tumor, oral intubation may not be possible; securing the airway nasally or by tracheostomy may be needed.

- Minimizing epistaxis with nasal intubation can be achieved with a softened, warmed ETT and application of vasoconstrictor to the nares.
- For nasal intubation, choices of endotracheal tubes include standard endotracheal tubes with a curved metal adaptor, nasal RAE tubes, or a reinforced armored tube.
- Blood entering the stomach may cause postoperative nausea and vomiting. A nasogastric tube will facilitate removal of blood prior to extubation and may remain in place in the postoperative phase.
- In some cases postoperative spontaneous/controlled ventilation through the ETT may be safer than immediate extubation, particularly with surgical flaps or where edema is a concern.
- The operating room table is sometimes turned away from the anesthesiologists, and appropriate circuit connections and intravenous extensions should be considered.
- Submandibular gland resection has the following associated complications: hemorrhage from the facial artery or the anterior facial vein, injury to the marginal mandibular branch of the facial nerve (resulting in lower lip depression), injury to the lingual nerve (resulting in sensory loss of the anterior two-thirds of the ipsilateral tongue) and hypoglossal nerve injury (causing ipsilateral tongue paralysis).
- Deliberate hypotensive anesthesia for orthognathic procedures is sometimes used to minimize blood in the operative field; the mean blood pressure is usually kept to around 60 mmHg.
- Facial edema may occur in such cases and can be managed with ice packs, corticosteroids and head elevation.

References

1. O'Rahilly R. Head and neck. In Gardner E, Gray D, O'Rahilly R, eds. *Anatomy*. Philadelphia: W.B. Saunders; 1975. pp. 558–9, 665–7.

2. Spiro RH, Strong EW, Shah JP. Maxillectomy and its classification. *Head Neck* 1997; **19**(4):309–14.

3. Carrau R. *Maxillectomy*. 2011; available from: http://emedicine.

medscape.com/article/1890955-overview. Accessed June 1, 2011.

4. Bhatki A, Goldberg A. Complications of surgery of the paranasal sinuses. In Eisele D, Smith R, eds. *Complications in Head and Neck Surgery*, 2nd edn. Philadelphia: Mosby/Elsevier; 2009. pp. 543–58.

5. Cooper RM. Extubation and changing endotracheal tubes. In

Hagberg C, ed. *Benumof's Airway Management*. Philadelphia: Mosby Elesevier; 2007. pp. 1146–80.

6. Lin HS, Wang D, Fee WE, Goode RL, Terris DJ. Airway management after maxillectomy: routine tracheostomy is unnecessary. *Laryngoscope* 2003;**113**(6):929–32.

7. Practice guidelines for cancer pain management. A report by the

American Society of Anesthesiologists Task Force on Pain Management, Cancer Pain Section. *Anesthesiology* 1996; **84**(5):1243–57.

8. Straker T. Pain Management for head and neck surgery. In Eisele D, Smith R, eds. *Complications in Head and Neck Surgery*, 2nd edn. Philadelphia: Mosby/Elsevier; 2009. pp. 189–94.

9. Martins TL, Kahvegian MA, Noel-Morgan J, *et al*. Comparison of the effects of tramadol, codeine, and ketoprofen alone or in combination on postoperative pain and on concentrations of blood glucose, serum cortisol, and serum interleukin-6 in dogs undergoing maxillectomy or mandibulectomy. *Am J Vet Res* 2010;**71**(9):1019–26.

10. Carpenter RL, Rauck RL. Refractory head and neck pain. A difficult problem and a new alternative therapy. *Anesthesiology* 1996;**84**(2):249–52.

11. Iwade M, Fukuuchi A, Kawamata M, *et al*. [Management of severe pain after extended maxillectomy in a patient with carcinoma of the maxillary sinus]. *Masui* 1996;**45**(1):82–5.

12. Little J, Bumpous J. Complications of maxillectomy. In Eisele D, Smith R, eds. *Complications in Head and Neck Surgery*, 2nd edn. Philadelphia: Mosby/Elsevier; 2009. pp. 577–80

13. Butt FY. Benign diseases of the salivary glands. In Lalwani AK, ed. *Current Diagnosis & Treatment in Otolaryngology – Head & Neck Surgery*, 3rd edn. McGraw-Hill; available from: http://accessmedicine.com/content.aspx?aid=55766963.

14. Lustig L, Schindler R. Ear, nose and throat disorders. In McPhee SJ, Papadakis MA, eds. *Current Medical Diagnosis and Treatment 2012*. McGraw-Hill; available from: http://accessmedicine.com/content.aspx?aid=2356.

15. Durso S. Oral manifestations of disease. In Fauci AS, Braunwald E, Kasper DL, eds. *Harrison's Principles of Internal Medicine*, 18th edn. 2011; available from: www.accessmedicine.com/content.aspx?aID=9097184.

16. Gillespie M, Easel D. Complications of surgery of the salivary glands. In Eisele D, Smith R, eds. *Complications in Head and Neck Surgery*. Philadelphia: Mosby/Elsevier; 2009. pp. 221–50.

17. Rassekh CH, Seikaly H. Oropharyngeal cancer. In Bailey BJ, Johnson JT, eds. *Head & Neck Surgery - Otolaryngology*, 4th edn. Philadelphia: Lippincott Williams & Wilkins; 2006. pp. 1686–7.

18. Lutcavage GJ, Finkelstein MW. Sarcomas of the jaw in oral and maxillofacial surgery. In Robert M, edr. *Oral and Maxillofacial Surgery*, 2nd edn. St. Louis: Saunders Elsevier; 2009. pp. 680–706.

19. Small RH, Ganzberg SI, Schuster AW. Unsuspected temporomandibular joint pathology leading to a difficult endotracheal intubation. *Anesth Analg* 2004;**99**(2):383–5.

20. Patane PS, Ragno JR Jr, Mahla ME. Temporomandibular joint disease and difficult tracheal intubation. *Anesth Analg* 1988; **67**(5):482–3.

21. Donlon W. Temporomandibular disorders and surgery. In Bailey BJ, Johnson JT, eds. *Head & Neck Surgery - Otolaryngology*, 4th edn. Philadelphia: Lippincott Williams & Wilkins; 2006. pp. 631–43.

22. Furst IM, Kryshtalskyj B, Weinberg S. The use of intra-articular opioids and bupivacaine for analgesia following temporomandibular joint arthroscopy: a prospective, randomized trial. *J Oral Maxillofac Surg* 2001;**59**(9): 979–83

23. Israel HA. Part I: The use of arthroscopic surgery for treatment of temporomandibular joint disorders. *J Oral Maxillofac Surg* 1999;**57**(5):579–82.

24. Tsuyama M, Kondoh T, Seto K, Fukuda J. Complications of temporomandibular joint arthroscopy: a retrospective analysis of 301 lysis and lavage procedures performed using the triangulation technique. *J Oral Maxillofac Surg* 2000;**58**(5): 500–5.

Anesthesia for face transplantation

Jacek B. Cywinski, Thomas Edrich and D. John Doyle

Introduction

Face transplantation (Figure 23.1) remains a very rare procedure. Only about 15 cases, including total and partial face transplantation, have been done worldwide at the time of writing this chapter. Each procedure has been unique with respect to indications and the nature and extent of the transplanted tissue. There has been one case report detailing the anesthesia management during face transplantation in the setting of coagulopathy [1]. However, there has been no systematic description of the anesthesia management for face transplantation. This chapter will outline anesthetic considerations for this unique and complex procedure based on the experience of two hospitals where the first face transplants in the United States took place as well as preliminary data from three international centers (personal communication).

Management of the donor during face tissue and multiorgan harvest

The details of anesthetic care for the multiorgan donor has been outlined in the literature [2–5]. Similar principles to conventional organ procurement apply, however, when consideration is given to the harvest of a composite facial graft, one has to keep in mind that due to the surgical complexity and long duration of procurement, harvesting of the facial graft should ordinarily be performed before other organs are retrieved. Maintenance of adequate tissue perfusion and donor hemodynamic stability during this long procurement period can have a significant impact on the quality of the graft and organs to be procured later [6].

Since each case of face transplantation is different, detailed planning of the harvesting strategy is extremely important: in many instances a practice "mock harvest" is performed in a cadaver lab to solidify the surgical approach. In order to avoid interference with the surgical field, a donor tracheostomy can be performed first [6]. Communication with the procurement team is very important during dissection of the graft: frequently a nerve stimulator is used to identify motor branches of the facial nerve. For this reason muscle relaxants need to be avoided until dissection and isolation of the nerves is completed. To achieve a motionless surgical field a combination of a volatile anesthetic and intravenous infusion of an opioid (for example, fentanyl, remifentanil or sufentanil) or total intravenous anesthesia (TIVA) can be used. Because of frequent hypotension in such a setting, circulatory function must often be supported with intravascular volume expansion and/or vasoactive drugs. However, it is important to realize that high doses of vasoconstrictors can make it difficult for the surgeon to identify small facial blood vessels during the tissue dissection and may also compromise tissue perfusion through vasoconstriction. Consequently, intravascular fluids infusion may be a better choice as a first-line approach to restore blood pressure. Not uncommonly brain-dead donors arrive in the operating room already on significant pharmacological circulatory support, which makes it even more challenging to maintain adequate perfusion pressure to avoid compromise to any other organs that are to be eventually procured during long dissection of the facial graft [6].

Preoperative assessment of the recipient

The anesthetic assessment of candidates for face transplantation is an important part of the pre-transplant

Anesthesia for Otolaryngologic Surgery, ed. Basem Abdelmalak and D. John Doyle. Published by Cambridge University Press.
© Cambridge University Press 2013.

(A)

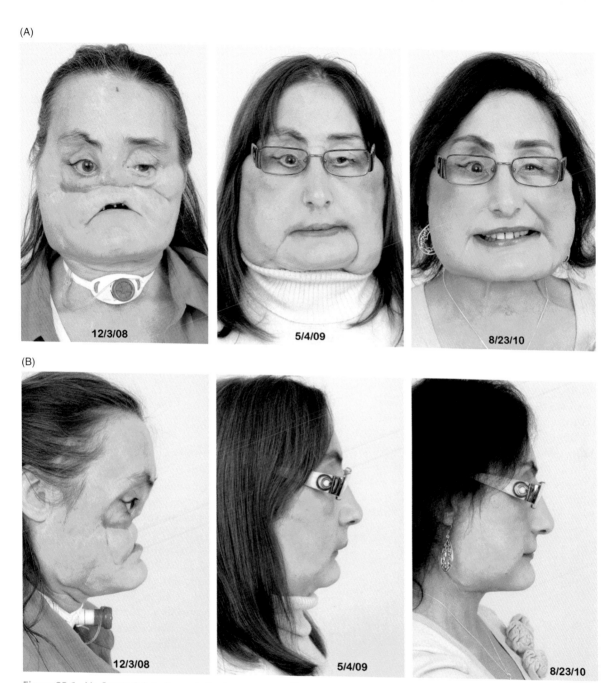

(B)

Figure 23.1. Ms. Connie Culp before and after the two stages of her face transplant at Cleveland Clinic. Stage 1 was carried out in December 2008 (lead surgeon: Dr. Maria Siemionow). Images courtesy of Cleveland Clinic. Reprinted with permission, Cleveland Clinic Center for Medical Art & Photography © 2012. All rights reserved.

process; similar to the evaluation of any other surgical patient, the major goal is to identify and optimize clinical conditions which might adversely impact postoperative outcomes [6]. Based on experience from different centers where face transplants have been performed, there is no uniform set of preoperative tests; each program tailors evaluation to each individual patient and his or her comorbid conditions. Universal criteria for approval or disqualification of the face transplant candidate do not yet exist;

221

however, there is a general consensus that the patient needs to be sufficiently fit to undergo a very prolonged anesthetic and surgery. Such a candidate should be free from any significant comorbidity, which could impact the perioperative course in a negative way.

Anesthetic evaluation begins with a comprehensive review of the medical history and physical examination: an identification of comorbid conditions helps to determine the patient's surgical risk as well as help tailor pre-transplant testing. Detailed evaluation of face injury and past reconstructive efforts is of utmost importance, because they may greatly influence airway management plans [6]. As most face recipients have undergone several general anesthetics during past reconstructions, close attention should be paid to the previous anesthesia records; in particular, details of the airway management during the past surgeries can be very helpful in developing a future anesthetic plan. Any past hemodynamic instability or cardiac complication should be clarified and investigated. Cardiac testing including echocardiography and stress testing may be necessary to exclude significant coronary or valvular disease. Some centers perform the same cardiac testing as for liver transplantation candidates [6]. Keeping in mind that facial transplantation must be considered an elective procedure, that is, not life-saving, the risk of proceeding in the presence of significant undetected cardiac comorbidity should be weighed carefully. Evaluation of respiratory function focuses on assessment of pulmonary reserve and may include chest radiographs and lung function testing.

Careful examination of a patient's airway is critical since it dictates intraoperative airway management plan. All candidates for face transplantation have significant facial disfigurement; this compromises the upper airway, making mask fit and positive-pressure ventilation through it after the induction of general anesthesia difficult or impossible. Oral awake fiberoptic intubation the best choice to secure the airway although one must keep in mind that the ability to topicalize oropharyngeal mucosa may be limited due to distorted anatomy. After oral intubation, the surgical team will proceed with tracheostomy, so that the endotracheal tube is out of the surgical field [6]. Some patients may present with a tracheostomy (with or without tracheostomy tube), which can be cannulated with a reinforced endotracheal tube sutured to the chest wall. A detailed review of head and neck imaging studies (computed tomography, magnetic resonance) may be helpful in defining airways anatomy and developing a plan for airway management. In selected patients flexible fiberoptic evaluation of the airway may be useful in revealing further pertinent anatomic details and plan the strategy of securing the airway during transplantation [6].

Intraoperative management

Monitoring

Since the majority of the face transplant candidates are free of significant comorbidities, in most cases standard ASA monitors [7] along with an arterial line and central venous access will be sufficient. Because maintenance of adequate intravascular volume is important in both the recipient and the donor in order to assure adequate graft perfusion central venous pressure trends and the response to fluid challenges can be very helpful in assessing fluid status. Although not yet reported in cases of face transplantation, monitoring of systolic pressure variation during the respiratory cycle of a mechanically ventilated patient to guide "goal-directed" therapy may be helpful as well [8].

Airway management

The donor will have an endotracheal tube in place (oral or nasal) at the time of tissue procurement [6]. However, a tracheostomy may be performed first to avoid interference with the surgical field. To prevent accidental kinking, a wire-reinforced endotracheal tube is often used in this setting. Airway management in the recipient is dictated by the extent and nature of the facial injuries; in many cases the patient presents with a tracheostomy and airway management is limited to the insertion of an appropriate reinforced endotracheal tube into the tracheal stoma [6]. If the tracheostomy has been decannulated and has started to close, extension under local anesthesia may be performed by the surgeon to fit the endotracheal tube. Recipient patients who do not have a tracheostomy may first require awake fiberoptic oral intubation, followed by a tracheostomy subsequently cannulated with a wire-reinforced endotracheal tube.

Vascular access

Face transplant procedures can be very lengthy in duration and entail significant blood loss necessitating transfusion of multiple blood products in a relatively short period of time. In a preliminary survey of five medical centers that have performed 13 face tranplants, the duration of surgery has ranged from 14 to 24 hours (average 19 hours). The blood loss has varied greatly depending on the underlying pathology of the recipient. Resuscitation has required between 2 and 60 packed red blood cell units (average 20.5 units) and zero to 60 fresh-frozen plasma units (average 14.5 units). Two centers placed large-bore central venous catheters to facilitate reliable high-volume resuscitation (personal communication with A. Gilton, M. Colomina, I. Lopez, J. Cywinski and T. Edrich). Alternatively, several large-bore peripheral intravenous catheters may serve as venous access for rapid resuscitation. A central line may be useful to monitor and trend central venous pressures and it may become necessary in the ICU if venous access is limited. The nature and extent of the facial injury, previous reconstructive procedures as well as planned planes of surgical dissection may help to predict the risk of intraoperative bleeding and the need for special vascular access. The location choice of the central line placement has to be discussed with the surgical team: a subclavian vein may be preferable to the internal jugular vein in order to avoid the surgical field. However, there is a valid concern that placement of a central venous catheter in the internal jugular vein or in the subclavian vein will compromise adequate venous outflow from the graft in case of venous thrombosis. The femoral vein in some cases may be the only central access site if conventional central venous access location is deemed to be inappropriate [6]. The strict sterile technique with central line insertion is extremely important, since after face transplantation immunosuppression is started immediately, so the risk of infection is increased [6,9]. Real-time ultrasound guidance should be used during central line insertion in order to limit unnecessary needle passes and diminish risk of complications (arterial puncture, pneumothorax) [6,10].

Choice of the anesthetic (volatile agent vs. TIVA)

Limited data is available in the literature regarding the best choice of anesthetic technique for long and extensive surgical procedures. Both volatile agents as well as total intravenous anesthesia (TIVA) have been successfully used; however, avoidance of nitrous oxide

with its adverse effects following prolonged administration [11] would seem to be justified, although there is no definitive evidence to quantify its risk. Muscle relaxants are part of the balanced anesthesia technique; however, during certain portions of the procedure, where nerve monitoring is required, they must be avoided [6]. The use of a remifentanil infusion can be helpful in reducing movement in these instances but, unfortunately, its use is often complicated by hypotension and bradycardia (at high infusion rates). Volatile anesthetic agents are believed to protect against intraoperative awareness more reliably than intravenous anesthetics used during TIVA. Since the electroencephalographic monitoring of depth of anesthesia may be impossible in patients undergoing face transplantation, the use of a volatile anesthetic agent may be advantageous. Finally, as noted below, anesthesia achieved with volatile anesthetics appears to improve peripheral tissue perfusion [6].

The choice of anesthetic agent for the transplant of composite tissue grafts may be quite important and affect the outcome of the graft. Experimental models demonstrated that some anesthetic agents improved blood flow in the microcirculation of free flaps and the flow through micro- and macrovascular anastomoses [12]. The effect of halothane on free flap microcirculation has been studied extensively in animal models, in particular its effect on postcapillary venules [13]. Since other halogenated volatile anesthetics have similar effects on microcirculation to halothane these laboratory findings can be extrapolated [14]. Based on experimental data, exposure to a halogenated volatile anesthetic may improve free flap survival by reducing the number of leukocytes flowing through microcirculation, as well as by decreasing the number of leukocytes adhering to the endothelium of vessel wall, and migrating outside the vessel. During reperfusion, these leukocytes can potentially cause tissue injury related to the release of proinflammatory mediators (via degranulation). The edema of endothelium related to the leucocyte degranulation process and the presence of leukocytes adhering to the endothelial wall of venules can cause decreased capillary blood flow due to impaired blood drainage. Other halogenated volatile anesthetics may offer a similar protective effect on microcirculation, although the effect may be smaller [6,13,15,16].

Propofol infusion in experimental models of free musculo-cutaneous flaps has been shown to cause significant endothelial edema, with a decrease in the

223

number of rolling leukocytes and lymphocytes passing through postcapillary venules [17]. Also, the numbers of leukocytes and lymphocytes adhering to the endothelial wall and migrating outside the postcapillary venule were significantly increased. Release of proinflammatory mediators from the leukocytes upon graft reperfusion potentiate the activity of free oxygen radicals and, for these reasons, prolonged propofol infusions may be less than ideal in patients undergoing composite tissue grafts. It is worth mentioning that experimental models propofol demonstrated immunomodulatory properties resulting in inhibition of lymphocyte activity [6,17,18].

Limited data from animal model experiments demonstrated that opioids decrease the diameter of the arterioles in skeletal muscle, which decreases blood flow in the free flap, which can be detected by increased velocities of the blood flow measured with Doppler flow meter [13,19].

Fluid management

The goals and principles of intraoperative fluid management in face transplantation are similar to any other long surgical procedure involving microvascular free flaps. Adequate graft perfusion is difficult to assess directly; however, careful monitoring of the patient's urine output, changes in central venous pressure, as well as changes in systolic pressure as a consequence of positive-pressure ventilation (pulse pressure variations) can guide intraoperative fluid management. The risk of impaired coagulation must be considered when using hetastarch formulations; however, other colloids (albumin) may be helpful to maintain adequate intravascular volume [20].

Transfusion of blood products

Although the general guidelines for the transfusion of blood components are well defined in the published literature; in the face transplant recipient, transfusion practice needs to be highly individualized and guided by the clinical situation [21–23]. In the general population, transfusion of red blood cells is not indicated in relatively healthy, asymptomatic individuals until the hemoglobin level drops below approximately 7 gm/dl. However, in the case of acute intraoperative blood loss (as has been reported in some of the face transplants – personal communication), appropiate blood products would be transfused before reaching this threshold to avoid excessive anemia and coagulopathy. In addition, in face transplant recipients the threshold for transfusion of red cells may be slightly higher to provide adequate oxygen-carrying capacity to the graft [6]. Excessive increases in hematocrit should be avoided because high hematocrit compromises the rheologic properties of blood and microcirculation as well. Coagulopathy can cause microvascular bleeding and hematoma formation, which are potentially devastating postoperative complications; therefore, coagulation status of the recipient must be closely monitored, especially in cases complicated by large blood loss (> one blood volume). Tests which provide whole blood clotting assessment, such as Thromboelastograph® (TEG) and Sonoclot®, can facilitate the decision on which blood clotting components need to be transfused in order to correct ongoing coagulopathy. In a general population, evidence-based data supporting administration of fresh frozen plasma in patients with INR values < 2.0 is lacking [22]; however, lower thresholds may be appropriate during the face transplantation, where the consequences of surgical bleeding from impaired coagulation could be disastrous. The need for administration of platelets should be driven by the assessment of the clinical situation rather then specific platelet count threshold; however, platelet transfusion is rarely indicated if the platelet count is greater than 100×10^9/liter [21]. Transfusion of the blood products is associated with well-defined risks and should be used judiciously: [23] transfusion-related acute lung injury (TRALI) is the most common life-threatening adverse effect, [24]; transfusion-associated graft-versus-host disease (TA-GVHD) and immunomodulation are other well-documented complications.

Pressors

Direct sympathetic α-receptor agonists (such as phenylephrine or norepinephrine) are commonly used in clinical practice to treat hypotension; however, in situations where microvascular surgery is involved (such as face transplant), they should be avoided because of the risk of vasoconstriction that can potentially compromise graft perfusion. Also, vasoconstriction can make it difficult for the surgeon to identify and handle small vascular structures in the graft-procurement phase of the operation [6].

Muscle relaxants

Muscle relaxation may be needed at various phases of both the donor and recipient operations; during construction of microanastomoses (blood vessels, nerves), a motionless surgical field is quite desirable. However, both the donor and recipient operations may at times require use of a nerve stimulator to identify various nerves and at that times conduction at the neuromuscular junction has to be restored. Shorter-acting muscle relaxants like rocuronium or atracurium are preferable to a longer-acting drug like pancuronium for this very reason. Communication with the surgical team is important to facilitate proper timing and dosing of the muscle relaxants [6].

Postoperative sedation

During the postoperative period the face transplant recipients are ventilated through a tracheostomy tube which replaces reinforced endotracheal tube at the end of the surgical procedure in the majority of cases. The need for postoperative sedation and ventilatory support is individualized: in some situations postoperative sedation is deemed necessary to avoid mechanical compromise of the graft from patient movement [6]. Adequate sedation can be achieved by a variety of means: an infusion of propofol in conjunction with an opiate such as fentanyl or an infusion of dexmethetomidine may be considered as well, depending on the anticipated duration of postoperative sedation and need for mechanical ventilation. Sedation should be gradually withdrawn to avoid agitation, coughing, and straining, all of which can potentially compromise graft tissue [6].

The anesthetic team

Anesthetic care for face transplant operations is usually provided by the anesthesia team, which consists of an attending anesthesiologist(s) in conjunction with a resident doctor(s) and/or certified registered nurse anesthetist(s) (CRNA). The long duration of the procedure and the unpredictable timing frequently require multiple teams to be involved. To ensure smooth and safe transfer of care from one team to the other, good communication and documentation are vital.

Providing anesthetic care to face transplant recipients for subsequent surgical procedures

Face transplant recipients may require subsequent surgical procedures, related or unrelated to the face transplant. Airway management in cases where the composite graft involves maxillary or mandibular structures may present a significant challange: the forces associated with direct laryngoscopy for intubation could conceivably cause damage to incompletely healed bony structures. Discussion with the surgical team which performed the face transplant can help to clarify the safest way to manage the airways. In some cases where the tracheostomy has healed over and the risk of the disruption of bony structures during direct laryngoscopy is high, reopening of the tracheostomy under local anesthesia may be considered. Alternatively, one can perform awake fiberoptic intubation [6].

Summary

Face transplantation is a quite rare procedure that is best approached by a collaborative team of anesthesiologists, surgeons and transplant coordinators. Previously performed transplants have required detailed planning that must be tailored to the specific patient. Often, airway access involves tracheostomy. The location and type of intravascular access line need to be balanced against the risk of rapid blood loss and the concern for complications such as impairment of the blood drainage from the facial graft causing venous stasis. Fluid management is especially important in ensuring good graft perfusion in both donor and recipient; avoidance of direct vasoconstrictors seems to be justified [6]. In addition, during some periods of donor and recipient operations, muscle relaxation should be avoided to facilitate nerve identification using electrical stimulation. The duration and complexity of the face transplant operation requires participation of multiple teams, including more than one anesthesia team.

Clinical pearls

- Although detailed criteria for approval do not yet exist, a general consensus exists that the patient must be sufficiently fit to undergo a very prolonged anesthetic and surgery in order to be considered for face transplantation. Additionally, facial transplantation must be considered to be an elective procedure that is not life-saving.

- Face transplant procedures can be very lengthy in duration and entail significant blood loss, necessitating transfusion of multiple blood products in a relatively short period of time.
- Oral awake fiberoptic intubation may be the best choice to secure the recipient airway in the absence of an existing tracheostomy. Following successful intubation, the surgical team will usually proceed with tracheostomy if one is not already present. In order to avoid interference with the surgical field, a donor tracheostomy can be performed first.
- Harvesting of the facial graft should be usually performed before other organs are retrieved. Maintenance of adequate tissue perfusion during the long procurement period can have a significant impact on the quality of the procured material. Intravascular volume expansion may be needed to restore blood pressure.
- Communication with the procurement team is very important during dissection of the graft: frequently a nerve stimulator is used to identify the facial nerves. For this reason muscle relaxants should be avoided until dissection of the nerves is completed.
- In most cases standard ASA monitors, an arterial line and central venous access will be sufficient.

A subclavian vein for the central venous access may be preferable over the internal jugular vein in order to avoid impinging on the surgical field. Strict sterile technique with these procedures should be applied, since after face transplantation immunosuppression is started immediately.

- While both volatile agents and TIVA are adequate as anesthetic technique, because electroencephalographic monitoring of the depth of anesthesia may not be feasible in these patients, the use of a volatile anesthetic agent may be advantageous. Given the long duration of the surgery, avoidance of nitrous oxide would seem to be justified.
- During certain portions of the procedure, where nerve monitoring is required, so muscle relaxant use must be avoided.
- Free flap perfusion-related issues, e.g., transfusion threshold, avoidance of pressors, and volume monitoring and resuscitation, apply to the face transplant recipient as well.
- Multiple anesthesia care teams may be involved; consequently good communication and documentation are vital when care is transferred from one team to another.
- Postoperatively, the majority of the face transplant recipients will be mechanically ventilated through a tracheostomy tube and may require sedation for some period of time in an intensive care setting.

References

1. Pomahac B, Pribaz J, Eriksson E, et al. Three patients with full facial transplantation. N Engl J Med 2011 Dec 28. [Epub ahead of print] PubMed PMID: 22204672.

2. Hevesi ZG, Lopukhin SY, Angelini G, et al. Supportive care after brain death for the donor candidate. Int Anesthesiol Clin 2006;44:21–34.

3. Venkateswaran RV, Patchell VB, Wilson IC, et al. Early donor management increases the retrieval rate of lungs for transplantation. Ann Thorac Surg 2008;85:278–86.

4. Shah VR. Aggressive management of multiorgan donor. Transplant Proc 2008;40:1087–90.

5. DuBose J, Salim A. Aggressive organ donor management protocol. J Intensive Care Med 2008;23:367–75.

6. Cywinski JB, Doyle DJ, Kusza K. Anesthetic care for face transplantation. In Siemionow MZ, ed. The Know How of Face Transplantation. London: Springer; 2011. pp. 95–102.

7. American Society of Anesthesiologists (2005) Standards for basic anesthetic monitoring. American Society of Anesthesiologists. http://www.asahq.org/publicationsAndServices/standards/02.pdf; available from http://www.asahq.org/publicationsAndServices/standards/02.pdf. Accessed May 14, 2010.

8. Marik PE, Cavallazzi R, Vasu T, et al. Dynamic changes in arterial waveform derived variables and fluid responsiveness in mechanically ventilated patients: a systematic review of the literature. Crit Care Med 2009;37:2642–7.

9. Maki DG, Kluger DM, Crnich CJ. The risk of bloodstream infection in adults with different intravascular devices: a systematic review of 200 published prospective studies. Mayo Clin Proc 2006;81:1159–71.

10. Gann M Jr, Sardi A. Improved results using ultrasound guidance for central venous access. Am Surg 2003;69:1104–7.

11. Renard D, Dutray A, Remy A, et al. Subacute combined degeneration of the spinal cord caused by nitrous

oxide anaesthesia. *Neurol Sci* 2009;**30**:75–6.

12. Adams J, Charlton P. Anaesthesia for microvascular free tissue transfer. *Br J Anaesth (CEPD Reviews)* 2003;**3**: 33–7.

13. Kusza K, Siemionow M, Nalbantoglu U, *et al.* Microcirculatory response to halothane and isoflurane anesthesia. *Ann Plast Surg* 1999;**43**:57–66.

14. Sigurdsson GH, Banic A, Wheatley AM, *et al.* Effects of halothane and isoflurane anaesthesia on microcirculatory blood flow in musculocutaneous flaps. *Br J Anaesth* 1994;**73**:826–32.

15. Hagau N, Longrois D. Anesthesia for free vascularized tissue transfer. *Microsurgery* 2009;**29**:161–7.

16. Liu X, Peter FW, Barker JH, *et al.* Leukocyte-endothelium interaction in arterioles after ischemia and reperfusion. *J Surg Res* 1999;**87**:77–84.

17. Kusza K, Blaszyk M, Siemionow M, *et al.* Alteration in peripheral microcirculatory haemodynamics of muscle flaps during propofol infusion anaesthesia. *Anesth Intens Care* 2002;**34**:187–93.

18. Holzmann A, Schmidt H, Gebhardt MM, *et al.* Propofol-induced alterations in the microcirculation of hamster striated muscle. *Br J Anaesth* 1995;**75**:452–6.

19. Brookes ZL, Brown NJ, Reilly CS. The dose-dependent effects of fentanyl on rat skeletal muscle microcirculation in vivo. *Anesth Analg* 2003;**96**:456–62.

20. Marx G, Schuerholz T. Fluid-induced coagulopathy: does the type of fluid make a difference? *Crit Care* 2010;**14**:118.

21. American Society of Anesthesiologists Task Force on Perioperative Blood Transfusion and Adjuvant Therapies. Practice guidelines for perioperative blood transfusion and adjuvant therapies: an updated report by the American Society of Anesthesiologists Task Force on Perioperative Blood Transfusion and Adjuvant Therapies. *Anesthesiology* 2006;**105**: 198–208.

22. Triulzi DJ. The art of plasma transfusion therapy. *Transfusion* 2006;**46**(8):1268–70.

23. American Society of Anesthesiologists Committee on Transfusion Medicine. *Questions and Answers About Blood Management*, 4th edn. American Society of Anesthesiologists; 2008; http://www.asahq.org/ publicationsAndServices/ transfusion.pdf.

24. Bux J. Transfusion-related acute lung injury (TRALI): a serious adverse event of blood transfusion. *Vox Sang* 2005; **89**(1):1–10

24

Anesthesia for airway panendoscopy

Louise Ellard and David T. Wong

Introduction

Procedure overview

Panendoscopy or "triple endoscopy" encompasses rigid laryngoscopy, bronchoscopy, and esophagoscopy. It is primarily used to evaluate the patient with head and neck cancer, in order to document the extent of a tumor, obtain a biopsy for tissue diagnosis, search for a synchronous primary tumor or to look for recurrence post treatment. Other indications include vocal cord lesions and pathology involving the pharynx, larynx or tongue.

Following induction of general anesthesia, the patient is placed in the "Jackson position" to maximize laryngeal exposure, with the neck flexed and the head extended. A shoulder roll assists with obtaining this position and a head ring stabilizes the head. If the neck cannot be extended due to arthritis or a fixed flexion deformity, or there is a contraindication to neck extension such as an unstable cervical spine or myelopathy, correct placement of the laryngoscope is hindered [1]. In these patients a flexible bronchoscope should be considered.

The eyes are covered and the upper dentition is protected with a mouth guard or folded gauze. The laryngoscope is inserted and the surgeon completes an examination of the pharynx and supraglottic larynx. The vocal cords are exposed and examined. Next, the laryngoscope is exchanged for a rigid bronchoscope, which is guided past the base of the tongue under the epiglottis and through the vocal cords into the trachea. Esophagoscopy usually proceeds next. Biopsies are deferred until after the examination as bleeding can render visualization more difficult [2]. Sometimes the laryngoscope is fixed in position by suspension so the surgeon's hands are free to operate, and the operating microscope can be brought in as necessary.

Equipment

The rigid laryngoscope consists of a metal tube, the working channel, with a light source attached to a fixed handle in an "L" or "C" shape configuration (Figure 24.1). The working channel is the access port for surgical instruments, suction and for jet ventilation. Many different laryngoscopes are available, which differ primarily in the shape, taper, and size of the working channel. The anterior commissure scope is one example.

The rigid bronchoscope is a tapered metal tube, longer (40 cm) and narrower than the rigid laryngoscope; standard adult sizes range between 7 and 9 mm in diameter. The proximal end usually has three openings – the working channel in line with the rest of the scope, a light source connection and a third port to connect the anesthetic circuit. A removable eyepiece on the working channel opens to allow passage of surgical instruments and closes to permit ventilation.

Anesthetic management

Preoperative assessment

The anesthesiologist should consider some specific questions for the patient presenting for panendoscopy:

1. What is the pathology?
2. Is there anticipated difficulty with ventilation, intubation or cricothyroid access?
3. Is there any coexisting disease?
4. What is the surgeon's preference for airway management?

The underlying pathology, if known, is of importance to the anesthesiologist. A supraglottic lesion can obstruct the airway, hinder ventilation and make visualization of the larynx difficult. A subglottic lesion may impede passage of the endotracheal tube or rigid

Anesthesia for Otolaryngologic Surgery, ed. Basem Abdelmalak and D. John Doyle. Published by Cambridge University Press.
© Cambridge University Press 2013.

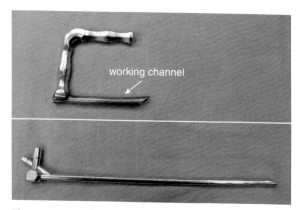

Figure 24.1. Rigid laryngoscope and bronchoscope Upper picture: Holinger anterior commissure laryngoscope. Lower picture: rigid bronchoscope size 7.5.

bronchoscope. Compression or invasion of the airway, vessels or nerves should be carefully noted.

More than 80% of laryngeal cancers are found in men 40–75 years old [3] and many patients presenting for panendoscopy will have a history of smoking and/or heavy alcohol intake. Pulmonary disease or obesity causing poor lung compliance may interfere with jet ventilation. Cardiovascular disease commonly coexists and can be exacerbated by the sympathetic stimulation that accompanies panendoscopy. Reflux history and potential for aspiration should be carefully noted. Liver disease, malnutrition and electrolyte abnormalities can be a consequence of heavy alcohol use or swallowing difficulty associated with oral tumors.

Intraoperative management

The choice of airway, method of ventilation and anesthetic technique are important considerations; however, no single airway device, ventilation technique or anesthetic method is ideal for all patients or pathologies.

During panendoscopy, the anesthesiologist and surgeon must share the airway, with different objectives. The anesthesiologist must deliver oxygen, remove carbon dioxide, provide anesthesia and protect the airway from soiling or aspiration. The surgeon requires an immobile, unobstructed surgical field and adequate time for diagnostic evaluation and intervention. Regardless of the chosen technique, continued communication with the surgeon throughout the procedure is vital.

Which airway?

The presence of a traditional endotracheal tube (ETT) during panendoscopy compromises visualization of and access to the larynx. The three airway options for panendoscopy are a tubeless technique, supraglottic airway or modified ETT (e.g. microlaryngeal tube.)

A tubeless technique implies ventilation using a bag and mask, or via the rigid laryngoscope. A supraglottic airway can be used prior to the commencement of surgery whilst the surgeon is preparing to insert the laryngoscope, or at the completion of surgery to facilitate smooth emergence [4]. A microlaryngeal tube (MLT) is a long polyvinyl chloride ETT with a high-volume, low-pressure cuff. Compared to a standard size 5 cuffed ETT, a size 5 MLT is longer (320 mm) and has the same internal (5.0 mm) and external diameter (6.9 mm) with a larger volume cuff, permitting tracheal occlusion in an adult. An MLT fits between the arytenoid cartilages leaving an unobscured view of the anterior two-thirds of the glottis and can be lifted anteriorly for visualization of the posterior glottis. However, even the small-diameter MLT can obscure the surgical field, especially the posterior commissure of the larynx [5] and when panendoscopy is combined with laser surgery, the presence of any endotracheal tube increases the risk of airway fire.

The difficult airway

There are three main options for the patient with a known or suspected difficult airway who presents for panendoscopy – awake intubation, prophylactic placement of a cricothyroid cannula or awake tracheostomy. A discussion with the ear-nose-and-throat surgeon and a preoperative nasal endoscopic examination of the upper airway may assist with this decision-making [6].

If an awake intubation is chosen, the carefully placed ETT will lie within the surgical field, hindering laryngoscopy and completely preventing rigid bronchoscopy. However, the surgeon can move the ETT anteriorly, posteriorly or side-to-side during surgery, so this should not be considered an absolute contraindication.

Another option is the elective placement of a transtracheal jet ventilation catheter prior to induction. Several specially designed cannulae are available, including the 13G Ravussin jet ventilation catheter [7] (VBM Medical, Germany) or the 15G Cook transtracheal jet ventilation catheter (Cook Critical Care,

Table 24.1. Advantages and disadvantages of ventilation methods for panendoscopy

Technique	Advantages	Disadvantages
Spontaneous ventilation	• Ideal surgical access	• No airway protection • ETCO$_2$ measurement inaccurate • Vocal cords may move unexpectedly • Difficult to control depth of anesthesia • Risk of laryngospasm
Intermittent apnea	• Unobstructed view of larynx • No need for jet ventilation • No movement of vocal cords	• Trauma from repeated intubations • Interrupted ventilation and surgery
Positive-pressure ventilation via MLT	• Familiar to all anesthesiologists • Control of ventilation • Protection against aspiration • ETCO$_2$ measurement • Ability to use volatile anesthesia without OR pollution	• Hindered surgical access • Risk of airway fire if laser used • May obscure a glottic lesion
Supraglottic jet ventilation	• Optimal access for the surgeon – especially for posterior commissure lesions	• Inability to measure ETCO$_2$ • Vocal cord movement with each jet • Risk of aspiration and barotrauma • Potential for tumor seeding • Need for TIVA
Subglottic jet ventilation	• Some ability to monitor ETCO$_2$ • More efficient than supraglottic ventilation • Minimal vocal cord movement	• Greater risk of barotrauma compared to supraglottic technique • Need for TIVA
Transtracheal jet ventilation	• Assists in management of difficult airway if placed prior to induction	• Catheter may kink, block or dislodge • Bleeding • Barotrauma • Tumor seeding
High-frequency jet ventilation	• Lower peak airway pressure • Less hemodynamic compromise than IPPV • Minimal movement of surgical field • Excellent surgical conditions • Laser compatible	• Requires specialized ventilators • Risk of gas trapping and barotrauma

Bloomington, IN), which is wire-reinforced and kink-resistant [8]. The jet ventilation catheter is inserted through the cricothyroid membrane using local anesthesia and placement is confirmed with capnography. The patient is then induced and if there is any difficulty with airway access or ventilation, the catheter allows temporary oxygenation whilst a more secure permanent airway, usually a surgical tracheostomy, is established. Disadvantages include risk of bleeding or the possibility of tumor seeding if the cannula is placed through underlying tumor. It is important to carefully secure the cannula to ensure it remains within the airway, to avoid subcutaneous emphysema.

Some patients requiring panendoscopy will present with critical airway obstruction and in these circumstances the safest approach is to proceed to elective tracheostomy under local anesthesia prior to any further endoscopic evaluation.

Which ventilation technique?

Ventilation techniques can be considered in terms of "open" and "closed" systems. A closed system implies ventilation via a cuffed ETT. An open system without an ETT is more commonly used for panendoscopy (Table 24.1).

Spontaneous ventilation

A spontaneously breathing patient negates the difficulty associated with providing artificial ventilation; however, this is a challenging technique to perfect. A deep plane of anesthesia is required to produce laryngeal immobility in an un-paralyzed patient, which can result in apnea or cardiovascular instability. This technique is usually most suitable for pediatric patients.

A standard intravenous induction or gaseous induction is performed before using direct laryngoscopy to apply lidocaine to reduce airway reactivity. A shortened ETT is placed via the nose into the nasopharynx, to allow insufflation of gases, or the anesthesia circuit can be connected to the side arm of the rigid bronchoscope for gas delivery. Alternatively, intravenous anesthesia can be titrated to maintain spontaneous ventilation.

A benefit of spontaneous ventilation is the ability to determine dynamic airway movement in order to assess vocal cord movement and tracheomalacia.

Positive-pressure ventilation

When using a microlaryngeal tube, positive-pressure ventilation can proceed in the usual manner. Alternatively, by connecting the anesthetic circuit to the side arm of the rigid bronchoscope, positive-pressure ventilation can be used; however, a large leak around the bronchoscope necessitates the use of high fresh gas flows. Additional leaks occur from the proximal end of the bronchoscope whenever the working channel is open.

Jet ventilation

Jet ventilation involves the delivery of high-pressure gas boluses through a narrow cannula or needle. When each bolus of gas is released, it entrains room air, increasing the volume of the bolus [5] and diluting the FiO_2 to approximately 0.8–0.9 [9]. The entrainment of ambient air is due to the drop in pressure that occurs as a gas stream exits a narrow tube, known as the Venturi effect. Central wall high-pressure oxygen at 50 psi is passed through a pressure-reducing valve and is further adjusted, by a regulator on a hand-triggered device, to 20–50 psi. Short tubing connects the hand piece to the jet ventilation cannula via a luer-lock connection. Manual depression of the nozzle or lever on the hand-held device expels a jet of gas (Figure 24.2). Two examples of hand-held jet

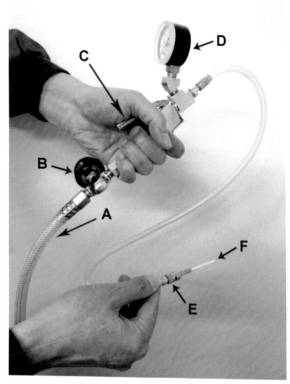

Figure 24.2. Manual jet ventilator Typical components of the manual jet ventilator: high-pressure oxygen tubing (A), pressure regulator (B), manual on/off trigger (C), pressure gauge (D), luer lock (E) and 14G cannula (F).

ventilators are the Sanders injector and the Manujet III. Adult ventilation is usually achieved with 20 psi pressure and it is prudent to start with the lowest possible pressure that achieves chest expansion.

Jet ventilation can be supraglottic, subglottic or transtracheal.

Supraglottic ventilation

Supraglottic ventilation is achieved by attaching the jetting cannula to the proximal end of the laryngoscope, via the side channel or clamped in such a way that the needle is directed along the long axis of the laryngoscope lumen [10]. A simpler set-up involves the anesthesiologist holding the jetting cannula in the proximal end of the working channel. It is important that the surgeon aligns the laryngoscope with the vocal cords and the anesthesiologist aligns the jetting cannula along the axis of the laryngoscope. Failure to do both of these things can result in ineffective ventilation or gastric distension [9]. The manual jet

231

injector trigger is depressed, ensuring bilateral chest expansion. Sufficient time must be allowed for full expiration prior to the next jet to avoid air-trapping.

Subglottic ventilation

To facilitate subglottic jet ventilation, a narrow tube is inserted 5–7 cm below the vocal cords using direct laryngoscopy. Several versions of this tube exist, including the Hunsaker monjet tube (Medtronic Xomed, Jacksonville, FL, USA) and the Ben-jet tube (Baldwin Medical, Melbourne, Australia.) The Hunsaker monjet tube is 33 cm long with an outside diameter of 2.9 mm, incorporating an integral line for monitoring end-tidal CO_2 [11]. The Ben-jet tube is 30 cm long with a proximal luer-lock connection. Both tubes have distal petals to keep them centered in the airway. Compared to supraglottic jet ventilation, there is less vocal cord movement hence less need to interrupt ventilation; however, there is an increased risk of gas trapping, particularly in patients with upper airway obstruction, as egress of air depends on a patent upper airway.

Transtracheal ventilation

Transtracheal jet ventilation can be facilitated using a jet ventilation catheter as discussed in management of the difficult airway.

High-frequency jet ventilation

High-frequency jet ventilation (HFJV) requires specialized ventilators capable of administering high respiratory rates that are not universally available within the OR setting. Typically, the high-frequency jet ventilator is set to a respiratory rate of approximately 100 breaths/min, a driving pressure of 30 psi and inspiratory time 30–50%. HFJV can be applied supraglottically by the side arm attachment of the rigid laryngoscope. Gas exchange during high-frequency jet ventilation occurs through several mechanisms, including molecular diffusion and cardiogenic mixing [9]. In addition, there is a difference in velocity between gas in the center of the airway and that close to the walls, which becomes exaggerated during HFJV, resulting in a spike of rapidly moving gas down the center of the airway [9].

Benefits of HFJV include minimal movement of the vocal cords and surgical field due to the use of small tidal volumes. It is also suitable for use in patients with poor lung compliance and can be

superimposed during resumption of spontaneous ventilation at the completion of surgery [12].

Disadvantages of jet ventilation include the need for specialized equipment and potential complications including pneumothorax, pneumomediastinum and subcutaneous emphysema. Gastric distension or rupture can occur if the catheter and/or laryngoscope are misaligned. Drying of airway mucosa occurs if humidification is not used. Gas exchange during low-frequency jet ventilation can be difficult in patients with poor chest wall or lung compliance. A mobile or pedunculated tumor can act like a ball-valve obstruction to expiration, resulting in gas trapping and barotrauma [10]. There is the potential for seeding of tumor or papilloma down the tracheobronchial tree.

Apneic ventilation

In this approach the surgeon and anesthesiologist take turns instrumenting the airway. The anesthesiologist intubates and hyperventilates the patient before extubating and handing the airway over to the surgeon. When ventilation is required again, the anesthesiologist reintubates, or returns to bag/mask ventilation and the cycle continues. This is preferred in some instances as there is an unobstructed, immobile surgical field during the apneic period. An obvious disadvantage is the potential for airway trauma due to repeated intubations.

Table 24.1 summarises the advantages and disadvantages of different methods of ventilation for panendoscopy.

Which anesthetic?

Panendoscopy is a brief yet highly stimulating procedure that requires deep anesthesia, obtunded hemodynamic reflexes, an immobile surgical field and rapid emergence with early return of protective airway reflexes. Prior to induction an antisialogogue (i.e. glycopyrrolate 0.2 mg IV or IM) can be given to minimize secretions. Typically a routine intravenous anesthetic induction is chosen with application of local anesthetic (i.e. lidocaine 4%) to the vocal cords prior to further airway manipulation. Confirm with the surgeon if local anesthesia will interfere with their planned procedure.

TIVA vs. volatile agents

If a closed system utilizing a microlaryngeal tube is chosen, volatile agents can be delivered via the anesthetic circuit. A spontaneously breathing patient can have volatile agents delivered via a shortened endotracheal tube placed through the nostril into the nasopharynx. Volatile anesthesia can also be used when ventilating via the side arm of the rigid bronchoscope, but in the latter two scenarios pollution of the operating room will occur. Depth of anesthesia can vary due to interrupted volatile delivery and there is a limited ability to measure end-tidal anesthetic concentrations.

A more reliable anesthetic for panendoscopy is a total intravenous technique using an intravenous hypnotic agent and opioid. Propofol in combination with alfentanil or remifentanil is an ideal choice. TIVA utilizing propofol with remifentanil resulted in a superior recovery profile compared with alfentanil-based TIVA [13]. Alfentanil was used with a loading dose of 50 µg/kg and a maintenance infusion of 1 µg/kg/min. For remifentanil a loading dose of 1 µg/kg and infusion rate of 0.25 µg/kg/min were used. Both groups were combined with propofol 2 mg/kg followed by infusion of 100 µg/kg/min [13].

The balance of hypnosis vs. analgesia has also been studied to see if the respective doses of propofol and remifentanil influenced recovery. "Propofol pronounced" anesthesia (100 µg/kg/min propofol + remifentanil 0.15 µg/kg/min) was compared with a "remifentanil pronounced" regime (50 µg/kg/min propofol + remifentanil 0.45 µg/kg/min.) Both regimes were satisfactory, with little difference between the groups [14].

The use of an Entropy (GE Healthcare, Helsinki, Finland) or Bispectral index (BIS, Aspect Medical Systems, Newton, MA, USA) monitor can assist with optimizing anesthetic depth and to reduce the risk of awareness.

Other agents, including local anesthetics and β-blockers, can be used to minimize the hemodynamic response. Lidocaine sprayed onto the larynx and upper trachea under direct laryngoscopy reduces the rise in BP and HR from baseline following the introduction of a rigid bronchoscope [15], and also reduces the risk of laryngospasm.

Short acting β-blocking agents such as esmolol have been shown to limit the increases in HR and BP throughout panendoscopy [16].

Muscle relaxants

Panendoscopy is very brief; however, muscle relaxation wearing off mid-way through the procedure can result in trauma. Succinylcholine is unlikely to have sufficient duration of action for all but the briefest of procedures; however, repeated doses of 0.3–0.5 mg/kg or a continuous infusion of 100 µg/kg/min can be used. A phase 2 block is unlikely if the total dose is < 4–6 mg/kg [17]. Alternatively, an intermediate-duration non-depolarizing muscle relaxant can be chosen, including mivacurium 0.25 mg/kg, rocuronium 0.6 mg/kg or cisatracurium 0.15–0.25 mg/kg.

When monitoring depth of neuromuscular blockade for panendoscopy, it is best to stimulate a peripheral nerve whose onset/offset characteristics more closely resemble that of the larynx. Orbicularis oculi has fast onset of neuromuscular blockade and is resistant, similar to the larynx, therefore is a good choice for monitoring [18].

Antiemetics and dexamethasone

Nausea and vomiting is a common reason for prolonged recovery room stay and prophylactic use of antiemetics should be considered. If dexamethasone is chosen, it has the additional benefit of reducing post-surgical airway swelling that can result from instrumentation.

"Tips and tricks"

- A reliable intravenous line on the side where the anesthesiologist is standing allows monitoring for patency and easy access, when using TIVA.
- Consider an arterial line if there is significant coexisting disease to permit closer hemodynamic monitoring and blood gas sampling to determine adequacy of ventilation. Transcutaneous CO_2 measurement is an alternative, if available.
- The anesthesiologist should position themselves to one side at the head of the bed, to deliver jet ventilation and watch the patient's chest for adequate excursion and expiration, with the anesthetic monitor easily visible (Figure 24.3).
- Delivery of propofol and remifentanil/alfentanil, ideally via infusion pumps, should be within reach for titration.
- Any additional medications that may be required – e.g., additional muscle relaxant – should be drawn up and within arm's reach.

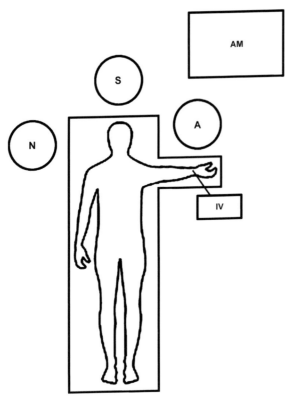

Figure 24.3. Typical panendoscopy set-up. AM: Anesthesia Machine; S: Surgeon; A: Anesthesiologist; N: Surgical nurse; IV: Intravenous pole and bag.

Postoperative care
Emergence phase
The emergence phase can be managed in several ways. At the completion of panendoscopy, muscle relaxation is reversed if non-depolarizing agents have been used and the intravenous or volatile anesthetic is stopped. The patient can be managed with bag/mask ventilation or by insertion of a supraglottic airway until spontaneous ventilation resumes.

Alternatively, in patients with a "difficult airway" the surgeon can pass a bougie or introducer via the laryngoscope/bronchoscope under direct vision [19]. The laryngoscope is then removed and an endotracheal tube is railroaded over the introducer to ensure a secure airway during emergence. If subglottic ventilation via a ben-jet or monjet tube has been used, this could be left *in situ* to facilitate subglottic ventilation if necessary. In extreme circumstances, an intraoperative tracheostomy may be performed to prevent postoperative

airway compromise when the airway is obstructed by tumor or other pathology.

If there is anticipation of postoperative pain, a small dose of longer-acting opiate, i.e. fentanyl 25–100 μg IV, is given. Often this is unnecessary and acetaminophen and anti-inflammatory medications could be substituted.

Complications
Complications of panendoscopy that present intraoperatively include arrhythmia, hypercarbia due to inadequate ventilation, and bleeding [17]. Direct trauma to the tracheobronchial tree including lacerations, hemorrhage or arytenoid dislocation can occur [1]. However, most complications become evident during emergence or the early postoperative period, including dental injury, eye trauma and injury to the lips and tongue. Surgical manipulation can result in edema or bleeding causing laryngospasm or airway obstruction [17]. Neurological injury related to neck extension, especially in patients with atlanto-axial instability, is a disastrous consequence. A postoperative chest X-ray should be performed if there is any suspicion of pneumothorax or pneumomediastinum [17].

Summary
Although usually brief, panendoscopy is not a trivial procedure and can be associated with pulmonary, cardiovascular or airway complications. It requires the anesthesiologist to be "hands-on", familiar with surgical needs, airway and ventilation techniques; proficient in maintenance of appropriate depth of anesthesia during surgical stresses; vigilant for the development of complications and in constant communication with the surgeon.

Case study
A 60-year-old man with a 6-month history of progressive hoarseness was booked for panendoscopy and vocal cord biopsy. He had a history of hypertension, smoking, and COPD. His medications included bisoprolol, ramipril, and inhaled salbutamol (albuterol). He was 175 cm tall, weighed 70 kg and had preoperative BP 160/100 and heart rate 64 bpm. Airway examination revealed a Malampatti score of 3, adequate mouth opening and thyromental distance and poor dentition. His ECG showed left ventricular hypertrophy and pulmonary function tests, an FEV_1/

FVC ratio 60% predicted. Nasal endoscopy by the ENT surgeon diagnosed a 4 mm lesion on the posterior third of the left vocal cord, suspicious for glottic carcinoma. A CT scan of the neck did not reveal any suspicious nodes or lesions.

Preoperative assessment is therefore summarized as a patient with an isolated left vocal cord lesion suspicious for carcinoma with no obvious spread and unlikely to present difficulties with intubation. The surgeon indicated a preference for no ETT, jet ventilation via the rigid laryngoscope, and immobility of vocal cords during the procedure.

In the operating room, standard monitors were placed and intravenous access obtained. Room air oxygen saturation of 94% improved to 100% with preoxygenation. Airway equipment including an LMA Classic™ (LMA), Glidescope® and a flexible bronchoscope were available. After intravenous induction with midazolam 1 mg, fentanyl 100 μg, propofol 150 mg, and rocuronium 35 mg, a size 4 LMA was inserted. Infusions of propofol 100 μg/kg/min and remifentanil 0.25 μg/kg/min were started. After 2 min of ventilation, the LMA was removed, the patient positioned using a shoulder roll to extend the head and a rigid laryngoscope was inserted with the tip just above the glottis. Wall-source oxygen at 50 psi was pressure-reduced to 20 psi via a hand-operated jet ventilator, connected to a 14G cannula. The patient was intermittently jet ventilated by holding the 14G cannula in the working channel of the rigid laryngoscope. Oxygen saturation was maintained between 92% and 100%. Propofol and remifentanil infusions were titrated according to hemodynamic changes. After bronchoscopy and esophagoscopy, four biopsies were taken from the left glottic lesion. Hemostasis was obtained. Prior to removal of the rigid laryngoscope, the surgeon sprayed 4% lidocaine onto the vocal cords to reduce the risk of laryngospasm.

After removal of the rigid laryngoscope, the LMA was re-inserted, and mechanical ventilation resumed. Nerve stimulation showed a train-of-four count of 4 with fade; neostigmine 2.5 mg and glycopyrrolate 0.4 mg were given and intravenous anesthesia was stopped. Dexamethasone 4 mg and granisetron 1 mg were given for antiemesis and reduction of postoperative swelling. The patient regained spontaneous ventilation and upon awakening the LMA was removed uneventfully. The patient returned home later that day.

Clinical pearls

- Although usually brief in duration, a panendoscopy is not a trivial procedure and can be associated with significant pulmonary, cardiovascular or airway complications.

- A supraglottic lesion can obstruct the airway, hinder ventilation and make visualization of the larynx extremely difficult. A subglottic lesion may impede passage of the endotracheal tube or rigid bronchoscope. Compression or invasion of the airway, vessels or nerves should be carefully noted.

- No single airway device, ventilation technique or anesthetic method is ideal for all patients or pathologies.

- The three airway options for panendoscopy are a tubeless technique (a bag and mask, or via the rigid laryngoscope), use of a supraglottic airway (can be used prior to the commencement of surgery whilst the surgeon is preparing to insert the laryngoscope, or at the completion of surgery to facilitate smooth emergence) or modified ETT (e.g., MicroLaryngeal Tube – MLT).

- If a closed system utilizing a MicroLaryngeal Tube is chosen, volatile agents can be delivered via the anesthetic circuit. A more popular anesthetic technique for panendoscopy is a total intravenous technique using an intravenous hypnotic agent (e.g., propofol) and opioid (e.g., remifentanil).

- A reliable intravenous line on the side where the anesthesiologist is standing allows monitoring for patency and easy access, an especially important consideration when using TIVA.

- Consider an arterial line if there is significant coexisting disease so as to allow close hemodynamic monitoring and blood gas sampling. Where available, transcutaneous CO_2 monitoring is a potential alternative.

References

1. Pereira K, Hessel A. Performance of rigid bronchoscopy. In Hagberg C, ed. *Benumof's Airway Management*, 2nd edn. Philadelphia: Mosby Elsevier; 2007. pp. 631–9.

2. Hillel A, Sie K. A reliable method to maintain an airway after bronchoscopy. *Laryngoscope* 1988;**98**:1353–5.

3. Feldman MA, Patel A. Anesthesia for eye, ear, nose and throat surgery. In Miller RD, ed. *Miller's Anesthesia*, 7th edn. Philadelphia: Churchill Livingstone/Elsevier; 2009. pp. 2357–88.

4. Nair I, Bailey PM. Review of uses of the laryngeal mask in ENT anaesthesia. *Anaesthesia* 1995;**50**:898–900.

5. Borland L. Airway management for CO$_2$ laser surgery on the larynx: venturi jet ventilation and alternatives. *Int Anesthesiol Clin* 1997;**35**:99–106.

6. Rosenblatt W, Ianus AI, Sukhupragarn W. Preoperative endoscopic airway examination provides superior airway information and may reduce the use of unnecessary awake intubation. *Anesth Analg* 2011;**112**:602–7.

7. McLellan I, Khawaja S, Thomas A. Percutaneous trans-tracheal high frequency jet ventilation as an aid to difficult intubation. *Can J Anaesth* 1988;**35**:404–5.

8. Rosenblatt W, Benumof J. Transtracheal jet ventilation via percutaneous catheter and high-pressure source. In Hagberg C, ed. *Benumof's Airway Management*, 2nd edn. Philadelphia: Mosby Elsevier; 2007. pp. 616–30.

9. Evans E, Biro P, Bedforth N. Jet ventilation. *CEACC Pain* 2007; 7:2–5.

10. Crockett D, Scamman F, McCabe B, *et al.* Venturi jet ventilation for microlaryngoscopy: technique, complications, pitfalls. *Laryngoscope* 1987;**97**:1326–30.

11. Vadodaria B, Cooper C. The anesthetic management of a case of severe upper airways obstruction due to an enlarging subglottic benign polyp. *Eur J Anaesthesiol* 2001;**18**:766–9.

12. Babinski M, Smith RB, Klain M. High-frequency jet ventilation for laryngoscopy. *Anesthesiology* 1980;**52**:178–80.

13. Wuesten R, Van Aken H, Glass P, *et al.* Assessment of depth of anesthesia and postoperative respiratory recovery after remifentanil-based versus alfentanil-based total intravenous anesthesia in patients undergoing ear-nose-throat surgery. *Anesthesiology* 2001;**94**:211–7.

14. Hackner, Detsch O, Schneider G, *et al.* Early recovery after remifentanil-pronounced compared with propofol-pronounced total intravenous anaesthesia for short painful procedures. *Br J Anaesth* 2003;**91**:580–2.

15. Gaumann D, Tassonyi E, Fathi F, *et al.* Effects of topical laryngeal lidocaine on sympathetic response to rigid panendoscopy under general anesthesia. *J Oto Rhino Laryngol Relat Spec* 1992;**54**:49–53.

16. Ayuso A, Luis M, Sala X, *et al.* Effects of anesthetic technique on the hemodynamic response to microlaryngeal surgery. *Ann Otol Rhinol Laryngol* 1997;**106**: 863–8.

17. Kaplan MJ, *et al.* Otolaryngology – head and neck surgery. In Jaffe R, Samuels SI, eds. *Anesthesiologist's Manual of Surgical Procedures*, 4th edn. Philadelphia: Lippincott Williams & Wilkins; 2009. pp. 173–85.

18. Donati F, Meistelman C, Plaud B. Vecuronium neuromuscular blockade at the adductor muscles of the larynx and adductor pollicis. *Anesthesiology* 1991;**74**:833–7.

19. Nekhendzy V, Simmonds P. Rigid bronchoscope-assisted endotracheal intubation: yet another use of the gum elastic bougie. *Anesth Analg* 2004;**98**:545–7.

Chapter
25
Anesthesia for ENT laser surgery

D. John Doyle

Introduction

Lasers are commonly used in otolaryngologic surgery (Table 25.1), in plastic surgery (for instance, in the removal of port wine birthmarks), in gynecologic surgery (for instance, in the treatment of endometriosis), in ophthalmic surgery (for instance, in retinal surgery) and elsewhere [1,2]. Depending on the clinical circumstances, various laser types producing light (photons) of different wavelength (color) are employed (Table 25.2).

The most widely utilized laser in ENT surgery is the carbon dioxide (CO_2) laser. It allows precise cutting with a particularly fine zone of coagulation that helps reduce surgical bleeding. It can be especially useful in the removal of obstructing laryngeal carcinomas, the removal of lingual tonsillar tissue, the ablation of hemangiomas, and the resection of small oropharyngeal malignant lesions. The carbon dioxide laser can be used either as a precision cutting instrument or as a tissue vaporizer depending on the extent to which the beam is focused. Tissue vaporization is particularly efficient with the carbon dioxide laser because of the excellent absorption of the produced far infrared photons (10 600 nm wavelength) by water present in tissue.

Another popular laser in ENT surgery is the Nd:YAG laser. This laser emits photons with a wavelength of 1064 nm. These photons are poorly absorbed by water and thus tend to penetrate tissue much more deeply than those from a carbon dioxide laser. In addition, light (photons) from a Nd:YAG laser can be transmitted through flexible quartz fibers that can be used in conjunction with a flexible fiberoptic bronchoscope for use in treating lesions in tracheobronchial structures.

Table 25.1. Some otolaryngologic clinical situations where laser techniques can be useful

Nose
  Turbinate reduction
  Septoplasty
  Removal of nasal obstructions, polyps, synechiae
  Treatment of rhinophyma
  Treatment of keloids and hypertrophic scars

Oropharynx/pharynx
  Vaporization of papillomas, leukoplakias and hemangiomas
  Tumor surgery (e.g., partial glossectomy)
  Laser-assisted uvulopalatoplasty
  Tonsillectomy

Larynx
  Removal of vocal cord polyps and granulomas
  Epiglottectomy
  Cordectomy
  Arytenoidectomy

Tracheobronchial tree
  Treatment of tracheal stenosis
  Removal of nodules, polyps, tumors and fibromas

Ear
  Surgery of the stapes
  Laser-assisted myringotomy
  Cholesteatoma

Anesthesia for Otolaryngologic Surgery, ed. Basem Abdelmalak and D. John Doyle. Published by Cambridge University Press.
© Cambridge University Press 2013.

237

Table 25.2. A sampling of various kinds of lasers available for clinical use

Type	Gas/solid	Wavelength (nm)	Color	Fiberoptic transmissible?
Helium/neon	Gas	633	Red	Yes
Argon	Gas	500	Blue-Green	Yes
CO_2	Gas	10 600	Invisible (far infrared)	No
Ruby	Solid	695	Red	Yes
Nd:YAG	Solid	1064	Invisible (near infrared)	Yes
KTP	Solid	532	Green	Yes

Wavelengths are given in nanometers (nm). There are 10^9 nm to a meter.
The argon laser produces blue-green coherent light at a number of wavelengths but most of the energy is at wavelengths 488 nm and 514 nm.
Nd:YAG is short for neodymium-doped yttrium aluminum garnet.
KTP is short for potassium titanyl phosphate.

Laser physics

The following is a capsule summary of basic laser physics. "Laser" is an acronym for **l**ight **a**mplification by **s**timulated **e**mission of **r**adiation. Lasers control the manner in which energized atoms release coherent monochromatic light (photons). While the concept dates back to Einstein, in 1960 the American physicist Theodore Maiman made the first working laser from a ruby rod.

Laser light is very different from the light that we experience every day [3,4]. Ordinary light consists of a number of colors, i.e., is polychromatic. In addition, ordinary light is noncoherent, that is, it contains multiple wave fronts and is multidirectional. Laser light is different from ordinary light in that (1) it is "monochromatic" (consisting of only one particular wavelength of light), (2) it is "coherent" (organized so that each photon moves in step with the others), and (3) it is directional, presenting a very tight beam that this does not widen significantly as it travels.

If we apply energy to an atom, electrons will leave the ground state energy level and go to an excited level. When the electrons subsequently move back to the ground state they do so by releasing energy as a photon – a particle of light. If the released photon encounters another atom that has electrons in an excited state, "stimulated" emission of another photon can occur; this newly emitted photon will vibrate with the same frequency and direction as the stimulating photon [3,4].

The laser type is named after the atoms that are energized (lasing medium). For example if it is carbon dioxide atoms that are energized, it is known as a CO_2 laser, and the photons emitted from this laser have a wavelength of 10 600 nm. This wavelength is in the far infrared region and is not visible. By contrast, a helium-neon laser emits photons with a wavelength of 633 nm, which appears red to the human eye. Because CO_2 laser beams are invisible, they often incorporate a helium-neon laser as an aiming beam. Table 25.2 lists various other kinds of lasers and their characteristics.

Laser safety

Surgical lasers involve high amounts of energy and have the potential for unintended tissue damage as well as for causing operating room fires. Instruments with a polished surface can reflect laser beams to an unintended destination and thus cause injury. To warn passersby that lasers are in use, one should place warning signs outside the operating room (Figure 25.1). Opaque coverings on any operating room windows will prevent stray laser beams from exiting. It is also customary to provide extra goggles for visitors near the entrance to the operating room (Figure 25.2).

Another concern is that stray laser beams can ignite surgical drapes. Since the presence of high levels of oxygen around the patient's face can facilitate ignition in this region, delivering supplementary oxygen by face mask or nasal cannula requires special vigilance. Fires can also occur within the airway itself; this is discussed in detail in Chapter 11.

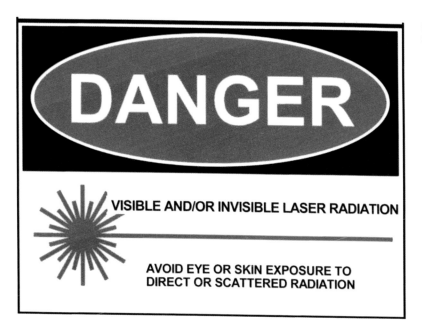

Figure 25.1. Typical warning sign for use with clinical lasers.

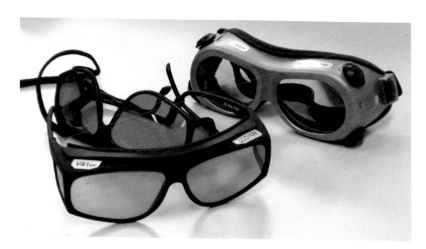

Figure 25.2. Example of three types of laser safety eyewear. Reproduced from: http://en.wikipedia.org/wiki/Image: Laser_goggles.jpg (Author Han-Kwang) under a Creative Commons Share Alike license.

Yet another concern is for possible ophthalmic injuries, since CO_2 lasers can cause serious corneal injuries, while Nd:YAG lasers can cause retinal damage. To mitigate such risks, the eyes of the patient can be protected by taping the eyelids and then applying moist dressings on top, while caregivers should wear protective goggles. Each kind of laser is associated with its own kind of protective eyewear that filters out photons having a wavelength associated with that kind of laser. For example, goggles absorbing radiation at 532 nm wavelength (KTP lasers) typically have an orange appearance, and would be relatively ineffective in protecting against an Nd:YAG laser emitting energy at 1060 nm. Protective eyewear for carbon dioxide lasers consists of material opaque to far infrared wavelengths. Note also that the energy of the photons making up a laser beam depends on their wavelength in that shorter-wavelength photons (toward the ultraviolet region) have more energy than longer-wavelength photons (toward the infrared region).

In addition to the dangers associated with stray laser beams that may produce eye injuries or burns, the clinician should be aware of the possibility of lasers igniting fires, as well as the possibility of inadvertently perforating organs or vessels or of causing a gas embolism.

Table 25.3. Some types of laser ETTs in clinical use

Name	Description	Intended use
Laser Flex	Airtight stainless-steel corrugated spiral with a PVC Murphy eye tip and double cuffs. More information is available at http://www.cardinal.com/us/en/distributedproducts/ASP/43168–45.asp	CO_2 or KTP lasers
Laser-Shield II	Silicone rubber tube wrapped with aluminum and wrapped over with Teflon. More information at http://www.medtronicent-techcomms.com/inserts-web/68E1503_B.pdf	CO_2 or KTP lasers
Lasertubus	Soft white rubber, reinforced with corrugated copper foil and an absorbent sponge. Double cuffed. More information at http://www.myrusch.com/images/rusch/docs/A20C.pdf	CO_2 or KTP lasers
Sheridan Laser-Trach	Red rubber design with embossed copper foil and outer covering designed to reduce damage to mucosal surfaces and vocal cords. More information at http://www.orsupply.com/product/Hudson-RCI-Sheridan-Laser-Trach-Endotracheal-Tubes/6951	CO_2 or KTP lasers

Finally, note that ANSI standard Z136.3 (Safe Use of Lasers in Health Care Facilities) provides additional information on this and related matters. EN 207 is the related European standard for laser safety eyewear.

Laser-safe endotracheal tubes

Not long after the advent of laser surgery clinicians came to realize the special dangers that could occur should a regular ETT ignite from a laser beam. In the past, metallic tapes applied in a spiral manner or the use of similar "guard" methods to prevent endotracheal tubes from igniting due to laser energy have been tried [3,4]. Today, however, a number of special-purpose [5] ETTs are available for this purpose (Table 25.3, Figure 25.3). It is common to fill cuffs of laser ETTs with saline to serve as an additional protection against fire. Some clinicians add small amounts of methylene blue to this saline to help detect cuff perforation. Note that the addition of fluid to the cuff will slightly prolong the cuff deflation time. Finally, carefully placed saline-soaked pledgets are occasionally applied to laser ETT cuffs for additional protection; these must be kept wet to avoid ignition and, of course, special care must be taken to retrieve all the pledgets at the end of the operation.

Anesthetic technique

The choice of anesthetic technique will depend on clinical circumstances. Total intravenous anesthesia (TIVA) techniques for laser ENT surgery are particularly popular, and are essential in cases where the

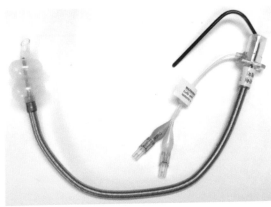

Figure 25.3. Laser-Flex laser-resistant endotracheal tube from Cardinal Health. Note the special double cuff arrangement. Some clinicians like to fill the cuffs with dilute methylene blue; in this way an ETT cuff rupture from a misdirected laser beam can be readily detected. Photo courtesy the author.

patients are unintubated and jet ventilation is used. When patients are intubated, a potent inhalational agent like sevoflurane is often used, although not infrequently an infusion of remifentanil is used as an anesthetic adjunct in such cases (typical rate: 0.05 to 0.1 µg/kg/min). More commonly total intravenous anesthesia (TIVA) is used and potent inhalational agents are avoided. Our traditional TIVA recipe consists of propofol 500 mg (50 ml) to which is added 1 mg of remifentanil in a single 60 ml syringe. Remifentanil, with its vagomimetic effect, is especially useful to limit the heart rate in the face of intense sympathetic stimulation from the effects of the suspension laryngoscope. After induction with midazolam, fentanyl, propofol and rocuronium, our usual starting dose of the propofol portion of this mixture is 100 µg/kg/min, followed by titration to clinical effect. Note that a dose of 100 µg/kg/min of propofol here produces a corresponding remifentanil dose of 0.2 µg/kg/min. While some clinicians prefer to use two separate infusion systems in such cases, with the possibility of controlling each infusion separately, we believe that our approach is simpler, has withstood the test of time, involves less chance for operator error, and requires less equipment and space.

Premedication is usually not used in these cases, although an antisialagogue like glycopyrrolate can often be helpful. Finally, to reduce the likelihood of airway fires, while lasers are in use nitrous oxide should not be used and the oxygen concentration should be limited to the lowest concentration necessary to maintain acceptable arterial oxygen saturation levels. For additional details see Chapter 11 on airway fires.

Airway management is without doubt a frequent challenge in many laser surgery cases. The importance of the surgeon and anesthesiologist working together to plan and implement a management strategy cannot be overemphasized. First, the presence of any airway pathology has the potential to make both ventilation and intubation difficult. One important issue here is whether general anesthesia should be preceded by awake intubation. Another issue is whether or not the procedure should be performed under general anesthesia with the patient breathing spontaneously, albeit with assistance, as is sometimes desirable in cases where an anterior mediastinal mass is present. The otolaryngology and anesthesia teams will find it necessary to discuss the advantages and disadvantages of the various clinical options in the light of the patient's condition, the available equipment and the preferences and training of the two clinical teams.

Muscle relaxation is often employed to help ensure an immobile surgical field. In the USA, where sugammadex is still not available (at the time of writing), succinylcholine is often used as an initial relaxant in patients with a potentially difficult airway because its short duration of action adds a measure of safety should the patient become impossible to intubate or ventilate following its administration. Many Europeans would instead be more comfortable using rocuronium as a relaxant, followed by a "sugammadex rescue" should the airway become unmanageable following relaxant administration. Many clinicians, however, simply intubate the patient awake whenever issues of this kind arise.

Extubation in these cases can sometimes be very challenging. Some cases will benefit from the administration of intravenous dexamethasone (Decadron ®) to reduce edema. Stridor is sometimes encountered after extubation; while this may require reintubation, we are often able to avoid this via the use of inhaled racemic epinephrine or the use of heliox, a mixture of helium (typically 70%) and oxygen. Extubation over a tube exchanger can be helpful in cases where the need for reintubation is a concern and would be expected to be challenging. Clinicians will vary in their estimation as to when conditions have improved sufficiently to allow "safe" extubation.

In some cases the entire surgical procedure is done without intubation. The advantages of this approach are a decreased risk of fire (no ETT to ignite) and improved access to airway structures. Disadvantages include the risk of aspiration with an unprotected airway and potential difficulties in ventilating the patient. Typically in such cases an anterior commissure laryngoscope or similar device is used in conjunction with TIVA and jet ventilation. In other cases the laryngoscope is used in conjunction with a small-diameter ETT (e.g., MLT size 5.0) with the procedure performed under brief periods of apnea in conjunction with intermittent removal of the ETT to allow unimpaired access to the glottic structures.

Atmospheric contamination issues

Laser vaporization of tissue, especially from CO_2 lasers, often results in a plume of smoke that can be annoying and sometimes even dangerous. The use of a smoke evacuator at the surgical site along with protective masks which filter out particulate material is often advised, especially when virus particles are present in the vaporized tissue (Figure 25.4).

Postoperative concerns

Even when patients are extubated conservatively following laser surgery cases, airway problems can arise later. In cases of immediate respiratory distress following laser cases, consider the following possibilities: (1) tissue edema (e.g., after Nd:YAG laser use), (2) residual muscle relaxant or anesthetic effects, (3) airway secretions, (4) pneumothorax, (5) bleeding, and (6) pneumomediastinum. Of course, delayed complications can also arise, such as infection and/or pneumonia from atelectasis or airway secretions, or from delayed onset edema (see Case study).

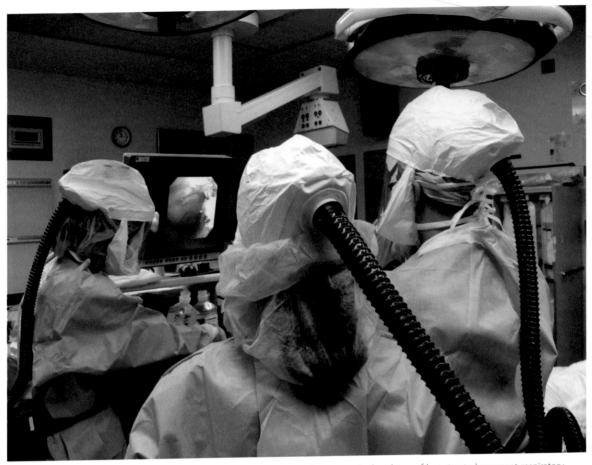

Figure 25.4. Concern that infectious human papilloma virus (HPV) may be present in the plume of laser-treated recurrent respiratory papillomatosis has led some clinicians to use battery-operated air-purifying hoods such as those as shown here. Such systems typically include a blower, battery, headpiece and a breathing tube, creating a decidedly eerie effect. Photo courtesy of the author.

Summary

Anesthesia for otolaryngologic laser surgery is fraught with special challenges, such as possible difficulties with intubation and ventilation, the need to prevent airway fires, the frequent need for total intravenous anesthesia (TIVA), and the need to protect clinicians against airborne viruses released as a result of papilloma surgery. Special laser endotracheal tubes are often employed. TIVA is usually carried out using a combination of propofol and remifentanil. Concerns about the possibility of tissue edema (especially after Nd:YAG laser use), pneumothorax, bleeding, and pneumomediastinum are also frequent postoperative issues.

Case study

Abdelmalak *et al.* [6] described a patient who developed respiratory arrest 4 hours after successful laser treatment of tracheal stenosis using a Nd:YAG (neodymium: yttrium-aluminum-garnet) laser. She had earlier been extubated at the end of the procedure without difficulty. Respiratory arrest was believed to be caused by delayed airway narrowing due to tissue edema from thermal injury by deep penetration of the laser beam. The following commentary is from their report:

> Two hours after surgery, the patient began coughing. One hour later, she developed stridorous breath sounds consistent with upper-respiratory obstruction, and she was treated with oxygen and bronchodilator

aerosol. Over the next hour, airway obstruction progressively became worse. Air exchange became inadequate, and the patient became obtunded over several minutes, oxyhemoglobin saturation decreased to 80%, heart rate decreased to 40 bpm, and arterial blood pressure decreased to 60/46 mmHg. Controlled ventilation via a mask was attempted, with much difficulty. To maintain adequate oxygenation, the trachea was intubated. An endotracheal tube, size 6.0 mm internal diameter, was passed with difficulty beyond the lasered area. With a fraction of inspired oxygen of 1.0, oxyhemoglobin saturation promptly increased to 100%. Heart rate and blood pressure returned to baseline levels. The patient was then admitted to the intensive care unit (ICU) for ventilatory support. She was given methylprednisolone 60 mg IV at 6-h intervals. The next day her trachea was exubated, and the following day she was discharged from the hospital.

Instructional videos

The following are some educational videos concerning otolaryngologic laser surgery that may be of interest to readers:

Laser resection of vocal cord nodules
http://www.youtube.com/watch?v=RGSU4i1O-P0
Arytenoidectomy surgery
http://www.youtube.com/watch?v=ZZvRp8KhbIM
Laryngeal papilloma – MGH voice center
http://www.youtube.com/watch?v=kRI9AVheKdQ
Nasal surgery laser
http://www.youtube.com/watch?v=Qio2cJIl1X0

Clinical pearls

- Surgical lasers emit high amounts of energy and have the potential for unintended tissue damage (for example, when accidently reflected from a polished surgical instrument).

- Lasers can accidently start operating room fires (e.g., a stray laser beam can ignite surgical drapes), especially when high levels of oxygen around the patient's face are used in unintubated patients.
- Yet another concern is for possible ophthalmic injuries, since CO_2 lasers can cause serious corneal injuries while Nd:YAG lasers can cause retinal damage. To mitigate such risks, the patient's eyes can be protected by taping the eyelids and then applying moist dressings on top, while caregivers should wear protective goggles.
- A number of special laser-safe ETTs are available. It is common to fill cuffs of laser ETTs with saline to serve as an additional protection against fire. Some clinicians add small amounts of methylene blue to this saline to help detect cuff perforation. Note that the addition of fluid to the cuff will slightly prolong the cuff deflation time.
- Total intravenous anesthesia (TIVA) techniques for laser ENT surgery are particularly popular; muscle relaxation is often employed to ensure an immobile surgical field.
- Some patients will benefit from the administration of intravenous dexamethasone (Decadron ®) to reduce edema. Be especially concerned about the possibility of delayed tissue edema after Nd:YAG laser use.
- Stridor is sometimes encountered after extubation; while this may require reintubation, we are often able to avoid this via the use of inhaled racemic epinephrine or the use of heliox, a mixture of helium (typically 70%) and oxygen. Extubation over a tube exchanger can be helpful in cases where the need for reintubation is a concern and would be expected to be challenging.

References

1. Rampil IJ. Anesthetic considerations for laser surgery. *Anesth Analg* 1992;**74**:424–35.
2. Sheinbein DS, Loeb RG. Laser surgery and fire hazards in ear, nose, and throat surgeries. *Anesthesiol Clin* 2010;**28**(3):485–96. PubMed PMID: 20850079.
3. Absten GT. Physics of light and lasers. *Obstet Gynecol Clin North Am* 1991;**18**(3):407–27. PubMed PMID: 1956663.
4. Van Der Spek AFL, Spargo PM, Norton ML. The physics of lasers and implications for their use during airway surgery. *Br J Anaesth* 1998;**60**:709–29.
5. Lai HC, Juang SE, Liu TJ, Ho WM. Fires of endotracheal tubes of three different materials during carbon dioxide laser surgery. *Acta Anaesthesiol Sin* 2002;**40**(1):47–51. PubMed PMID: 11989049.
6. Abdelmalak B, Ryckman JV, AlHaddad S, Sprung J. Respiratory arrest after successful neodymium:yttrium-aluminum-garnet laser treatment of subglottic tracheal stenosis. *Anesth Analg* 2002;**95**(2):485–6. PubMed PMID: 12145077.

Chapter

26

Anesthesia for laryngoplasty

Michael S. Benninger and Tatyana Kopyeva

Introduction

Laryngeal framework surgery (LFS) is a very dynamic, rapidly expanding area of phonosurgery (PS), which is intended primarily to improve or restore voice. The concept of LFS was systematically developed by Isshiki in the 1970s. The acceptance of the procedures and further new developments in the field made it confusing even for the specialists with regard to terminology, types of surgery, and classification, which in turn made it difficult to compare results between different institutions and authors. Attempts have been made to establish a practical classification system for PS and a more precise list of definitions [1,2].

In 2001 the Phonosurgery Committee of the European Laryngological Society published a proposal for classification and nomenclature in LFS [1]. A few terms are often used describing LFS [1,2]: laryngeal framework surgery, laryngoplasty and thyroplasty. LFS is the general term for the phonosurgical procedures modifying the supporting structures of the larynx and aiming at functional improvement. Laryngoplasty (LPL) is often used as a synonym to LFS and may be more suitable to use in daily practice, though it is not as inclusive as LFS. "Injection laryngoplasty" refers to some injection techniques for augmentation of the vocal fold, but it is not true LFS and is described elsewhere. Thyroplasty (TPL) is a specific subgroup of LPL (or LFS) and includes the procedures which alter or modify the thyroid cartilage in order to change the position or the length of the vocal folds.

In general, LFS can be divided into four major groups [1,2] according to intended purpose:

- approximation laryngoplasty (correction of insufficient glottic closure): injection laryngoplasty, medialization thyroplasty; arytenoid adduction, arytenopexy

- expansion laryngoplasty (correction of vocal fold hyperadduction or bilateral vocal fold paralysis): lateralization thyroplasty; vocal fold abduction
- relaxation laryngoplasty (procedures for pathologically tightened vocal folds or too high-pitched voice): shortening thyroplasty
- tensioning laryngoplasty (procedures for pathologically lax vocal folds or too low-pitched voice): cricothyroid approximation; elongation thyroplasty.

During the above procedures, position and/or tension of the vocal folds is changed to improve vibratory movements of the vocal folds, reduce turbulent phonatory airflow or alter vocal pitch [1,2]. The different types of LPL are often combined to achieve optimal functional results.

The most common procedures performed are glottal narrowing procedures (approximation LPL) for glottic insufficiency with dysphonia and/or aspiration. Injections are the most common procedures to medialize the vocal folds, although for the most part injectables are temporary. Different techniques and implants (Silastic, Gortex, hydroxylapatite, titanium, cartilage) can be used to achieve the glottic approximation [3–5].

Unilateral vocal fold paralysis (UVFP) is the most frequent reason for laryngoplasty (medialization thyroplasty type I with/without arytenoid adduction or arytenopexy). It results in incomplete glottic closure, compromising the vocal function and increasing the risk of aspiration. Most often the reason for UVFP is neural injury to vagal or recurrent laryngeal nerve. Incomplete glottic closure can also be caused by atrophy, scarring, or cricoarytenoid joint fixation. Symptoms may include hoarseness, dysphagia, aspiration, poor cough production, and frequent pneumonia. In

Anesthesia for Otolaryngologic Surgery, ed. Basem Abdelmalak and D. John Doyle. Published by Cambridge University Press.
© Cambridge University Press 2013.

the etiology of unilateral vocal fold paralysis neoplastic process has the major role, with nonlaryngeal malignancy being the leading cause (pulmonary, mediastinal malignancies, neoplasms of the base of the skull and brain metastases, neck neoplasms). Surgery (thoracic, cardiac, thyroidectomy and neck surgeries) is the second leading cause of the UVFP, but it is the first leading cause for bilateral vocal fold paralysis. Idiopathic paralysis, which is a diagnosis of exclusion, when no apparent reason for vocal fold paralysis can be found, is also a cause of UVFP in a good number of patients as well as traumatic injury (including intubation injury), cerebrovascular accidents, and infection [6,7].

Preoperative evaluation

Preoperative evaluation by the surgeon of a patient with vocal fold paralysis includes assessment of many factors and is done with subjective and objective methods. Objective tests for evaluation of voice quality may include measurement of phonatory airflow, acoustic parameters, perceptual voice analysis, and assessment of maximum phonation time (MPT). MPT is a very simple test to perform and gives very good evaluation between pre- and postoperative results in an individual patient and can be done during the surgery under light sedation.

Laryngeal videostroboscopy is an essential part of evaluation of vocal fold pathology and helps to evaluate anatomy, position, vibration and function of the vocal fold. With the advent of distal "chip-in-tip" endoscopes an assessment can be made of motion in running speech and vibration in the same examination.

Laryngoplasty is a permanent procedure and usually is reserved for the patients in whom the potential for functional recovery of the vocal fold is very small. Laryngeal EMG is currently the best method to evaluate the vocal fold innervation and determine the prognosis for recovery and is also used in preoperative evaluation of patients with vocal fold paralysis. Laryngeal EMG can help to distinguish between neural and other causes of paralysis. Even with an EMG that suggests a good prognosis, if there is no clinical evidence of recovery at 1 year following onset or injury, motion is very unlikely to return.

Preoperative subjective evaluation with different quality-of-life surveys plays an important role since LPL is a functional surgery and many patients base their decision to undergo the surgery on the level of disability they experience as a result of a voice disorder. One of the very widely used questionnaires is the Voice Handicap Index (VHI), which consists of 30 statements divided into three subgroups (functional, emotional, and physical). It is useful for comparison of results pre- and post-intervention in the same patient as well as the results of different studies [8].

Surgical procedure (medializaton laryngoplasty (thyroplasty) with/without arytenoids adduction or arytenopexy)

This surgery is performed with the patient in the supine position with the neck slightly extended. Typically, the patient is given dexamethasone (10 mg) and an antibiotic at the beginning of the procedure. Oxygen can be delivered via a mask or a nasal cannula placed in the mouth. Local anesthetic is used to anesthetize the skin at the incision and soft tissues down to the thyroid cartilage. One of the most common local anesthetics used is a mixture of 1% lidocaine with 1:100 000 of epinephrine and 0.25% bupivacaine (50:50 mixture). Nasal mucosa is topicalized with 4% lidocaine after spraying it with oxymetazoline, a nasal decongestant. A flexible videolaryngoscope can be used during the procedure either continuously or intermittently. The flexible videolaryngoscope is passed through the nose on the opposite site from the paralysis if possible and is suspended if being used to visualize the larynx through the entire case (Figure 26.1).

Incision is made horizontally at about the midpoint of the thyroid cartilage and begins just lateral to the midline on the non-involved side and extends laterally on the involved side to about the lateral aspect of the thyroid cartilage (7–8 cm long) (Figure 26.2). After dissection is done and thyroid cartilage is exposed, a window in the anterior cartilage is created with the preservation of the inner perichondrium (it is just elevated in all directions, the most being in the posterior direction). Carving the Silastic prosthesis is the most critical part of the procedure and requires significant experience. The determination whether the prosthesis is appropriate is made with a combination of intraoperative assessments: the size and angle of the thyroid cartilage, the quality of the patient's voice, the laryngoscopic appearance of the position of the

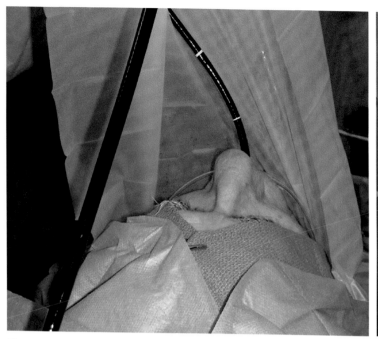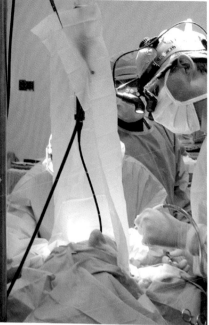

Figure 26.1. The fiberoptic scope is inserted nasally with the help of topical anesthesia and is positioned hanging from an IV pole. This arrangement allows for laryngeal visualization during the surgery. Images courtesy of Drs. B. Abdelmalak and R. Lorenz of Cleveland Clinic Reprinted with permission, Cleveland Clinic Center for Medical Art & Photography © 2011–2012. All rights reserved.

prosthesis and the amount of medialization of the vocal fold, and the MPT. An excellent voice may not occur immediately in the operating room even with a good prosthesis since many patients have developed compensatory, hyperfunctional voice behaviors that they may need to correct. Patients who have a vocal fold paralysis from lung surgery or have simply reduced pulmonary reserve may not be able to support the voice in the surgical position. In such cases, a midline position of the vocal fold and a dramatic improvement in MPT would predict good long-term results.

In cases of small defects Gortex can be used for the medialization of the vocal fold. Gortex has less long-term predictability as it is compressible and may shift over time. High or overcorrected Gortex implants may result in extrusion and require revision.

If an arytenoid adduction is to be performed at the same time as the medialization thyroplasty, the prosthesis is removed and a posterior window is created in the thyroid cartilage so that a stitch can be placed and pulled forward to allow the vocal process of the arytenoid to rotate medially in a vertical plane which is at the same level as on the other side. The prosthesis is then replaced and the position of the vocal fold is verified.

The wound is closed, and a small drain (rubber band) and a light pressure dressing are applied. Such surgeries are done almost exclusively as outpatient procedures unless there is a medical indication to admit the patient. They are re-evaluated with flexible laryngoscopy 3 hours after the procedure to ensure there is no bleeding or hematoma and discharged to be seen the next day for drain removal.

Monitored anesthesia care for laryngoplasty

Laryngoplasty is a functional surgery and as such it is important to have a patient who is able to cooperate during the procedure and be able to verbalize at the surgeon's request. Although the surgery can be done under sole local anesthesia performed by the surgeon, many patients find it uncomfortable and require some form of sedation, particularly during the initial injection. Most patients tolerate the entire procedure well with minimal sedation with a brief period of propofol-induced deep sedation at the time of the local anesthetic injection. They are then weaned off the sedation in order to maximize their cooperation with the surgeon. This is the preferred technique.

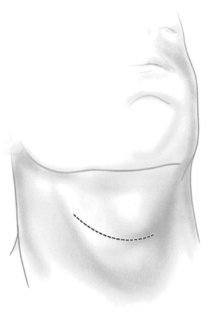

Figure 26.2. Location of the incision at the midpoint of the thyroid cartilage, extending from just lateral to the midline on the uninvolved side and then extending 5–7 cm in length. Reprinted with permission, Cleveland Clinic Center for Medical Art & Photography © 2011–2012. All rights reserved.

Those rare patients who require more sedation may provide a number of challenges for the anesthesiologist: provision of adequate sedation, patient comfort and anxiolysis, adequate airway control with the challenge of a shared airway, requirement for a patient to remain cooperative and be able to phonate or rapid reversibility of sedation when needed.

Traditionally the procedure has been done using opioids, benzodiazepines, propofol (as boluses or an infusion) [3,9,10]. These combinations may be difficult to titrate, often producing under-sedation or over-sedation and making it difficult to achieve the degree of cooperation needed to maximize the voice outcome or even risking airway collapse or apnea in some cases.

Dexmedetomidine, an α_2-adrenoreceptor agonist, has been successfully used for sedation during LFS [11–13]. It has unique properties of anxiolysis, sedation, analgesia and some amnestic properties with minimal respiratory depression and thus significantly reduced risk of airway collapse. The sedation with dexmedetomidine is similar to natural sleep and provides a comfortable, sleeping patient, who is easily aroused when needed and able to verbalize [14–17].

Jense et al. [11]. reported the use of dexmedetomidine as a sole agent in 14 patients during LFS. Twelve out of 14 patients received a bolus of dexmedetomidine (0.2–1 µg/kg), followed by an infusion; the remaining two had an infusion started without a bolus. On average, each patient received an additional three boluses of dexmedetomidine of 0.32 µg/kg during the duration of the surgery.

Abdelmalak et al. [13] reported the use of dexmedetomidine in one patient for LFS and it was used in a more conventional way with an initial bolus of 1 µg/kg, followed by an infusion 0.6 µg/kg/h titrated to the effect.

Another three patients in whom dexmedetomidine was used for sedation for LFS were reported by Busick et al. [12]. In all patients sedation was supplemented with opioids and midazolam and in two of them additional propofol infusion was used.

Few minor negative side effects were reported in all 18 patients: one patient had an episode of tachycardia and three patients had bradycardia. All episodes were self-limiting and asymptomatic. One patient in the Busick et al. report, where dexmedetomidine was used in combination with opioids, midazolam and low-dose propofol infusion, developed mild hypotension and bradycardia towards the end of the procedure, although it did not require any intervention. In the study, three additional patients developed brief episodes of airway obstruction resolved with a chin lift or lightening of sedation.

Although the published experience in dexmedetomidine use in LFS is limited, it appears to be close to an ideal agent for use in laryngoplasty due to its unique sedation profile and lack of respiratory depression.

General anesthesia for laryngoplasty

General anesthesia is considered by many of the surgeons unacceptable for laryngoplasty due to the need for the patient to verbalize during the procedure for better results. In over 1000 cases performed by the first author, not one patient has required a general anesthetic in order to complete the procedure. Nonetheless, there may be rare patients who cannot tolerate the procedure under sedation and may require general anesthesia. General anesthesia has some advantages, providing a quiet operative field with no laryngeal, cough or swallowing reflexes.

The most common procedure reported done under general anesthesia is medialization thyroplasty

(thyroplasty type 1) [18–22], with few reports describing arytenoid adduction with or without thyroplasty [23–25].

Different general anesthesia techniques were used in reported cases. Bielamowicz *et al.* [23] published their experience with 26 patients with a vagal nerve paralysis after skull base surgery who underwent early arytenoids adduction for aspiration prophylaxis under general endotracheal anesthesia.

In the majority of the other reported cases or case series a laryngeal mask was used during general anesthesia for medialization thyroplasty alone. The Pro-Seal LMA may be used in cases where esophageal reflux is a concern. The choice of anesthetic was sevoflurane or total intravenous anesthesia with propofol (with intermittent boluses of opioids or with a remifentanil infusion). Patients were either spontaneously breathing or provided with positive-pressure ventilation. Continuous flexible fiberoptic laryngoscopy was used in all cases creating a potential challenge of a shared airway. A bronchoscopic swivel connector with a diaphragm can be used to accommodate a fiberoptic scope for continuous laryngoscopy while maintaining ventilation.

Griffin *et al.* [19] and Sproson *et al.* [20] used "interrupted" general anesthesia: when the surgeon was ready to site the implant, the anesthetic was discontinued and the patient was allowed to wake up, the laryngeal mask was removed and the patient phonated at the surgeon's request. Sedation with a propofol infusion was then reinstated until the end of surgery.

The use of a laryngeal mask for procedures involving arytenoid adduction may not be suitable depending on the surgical technique: if dissection in the piriform fossa or the removal of the posterior part of thyroid cartilage is required during the surgery, the inflated cuff of the laryngeal mask may make it difficult for the surgeon to get adequate exposure. Stow *et al.* [25] suggested deflating the laryngeal mask cuff temporarily during dissection in the piriform fossa.

The question remains largely unanswered whether the results of laryngoplasty done under general anesthesia are comparable with the results when surgery is done under local anesthesia with or without sedation. Buckmire *et al.* [26] compared two surgical techniques: laryngoplasty under local anesthesia (16 patients) and laryngoplasty performed under general anesthesia with a laryngeal mask airway (four patients).

Surprisingly, the LMA subgroup demonstrated a greater degree of improvement for all measured subjective parameters (grade, roughness, breathiness, asthenia, strain of the voice; GRBAS) assessed by a skilled listener, glottal function index (GFI), and voice-related quality of life (VRQOL) than did the more standard local anesthetic subgroup. These data go against the conventional reliance on intraoperative voice testing for better functional results, but are probably biased by the small numbers, and the apparent reluctance of the surgical team in performing these cases under local anesthesia, since 1 in 4 of their patients required a general anesthetic. In addition, the use of temporary injection laryngoplasty to provide a laryngoscopic reference for the proper degree of vocal fold augmentation in the LMA group (laryngoscopic images were acquired in a clinic at a period deemed by the patient to be his/her "best postinjection voice" and used intraoperatively to guide the proper vocal fold position) may have influenced the results. Larger studies are needed to evaluate the relative vocal outcomes of type I laryngoplasty under general anesthesia.

In contrast, both the expansion laryngoplasty and relaxation thyroplasty may be performed equally well under local or general anesthesia with either jet ventilation or laryngeal mask [27] as reported by Remacle *et al.*, because the posterior displacement of the anterior cartilage segment cannot be adjusted incrementally under phonation control as is the case during medialization thyroplasty. In such cases, visual control of the airway remains very important.

Complications of laryngoplasty
Early complications

In the earlier report by Tucker *et al.* [28] 10% of the patients (six out of 60) who underwent medialization thyroplasty had significant complications. All six of these patients developed some degree of airway obstruction due to hematoma, in one patient requiring urgent tracheostomy. Only two instances of obstruction occurred in the first 24 hours, while the later four (4–7 days after the surgery) were just observed (unfortunately, the authors did not elaborate on any other non-surgical interventions). In addition, one patient had a prosthesis extrusion on the fifth postoperative day.

Another group of researchers (Cotter *et al.* [29]) did not encounter any major airway obstruction after medialization thyroplasty for unilateral vocal fold paralysis. However, they reported an 8.6% rate of major complications, mainly due to prosthesis extrusion. Minor vocal fold hematoma without airway obstruction was observed in 24% of the patients. The relatively high complication rates that are noted in these early reports are encountered much less frequently over time with refinement of technique and increased experience. In our experience in over 1000 cases of medicalization laryngogoplasty with Silastic, there have been no episodes of acute hematoma requiring surgical drainage and only three cases of edema that required admission for observation. Most patients will have bruising of the vocal folds, but without noticeable edema or swelling.

It appears that the complication rate is higher after medialization thyroplasty with arytenoid adduction/fixation or bilateral medialization thyroplasty as compared with medialization thyroplasty alone [30,31], most likely due to more extensive dissection throughout the former. Because of this, it is often recommended that patients be admitted following these procedures. Despite the very rare occurrences of an airway complication, the surgical and anesthesia teams should be prepared to establish an airway if needed. Severe airway obstruction requiring tracheostomy may occur within 24 hours after the surgery secondary to hematoma and edema. The relatively slow onset of airway obstruction makes it reasonable to use conservative measures first before proceeding with tracheostomy: racemic epinephrine, intravenous dexamethasone (8–16 mg). Heliox (a mixture of helium and oxygen) may be useful as it has reduced gaseous density and decreases work of breathing; the use of Heliox is discussed in detail in Chapter 10.

In cases of stridor and respiratory distress after medialization thyroplasty conservative measures (as above) usually suffice [30,32]. Occasionally severe vocal fold edema may develop during the surgery, necessitating termination of the procedure [22].

A different mechanism of severe dyspnea was observed by Yumoto et al. [33] in two cases requiring emergency tracheostomy in patients 1–2 days after completion of arytenoid adduction combined with type I thyroplasty (medialization). Both patients had a history of prior esophagectomy with reconstruction of the esophagus using a gastric tube. Laryngeal closure reflex triggered by esophageal regurgitation during or after taking a meal was considered to be the most probable cause of severe dyspneic attacks after a thorough evaluation.

Because of possible severe airway compromise in patients after laryngoplasty the decision to have these surgeries done as outpatient procedures needs careful consideration. Some surgeons routinely observe all patients overnight, some – in cases of unilateral medialization thyroplasty without arytenoid adduction – discharge patients the same day after re-examination of the airway 2–3 hours after the procedure. Our experience is that less than 1% of patients undergoing a medialization with Silastic or Gortex alone require admission, and we have been performing these as outpatient surgeries for over 20 years.

Late complications

The aims of medialization thyroplasty for unilateral vocal fold paralysis with or without arytenoid adduction are augmentation and median fixation of the immobile vocal fold and the postoperative glottic aperture may become narrower. Therefore, some degree of subclinical extrathoracic airway compromise may ensue after the surgery. Since it is fixed extrathoracic obstruction it affects inspiratory flow more and may not correlate with pulmonary function testing [34–36]. Flow-volume loops may demonstrate the flattening of inspiratory and expiratory portions of the loops compatible with fixed extrathoracic obstruction. As reported by Yumoto et al. [36], an increase in the index of $FEV_1/PEFR$ is also expected when upper airway obstruction is present: in upper airway obstruction a large reduction of expiratory flow occurs at high lung volumes only, so that the PEFR (peak expiratory flow rate) decreases while the FEV_1 (forced expiratory volume in 1 second) remains almost unchanged. It appears that arytenoid adduction may potentially cause more significant airway obstruction compared to medialization thyroplasty alone.

Overall, symptomatic airway obstruction is uncommon after laryngoplasty, possibly because the majority of the patients are not very active and their ventilatory demand is relatively low.

Since the glottic aperture becomes smaller, patients after medialization thyroplasty are more susceptible to airway edema after airway management for procedures unrelated to the airway [37]. Stridor may occur in the operating or recovery rooms, requiring nebulized racemic epinephrine, intravenous steroids, or in severe cases urgent tracheostomy. Airway instrumentation may also cause displacement of a thyroplasty implant [38], which may also happen spontaneously, even many months or years after the thyroplasty [28,29,39].

Any anesthesiologist must be aware of possible airway complications in such patients (fortunately, these occur rarely). To minimize the risk of airway trauma, atraumatic intubation with a small endotracheal tube should be considered if feasible, and extubation should be performed smoothly, with fully deflated cuff. Patients need close observation in the postoperative period [40].

Summary

Laryngeal frame surgery is a very dynamic and rapidly developing field. Communication with the surgeon is of utmost importance to understand the proposed procedure and better prepare for the anesthetic management.

Since it is functional surgery many surgeons prefer to operate under local anesthesia with or without sedation for the patient to be able to phonate for better surgical results.

General anesthesia may be reserved for the rare patients in whom sedation is not an option. Different techniques exist, with the laryngeal mask being the preferred airway device, if intubation is not required, allowing continuous laryngoscopy.

Anesthesiologists should be aware of rare, but possibly severe, airway complications which may happen in the recovery room as well as on the ward. In patients requiring endotracheal intubation after laryngoplasty for unrelated procedures the anesthesiologist must be extremely cautious and gentle during the airway management and in the postoperative period.

Case study

The patient was a 66-year-old male, 185.4 cm in height and weighing 79 kg, with a history of right vocal fold paralysis for 1.5 years. During evaluation for unilateral vocal fold paralysis he was found to have right posterior fossa meningioma with brain stem compression and so underwent debulking of the meningioma 1 month after the diagnosis. He later had two vocal fold injections for paralysis, the last one over a year before his current presentation. Although he had some improvement with the injections he still felt that he had significant voice fatigue. VHI score was 65. Stroboscopy showed right vocal fold immobility. The right vocal fold appeared to be in a near midline position, flaccid with phonation, with incomplete glottic closure. The CT of the head showed bulky residual posterior fossa meningioma with brainstem compression, post craniectomy, unchanged since the previous CT.

He was scheduled for a right medialization thyroplasty with Silastic prothesis.

Preoperative evaluation

Comorbidities: hyperlipidemia, GERD, PE post craniectomy (stopped coumadin 5 days before the scheduled surgery), mild to moderate OSA, improved since he lost 12 kg of his weight after the initial surgery.

Airway: MP II airway, thyromental distance of 3 finger breadths, no overbite, limited neck extension. History of easy ventilation and intubation for his brain surgery.

Anesthesia management

On the day of surgery the patient had been NPO for more than 8 hours. He appeared to be anxious, and stated that he had difficulty lying flat due to frequent cough. The ENT surgeon prefers the patient to be awake for voice control. MPT was checked by the surgeon preoperatively and was 4 seconds.

The patient was positioned supine and the, operative bed in reverse Trendelenburg position for patient comfort.

After applying standard ASA monitors, the patient was premedicated with 2 mg of midazolam IV, dexamethasone 10 mg IV, and cefazolin 1 g IV. Oxygen was delivered via MAC Safe® nasal cannula at 4 l/min.

The surgeon prepped and draped the neck and injected 20 ml of a mixture of lidocaine 1% with epinephrine 1:100 000 and 0.25% bupivacaine (50:50) after a propofol 40 mg IV bolus was given to the patient. Then the left side of the nose was topicalized with 4% lidocaine and a fiberoptic scope was passed to visualize the glottic opening (Figures 26.1 and 26.2). Before the incision the patient was fully awake and cooperative.

The surgery proceeded. After the dissection was completed and the Silastic implant carved and placed, the patient was asked to phonate and MPT was checked and the position of the vocal folds checked again. The prosthesis required some adjustment. After the position of the prosthesis was judged satisfactory, the wound was irrigated with normal saline and closed. A drain was left in place. During the procedure the patient was given only small doses of fentanyl for comfort (total of 50 µg), which was possible because of the careful use of local anesthesia and patient padding/positioning. His final MPT was 42 s and his voice improved significantly.

The patient was admitted to PACU for phase II recovery and shortly after was admitted to the hospital for overnight observation.

Potential complications

Airway edema
Hematoma
Early implant extrusion

Clinical pearls

- Unilateral vocal fold paralysis (UVFP) is the most frequent reason for laryngoplasty. It results in incomplete glottic closure, compromising the vocal function and increasing the risk of aspiration.

- Typically, the patient is given dexamethasone (10 mg) and an antibiotic at the beginning of the procedure. Oxygen can be delivered via a mask or a nasal cannula placed in the mouth.

- Local anesthetic is used to anesthetize the skin at the incision and soft tissues down to the thyroid cartilage.

- A flexible videolaryngoscope can be used during the procedure either continuously or intermittently. The flexible videolaryngoscope is passed through the nose on the opposite side from the paralysis if possible and is suspended if being used to visualize the larynx through the entire case.

- Laryngoplasty is a functional surgery and as such it is important to have a patient who is able to cooperate during the procedure and be able to verbalize at the surgeon's request. Most patients tolerate the entire procedure well with minimal sedation following a brief period of propofol-induced sedation at the time of the local anesthetic injection.

- General anesthesia with a supraglottic airway can be utilized in rare instances.

- A rare but serious early complication is varying degrees of airway obstruction secondary to hematoma; this requires the immediate attention and intervention of both the anesthesia and surgical teams.

References

1. Friederich G, de Jong FICRS, Mahien HF, Benninger MS, Isshiki N. Laryngeal framework surgery: a proposal for classification and nomenclature by the Phonosurgery Committee of the European Laryngological Society Eur. *Arch Otorhinolaryngol* 2001;**258**: 389–96.

2. Friederich G, Remacle M, Birchall M, Marie JP, Arens C. Defining phonosurgery: a proposal for classification and nomenclature by the Phonosurgery Committee of the European Laryngological Society (ELS). *Eur Arch Otorhinolaryngol* 2007;**264**: 1191–200.

3. van Ardenne N, Vanderwegen J, Van Nuffelen G, De Bodt M, Van de Heyning P. Medialization thyroplasty: vocal outcome of silicone and titanium implant. *Eur Arch Otorhinolaryngol* 2011;**268**:101–7.

4. Hendricker RM, de Silva BW, Forrest LA. Gore-Tex medialization laryngoplasty for treatment of dysphagia. *Otolaryngol Head Neck Surg* 2010;**142**:536–9.

5. Mesallam TA, Khalil YA, Malki KH, Farahat M. Medialization thyroplasty using autologous nasal septal cartilage for treating unilateral vocal fold paralysis. *Clin Exp Otorhinolaryngol* 2011;**43**:142–8.

6. Rosenthal-Swibel L, Benninger MS, Deeb RH. Vocal Fold Immobility: A Longitudinal Analysis of Etiology over 30 Years. *Laryngoscope* 2007; **117**:1864–70.

7. Ramadan HH, Wax MK, Avery S. Outcome and changing cause of unilateral vocal cord paralysis. *Otolaryngol Head Neck Surg* 1998;**118**:199–202.

8. Jacobson BH, Johnson A, Grywalski C, *et al.* The Voice Handicap Index (VHI): development and validation. *Am J Speech Lang Pathol* 1997;**6**(3): 66–70.

9. Santhanam S, Templeton L. Superficial cervical plexus block

for vocal cord surgery in an awake pediatric patient. *Anesth Analg* 2004;**98**:1656–57.

10. Donnelly M, Browne J, Fitzpatrick G. Anaesthesia for thyroplasty. *Can J Anaesth* 1995;**42**(9):813–5.

11. Jense RJ, Souter K, Davies J, Romig C, Panneerselvan A, Maronian N. Dexmedetomidine sedation for laryngeal framework surgery. *Ann Otol Rhinol Laryngol* 2008;**117**(9);659–64.

12. T. Busick, Kussman M, Scheidt T, Tobias JD. Preliminary experience with dexmedetomidine for monitored anesthesia care during ENT surgical procedures. *Am J Therapeutics* 2008;**15**;520–7

13. Abdelmalak B, Guttenberg L, Lorenz RR, *et al.* Dexmedetomidine supplemented with local anesthesia for awake laryngoplasty. *J Clin Anesth* 2009;**21**(6):442–3.

14. Kamibayashi T, Maze M. Clinical uses of alpha 2-adrenergic agonists. *Anesthesiology* 2000;**93**:1345–9.

15. Hall JE, Uhrich TD, Barney JA, Arain SR, Ebert TJ. Sedative, amnestic, and analgesic properties of small-dose dexmedetomidine infusions. *Anesth Analg* 2000;**90**:699–705.

16. Ramsay MA, Luterman DL. Dexmedetomidine as a total intravenous anesthetic agent. *Anesthesiology* 2004;**101**:787–90.

17. Nelson LE, Lu J, Guo T, *et al.* The alpha 2-adrenoreceptor agonist dexmedetomidine converges on an endogenous sleep-promoting pathway to exert its sedative effects. *Anesthesiology* 2003;**98**:428–36.

18. Grunler S, Stasey MR. Thyroplasty under general anesthesia using a laryngeal mask airway and fiberoptic

bronchoscope. *Can J Anesth* 1999;**46**(5):460–3.

19. Griffin M, Russel J, Chambers F. General anaesthesia for thyroplasty. *Anaesthesia* 1998;**53**:1202–4.

20. Sproson E, Nightingale J, Puxeddu R. Thyroplasty type I under general anaesthesia with the use of the laryngeal mask and a waking period to assess voice. *Auris Nasus Larynx* 2010;**37**: 357–60.

21. Karmarkar A, Wisely NA, Wooldridge W, Jones P. Thyroplasty under total intravenous anaesthesia with intermittent positive pressure ventilation. *Eur J Anaesthesiol* 2007;**24**(12):1041–4.

22. Razzaq I, Woolridge W. A series of thyroplasty cases under general anaesthesia. *Br J Anaesth* 2000; **85**(4):547–9.

23. Bielamowicz S, Gupta A, Sekhar LN. Early arytenoid adduction for vagal paralysis after skull base surgery. *Laryngoscope* 2000; **110**(3 Pt 1):346–51.

24. Tokashiki R, Hiramatu H, Tsukahara K, *et al.* A new procedure of arytenoids adduction combined with type I thyroplasty under general anesthesia using a laryngeal mask. *Acta Oto-Laryngol* 2007;**127**:328–31.

25. Stow NW, Lee JW, Cole I E. Novel approach of medialization thyroplasty with arytenoid adduction performed under general anaesthesia with a laryngeal mask. *Otolaryngol Head Neck Surg* 2012;**146**:266–71.

26. Buckmire RA, Bryson PC, Patel MR. Type I Gore-Tex laryngoplasty for glottic incompetence in mobile vocal folds. *J Voice* 2011;**25**(3):288–92.

27. Remacle M, Matar N, Verduyckt I, Lawson G. Relaxation

thyroplasty for mutational falsetto treatment. *Ann Otol Rhinol Laryngol* 2010;**119**(2): 105–9.

28. Tucker HM, Wanamaker J, Trott M, Hicks D. Complications of laryngeal framework surgery (phonosurgery). *Laryngoscope* 1993;**103**:525–8.

29. Cotter CS, Avidano MA, Crary MA, Cassisi NJ, Gorham MM. Laryngeal complications after type I thyroplasty. *Otolaryngol Head Neck Surg* 1995;**113**:671–3.

30. Abraham MT, Gonen M, Kraus DH. Complications of Type I thyroplasty and arythenoid adduction. *Laryngoscope* 2001;**111** (8):1322–9.

31. Weinman EC, Maragos NE. Airway compromise in thyroplasty surgery. *Laryngoscope* 2000;**110**(7):1082–5.

32. Zhao X, Roth K, Fung K. Type I thyroplasty: risk stratification approach to inpatient versus outpatient postoperative management. *J Otolaryngol Head Neck Surg* 2010;**39**(6):757–61.

33. Yumoto E, Samejima Y, Kumai Y, Haba K. Esophageal regurgitation as a cause of inspiratory distress after thyroplasty. *Am J Otolaryngol* 2006;**27**(6):425–9.

34. Janas JD, Swenson ER, Waugh P, Hillel A. Effect of thyroplasty on laryngeal airflow. *Ann Otol Rhinol Laryngol* 1999;**108**(3): 286–92.

35. Schneider B, Kneussl M, Denk DM, Bigenzahn W. Aerodynamic measurements in medialization thyroplasty. *Acta Otolaryngol* 2003;**123**(7):883–8.

36. Yumoto E, Minoda R, Toya Y, Miyamaru S, Sanuki T. Changes in respiratory function after thyroplastic surgery. *Acta Otolaryngol* 2010;**130**(1):132–7.

37. Lin HW, Bhattacharyya N. Incidence of perioperative airway complications in patients with previous medialization thyroplasty. *Laryngoscope* 2009;**119**(4):675–8.

38. Ayala MA, Patterson MB, Bach KK. Late displacement of a montgomery thyroplasty implant following endotracheal intubation. *Ann Otol Rhinol Laryngol* 2007;**116**(4):262–4.

39. Rosen CA, Murry T, DeMarino DP. Late complications of type I thyroplasty: a case report. *J Voice* 1999;**13**(3):417–23.

40. Friedlander P, Aygene E, Kraus DH. Prevention of airway complications in thyroplasty patients requiring endotracheal intubation. *Ann Otol Rhinol Laryngol* 1999;**108**(8): 735–7.

Chapter 27

Anesthesia for tracheotomy

Onur Demirci and Marc Popovich

Introduction

Over the past decade, the role of anesthesiologist during tracheotomies has evolved. Though surgical tracheotomies performed in the operating room are the norm, there is a growing trend of performing bedside percutaneous dilatational tracheotomies in the intensive care unit. For anesthesiologists the provision of care for patients undergoing tracheotomies in the operating room is a routine matter; however, with published studies finding decreased morbidity with bedside-performed percutaneous dilatational tracheotomies, anesthesiologists are challenged outside their comfort zone in the traditional operating rooms to support surgeons at the bedside in the ICU, thus adding another so-called "remote anesthesia service location". Furthermore, some intensive-care-trained anesthesiologists are opting to perform their own patients' percutaneous tracheotomies, which blurs the boundaries between a surgeon's role and that of the intensivist anesthesiologist.

The cricothyrotomy and the tracheotomy are both procedures that create a subglottic surgical airway. A cricothyrotomy is an emergency procedure that is performed with a stab incision through the cricothyroid membrane, whereas a tracheotomy usually requires a more meticulous and lengthy dissection of the neck tissues before entering the trachea between the second and third tracheal rings. Therefore most tracheotomies are performed in a more controlled environment and are considered elective or urgent procedures.

Although tracheo*tomy* and tracheo*stomy* are used interchangeably by most healthcare professionals, based on their Greek roots, the former refers to the surgical procedure of "cutting" the trachea whereas the latter refers to the "mouth" or the opening that has been created.

With references dating back to 2000 BC in the sacred Hindu scripture of Rig Veda, tracheotomies have a long history. Practitioners have been securing airways with tracheotomies long before endotracheal devices were utilized [1]. The procedure gained more acceptance in the early nineteenth century as a life-saving measure in patients with diphtheria [1]. The currently-used technique of "low" tracheotomy was advocated and standardized by Dr. Chevalier Jackson in 1932 [1]. Although the percutaneous tracheotomy was first described in 1957 by Shelden *et al.* [2], it gained popularity after two papers published by Dr. Ciaglia, a surgeon from New York, and Dr. Griggs, an intensivist from Australia, in the late 1980s [3,4]. These methods, with some modifications, led to the modern-day bedside techniques with commercially available kits including the commonly used "Blue Rhino"™ [5].

Surgical procedure

While the indications for a tracheotomy are many, they can be categorized into five groups:

1. Acute or chronic upper airway obstruction (Ludwig's angina, retropharyngeal abscess, obstructive sleep apnea).
2. Risk of or presence of chronic aspiration (stroke patients).
3. Chronic respiratory failure (ICU patients with endotracheal tubes).
4. Retention of bronchial secretions (weak cough, cystic fibrosis, severe pneumonia).
5. Elective during surgical procedures involving the head or neck (cancers of the tongue, oral cavity or the upper airways, laryngectomy).

Although there are no absolute contraindications, three instances that constitute a relative contraindication should be mentioned:

1. Uncorrected coagulopathy or thrombocytopenia (INR > 1.5 or platelet count < 50 000).
2. Presence of a laryngeal cancer (to avoid manipulation before a laryngectomy because of a possibility of stomal recurrence).
3. Hemodynamic instability in the setting of elective tracheotomy.

A surgical tracheotomy requires a vertical or transverse incision to be made approximately 2–3 cm above the sternal notch. This skin incision is carried through the subcutaneous tissue and the platysma. Once the strap muscles are retracted and the thyroid isthmus is divided, if necessary, the trachea with its rings is visualized. Depending on the surgeon's preference, the trachea is entered either through a horizontal incision between the second and third or third and fourth tracheal rings or by using an inferiorly based flap with the corresponding tracheal ring. If desired, stay sutures are placed to facilitate reintubation in case of accidental removal of the tracheotomy tube. Once the tube has been placed, it is secured using skin sutures and a circumferential tie.

Device manufacturers cite decreased procedure times and reduced hospital costs as benefits of percutaneous dilatational tracheotomies performed at the bedside in the intensive care unit [5]. However, given the relatively blind entry into the trachea, patient selection for percutaneous dilatational tracheotomy requires more stringent assessment criteria to prevent complications that might be fatal outside the controlled environment of the operating room. Therefore patients with neck masses, prior neck surgery, prior neck radiation or obese patients with large neck circumference are best served with a surgical tracheotomy.

When compared to the surgical tracheotomy, the minimally invasive percutaneous dilatational tracheotomy using a commercially available kit requires a smaller skin incision and a less involved blunt dissection of the surrounding tissues. The trachea is transilluminated between the second and third or third and fourth tracheal rings with the bronchoscope introduced through the endotracheal tube, and the trachea is entered at this site with an introducer needle. A guide wire is placed and the tract is dilated using serial dilators using a Seldinger technique. The tracheotomy tube is then placed under direct visualization with the bronchoscope and secured in a fashion similar to the surgical tracheotomy.

Finally, mention should be made of permanent tube-free tracheostomy. This is a surgical technique to create a skin-lined, non-collapsing, non-stenosing and self-sustaining stoma that does not require a cannula to keep the tract open [6].

Anesthetic management

Preoperative evaluation

It is the anesthesiologist's obligation to ensure a safe and smooth procedure. Given the multitude of indications for tracheotomy, the patients' severity of medical conditions can vary greatly. For example, the patient undergoing elective surgical tracheotomy before a glossectomy would most likely have fewer comorbid conditions than the ICU patient undergoing a percutaneous dilatational tracheotomy. Therefore a thorough history and physical examination, including the patient's current medications, infusions, and ventilator settings, if intubated, are of utmost importance. Based on these finding an appropriate laboratory workup should be ordered.

Besides the usual pre-anesthetic evaluation, some common comorbidities and problems associated with them are outlined below.

Neurological system

A full neurological exam should be performed and any deficits should be carefully recorded.

Respiratory system

History of previous neck surgery or radiation should be communicated to the surgeon due to the possibility of complications during the tracheotomy.

Patients who do not have a secure airway before the procedure should undergo a thorough airway evaluation since most of them do have an underlying anomaly of the oral cavity or upper airway. If a difficult airway is expected, the anesthesiologist must decide whether an airway should be obtained using an awake intubation technique (e.g., fiberoptic) or an awake tracheotomy.

ICU patients already intubated and mechanically ventilated should be assessed for the ventilator mode, FiO_2 and PEEP requirements. Certain ventilator modes, such as inverse ratio or bilevel, cannot be provided by most of the operating room anesthesia machines and will require an ICU ventilator. Patients on these ventilator modes as well as patients on high PEEP (especially if over 15 cmH$_2$O) should be considered for a bedside tracheotomy to prevent complications associated with patient transport.

Cardiovascular system

All patients should be evaluated for cardiac risk factors and further workup should be obtained as indicated.

When ICU patients are hemodynamically stable on pressor or inotropic support, anesthesia for tracheotomy can be safely provided in most instances. However, if hemodynamic stability is a concern, further invasive monitoring should be obtained or the case should be postponed until the patient is more stable.

Gastrointestinal system

NPO status of the patient should be verified, especially if the patient is receiving tube feeding. To achieve complete gastric emptying, tube feeds should be stopped at least 6 hours before the procedure unless the feeding tube is post-pyloric.

Coexisting ileus or small bowel obstruction might pose an aspiration risk even in intubated patients, since the cuff of the endotracheal tube will be deflated during the placement of the tracheotomy tube.

Urinary system

ICU patients have a high incidence of acute kidney injury requiring renal replacement therapy [7]. If a patient has completed a recent intermittent hemodialysis session, a period of 6 hours should elapse before proceeding with elective tracheotomy to allow equilibration of the electrolytes. Cardiac arrhythmias due to electrolyte shifts and hypotension in the immediate post-dialysis period are common.

Hematological system

The incidence of coagulopathy and thrombocytopenia in ICU patients has been reported as high as 28% and 44%, respectively [8]. Similarly, patients with malignancies who are undergoing chemotherapy have a higher risk of bleeding diathesis. Therefore, a coagulation panel and platelet count should be obtained the day of the planned procedure. If any abnormalities are detected, fresh frozen plasma and platelet concentrates might be needed to achieve an INR < 1.5 or platelet count > 50 000.

Uremic ICU patients might have abnormal platelet function despite adequate platelet counts. To investigate further, nursing staff can be asked about increased bleeding during IV starts and nasogastric tube insertion; however, a platelet function test is rarely indicated.

Laboratory tests

As mentioned above, at a minimum, a coagulation panel, complete blood count with platelets and a metabolic panel should be drawn the day of surgery. Other laboratory values might be needed as indicated by the history and physical exam.

Premedication

For awake tracheotomies, an anxiolytic like midazolam with the addition of a potent opiate like fentanyl should be used.

In critically ill patients or if there is a concern for difficult airway or impeding acute upper airway obstruction, premedication should be used very judiciously or avoided all together.

Patients receiving steroids may benefit from stress dose steroids, e.g., hydrocortisone 100 mg IV every 8 hours for three doses, if the tracheotomy will be performed under general anesthesia.

The surgeon should be consulted about the preference for preoperative antibiotic. Usually a first-generation cephalosporin (e.g., cefazolin 1 g IV) to cover the skin flora will be administered before incision.

Intraoperative management

Blood loss is usually minimal; therefore a functioning 18-gauge IV for access is sufficient. The majority of the ICU patients will have a central line in place, which can be used intraoperatively.

An isotonic crystalloid solution (0.9% saline or lactated Ringer's) at 2 ml/kg/h should be used as maintenance fluid; however, since most ICU patients have different maintenance fluid requirements due to coexisting conditions (e.g 5% dextrose in water for patients with hypovolemic hypernatremia or no maintenance fluids for patients who are hypervolemic), a discussion with the intensive care team preoperatively would help determine the selection and rate of maintenance fluids for these patients.

In addition to the standard ASA monitors [9], all other monitoring should be continued for ICU patients (e.g., intracranial pressure monitors, invasive cardiac index monitors, etc.).

The patient will be positioned supine. A shoulder roll to extend the neck for better surgical access will most likely be utilized by the surgeon.

Awake tracheotomies will require local anesthetic to be injected to the incision site and deeper tissues by the surgeon. It is important to communicate with the surgeon in order to avoid exceeding the toxic dose for the local anesthetic used. The procedure will be completed under monitored anesthesia care with minimal sedation until the surgeon secures the airway. If local anesthesia alone is not sufficient due to patient factors (e.g., preexisting anxiety disorder), intravenous sedation with dexmedetomidine infusion can be attempted. Another described approach was to convert scheduled awake tracheotomy to asleep tracheotomy, utilizing a carefully planned topicalization and sedation technique dependent mainly on a respiratory sparing sedative like dexmedetomidine [10]. Awake tracheostomy is somewhat stressful to patients, surgeons and anesthesiologists; asleep tracheotomy is a much preferred technique if feasible.

If the tracheotomy will be done under general anesthesia and the airway exam reveals possible airway difficulty, an awake fiberoptic intubation should be performed.

If no airway difficulty is expected, the patient can be induced using propofol IV titrated to blood pressure or etomidate IV, if the patient requires pressor or inotrope support.

Maintenance of anesthesia can be provided with inhaled anesthetics or total intravenous anesthesia, especially if the procedure is being performed at the bedside in the intensive care unit.

Pharmacological muscle relaxation is required to facilitate endotracheal intubation. However, while it is not required otherwise, it is preferred as it provides a motionless patient, which might contribute to ease of the procedure, and potentially less bleeding and safe cannulation of the newly formed tracheotomy.

When the surgeon is ready to incise the trachea, the FiO_2 should be decreased to less than 30%, if feasible. Next, the endotracheal tube should be advanced further into the trachea, so the incision can be made above its cuff. Once the tracheotomy is completed FiO_2 should be increased to 100% for a couple of minutes to provide an appropriate pre-oxygenation to allow time for managing the airway in case of failure to intubate the trachea through the newly created tracheotomy. Once the trachea has been entered, the cuff will be deflated (do not forget to suction orally above the cuff before deflating the cuff to avoid aspiration of pooled secretions) and the endotracheal tube will be slowly withdrawn. A sterile anesthesia circuit extension will be passed onto the surgical field to be attached to the newly placed tracheotomy tube. After the tracheotomy tube placement has been verified with the presence of end-tidal CO_2, the endotracheal tube can be removed.

Percutaneous dilatational tracheostomies will require similar intraoperative management. A swivel adapter will be attached to the endotracheal tube to allow simultaneous mechanical ventilation and visualization of trachea with the flexible broncho-scope. Rather than advancing the endotracheal tube before the trachea is entered, it must be withdrawn proximally to an immediate subglottic position to transilluminate the expected tracheotomy site. The anesthesiologist might be requested to maneuver the flexible bronchoscope in certain instances.

Postoperative management

Most patients will require mechanical ventilation and ICU admission in the immediate post-tracheotomy period. Therefore necessary monitoring and equipment to transfer the patient to the ICU should be readily available. Intravenous sedation should be continued during transport.

The anesthesia provider should be vigilant for the complications that might occur in the early postoperative period as described below. Tube dislodgement during patient transport can be especially disastrous. An endotracheal tube and a laryngoscope or a portable videolaryngoscope should be brought along for transport to secure the airway.

Although a chest X-ray has been performed customarily after all tracheotomies, it has been suggested that chest X-rays are not necessary in routine surgical tracheotomies or percutaneous dilatational tracheotomies [11,12]. Therefore chest X-rays should be obtained only after emergency or difficult procedures, or in patients suspected of having pneumothorax (symptomatic ones are mostly diagnosed clinically and managed expeditiously, as the clinical condition might be deteriorating very fast, not allowing time to obtain a chest X-ray).

The tracheotomy is a relatively painless procedure and low-dose intermittent IV narcotics can be used for postoperative analgesia.

Other considerations

Central lines placed in the internal jugular veins might pose a higher infection risk in patients with tracheotomies. It has been recommended to replace these central lines with lines in the subclavian or even femoral veins, since they have been shown to decrease the risk of catheter-related bloodstream infections in this patient group [13].

Complications

Tracheotomies are one of the most frequently performed invasive procedures among critically ill patients and carry a relatively low complication rate. Most common complications are wound infections and bleeding, with an incidence of 6.6% and 5.7%, respectively [14].

Based on the time of occurrence tracheotomy complications can be classified as intraoperative, early postoperative and late [1,15].

Intraoperative complications

Most intraoperative complications are due to close proximity of the surgical site to other major structures in the neck and thoracic cavity.

Bleeding

Although preoperative coagulopathy is a common cause of bleeding during tracheotomies in ICU patients, surgical bleeding through the anterior jugular veins and thyroid isthmus is also a common culprit. Injuries to the internal jugular veins and carotid arteries are possible but rare.

Airway fire

This feared complication during airway surgeries can be prevented by limiting $FiO_2 < 30\%$ when cautery is being used; however, this might present a challenge in patients with moderate to severe ARDS who already have a higher FiO_2 requirement. Although the American Society of Anesthesiologists' Practice Advisory recommends removing the endotracheal tube during an airway fire [16], the benefits of leaving the endotracheal tube in place for a patient who was a difficult intubation may outweigh the risks [17].

Pneumothorax and pneumomediastinum

This complication is especially concerning in children due to high pleural domes. In addition, patients with hyperinflation of the lungs due to emphysematous changes are at high risk. Both may manifest as cardiopulmonary arrest in an otherwise stable patient.

Air embolism

This may occur secondary to injury to the internal jugular vein.

Injury to nearby structures

The posterior wall of the trachea, cricoid cartilage and first tracheal ring are potential injury sites. These injuries could result in tracheal stenosis as well as in the formation of a tracheoesophageal fistula. Recurrent laryngeal nerve and vagus nerve can also be injured if the dissection is carried lateral to the trachea.

Early postoperative complications
Subcutaneous emphysema

This occurs if air is allowed to escape into the subcutaneous tissue due to an incorrectly sized tracheotomy tube. The emphysema will be reabsorbed quickly after replacing the tube with a properly fitting one, unless the tube is displaced in a false tract (see below).

Tube displacement

Any attempt to replace a displaced tracheotomy tube within the first postoperative week (before the tract has been epithelialized (mature tracheostomy)) should be done under direct visualization using a flexible bronchoscope due to the risk of creating a false lumen. If any difficulty is encountered while doing this, the patient should be reintubated orally or nasally using direct laryngoscopy and the tube replacement should be delayed until it can be done in the controlled environment of the operating room. In the case of unsuccessful endotracheal intubation attempts, bag-mask ventilation or placement of an LMA while holding pressure on the tracheal stoma to avoid air escape can prevent hypoxemia and potential catastrophic anoxia.

Tube blockage

By using humidified oxygen, tube blockage can be easily avoided. If a blockage is suspected, the inner cannula of the tracheotomy tube should be removed and inspected for any inspissated material. Further attempts to loosen and remove the blockage can be made by using saline or bicarbonate flushes along with suctioning, with either a medium-bore suction catheter or a flexible bronchoscope.

Bleeding

Minor bleeding from the skin edges should be differentiated from a more catastrophic bleeding secondary to erosion into a large vessel, such as the innominate artery. Therefore, any bleeding during the first 2 weeks warrants a thorough inspection of the wound by the surgeon.

Wound infection

Self-limiting skin infections due to skin and respiratory flora are common and usually do not require treatment; however, necrotic skin due to excessive pressure on the wound edges and prolonged use of surgical packing for bleeding will provide an excellent breeding medium for more virulent organisms and should be avoided. Extension of a superficial infection can cause tracheitis, perichondritis or even paratracheal abscess [18].

Late postoperative complications

Tracheoesophageal fistula

This complication is caused either by direct trauma to the posterior wall of the trachea during initial tracheotomy or by pressure necrosis. The patient may present with increasing oxygen requirements, signs of infection and aspiration, as well as "bubbling" from the mouth. Avoidance of high cuff pressures and large-bore feeding tubes in the esophagus will help prevent this complication. The use of fiberoptic bronchoscopy during percutaneous tracheotomies minimizes injuries to the posterior tracheal wall and therefore decreases the incidence of this complication.

Tracheal stenosis

This is mostly surgical technique related (damage to the first tracheal ring or cricoid cartilage).

Granuloma formation

Usually due to the tracheotomy tube causing irritation in the trachea, granuloma formation may manifest as bleeding during suctioning and difficulty in passing a suction catheter. This condition rarely needs treatment and can be prevented by avoidance of constant rubbing of an inappropriately fitting tracheotomy tube against the trachea.

Despite the somewhat widely spread belief that percutaneous dilatational tracheotomies have higher complication rates, a systematic review and meta-analysis published in 2006 concluded that the percutaneous dilatational tracheotomy reduces the overall incidence of wound infection, may further reduce clinically relevant bleeding and mortality when compared with surgical tracheotomy and should be considered the procedure of choice for performing elective tracheotomies in critically ill adult patients [14]. Although the decreased complication rate can be attributed to less surgical trauma to the surrounding tissue, it should be kept in mind that careful patient selection plays an important role as well.

Summary

With the increasing number of ICU admissions globally, anesthesiologists will most likely encounter more patients with chronic respiratory failure and therefore more patients requiring tracheotomies as part of their hospital course. Anesthesiologists need to have the knowledge and skills to provide care for the special needs of these patients.

Although tracheotomies are considered relatively safe procedures due to low complication rates, one should always keep in mind that there is a potential risk of losing the airway with catastrophic consequences. Therefore being prepared for any difficult or lost airway situation in terms of having well-equipped difficult-airway carts (including LMAs, intubating stylets, tube exchangers and flexible bronchoscopes) and thorough knowledge of the American Society of Anesthesiologists' difficult airway algorithm [19] can potentially improve airway management outcomes.

Case study

"Tracheotomy saves the night"

A 74-year-old female, 5′3″ (160 cm) in height and weighing 72 kg, has a history of hypertension, hyperlipidemia, hypothyroidism, peripheral vascular disease, remote tobacco use and previous cerebrovascular accident resulting in mild right-sided residual weakness.

She was admitted to the hospital for an elective left-sided carotid endarterectomy. Her pre-anesthetic evaluation revealed a small mouth opening, a limited neck range of motion and a slightly recessed chin, all of which were relatively minor. As a precaution the anesthesiologist decided to use a GlideScope Video Laryngoscope (by Verathon), which he is most experienced with. Although her larynx was noted to be anterior, a 7.0 endotracheal tube was placed without difficulty. The remainder of her intraoperative course was uneventful; she was extubated in the operating room and admitted to the intensive care unit in stable condition.

However, on postoperative day 3, she developed a new-onset right-sided hemiparesis and aphasia. An emergency CT angiogram of her brain showed a subtotal occlusion of the left-middle cerebral artery, for which she was taken to the neuroradiology suite. She underwent CT-guided revascularization with mechanical clot aspiration under monitored anesthesia care. In despite of this intervention, her hemiparesis and her aphasia did not resolve.

On the night of postoperative day 4, she was noted to be more lethargic. An arterial blood gas obtained at that time showed severe respiratory acidosis with marginal oxygenation while receiving 50% oxygen via a facemask. Although the hypercarbia was believed to be secondary to excessive narcotic administration, the intensive care physician voiced concerns of possible pneumonia due to ongoing micro-aspiration. He decided to electively intubate the patient before she deteriorated further. He notified the anesthesiologist on-call as backup after reviewing the anesthetic record from her initial surgery. He chose not to administer any sedatives or muscle relaxants, since the patient was already lethargic and made an initial attempt at direct laryngoscopy with a MAC 3 laryngoscope. This attempt was unsuccessful due to a very anterior larynx and copious thick oropharyngeal secretions. The on-call anesthesiologist made a second unsuccessful attempt using a Miller 2 laryngoscope, which was followed by a third unsuccessful attempt using a GlideScope Video Laryngoscope. At this time a flexible bronchoscope was brought to the bedside for another attempt. Unfortunately, the laryngeal structures could not be visualized due to excessive swelling and presence of blood after previous intubation attempts. The patient was easy to bag-mask ventilate throughout this episode. The anesthesiologist chose to place an LMA #4 and to notify the ENT surgeon for an urgent tracheotomy.

The patient was transferred to the operating room while being bag-ventilated through the LMA. Upon arrival at the operating room, she was placed on the operating room table in supine position and general anesthesia was administered with 0.6 MAC of sevoflurane. Any further narcotics were avoided. A shoulder roll was placed underneath the patient's shoulders and her neck was prepped and draped in sterile fashion. The ENT surgeon administered 10 ml of 0.5% bupivacaine with 1:200 000 epinephrine to achieve local anesthesia as well. Her trachea was visualized after a quick dissection; an 8.0 Shiley tracheotomy tube was placed through an incision between the third and fourth tracheal rings. After successful ventilation and verification of end-tidal carbon dioxide with capnography, the tracheotomy tube was secured with sutures. The patient was transferred back to the intensive care unit in guarded condition and placed on mechanical ventilation.

The next morning, the patient was noted to be awake and following commands, with no new neurologic sequelae from the previous night's events. On postoperative day 7 she was successfully weaned off the ventilator, but the tracheotomy was left in place for better pulmonary hygiene.

She was discharged to a skilled nursing facility on postoperative day 8 for further care and rehabilitation.

Clinical pearls

- Although tracheotomy and tracheostomy are used interchangeably by most healthcare professionals, based on their Greek roots the former refers to the surgical procedure of "cutting" the trachea whereas the latter refers to the "mouth" or the opening that has been created.
- Although there are no absolute contraindications, three circumstances constitute a relative contraindication for elective tracheostomy:
  (1) uncorrected coagulopathy or thrombocytopenia
  (2) presence of a laryngeal cancer (to avoid manipulation before a laryngectomy because of the possibility of stomal recurrence)
  (3) hemodynamic instability.
- Emergency tracheostomy can be performed under local anesthesia with no to minimal sedation; however, if time, equipment and expertise allow, awake intubation should be attempted to allow the procedure to proceed under general anesthesia.

261

- When the surgeon is ready to incise the trachea, the oxygen concentration should be decreased to 30% or less, where feasible. Next, the endotracheal tube should be advanced further into the trachea, so the incision can be made above its cuff. Once the tracheotomy is completed the oxygen concentration should be increased to 100% for a couple of minutes in case subsequent difficulties are encountered.
- Chest X-rays are not necessary in routine surgical tracheotomies or percutaneous dilatational tracheotomies, but should be obtained after

emergency or difficult procedures, or in patients suspected of having a pneumothorax.

- Central lines placed in the internal jugular veins might pose a higher infection risk in patients with tracheotomies.
- Airway fires and failure to cannulate the trachea are among the most feared complications during tracheostomy.
- Though surgical tracheotomies performed in the operating room are the norm, there is a growing trend of performing bedside percutaneous dilatational tracheotomies in the intensive care unit (ICU).

References

1. Bailey BJ, Johnson JT, Newlands SD. *Head & Neck Surgery – Otolaryngology*, 4th edn. Philadelphia: Lippincott Williams & Wilkins; 2006. pp. 786–801.

2. Shelden CH, Pudenz RH, Tichy FY. Percutaneous tracheotomy. *J Am Med Assoc* 1957; **165**(16):2068–70.

3. Griggs WM, Worthley LI, Gilligan JE, Thomas PD, Myburg JA. A simple percutaneous tracheostomy technique. *Surg Gynecol Obstet* 1990;**170**(6):543–5.

4. Ciaglia P, Firsching R, Syniec C. Elective percutaneous dilatational tracheostomy. A new simple bedside procedure; preliminary report. *Chest* 1985;**87**(6):715–9.

5. Cook Medical Ciaglia Blue Rhino® G2 Product Feature. 2011; available from: http://www.cookmedical.com/cc/datasheetFeature.do?id=4888. Accessed August 17, 2011.

6. Akst LM, Eliachar I. Long-term, tube-free (permanent) tracheostomy in morbidly obese patients. *Laryngoscope* 2004; **114**(8):1511–2; author reply 1512–3. PubMed PMID: 1528073.

7. Weisbord SD, Palevsky PM. Acute renal failure in the intensive care unit. *Semin Respir Crit Care Med* 2006;27(3):262–73.

8. Levi M, Opal SM. Coagulation abnormalities in critically ill patients. *Crit Care* 2006; **10**(4):222.

9. American Society of Anesthesiologists. Standards for Basic Anesthetic Monitoring. 2011; available from: http://www.asahq.org/For-Healthcare-Professionals/~/media/For Members/documents/Standards Guidelines Stmts/Basic Anesthetic Monitoring 2011.ashx. Accessed August 20, 2011

10. Abdelmalak B, Makary L, Hoban J, Doyle DJ. Dexmedetomidine as sole sedative for awake intubation in management of the critical airway. *J Clin Anesth* 2007;**19**: 370–3.

11. Smith DK, Grillone GA, Fuleihan N. Use of postoperative chest x-ray after elective adult tracheotomy. *Otolaryngol Head Neck Surg* 1999;**120**(6): 848–51.

12. Hoehne F, Ozaeta M, Chung R. Routine chest X-ray after percutaneous tracheostomy is unnecessary. *Am Surg* 2005;**71**(1):51–3.

13. Lorente L, Jimenez A, Naranjo C, *et al.* Higher incidence of catheter-related bacteremia in jugular site with tracheostomy than in femoral site. *Infect Control*

Hosp Epidemiol 2010; **31**(3):311–3.

14. Delaney A, Bagshaw SM, Nalos M. Percutaneous dilatational tracheostomy versus surgical tracheostomy in critically ill patients: a systematic review and meta-analysis. *Crit Care* 2006; **10**(2):R55.

15. Russell C, Matta B. *Tracheostomy: A Multiprofessional Handbook*. Cambridge: Cambridge University Press; 2004. pp. 51–7.

16. Caplan RA, Barker SJ, Connis RT, *et al.* Practice advisory for the prevention and management of operating room fires. *Anesthesiology* 2008;**108**(5): 786–801.

17. Chee WK, Benumof JL. Airway fire during tracheostomy: extubation may be contraindicated. *Anesthesiology* 1998;**89**(6):1576–8.

18. Cole AG, Kerr JH. Paratracheal abscess after tracheostomy. *Intensive Care Med* 1983;9(6):345–7.

19. Practice guidelines for management of the difficult airway: an updated report by the American Society of Anesthesiologists Task Force on Management of the Difficult Airway. *Anesthesiology* 2003; **98**(5):1269–77.

Chapter

28

Anesthesia for the management of subglottic stenosis and tracheal resection

John George III and D. John Doyle

Introduction

Subglottic stenosis (Figure 28.1) can be divided into two broad categories: congenital and acquired. The congenital causes of subglottic stenosis account for a small proportion of the disease. While inflammatory diseases such as Wegener's granulomatosis are a common cause of subglottic strenosis, a great many cases of subglottic stenosis are the result of prolonged endotracheal intubation. In the pediatric population, incidence rates as high as 24% occurred during the 1960s in association with prolonged endotracheal intubation. As familiarity with the technique and advances in the care of the disease progressed, the incidence of subglottic stenosis cited most commonly is 1–8%, with an incidence less than 1% if infants weighing less than 1500 g are excluded [1]. Similarly, the incidence in the adult population ranges from 1% to 8%.

Anatomy

Infant airway anatomy differs from the airway in the adolescent and adult. When considering the larynx specifically, four distinctions can be made: (1) the infant larynx is approximately one-third the size of the adult larynx; (2) the vocal cords are angled and the vocal process of the arytenoids comprises a larger portion of the length of the vocal cords in infants; (3) the cricoid in infants is located about the fourth cervical vertebra while in the adult it is roughly at the sixth vertebral level; and (4) the narrowest portion of the airway in adults is the glottic opening while in infants it is at the cricoid ring of the subglottis. Various tissues in the infant, in general, seem to have more elasticity than in the adult. It is this increased elasticity in association with less fibrous

tissue and the airway differences noted above that predispose infants to a greater incidence of airway narrowing from edema.

Etiology

Congenital causes of subglottic stenosis overwhelmingly occur in utero and result from malformation of the cricoid cartilage. The diagnosis is considered to be congenital if the patient has not had a history of endotracheal intubation and has an absence of other potential causes of stenosis. Severe conditions typically present during childhood, while milder forms can present in adolescence or even in adult life.

Acquired forms of subglottic stenosis most commonly occur from trauma to airway tissue, with 90–95% a result of endotracheal intubation. The factors that are consistently cited as causative include the duration of intubation, the size of the endotracheal tube, frequent manipulation of the endotracheal tube, and repeated intubations, with the duration of intubation being the most important factor. While reports of severe injury have been reported in periods less than 24 hours, a 7–10-day period of endotracheal intubation in the ICU is considered acceptable, with increasing potential for injury beyond that time frame. A variety of other factors can also contribute to the formation of subglottic stenosis as shown in Table 28.1.

Pathophysiology

As mentioned previously, the main cause of acquired subglottic stenosis is prolonged endotracheal intubation. The use of a tube too large for the airway, a tube with an overinflated cuff, or a tube surrounded by an edematous airway can lead to mucosal

Anesthesia for Otolaryngologic Surgery, ed. Basem Abdelmalak and D. John Doyle. Published by Cambridge University Press.
© Cambridge University Press 2013.

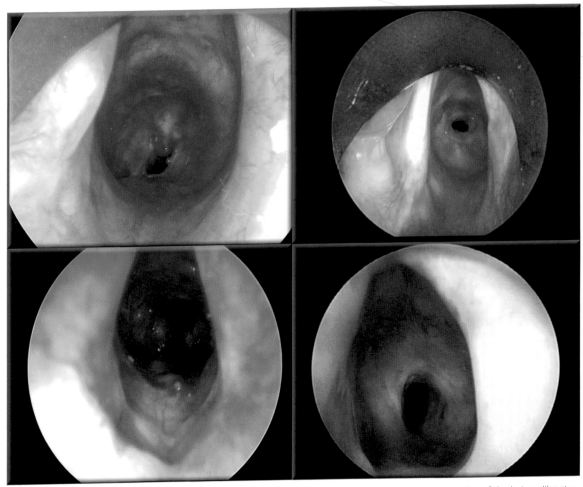

Figure 28.1. Examples of laryngotracheal stenosis. Treatment may involve expectant management, laser excision of the lesion, dilatation using a rigid bronchoscope or high-pressure inflatable balloon, and tracheal reconstruction. Reused from http://upload.wikimedia.org/wikipedia/commons/d/de/Laryngotracheal_stenosis_001.jpg, author rncantab under a Creative Commons license.

Table 28.1. Factors that contribute to the formation of subglottic stenosis

Iatrogenic causes	Autoimmune diseases
Past surgery	Polychondritis
Radiotherapy	Sarcoidosis
Tracheostomy	Wegener's
	granulomatosis
Bacterial conditions	Neoplasms
Mycobacterium	
tuberculosis	
External injury	

compression. Persistent compression leads to ischemia, and ultimately ulceration. This ulceration potentially leads to perichondritis and chondritis, which after healing by secondary intention results in scar tissue and weakened cartilage [2].

Gastroesophageal reflux disease is well known not only for its debilitating effects on the esophagus, but also for its role in many respiratory disease processes. Many patients with subglottic stenosis have a coexisting history of gastroesophageal reflux disease. Not only has it been implicated as the causal source of subglottic stenosis in those patients presenting without a history of endotracheal intubation, but it also may be the cause of restenosis after laryngotracheal reconstruction/repair (LTR) [2].

Disease classification

While subglottic stenosis (or laryngotracheal stenosis, to use the broader term) can affect all age groups, most experts differentiate the disease and its process based on a pediatric or adult presentation. The same is true for classifying the disease. Myer *et al.* [3] revised the original Cotton grading system for assessing severity of pediatric laryngotracheal stenosis. The system uses endotracheal size as a measure of airway diameter. Comparing the largest-size endotracheal tube that permits an audible leak pressure between 10 cm and 25 cm in an age-matched pediatric patient with and without the disease is how the stenotic percentage is calculated [3]. It consists of four grades: grade 1 is no obstruction to 50% obstruction, grade 2 is 51% obstruction to 70% obstruction, grade 3 is 71% obstruction to 99% obstruction, and grade 4 is no detectable lumen. While this system is a useful tool to assess the grade of subglottic severity and to predict the success rate of decannulation of pediatric tracheostomy patients, it does have limitations. The system probably has less value as a prognostic indicator in patients with multiple sites of airway disease, or with airway inflammation, or in the case of trauma from multiple intubation attempts [3]. Using cross-sectional area as a guide to consistently determine successful decannulation in the adult population is challenging at best, and therefore the McCaffrey system [4] for adults was created.

Defining treatment success as time to decannulation, McCaffrey collected data on age, sex, etiology, site of stenosis, length of stenosis, diameter of stenosis, and the surgical technique. Of these, only site and diameter of the stenosis had independent effects on the time to decannulation [4]. Based on this finding, he developed the four-stage system used to classify adult laryngotracheal stenosis. Stage 1 lesions are confined to the subglottis or trachea and are less than 1 cm, stage 2 lesions are subglottic stenoses longer than 1 cm within the cricoid ring and not extending to the glottis or trachea, stage 3 lesions are subglottic stenoses that extend into the upper trachea but do not involve the glottis, and stage 4 lesions involve the glottis and cause fixation or paralysis of one or both of the vocal cords.

Surgical management

No definitive medical therapies have been found to treat the disease process found in subglottic stenosis.

Steroids and antibiotics have been shown to limit the extent of granulation tissue in animal studies, but exact doses and duration of treatment in humans is unknown. Underlying medical causes (such as infectious or inflammatory causes) should be treated. Gastroesophageal reflux disease should also be aggressively treated to aid positive surgical results as well as to minimize potential restenosis that can occur following surgical repair. Ultimately, surgical correction is the definitive therapy.

Initial surgical approaches typically consist of endoscopic procedures, especially for mild disease. Two of the more common endoscopic procedures performed are dilatation and/or use of a carbon dioxide laser. Either procedure can be performed with or without the use of steroids or mitomycin therapy. Mitomycin, an antineoplastic agent, limits fibroblast growth and activity. It ideally aids endoscopic results by minimizing scar reformation. Severer forms of subglottic stenosis require a more invasive approach to treatment, namely open surgical reconstruction.

While various forms of reconstruction exist, there are four main procedures (each with multiple variations): (1) anterior cricoid split; (2) a single-stage approach using auricular, costal, or thyroid cartilage; (3) a multistage procedure involving various combinations of anterior and posterior cartilaginous grafting and stenting; and (4) cricotracheal resection. Of these, laryngotracheal reconstruction and cricotracheal resection are the procedures more routinely performed. The goal and measure of success of open surgical procedures is the decannulation rate. While a logical conclusion of which surgical procedure to use would be the one that offers the highest decannulation rate, no studies to date have compared matched patients to each of the surgical procedures. Laryngotracheal reconstruction has the advantage of being less invasive, but they have similar decannulation rates in patients with severe forms of subglottic stenosis (severe grade 3 and grade 4). Despite this observation, cricotracheal resection is typically the preferred surgical option for patients with severe grade 3 or grade 4 stenosis while laryngotracheal reconstruction is chosen for grade 2 and less severe grade 3 patients. The rationale is that while the decannulation rates are similar with severe stenosis and LTR is a less invasive procedure, comparatively more patients treated with LTR require a second surgery to achieve decannulation [1].

Use of stents

While the first reports of the use of airway stents were in 1915 and concerned stents made of rubber, the first mainstream stents were made of silicone. Today, stent selection includes not only silicone, but also self-expanding metal stents. Newer stent design allows stents to be retrievable, which is a very attractive feature for benign airway disease in particular. Silicone stents are easier to remove, and resist tumor ingrowth and granulation tissue accumulation. The disadvantages of using them are the potential for stent migration and the elimination of mucociliary clearance in the stented segment [5]. Metal stents are nitinol- or alloy-based. They can be deployed with smaller sheaths or over flexible bronchoscopes with minimal impact on mucociliary clearance. These stents too have the potential for migration, but a greater disadvantage is an eventual build-up of granulation tissue, particularly on the edges of these stents. Additional complications of either stent used are pneumothorax, pneumonitis, empyema, stent fractures, or hemoptysis due to erosion of a stent into blood vessels.

The airway stents currently used are designed for use in benign airway disease, preoperatively to restore airway patency prior to surgical treatment, and for malignant airway disease prior to chemoradiation, with malignancy being the most common indication for their use. The benign airway diseases or problems for which stents are commonly used are post-lung transplant strictures, radiation-induced airway stenosis, relapsing polychondritis, granulomatous disease such as Wegener's, congenital disease, and strictures from prolonged intubation to name a few. Airway stents for benign diseases, as mentioned previously, pose great challenges due to poor long-term patency due to the build-up of granulation tissue, and as a consequence patients with benign diseases require multiple procedures to maintain stent patency. Studies report the rate of granulation tissue formation on metal stents to be as high as 18%, while the need for repeat interventions to maintain airway patency ranges from 41% to 87% [5,6]. The average functional life of metal stents is around 12 months [6]. It is because of these problems that most advocate stent placement for benign conditions in only a select group of patients. Selection criteria recommendations include patients who have failed endoscopic management, are medically unsuitable for open procedures, and are not candidates for T-tube use or for frequent screening and therapeutic endoscopies.

Anesthetic management

Because managing the airway in these patients is often associated with great difficulty, collaboration amongst both the anesthesia and surgical teams should take place prior to the surgery. Special equipment such as multiple sizes of endotracheal tubes (ETT) or emergency tracheotomy kits should be readily available. An anesthetic plan should also be formulated which takes into account avoidance of airway irritants that may cause coughing or lead to total airway occlusion. Preoperative medications to limit or prevent gastroesophageal reflux are often given. The decision whether to premedicate with drugs such as benzodiazepines or opiates is controversial. A patient with imminent total airway occlusion might best be promptly brought to the operating room without sedation where equipment and personnel to perform an emergency surgical airway are available. Alternatively, pharmacologic anxiolysis may improve respiratory conditions in a patient without airway obstruction who may have some respiratory compromise due to the stress of the perioperative period. Ultimately, the decision should be made according to the clinical picture at hand.

Intravenous access typically consists of two peripheral IV lines (one in each upper extremity). If central venous access is being considered, location of its placement should be carefully considered, as the location must avoid compromising the surgical field. Standard ASA monitors are used. Blood pressure monitoring is most effectively accomplished with the use of an arterial line; not only does it provide continuous blood pressure monitoring, but it also provides a means for sampling blood in order to assess oxygenation, ventilation, and any electrolyte abnormalities. A left radial arterial line is the preferred site as confusion about a hypotensive state by inadvertent surgical compression of the innominate artery can be avoided. Along the same reasoning, the pulse oximeter should be placed on the right hand to alert to the presence of innominate artery compression.

The anesthetic intraoperative course for open surgical correction of this disease can be divided into five phases: (1) induction and intubation, (2) surgical dissection, (3) open airway, (4) surgical closure, and (5) emergence and extubation [7]. Of these, induction and intubation, open airway, and the emergence and extubation phases present the most challenging portion of the procedure for the anesthesiologist.

One of the main challenges during induction is establishing an airway in the face of a potentially severely stenotic airway with the possibility of a total airway occlusion. Additionally, a confounding complicating factor is the inability to utilize options typically available in the difficult airway algorithm such as transtracheal ventilation, tracheostomy, or other surgical airways due to the pathology found in subglottic stenosis. Based on these findings, an inhalational induction is sometimes chosen. The advantages of an inhalational induction are preservation of spontaneous ventilation and maintaining a patent airway with minimal airway irritation (due to the use of sevoflurane or halothane). The disadvantages include a prolonged passage through the excitement phase due to airway narrowing, and hypotension from the deep inhalational induction levels required for airway manipulation and intubation [5].

The second technique for induction that is more commonly used is total intravenous anesthesia (TIVA). This technique offers a rapid onset of induction and ease of titration during maintenance of anesthesia, facilitating smooth emergence and extubation. While TIVA has the advantage of avoidance of the problems found with an inhalational induction the technique has the potential to abolish spontaneous ventilation, potentially leading to total airway obstruction.

Bronchoscopy usually follows induction. Dilatation of the airway is performed first if the stenotic segment is roughly 5 cm or less. Serial dilatations are performed with dilators and pediatric bronchoscopes. Reports of the use of an esophageal bougie have also been published and potentially this may be less traumatic [8]. Following bronchoscopy, the intubation is performed. Depending upon the location of the lesion, an ETT can be placed above the lesion or through the lesion with a small (6 mm outside diameter) ETT if a proximal lesion is present. A cuffed 6 mm ETT is usually the smallest-size tube required, but an uncuffed tube may sometimes be required for severe stenotic lesions. Great care should be exercised on intubation attempts as tissue dislodgement, bleeding, and edema can quickly occur. Once a secure airway is established, maintenance of anesthesia usually consists of a TIVA approach. While excessive use of narcotics should be avoided in order to obtain prompt extubation at the conclusion of the surgery, propofol combined with remifentanil works well

for producing amnesia and providing intraoperative pain relief. An intermediate-acting muscle relaxant can be used sparingly throughout the case to prevent inadvertent patient movement, which is especially important during the open airway portion of the procedure. The open airway portion of the procedure poses the second major concern for the anesthesiologist. Gas exchange during this portion can be performed in one of four ways: (1) jet ventilation, (2) distal tracheal intubation and intermittent positive pressure ventilation, (3) spontaneous ventilation, and (4) cardiopulmonary bypass.

Multiple case reports have been written on the use of high-frequency jet ventilation (HFJV) for tracheal resection. The jet ventilation catheter is inserted through the ETT and passed into the distal trachea. Some of the advantages reported for HFJV are a simple approach to airway management, a surgical field unobstructed by the ETT, adequate control of gas exchange, and continuous gas flow coming out of the trachea [9]. One of the major risk factors of HFJV is barotrauma, and great care must be taken to limit excessive intrathoracic pressures. An additional drawback is the potential for hypercarbia due to hypoventilation.

The distal tracheal intubation technique is probably the most common method of ventilating during the open airway phase of the surgery. With this technique, the ETT is pulled back above the lesion (if not already in that location), and the distal trachea is intubated with a new ETT sterilely inserted by the surgeon. The tip of this tube rests in the trachea in high and mid-tracheal lesions, whereas for low tracheal or carinal lesions the tip can be placed in either mainstem bronchus, allowing one lung ventilation. Prior to anastomosis, the trachea must again be intubated. Reintubation typically consists of the surgeon pulling either the proximal ETT or a new one into the trachea past the anastomotic site.

Only a couple of reports have been published which document spontaneously breathing patients throughout the procedure. Two reports were of patients who were endotracheally intubated above the lesion and allowed to breathe spontaneously with oxygen flowing through the endotracheal tube. The other was a patient with a patent tracheal stoma allowed to breathe spontaneously with oxygen delivered through a catheter passed through the stoma [6]. Currently, novel approaches are being described and used in clinical practice making use of cervical epidural anesthesia. The epidural in these patients not only allows a patient to breath spontaneously throughout the case, but the patients are also awake for the airway surgery [10].

Cardiopulmonary bypass (CPB) and extracorporeal membrane oxygenation (ECMO) have both been described and used for tracheal surgery. They allow gas exchange while completely bypassing the stenotic lesion. While CPB can be a life-saving maneuver as a last resort for near or total tracheal occlusion, the potential risk of excessive bleeding due to anticoagulation requirements is present. Tracheal resection can therefore be done completely under CPB or only to establish an airway on induction [11,12].

Extubation at the conclusion of the procedure is most often the goal due to the potential for stress and potential disruption of the anastomosis from mechanical ventilation. Additionally, prolonged intubation is not only a common cause of subglottic stenosis, it also can predispose to an increased restenosis rate, which is another reason for early extubation. The neck is usually placed in flexion during the closure and a chin stitch placed. Maintaining this position during emergence is important as well as reminding the patient during emergence and after extubation to keep the neck flexed. Although the absence of significant airway swelling should be assessed prior to extubation by noting an air leak with ETT cuff deflation, it can still be present. Airway swelling can be temporarily treated by elevating the head of the bed until a more definitive treatment with racemic epinephrine can be obtained. Immediately following extubation, hearing the patient speak is important in order to exclude potential unilateral or bilateral recurrent nerve injury.

Postoperative management

Because the immediate postoperative period is such a tenuous time in terms of airway compromise for these patients, they are typically admitted to the intensive care unit (ICU) for postoperative management. While the goal for the majority of these patients is prompt extubation, concerns over airway edema or the need for continued ventilator support may warrant mechanical means of controlling the airway beyond that done in the operating room. This can be in the form of a small endotracheal tube, tracheostomy tube, or a T-tube. Regardless of the presentation to the ICU, all of these patients are started on humidified oxygen in

Table 28.2. Complications of tracheal surgery

Mucus plug occlusion

Wound infection or abscess formation

Granulation tissue formation

Bleeding/hematoma

Subcutaneous emphysema

Pneumothorax and/or pneumomediastinum

Stent problems (e.g., migration, breakage)

Re-formation of stenosis

Injury to recurrent or superior laryngeal nerves

Airway obstruction

Death

an attempt to minimize the risk of anastomotic disruption.

Potential complications of tracheal surgery are numerous, and can be found in Table 28.2. The need for reintubation because of any of these complications poses a serious problem. If required, an uncuffed 6 mm ETT is a reasonable first option, and care should be taken to avoid disruption of the anastomosis. While direct laryngoscopy may be possible, fiberoptic intubation is likely to be a better choice. Once reintubated, visualization of the tip of the ETT below the anastomosis should be verified.

Summary

While tracheal resection for subglottic stenosis has a relatively low occurrence rate, appropriate planning must be undertaken for those few surgeries. A well-thought-out anesthetic plan involves not only the anesthesiologist but also close collaboration and communication with the surgeon throughout the entire perioperative period. While this is true of most surgeries it is even more of a reality during these surgeries due to abnormal anatomy, potential for loss of the airway, and because the airway is shared by both anesthesiologist and surgeon. The main goals for the anesthesia provider during these cases should be having a variety of options for gaining and maintaining control of the airway, providing adequate anesthesia while maximizing surgical field exposure, and being able to extubate the patient at the end of the procedure.

Case study

The patient was a 33-year-old woman, 60 kg and 170 cm tall, who had suffered from Wegener's granulomatosis for almost a decade. Complications from the condition included structural damage to the nose (chondritis), past periods of renal insufficiency, as well as tracheal stenosis. Treatment included prednisone and cyclophosphamide.

The nose had previously been repaired using a bone graft while the trachea had been dilated a number of times previously. Each time when her breathing became difficult again she would be brought to the operating room for dilatation. Here, standard monitors were applied, followed by induction of anesthesia with propofol, fentanyl, midazolam and rocuronium. A size 5.0 ID MLT endotracheal tube was inserted effortlessly and positive-pressure ventilation with air/oxygen was achieved without difficulty. For maintenance of anesthesia the patient received TIVA, consisting of propofol 500 mg and remifentanil 1 mg mixed in a 60 ml syringe, starting at around 100 µg/kg/min of propofol. The surgeon than placed a suspension laryngoscope and removed the ETT while the patient was ventilated using the jet ventilation adapter to the suspension laryngoscope. The chest was seen to rise appropriately with each breath (30 psi of driving pressure in an initial pattern of 1 second on – 3 seconds off). Using the suspension laryngoscope and a long knife, the surgeon then made radial cuts through the stenosis, followed by balloon dilatation and the application of mitomycin. Following this the patient was reversed and allowed to wake up from anesthesia using an anesthesia face mask. Postoperatively she described her breathing as "much better".

Two years later, the patient returned again with severe tracheal stenosis, but this time she had become refractory to the above previously successful procedure due to excessive scarring. A decision was thus made to perform a formal tracheal resection (excision of the involved tracheal segments).

This time general anesthesia was induced as above, and an MLT size 4 ETT was inserted orally deep into the trachea, passing through the tracheal resection site and ending up with the tip immediately above the carina. A radial arterial line was inserted. The surgeon began exposing the trachea. When the tracheal incision was performed, the ETT cuff was deflated and the ETT retracted back above the incision site, then left in place. A transfield reinforced ETT size 5 was then inserted into the distal trachea. When the resection was completed and the end-to-end anastomosis was near completion, the transfield ETT was removed, and the original tube was pushed down the trachea under direct vision to its original position. The tracheal anastomosis was then completed. At all critical times the patient was ventilated with 100% oxygen, while at other times the oxygen levels were kept in the 30–40% range to reduce the chance of an airway fire. For the most part, scissors and blades were used to accomplish the tracheal resection, although when bleeding was anticipated or encountered electrocautery was used with the above-noted fire precautions. At the end of the surgery the patient was woken up very gently, and then extubated. She was then admitted to PACU for a standard recovery, and then to a step-down unit specialized in managing airway patients.

Clinical pearls

- Many patients with subglottic stenosis without a history of endotracheal intubation have a history of gastroesophageal reflux disease causing the subglottic stenosis; this also may be the cause of restenosis after laryngotracheal reconstruction.
- Silicone stents are easier to remove, and resist tumor ingrowth and granulation tissue accumulation. The disadvantages of using them are the potential for stent migration and the elimination of mucociliary clearance in the stented segment.
- Metal stents can be deployed via flexible bronchoscopes and have minimal impact on mucociliary clearance. These too have the potential for migration, but a greater disadvantage is an eventual build-up of granulation tissue.
- Patients with tracheal or subglottic stenosis are usually not difficult to mask ventilate (in the absence of other causes of the same) once general anesthesia is induced and a muscle relaxant has been administered.
- Multiple sizes of endotracheal tubes (ETT) and emergency tracheotomy kits should be readily available in managing tracheal stenosis patients.
- A left radial arterial line is the preferred site because inadvertent surgical compression of the innominate artery will produce false pressure readings in the right arm. Similarly, the pulse

oximeter should be placed on the right hand to alert to the presence of innominate artery compression.

- During the open airway portion of tracheal resection, gas exchange can be performed in one of four ways: (1) jet ventilation, (2) distal tracheal intubation and intermittent positive pressure ventilation, (3) spontaneous ventilation, and (4) cardiopulmonary bypass.

- Extubation at the end of the procedure is most often the goal to avoid the potential disruption of the anastomosis from mechanical ventilation. The neck is usually placed in flexion during the closure and a chin stitch placed to maintain this position during emergence and after extubation as well.

- Postoperatively these patients are typically admitted to the intensive care unit (ICU) for postoperative management.

References

1. Hartley BEJ, Cotton RT. Pediatric airway stenosis: laryngotracheal reconstruction or cricotracheal resection? *Clin Otolaryngol* 2000;**25**:342–9.

2. Eid EA. Anesthesia for subglottic stenosis in pediatrics. *Saudi J Anaesth* 2009;**3**(2):77–82.

3. Myer CM 3rd, O'Connor DM, Cotton RT. Proposed grading system for subglottic stenosis based on endotracheal tube sizes. *Ann Otol Rhinol Laryngol* 1994;**103**(4 Pt 1):319–23.

4. McCaffrey TV. Classification of laryngotracheal stenosis. *Laryngoscope* 1992;**102**:1335–40.

5. Walser, EM. Stent placement for tracheobronchial disease. *Eur J Rad* 2005;**55**:321–30.

6. Eller RL, Livingston WJ 3rd, Morgan CE, *et al.* Expandable tracheal stenting for benign disease: worth the complications? *Ann Otol Rhinol Laryngol* 2006;**115**(4):247–52.

7. Sandberg W. Anesthesia and airway management for tracheal resection and reconstruction. *Int Anesthesiol Clin* 2000;**38**(1): 55–75.

8. Pinsonneault C, Fortier J, Donati F. Tracheal resection and reconstruction. *Can J Anesth* 1999;**46**(5):439–55.

9. Magnusson L, Lang FJW, Monnier P, Ravussin P. Anaesthesia for tracheal resection: report of 17 cases. *Can J Anaesth* 1997;**44**(12):1282–5.

10. Macchiarini P, Rovira I, Ferrarello S. Awake upper airway surgery. *Ann Thorac Surg* 2010;**89**:387–91.

11. Chiu CL, Teh BT, Wang CY. Temporary cardiopulmonary bypass and isolated lung ventilation for tracheal stenosis and reconstruction. *Br J Anaesth* 2003;**91**(5):742–4.

12. DeWitt RC, Hallman CH. Use of cardiopulmonary bypass for tracheal resection: a case report. *Tex Heart Inst J* 2004;**31**(2):188–90.

Anesthesia for otologic and neurotologic surgery

Vladimir Nekhendzy

Introduction

Ear surgery can be organized around two broad categories: otologic and neurotologic surgery; some of the most commonly performed procedures are summarized in Table 29.1. Over the last decade, the patient outcomes after otologic and neurotologic surgery have become favorably affected by a plethora of technological advances, such as the introduction of high-magnification operating microscopes, the use of powered instrumentation with integrated irrigation-suction capability, the use of sophisticated endoscopic and navigation image-guided surgery, and improved intraoperative neurophysiologic monitoring [1–3].

Table 29.1. Categories of ear surgery, and most commonly performed surgical procedures

Otologic surgery	Neurotologic surgery

External auditory canal
  Exostoses resection
  Ear canal reconstruction
  (canalplasty)
	Temporal bone
	  Limited and radical
	  resection

Middle ear
  Myringotomy/
  myringoplasty
  Tympanoplasty
  Mastoidectomy/
  tympanomastoidectomy
  Stapes surgery
  Ossicular chain
  reconstruction
	Cranial nerves, skull base,
	cranial fossae
	  Restoration of facial
	  nerve function
	  Glomus tumors
	  Acoustic neuromas
	  Dural defects surgery

Inner ear
  Labyrinthectomy
  Endolymphatic sac
  surgery
	Restoration of hearing
	  Bone-anchored hearing
	  aids (BAHA)
	  Cochlear implantation
	  Auditory brainstem
	  implantation

Otologic and neurotologic surgery is performed for a wide spectrum of disorders, including congenital malformations, and infectious, traumatic, and neoplastic diseases. Patients of both sexes are equally affected, and the surgical procedures span across all age groups. However, the young adult patient population (aged 18–65 years old) tends to predominate [2,4].

This chapter focuses on the fundamental principles and details of anesthesia management of adult patients presenting for selected, most common otologic and neurotologic surgical procedures, such as middle ear surgery, skull base surgery, resection of acoustic neuroma, and cochlear implantation. Significant overlap in such principles exists for both otologic and neurotologic surgery, and knowledge of such principles by the anesthesiologist can help greatly in caring for such patients and may positively impact their outcomes.

Surgical considerations
Otologic surgical procedures [2,5–7]

Most otologic surgical procedures are performed via either a transcanal approach (through the natural meatus of the external ear), a retroauricular incision, or a combination of the two.

Depending on the extent of the disease, surgery involving the external auditory canal may require additional resection of adjacent tissues and skin grafting; graft may be harvested from the retroauricular region, the inner aspect of the patient's arm, or from the hip or thigh. Middle ear procedures are usually undertaken to control recurrent or chronic ear infections. A simple myringotomy is most commonly performed in pediatric patients, while myringoplasty involves the repair of a persistent tympanic membrane (TM) perforation, usually using autologous graft. Combined with repair of chronic middle ear changes, the latter procedure is termed a tympanoplasty.

A simple mastoidectomy, performed for removing loculated infection and diseased tissue from the air-filled cavities of the mastoid bone, is often combined with tympanoplasty (tympanomastoidectomy) to address the changes from chronic infection. This represents the standard surgical approach for resection of a cholesteatoma, a keratin-containing epithelial cyst originating from the TM that has grown into the middle ear and mastoid cavity. When the posterior bony wall of the external auditory canal is left in place to keep the mastoid cavity anatomically separated from the external auditory canal, the procedure is called a canal-wall-up tympanomastoidectomy. In contrast, a canal-wall-down tympanomastoidectomy, performed for more aggressive disease, exteriorizes the mastoid cavity into the external auditory canal. The complete removal of mastoid and middle ear contents is frequently referred to as a radical mastoidectomy.

Ossicular chain reconstruction involves rebuilding or replacing the bones of hearing (malleus, incus, and stapes) with either the patient's own tissues, or with alloplastic prostheses, and may be performed either in conjunction with other tympanomastoid surgery, or as an independent procedure. A stapedectomy (stapedotomy) is typically performed in patients suffering from otosclerosis that has resulted in the progressive fixation of the stapes to the surrounding bone and conducting hearing loss; the stapes is replaced by a prosthesis to restore more normal continuity of sound conduction.

Neurotology and skull base surgery [2,8–10]

The skull base can be divided into anterior, middle, and posterior fossae, and is formed by the frontal, ethmoid, sphenoid, temporal, and occipital bones. The term skull base surgery can be viewed as a misnomer, as the majority of lesions treated are located adjacent to the brainstem and not intrinsic to the skull base itself. Neurotologists primarily deal with lesions in the posterior fossa, which is bordered by the clivus (anterior), temporal bone (lateral), and occipital bone (posterior) (Figure 29.1). Removal of the skull base bone allows exposure to these lesions while minimizing cerebral and cerebellar retraction.

Vestibular schwannomas (acoustic neuromas) are removed via three surgical approaches: translabyrinthine, retrosigmoid, and middle fossa. The translabyrinthine approach uses a post-auricular incision to access the temporal bone (Figure 29.2). Retraction of the temporal lobe and cerebellum is minimized as the entire mastoid and labyrinth is removed to create access. This approach results in complete sensorineural hearing loss and is most commonly used in patients with large tumors and/or non-salvageable hearing. In other cases, a hearing-conservation approach (retrosigmoid or middle fossa) to the tumors is usually chosen. The retrosigmoid (suboccipital) approach uses a more posterior craniotomy between the sigmoid and transverse sinuses; the cerebellum is retracted posteriorly away from the petrous face of the temporal bone (Figure 29.3). Disadvantages include the need for rigid skull fixation (e.g., Mayfield head frame), the increased incidence of postoperative headache, and a somewhat higher incidence of cerebrospinal fluid (CSF) leakage. The middle fossa approach places the craniotomy above the ear and requires superior retraction of the temporal lobe (Figure 29.4). This approach has the highest rate of hearing conservation, but can only be used in smaller tumors without increasing the risk of postoperative facial palsy. The anatomy of the middle cranial fossa is variable, dural elevation can be difficult, and full appreciation of the three-dimensional anatomy of the temporal bone by the surgeon is crucial.

Another commonly approached area in neurotology is the jugular foramen (JF), which lies at the junction of the petrous apex and occipital bone. Glomus jugulare tumors originating in this region are highly vascular, and patients undergo preoperative embolization before surgery. A lateral transjugular craniotomy, which is similar to the translabyrinthine approach, exposes the entire jugular fossa and involves resection of the involved sigmoid sinus and jugular vein (Figure 29.5). In addition, a limited neck dissection is performed in order to gain proximal vascular control of the jugular vein and carotid artery.

Cochlear implantation is an option to address severe or profound inner ear hearing loss ("sensorineural hearing loss"). During implantation, a retro-auricular incision and mastoidectomy are performed to provide a pathway for device placement into the inner ear. A receiver-stimulator is placed under the

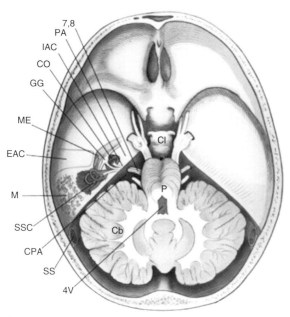

Figure 29.1. An axial view of the skull through the level of the internal auditory canal and cerebellopontine angle [2]. 5, Trigeminal nerve; 7, facial nerve; 8, audiovestibular nerve; PA, petrous apex; IAC, internal auditory canal; CO, cochlea; GG, geniculate ganglion of the facial nerve; ME, middle ear; EAC, external auditory canal; M, mastoid air cell system; SCC, semicircular canals; CPA, cerebellopontine angle; SS, sigmoid sinus; 4V, fourth ventricle; Cl, clivus; P, pons; Cb, cerebellum. Reproduced with permission from: Jackler RK. *Atlas of Neurotology and Skull Base Surgery*. St. Louis: Mosby-Year Book: 1996. Copyright Dr. R. K. Jackler © 2007.

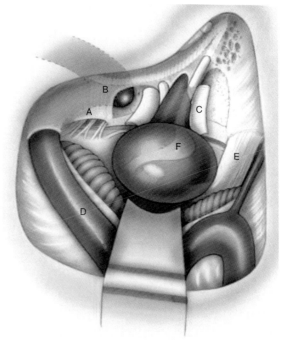

Figure 29.2. Typical left translabyrinthine posterior fossa craniotomy exposure of a medium-sized tumor [2]. Inferiorly, the lower cranial nerves (A) are visible and the jugular bulb (B) has been identified. Troughs have been drilled above and below the IAC, and the dura (C) has been reflected off the tumor surface. The sigmoid sinus (D) and cerebellum are gently retracted posteriorly. The trigeminal nerve (E) is located superiorly. The facial nerve (F) takes a variable and often serpentine course across the medial side of the tumor. Reproduced with permission from: Jackler RK. *Atlas of Neurotology and Skull Base Surgery*. St. Louis: Mosby-Year Book: 1996. Copyright Dr. R. K. Jackler © 2007.

skin behind the ear, and a flexible electrode array is threaded into the turns of the cochlea to later be used for stimulating the cochlear nerve directly, thereby bypassing the dysfunctional inner ear. The devices are usually activated several weeks following placement, at which time hearing function is expected to increase.

Intraoperative complications [2,7,11]

Although the internal carotid artery and jugular bulb pass through the middle ear (Figure 29.6), significant vascular injury happens infrequently, and most if not all bleeding can be readily controlled acutely with packing within the surgical field. An internal carotid artery (ICA) injury may require additional neuroradiologic or neurosurgical intervention; however, clinically significant hemorrhage is rare, and can usually be avoided with prompt packing.

Venous injury, such as laceration of the sigmoid sinus during mastoidectomy, can usually be controlled

using bone wax or with other hemostatic materials held with pressure against the site of bleeding. The walls of the sigmoid sinus are non-collapsible, and extensive surgical intervention aimed at obliteration of the sinus both above and below the laceration may be required if bleeding is severe. In the case of a large venous injury, a venous air embolism can potentially result, and timely communication between the surgical and anesthesia teams can facilitate its identification and treatment.

The temporal bone abuts the dura of the middle fossa above, and the posterior fossa behind, and dural violation may happen either as the result of pathology, from dissection of adjacent tissues, or due to direct dural trauma caused by indiscriminate cauterization of the dural vessels, or the use of the otologic drills. When this occurs, the surgeon can usually close the defect and control the cerebrospinal fluid (CSF) leak using autologous tissues, and administration of a

Valsalva maneuver may be requested to check the integrity of the repair.

General considerations and anesthesia objectives

The density and complexity of the microanatomy of the middle ear and the temporal bone (Figure 29.6) dictate the extremely delicate nature (and prolonged duration) of many otologic/neurotologic procedures, and hence many of the anesthetic requirements [2,5]. The essential requirements for precision otologic and neurotologic surgery include a clear, dry surgical field, absence of patient movement, preservation of facial/cranial nerve function, and non-stimulating emergence from anesthesia [2,4,5,7,12,13].

Maintenance of clear surgical field is extremely important in the majority of cases, as even a small amount of bleeding can have a significant impact on intraoperative exposure [2,12,13]. In addition to maintenance of controlled hypotension by the anesthesiologist (see "Anesthesia induction and maintenance" in "Anesthetic management of otologic surgical procedures" section), mixtures of local anesthetic-epinephrine containing solutions (e.g., 1% lidocaine with 1:100 000 epinephrine) are commonly used by the surgeon to improve hemostasis and facilitate quiet surgical field [2,7]. The anesthesiologist should be made aware of such use, and closely observe (and treat, where appropriate) the ensuing patient hemodynamic responses.

Smooth emergence from anesthesia, devoid of bucking and/or coughing on the *in situ* endotracheal tube (ETT) is necessary, and is essential after reconstructive surgery of the middle or inner ear, facial nerve, or closure of cranial base/dural defects [2,4]. Avoidance of protracted straining or retching associated with postoperative nausea and vomiting (PONV) is equally critical in that regard, and adequate pharmacological PONV prophylaxis should be routine [2,4,12,13].

Intraoperative patient positioning

Postauricular or temporal surgical incision is used, with possible extension into the neck for GT, as discussed above [2]. For the majority of the otologic and neurotologic procedures, the patient is positioned supine, with the head turned 45° away from the side of the surgery. Extreme rotation of the patient's head should be avoided, especially in elderly patients and those

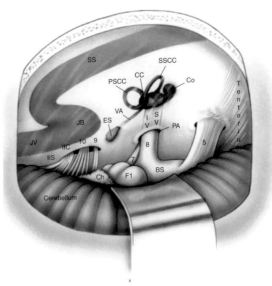

Figure 29.3. Anatomical relationships of the cerebellopontine angle shown through a retrosigmoid posterior fossa craniotomy [2]. JV, jugular vein; JB, jugular bulb; SS, sigmoid sinus; 11S, spinal component of the accessory nerve; 11C, cranial component of the accessory nerve; 10, vagus nerve; 9, glossopharyngeal nerve; Ch, choroid plexus emanating from the lateral recess of the fourth ventricle; F1, flocculus; BS, brainstem surface (pons); 5, trigeminal nerve; 7, facial nerve; 8, audiovestibular nerve; PA, porus acousticus; IV, inferior vestibular nerve; SV, superior vestibular nerve; ES, endolymphatic sac; VA, vestibular aqueduct; PSCC, posterior semicircular canal; CC, common crus; SSCC, superior semicircular canal; Co, cochlea. Reproduced with permission from: Jackler RK. *Atlas of Neurotology and Skull Base Surgery.* St. Louis: Mosby-Year Book: 1996. Copyright Dr. R. K. Jackler © 2007.

with cervical spine disease [4]. If necessary, a small roll placed under the shoulder on the side of the surgery can further facilitate surgical exposure. Once positioned, the patient's head is not usually moved until the surgery has been completed. Mayfield rigid fixation is used in retrosigmoid craniotomies or for very large tumors extending towards the brain stem [2].

The operating room (OR) table is typically turned 180° away from the anesthesiologist, to allow for the use of the operating microscope and to facilitate unrestricted access of the surgical team to the surgical field. As a result, immediate access to the patient's head becomes difficult or impossible for the anesthesiologist. The dedicated artificial airway must be diligently taped, and all the anesthesia circuit connections must be checked to prevent accidental disconnection under the surgical drapes. Steep lateral OR table rotation is frequently used intraoperatively, and the patient's body must be securely strapped. The patient's

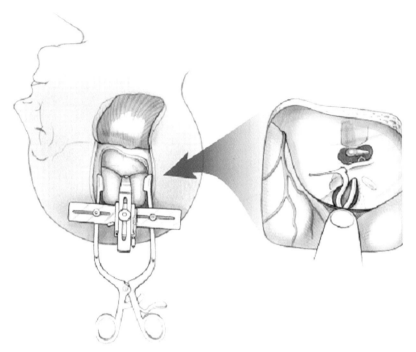

Figure 29.4. Middle fossa exposure of a small right-sided tumor [2]. The retractor is engaged over the posterior lip of the petrous bone and retracts the temporal lobe. Bone has been removed around the IAC, and the dura has been opened to expose the tumor. The facial nerve typically courses across the superior aspect of the tumor surface. Reproduced with permission from: Jackler RK. *Atlas of Neurotology and Skull Base Surgery.* St. Louis: Mosby-Year Book: 1996. Copyright Dr. R. K. Jackler © 2007.

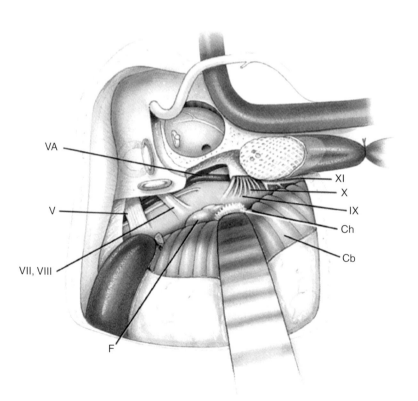

Figure 29.5. Transjugular craniotomy illustrating the degree of intracranial exposure obtained following resection of the sigmoid-jugular system and wide opening of the posterior fossa dura [2]. Note the multiple small rootlets of the lower cranial nerves emanating from the lateral surface of the medulla. In contrast to extracranial procedures, the sigmoid sinus is ligated proximally rather than packed extralumenally. While this illustration depicts anterior rerouting of the facial nerve, this is not necessary in most intracranial jugular foramen tumors. The sigmoid sinus has been controlled with a suture ligature just distal to the transverse-sigmoid junction. VA, vertebral artery; F, flocculus; Ch, choroid; Cb, cerebellum; V, trigeminal nerve; VII, facial nerve; VIII, audiovestibular nerve; IX, glossopharyngeal nerve; X, vagus nerve; XI, accessory nerve. Reproduced with permission from: Jackler RK. *Atlas of Neurotology and Skull Base Surgery.* St. Louis: Mosby-Year Book: 1996. Copyright Dr. R. K. Jackler © 2007.

(A)

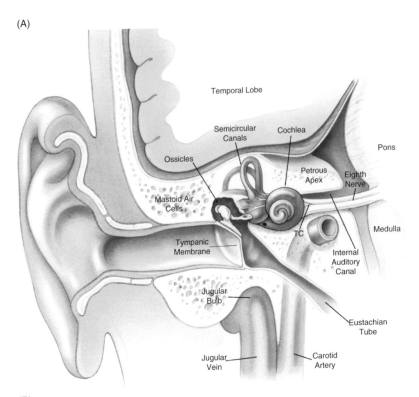

(B)

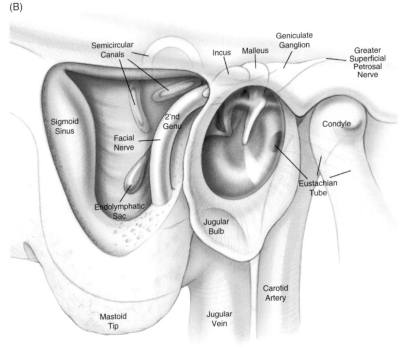

Figure 29.6. Multiple vital neurovascular structures interrelate in a small confined space. These include the organs of hearing and balance, the facial nerve, the carotid artery, jugular vein, sigmoid sinus, and the delicate mechanisms of the middle ear [2]. (A) Coronal representation of the anatomy of the ear and temporal bone TC: transverse crest. (B) Lateral view of the ear and temporal bone anatomy following a simple mastoidectomy. Reproduced with permission from: Jackler RK, Driscoll CLW, eds. *Tumors of the Ear and Temporal Bone*. Philadelphia: Lippincott Williams & Wilkins; 2000. Copyright Dr. R. K. Jackler © 2007.

pressure points and both arms must be well padded and secured to prevent any positioning-related complications [2,14], especially in view of the lateral OR table shifts. The patient's eyes must be properly protected to avoid accidental corneal abrasion caused by heavy instrumentation around the patient's face.

Immobility of the surgical field

Any intraoperative adjustment of equipment or position can have profound consequences during microdissection [2]. Under the microscope, the surgeon's attention is fully and continuously directed to the performance of gentle and careful microsurgical dissection, making it critical to avoid any external motion interference with the surgical field [2]. The noninvasive blood pressure (NIBP) cuff should be positioned on the patient's arm opposite to the surgeon, to eliminate the possibility of triggering sudden surgical tremor during cuff inflation (the pre-induction intravenous (IV) line is usually secured on the side of the procedure).

Situational awareness is required on the part of the anesthesiologist at all times to avoid any inadvertent action that may result in accidental movement of the OR table. The surgeon must be informed of any plans that may result in patient motion – even those that would otherwise seem insignificant [2]. Manipulation of OR table control by the anesthesiologist should be closely coordinated with the surgeon, who must first steer clear of the surgical field.

Avoidance of any active patient movement constitutes a challenging task. Deeper planes of anesthesia are frequently required to avoid sudden patient motor responses, because maintenance of intraoperative neuromuscular blockade (NMB) is usually contraindicated (see "Anesthesia induction and maintenance" in "Anesthetic management of otologic surgical procedures" section).

Preservation of facial/cranial nerve function

Intraoperative identification and preservation of the facial nerve constitutes one of the most important goals during otologic and neurotologic surgery [2,5,7,10,11]. The incidence of iatrogenic facial paralysis may reach nearly 4%, and can be as high as 10% during revision cases [11]. Administration of the NMB agents is best avoided intraoperatively to allow for adequate neural monitoring (see "Anesthesia induction and maintenance" in "Anesthetic management of otologic surgical procedures" section). When

full neurophysiological monitoring is used during cranial base surgery (e.g., acoustic neuroma resection), the selected anesthetic technique should also result in facilitation of such monitoring for best preservation of cranial nerve function (see "Anesthesia induction and maintenance" in "Anesthetic management of neurotological surgical procedures and skull base surgery" section).

The essential anesthetic considerations and requirements are summarized in Table 29.2.

Anesthetic management of otologic surgical procedures

Patient preoperative evaluation and preparation

Adult patients presenting for ear surgery are generally young and healthy (with the possible exception of those presenting for cochlear implantation), and most otologic procedures are performed on an outpatient basis. Presence of significant cardiovascular, cerebrovascular, and/or chronic renal disease may preclude the use of controlled hypotension (see "Anesthesia induction and maintenance" in "Anesthetic management of otologic surgical procedures"

Table 29.2. Essential anesthesia requirements for otologic and neurotologic surgery

Maintenance of stable, adequate plane of anesthesia at all times

Maintenance of moderate controlled hypotension

Secure patient positioning on the OR table (three straps)

Avoidance of iatrogenic external motion interference with microsurgical dissection

Absence of patient movement

Avoidance of intraoperative neuromuscular blockade

Facilitation of intraoperative monitoring of the facial nerve/cranial nerves

Smooth emergence from anesthesia, without bucking, coughing, straining

Rapid awakening, to facilitate early assessment of the facial/cranial nerve function

Avoidance of postoperative nausea and vomiting

Fast-tracking patients for discharge from the recovery room, where appropriate

Table 29.3. Advantages of the laryngeal mask airway (LMA) over the endotracheal tube (ETT)

Adverse event	ETT (%)	LMA (%)	ETT:LMA
Clinically significant problems	3.4	0.9	3.7
Laryngeal spasm	0.38	0.12	3.2
Aspiration	0.017	0.02	0.85
Sore throat	50	10	5
Laryngeal trauma	6.2	? (< 1)	> 6
Coughing on emergence	60	2	30

Modified from Brimacombe JR, Brain, AJ. *The Laryngeal Mask Airway. A Review and Practical Guide.* London: Saunders; 1997.

section), which is frequently required intraoperatively. Appropriate preoperative laboratory and diagnostic studies should be obtained in these patients.

During the preoperative visit, the anesthesiologist should allow sufficient time to establish rapport with the patient and the patient's family. Preoperative communication with the patients may be difficult due to their decreased hearing ability, and written communication may be required. Patients should be allowed to wear hearing aids for as long as possible, which must then be removed before induction of anesthesia to prevent intraoperative pressure injury to the external ear [2]. The hearing aid can be replaced before emergence to help minimize anxiety and facilitate communication [4]. The debilitating symptoms of the primary otologic disease and frequent revision surgeries may leave a long-standing negative psychological impact on the patient [5,7] and result in patient depression, anxiety, and irritability. Although a significant number of patients presenting for revision surgery may be taking antidepressant medications preoperatively [15], chronic ear pain requiring longstanding analgesic treatment is rare.

Preoperative airway compromise is rarely observed, with the possible exception of patients presenting with persistent trismus caused either by involvement of the temporomandibular joint (TMJ) in the primary disease process (e.g., malignancies of the temporal bone), or by post-radiation fibrotic changes involving the TMJ and/or muscles of mastication.

Conventional and alternative airway management options

Although some well-motivated patients can undergo selected, uncomplicated procedures under local anesthesia with sedation [4], general anesthesia is used most frequently. Tracheal intubation is most commonly performed; however, absent contraindications, the use of supraglottic airway (SGA) devices and, specifically, the laryngeal mask airway (LMA; LMA North America, Inc., San Diego, CA, USA) should be given consideration, and represents the author's first choice.

Prospective randomized studies by Webster et al. [16] and Atef et al. [17] have shown that LMA use in endoscopic ENT surgery was associated with better cardiovascular stability during airway management on induction and emergence, superior maintenance of a stable plane of anesthesia and controlled hypotension, improved quality of surgical field, smooth emergence from anesthesia, and faster awakening time. Large retrospective studies by Ayala [18] and Taheri [19] on LMA use in otologic surgery corroborate these findings, indicating improved intraoperative hemodynamic stability, reduced usage of anesthetic drugs, shortened operative time, and decreased incidence of adverse respiratory events. Furthermore, the use of the LMA does not require administration of NMB, facilitates the resumption of spontaneous ventilation, and is associated with the decreased likelihood of the airway reflex stimulation (Table 29.3).

When used appropriately in selected patients, absence of immediate access to the patient's airway should not be considered a deviation from the standard of care of the LMA use in the modern era [4,20]. Selection of the LMA devices that possess greater ventilating capability and provide gastric access (e.g., the LMA-Proseal™, the LMA-Supreme™) will increase the margin of safety (see "Case study: anesthesia for middle ear surgery" section). The new SGAs, such as i-gel™ (Intersurgical Ltd, Wokingham, Berkshire, UK) and air-Q™ Cookgas

Intubating Laryngeal Airway (ILA; Mercury Medical, Clearwater, FL, USA) also show some promise [21–26]; however, their ventilatory performance in prolonged surgical cases awaits formal evaluation.

With the LMA in place, either spontaneous or controlled ventilation can be maintained intraoperatively [4,16–20]. The author's experience corroborates that of others [20] that early institution of pressure support ventilation through the LMA is frequently required in anesthetized, spontaneously breathing patients. A combination of anesthesia-induced paradoxical diaphragmatic and rib cage movement [27] and increased patient inspiratory effort frequently results in a rocky respiratory pattern, which causes motion interference with the microsurgical dissection. The associated reduction in tidal volume and changes in intrapulmonary gas exchange can be further exacerbated by chest wall restriction due to positioning (chest straps) and deeper planes of anesthesia (see "Anesthesia induction and maintenance" in "Anesthetic management of otologic surgical procedures" section), resulting in alveolar hypoventilation, and therefore the use of controlled ventilation may be preferred from the outset.

If the LMA is used, meticulous attention must be directed to the confirmation tests of the proper placement of the device, and ensuring the full separation between the respiratory and gastrointestinal tracts (see section VII, below). Adequacy of the LMA positioning and effectiveness of controlled ventilation should be continuously monitored intraoperatively by observing the expired tidal volume (V_t), pulse oximetry and EtCO$_2$ values, EtCO$_2$ wave form, total leak fraction, total compliance, and by visually assessing the flow–volume and pressure–volume loops, if available. Sudden changes, such as increased leak fraction, decreased total compliance, and (depending on the mode of ventilation used) either decreased V_t or increased peak inspiratory pressure (PIP) will represent early signs of the lighter planes of anesthesia. With the LMA use, these changes typically precede the patient's hemodynamic and motor responses, thereby facilitating hypnotic monitoring and allowing for prompt deepening of anesthesia.

These advantages notwithstanding, future prospective randomized trials are needed to better define the role of the LMA in otologic surgery. Until then, the choice about the use of the LMA or the ETT as a primary ventilatory device will be largely based upon each individual practitioner's experience, preference, and clinical judgment.

Premedication and monitoring

Standard premedication with short-acting benzodiazepine (e.g., midazolam) is generally indicated, and may also decrease the incidence of PONV [28]. Antibiotic prophylaxis (e.g., cefazolin) is typically administered in the majority of cases. Routine monitoring is usually sufficient, even if controlled hypotension is used intraoperatively. The use of invasive blood pressure monitoring (A-line) should be dictated by the patient's medical history. Before induction, temporary removal of a surgical mask may be needed to allow patients to lip read the anesthesiologist's instructions in the OR [2].

Anesthesia induction and maintenance

Standard IV induction with propofol is used most often, although there is little evidence to support propofol's beneficial antiemetic effect if total intravenous anesthesia (TIVA) is not used intraoperativly [29,30]. If general endotracheal anesthesia (GETA) is planned, a single intubating dose of an intermediate-acting non-depolarizing NMB (e.g., rocuronium) is usually inconsequential with regard to the planned intraoperative electromyography (EMG) monitoring of the facial nerve [2]. In the absence of contraindications, succinylcholine can also be safely administered for tracheal intubation. A combination of remifentanil 2 µg/kg IV, propofol 2 mg/kg IV, lidocaine 1.5 mg/kg IV, and only half of an intubating dose of rocuronium (0.3 mg/kg) IV can also be used, and will achieve intubating conditions similar to administration of IV succinylcholine 1.5 mg/kg [31]. Co-administration of IV remifentanil bolus 3–4 µg/kg (or alfentanil 40–60 µg/kg) given over 90 s, and propofol IV bolus 2–2.5 mg/kg, will provide excellent intubating conditions without the need for NMB in the majority of patients [32–34].

Maintenance of NMB is usually contraindicated intraoperatively (see "Facial nerve monitoring", below), and sufficiently deep planes of anesthesia are frequently required to prevent sudden patient movement, which may lead to disastrous consequences [4,13]. Monitoring of the hypnotic state of anesthesia (e.g., processed electroencephalogram activity) may be advisable to maintain adequate anesthetic depth at all times, especially when TIVA is used. Overly deep planes of anesthesia may provoke hemodynamic instability, requiring appropriate volume loading, as well as judicious use of vasopressors.

Inhalational anesthesia, balanced inhalational anesthesia, TIVA, and even "sandwich" propofol-inhalational anesthetic have all been successfully used for maintenance [12,35–39]. Compared to other inhalational anesthetics, sevoflurane may be preferred for the outpatient surgery: it improves the quality of postoperative patient recovery, shortens the discharge time, is associated with reduced incidence of coughing and postoperative agitation compared to desflurane [40,41], and produces less somnolence and PONV compared to isoflurane [41,42]. However, Jellish *et al.* [12] were unable to demonstrate significant clinical difference between sevoflurane and desflurane during otologic surgery, whereas both drugs produced better emergence profile compared to isoflurane. Desflurane appears to cause a greater systemic and intrapulmonary pro-inflammatory response than sevoflurane during ear surgery [43], but clinical significance of this finding awaits further investigation.

TIVA with propofol and an opioid (most commonly, remifentanil or alfentanil) is frequently used for induction and maintenance of anesthesia for otologic surgery [12,35,37,44–47]. A propofol-based anesthetic results in profound depression of pharyngeal and laryngeal musculature and reflexes, suppresses hormonal stress response to ENT surgical procedures, and effectively blocks the catecholamine release and associated hyperdynamic cardiovascular responses, thereby facilitating maintenance of induced hypotension (see "Controlled hypotension", below) [35,44,46–54]. Most prospective studies demonstrate that, compared to inhalational and balanced inhalational techniques, TIVA offers many practical advantages, such as superior intraoperative hemodynamic stability, quicker recovery times, faster return of cognitive function, decreased incidence of PONV, and improved patient satisfaction [12,36,37,39,41,44,45,48–51,55–57].

Pain scores associated with otologic surgery are low [58], and the use of large doses of fentanyl or highly potent opioids, such as sufentanil, is usually not warranted with either anesthetic technique. In the author's experience, a total intraoperative dose of fentanyl can be safely limited to 2–3 µg/kg in the majority of patients, especially when remifentanil is used intraoperatively. During TIVA, the full synergistic effect of propofol with rapidly acting opioids, such as remifentanil or alfentanil, allows quick titration of anesthetic to the desired clinical effect

[37,39,49,59–61]. Continuous IV infusions of opioids offer advantages over intermittent boluses, resulting in decreased total dose, greater hemodynamic stability, more rapid recovery of consciousness, less pain in the immediate postoperative period, and decreased discharge times from the recovery room [61–64]. Remifentanil has been shown superior to both fentanyl [65] and alfentanil [37,39,42,46] in promoting intraoperative hemodynamic stability, improving respiratory and general patient recovery, and facilitating patient discharge after outpatient surgery [42,66–69]. The recommended induction doses are remifentanil IV bolus 0.5–2 µg/kg and IV bolus dose of propofol 1–2 mg/kg, followed by continuous maintenance infusions of propofol 80–200 µg/kg/min and remifentanil 0.1–0.5 µg/kg/min [35,37,46,49, 55,61,65]. At times, remifentanil infusion rates as high as 1.0 µg/kg/min have been used without untoward sequela [39]. Commonly used doses of alfentanil are IV induction bolus 20–30 µg/kg, followed by continuous maintenance infusion 0.25–1 µg/kg/min [37,42,46,64].

Compared to conventional weight-based manual infusions, target controlled infusions (TCI) allow easier and more rapid titration of anesthetic drugs to the individual patient's responses, therefore avoiding overshoot, improving the time course of the drug effects, facilitating perioperative hemodynamic control [70–72], and possibly improving the recovery profile after otologic surgery [73]. Targeting propofol concentration 3–3.5 µg/ml and remifentanil concentration 2–5 ng/ml should probably be sufficient for the majority of otherwise young (age 18–65 years) and healthy (ASA I–II) patients during the maintenance stage of anesthesia, especially if the LMA is used [64,70,73–76].

The use of nitrous oxide (N_2O) should be discouraged, especially during revision otologic surgery, as it may not only interfere with the graft placement, but also provoke graft dislodgement and even disarticulation of stapes upon N_2O discontinuation [4,13,77]. A recent ENIGMA trial found that in addition to severe PONV, the use of N_2O is also associated with a higher incidence of wound infection, pneumonia, atelectasis or any other pulmonary complications [78].

Controlled hypotension

Maintenance of moderate controlled hypotension (systolic blood pressure, SBP, below 100 mmHg; mean arterial pressure, MAP, 60–70 mmHg) is essential for maintaining optimal operating conditions during otologic surgery [12,75,79–81]. A variety of pharmacological approaches, such as the use of IV sodium nitroprusside, IV β-blockers (esmolol, labetalol, metoprolol), IV calcium channel blockers (nicardipine), IV α$_2$-adrenoreceptor agonists (dexmedetomidine), IV magnesium sulfate, and the use of potent inhalational agents and IV opioids have been successfully employed for this purpose, all producing comparable improvement in the operating conditions and quality of the surgical field [4,75,79–82].

The author's experience, as that of others [79], has shown that the use of remifentanil seems to be particularly effective in that regard due to the drug's superior potency and titratability. Maintenance of induced hypotension with remifentanil during otologic surgery rarely requires additional pharmacological supplementation, and is equally effective with both inhalational and TIVA techniques [39,79,81]. The incidence of rebound hypertension and tachycardia with the use of remifentanil appears to be low, and prophylactic administration of labetalol IV bolus 0.1–0.3 mg/kg at the end of surgery is usually effective in patients with preexisting cardiovascular disease.

Intraoperative use of esmolol 0.5–1 mg/kg IV bolus, followed by continuous IV infusion 100–300 μg/kg/min, titrated to the desired hemodynamic endpoint [82,83] represents another attractive therapeutic option. The potentiation of action of opioids and anesthetic agents by esmolol [84–86] further facilitates emergence from anesthesia, and results in decreased postoperative opioid analgesic requirements and shorter discharge time after outpatient surgical procedures [87–89].

Controversy exists with regard to the effect of induced hypotension on maintenance of cochlear blood flow and overall tympanometric stability with different anesthetic techniques. Albera et al. [90] demonstrated a protective effect of sevoflurane, but not propofol-based anesthetic, on inner ear microcirculation. However, propofol was administered by intermittent boluses in this study, and the repeated high peak concentrations may have negatively affected cochlear blood flow and homeostasis. Conversely, Preckel et al. [91] illustrated the preservation of cochlear autoregulation and function with TIVA rather than isoflurane-based anesthetic. The clinical significance of these findings has yet to be determined.

Facial nerve monitoring

Intraoperative facial nerve evoked EMG monitoring represents the current standard of surgical care during otologic and neurotologic surgery, and facilitates facial nerve preservation [2,55]. Maintenance of NMB should be avoided, although some studies suggest that a moderate ($\leq$ 50%) degree of NMB does not interfere with facial EMG responses [92–94]. Nevertheless, any consideration for instituting intraoperative NMB should be discussed and closely coordinated with the surgeon. Even if partial NMB is used intraoperatively, full immobility cannot be guaranteed during highly stimulating parts of the procedure, and close attention to maintenance of an adequate plane of anesthesia is required at all times. The use of remifentanil as part of the anesthetic technique (see above) greatly facilitates maintenance of a stable plane of anesthesia and patient immobility, without affecting the quality of neural monitoring [55]. Useful information can be drawn from the facial nerve audible EMG responses by the anesthesiologist, as increased activity of upper facial muscles usually indicates enhanced patient responsiveness [55,95]. Jellish et al. [55] found that large increases in such activity better predicted sudden movement in patients undergoing neurotologic surgery than the BIS monitor, thereby providing the anesthesiologist with advanced opportunity to expeditiously deepen the anesthesia [55].

Emergence from anesthesia

If GETA was used, deep stages of anesthesia are required until the very end of the procedure, to blunt the patient's laryngotracheal responses and avoid bucking and coughing associated with the patient's head movement during a dressing application [2,12]. The use of the LMA in lieu of the ETT will facilitate smooth patient awakening and allow for safe reduction of the level of anesthesia towards the end of the surgery (see "Conventional and alternative airway management options" section above and Table 29.3). Maintaining a very low-dose remifentanil IV infusion (e.g., 0.02 μg/kg/min) until the patient is fully awakened and the LMA is removed may be beneficial, particularly if the total intraoperative dose of IV fentanyl has been significantly reduced (see "Premedication and monitoring" section above). In the author's experience, this virtually eliminates the emergence-related events, such as patient agitation, coughing, uncontrolled head movements, and post-extubation laryngospasm, if the LMA was used.

If endotracheal intubation is utilized, smooth emergence from anesthesia may constitute a challenge in many patients. Among the strategies that can be used to facilitate smooth tracheal extubation, three deserve further discussion. First, the patient's trachea can be extubated at a deep plane of anesthesia, and the patient's airway supported by a mask, until the patient resumes spontaneous ventilation and emerges from anesthesia. For otologic surgery, this does not constitute a viable option because of the increased risk of post-extubation laryngospasm and overall increased need for airway support required on the part of the anesthesiologist. Application of PPV or continuous positive airway pressure (CPAP) is contraindicated on emergence, since the pressure transmitted through the eustachian tubes may unseat the tympanic membrane graft or disrupt other repairs [2]. The second approach (Bailey maneuver) [96] involves insertion of a SGA (usually the LMA) behind the existing ETT and removal of the ETT with the patient still anesthetized, followed by administration of supraglottic ventilatory support until the patient resumes spontaneous ventilation and awakens from anesthesia. The third, pharmacological, approach relies on a low-dose remifentanil infusion to blunt the tracheal responses and promote smooth extubation. Remifentanil provides a predictable, rapid, and almost simultaneous recovery of consciousness and protective airway reflexes [97]. Current data indicate that maintenance of remifentanil IV infusion 0.05–0.06 µg/kg/min (target concentration 1.5 ng/ml) during emergence can be effective for this purpose, since this dose effectively suppresses cough reflex in the majority of awake intubated patients [98,99].

Antiemetic prophylaxis should be routine (see "General considerations and anesthesia objectives" section), as the incidence of PONV may reach as high as 50–80% after otologic surgery [4,28]. The use of TIVA and avoidance of N_2O are highly advisable (see "Premedication and monitoring" section).

The optimal antiemetic drug combination has been a subject of intense investigations over the years [28], and is most commonly achieved by IV administration of a 5HT-3 antagonist (e.g., IV ondansetron 4–8 mg) [2,14]. A combination of a 5HT-3 receptor blocker with IV dexamethasone (8–10 mg) appears to be safe and highly effective [28,100], and may lead to improved patient outcome [28]. Multimodal PONV

prophylaxis (e.g., the addition of transdermal scopolamine patch) is warranted in high-risk patients [28].

Immediate post-anesthesia recovery period

Most common intraoperative complications include facial nerve injury and/or dural defects (see "Intraoperative complications" section above). Patients who have undergone stapedectomy are frequently positioned with the operated side up through their postoperative recovery, to allow a blood clot to form around the open inner ear [2]. Middle and inner ear surgery is frequently associated with postoperative vertigo; a combination of standard antiemetics and vestibular suppressants (e.g., benzopiazepines) is usually effective in controlling these symptoms [2].

Immediate postoperative pain associated with otologic surgery is usually low (see "Anesthesia induction and maintenance" section above), with the possible exception of radical mastoidectomy, where it can be moderate to severe. Intermittent IV bolus doses of fentanyl, in combination with standard oral analgesics, are usually sufficient for pain control and fast-tracking patients for discharge [2]. A multimodal analgesic regimen, incorporating the perioperative use of a selective cyclooxygenase-2 inhibitor (e.g., celecoxib) and either acetaminophen or ibuprofen, can further decrease postoperative pain, and improve the quality of recovery and patient satisfaction after outpatient otolaryngologic surgery [101,102].

Remifentanil-induced hyperalgesia has not been an issue in the author's experience, possibly because of the relatively low remifentanil IV infusion rates typically required intraoperatively (0.1–0.3 µg/kg/min). Should acute opioid tolerance be suspected, adequate doses of fentanyl and/or long-acting opioid analgesics (e.g., morphine) can be effectively and safely administered [103].

Anesthetic management of neurotologic surgical procedures and skull base surgery

General surgical and anesthesia considerations for neurotologic procedures have been discussed (see "Surgical considerations" and "General considerations and anesthesia objectives" sections). Anesthetic evaluation and management of uncomplicated neurotologic procedures aimed at restored hearing, such as BAHA or cochlear implantation (see Table 29.1), generally follows the same path as anesthesia for otologic surgery (see "Anesthetic management of otologic surgical procedures" section). Patients with the tumors involving the anterior skull base, jugular foramen and CPA present some of the unique anesthetic challenges.

Patient preoperative evaluation and preparation

The anterior skull base is a common location of many intradural and extradural cranial and/or facial pathologies [104]. Effective skull base surgery requires an established multidisciplinary team that involves otolaryngologist head and neck surgeons, neurotologists, neurosurgeons, plastic surgeons, specialized operating room nurses, neuroradiologists, neurophysiologists, a dedicated anesthesia team, medical oncologists, radiation oncologists, prosthodontists, and other supporting physicians and allied health professionals [10,105]. The anesthesiologist can help improve postoperative outcomes and reduce patient morbidity, provided (s)he is well familiar with the principles of neuroanesthesia, and possesses full preoperative details about the pathological process involved and the planned surgical approach [14].

Tumors that may require anterior skull base resection include selected malignant tumors of the paranasal sinuses that extend superiorly through the cribriform plate, ethmoid roof, and planum sphenoidale or posteriorly through the posterior wall of the frontal sinus; benign and malignant meningiomas that involve the same area; and selected benign processes such as orbital apex schwannomas, occasional encephaloceles and mucoceles, and selected large benign tumors including juvenile angiofibromas and inverted papillomas [105]. Preoperative surgical evaluation includes high-quality MRI, and is almost always supplemented by CT imaging to assess the integrity of bony structures [105]. Depending on the nature and the location of these lesions, a variety of surgical approaches can be utilized, such as craniofacial, endoscopic, bifrontal craniotomy, or a combination of the above [105]. Free muscle flap reconstruction of the cranial base may be required for large postoperative defects [104,106].

Highly vascular tumors are usually embolized during preoperative neuroangiography, particularly if the internal maxillary artery is the major contributor to the tumor's blood supply [105]. If the tumor's blood supply is from the anterior and posterior ethmoidal arteries, which are branches of the ophthalmic artery, then these vessels cannot be safely embolized unless vision has already been lost [105]. A preoperative ICA balloon occlusion test is performed during angiography, if the ICA is involved or encased [106], providing the anesthesiologist with valuable information for management. Dissection near the ICA and optic chiasm is often aided by intraoperative surgical navigation [105].

The cerebellopontine angle (CPA) is a fluid-filled space containing the facial nerve (VII) and vestibulocochlear nerve (VIII) coursing laterally towards the internal auditory canal [2]. A depiction of the CPA and associated cranial nerves is shown in Figure 29.3. This is one of the most commonly approached areas in skull base surgery; lesions include vestibular schwannomas (91.3%), meningiomas (3.1%), epidermoids (2.4%), non-vestibular schwannomas (1.4%), and arachnoid cysts (0.5%) [2,9,10]. Although most of the symptoms associated with vestibular schwannomas (acoustic neuromas) are related to hearing and vestibular dysfunction, large tumors can compress the brainstem, cause preoperative cranial nerve deficits, and occasionally produce symptoms of increased intracranial pressure (ICP). Anesthetic management in the setting of intracranial hypertension secondary to tumor extension should follow the same general principles as for other intracranial mass lesions [107].

The jugular foramen (JF) region is a complex area of the cranial base that can be invaded by several types of tumors, both benign and malignant [108]. The JF connects the intracranial compartment to the neck and contains the glossopharyngeal nerve (IX), vagus nerve (X), accessory nerve (XI), jugular bulb, and inferior petrosal sinus [2,8]. Immediately outside the foramen, the ICA, the jugular vein, and the cranial nerves are surrounded by a common connective tissue sheath [108]. Glomus tumors (GT) are the most common locally aggressive benign tumors (paragangliomas) of the temporal bone that principally originate around the jugular bulb; of less common occurrence are the meningiomas, schwannomas, and chondrosarcomas [2,8,9,106,108]. In advanced cases the GT grow in a variety of directions, and may involve the jugular bulb, ICA, and also spread transdurally/intracranially [2,8,9,106]. In rare cases, paragangliomas may originate in the tympanic branch of the IX cranial nerve (Jacobson's nerve) and the auricular branch of the X cranial nerve (Arnold's nerve) [9,108].

Paragangliomas are divided into two groups: (1) adrenal paragangliomas (pheochromocytomas), and (2) extraadrenal paragangliomas located in the abdomen, chest, and head and neck regions [2]. Less common pathologies in the JF area include meningiomas and lower cranial nerve schwannomas [2]. Large GT are capable of secreting catecholamines and (less commonly) serotonin, presenting significant anesthetic challenges associated with symptoms and signs of pheochromocytoma (e.g., hypertension, sweating, cardiovascular instability) or carcinoid syndrome [107]. Urine and plasma catecholamine levels should probably be routinely checked preoperatively for all extensive GT, even if the patient is asymptomatic [107]. Significant elevations of urine or serum catecholamines or their metabolites will require the same preoperative pharmacologic stabilization as for the patients with a pheochromocytoma (i.e., α- and β-blockers, calcium channel blockers, etc.) [107]. The reader is referred to comprehensive texts discussing the details of anesthetic management of these patients.

Determining a preoperative plasma serotonin level in the absence of clinical symptoms for serotonin excess (e.g., diarrhea, flushing, headaches) is probably unnecessary [107]. If serotonin-secreting GT are identified, dehydration and/or electrolyte abnormalities should be corrected preoperatively [107]. Intraoperatively, the release of histamine and bradykinin can cause bronchospasm, tachycardia, and both hypotension and hypertension [107].

Large GT can cause preoperative cranial nerve IX, X, XI, and XII palsies, with the vagal nerve dysfunction being the most common [108]. Cranial nerve IX, X, and XII deficits can predispose to airway compromise, either by obstruction or by aspiration (the risk of aspiration caused by gastroparesis is increased in these patients) [107,108]. Careful history and preoperative airway examination are required. In the majority of cases, vocal cord function will be comprehensively evaluated by the surgeons preoperatively.

Appreciating the nature of the lesion(s) and the pathological process involved will guide the anesthesiologist's preparation for possible significant blood loss. This especially concerns tumors that it was not possible to embolize preoperatively, and highly vascular neoplasms, such as GT and meningiomas [14,106]. Tumor involvement and extension into cranial sinuses (e.g., sigmoid sinus, the inferior petrosal sinus), ICA and its branches increases the likelihood

of substantial blood loss [14,106,107]. Preoperative embolization of the vascularized tumors should be done whenever possible, and will diminish intraoperative blood loss, decrease operation time, and permit one-stage operation [14,106,107]. Intraoperative blood loss can be in excess of 1 liter in these cases, and 2–4 units of cross-matched blood should be readily available (1 unit of cross-matched or autologous blood is usually sufficient for other skull base surgery) [2].

Conventional and alternative airway management

Preoperative airway compromise is rare. In patients with preexisting significant facial nerve paralysis mouth opening can be asymmetric and limited, but this does not interfere with direct laryngoscopy after induction of anesthesia. Rapid sequence induction should be considered in patients at increased risk of aspiration of gastric contents. Preoperative tracheostomy is rarely performed, but may be required postoperatively in selected patients (see "Emergence from anesthesia" section below).

Standard GETA is used in the majority of cases. Patients with the GT or other lesions extending into the JF or upper neck or skull-base brainstem-compressing lesions may require intraoperative identification and functional monitoring of the vagus nerve [109]. In these patients, placement of the specialized ETT (e.g., Xomed ETT, Medtronic Xomed Inc., Jacksonville, FL USA) to record and monitor the electromyography (EMG) activity of the vocal cords can be requested by the surgeon.

Premedication and monitoring

Standard premedication with short-acting benzodiazepine (e.g., IV midazolam) is warranted in the majority of cases, but should be done with caution or avoided if symptoms of increased ICP are present. IV antibiotics with good CSF penetration (e.g., IV ceftriaxone 2 g) are almost uniformly used [2,10]. Corticosteroids (e.g., IV dexamethasone 10–12 mg) are not routinely given, except in patients with large (> 3 cm) tumors or those with peritumoral brain edema [10].

Operations on the skull base can easily last up to 12 hours or longer [2], and meticulous attention should be directed to proper patient positioning before the surgery commences. Jellish *et al.* [14] recorded a 9% incidence of brachial plexus injury after skull base surgery, with over 60% of injuries occurring on the side of surgery. With rigid head fixation in place, excessive neck torsion should be avoided to prevent cervical injury, as well as to reduce the risk of cerebellar swelling secondary to compromised blood flow through the vertebral venous system [7,9,10].

The most critical aspect during operations on the skull base is identification and preservation of the cranial nerves [7,9,10]. Intraoperative neurophysiological monitoring (INM) immediately alerts the surgeon about the risk of nerve injury, helps trace the course of the nerve(s) when anatomy is distorted, and therefore facilitates tumor resection while achieving cranial nerve preservation [110]. INM is utilized most often when the tumors are located at the cervicomedullary junction, CPA, JF, and the upper clivus, when the tumors are large, and during revision surgeries [110]. Cranial nerves VII, IX, X, XI, and XII are most commonly monitored. Standard INM may involve, in part or in combination, EMG recordings, somatosensory and motor evoked potentials (SSEP and MEP), and brainstem auditory evoked responses (BAER) to monitor cochlear nerve (VIII) function [110,111].

Standard monitors are usually used for induction. Large-bore IV access and A-line monitoring are secured prior to the beginning of surgery. The use of CVP is rarely indicated and should be guided by the patient's medical history; however, it should be considered if significant blood loss is anticipated. The Foley catheter is used in all cases.

Anesthesia induction and maintenance

Intravenous induction with propofol may be preferred due to its rapid redistribution and facilitation of the baseline INM assessment. Intravenous barbiturates cause reduction in amplitude and increased latency of the evoked potentials [111]. Intravenous ketamine and etomidate have the unusual effect of increasing the SSEP amplitude, and etomidate also may increase the latency of the cortical SSEP [111].

The use of intermediate-acting non-depolarizing NMB will facilitate tracheal intubation, and also allow for non-hurried, careful patient positioning. In patients with increased ICP, standard induction precautions should be observed. With large tumors, a lumbar drain will be placed after the patient is anesthetized, to decompress CSF and to reduce the risk of

operative complications through minimizing surgical brain retraction [105]. It may also be used to reduce the risk of CSF fistulization, when extensive peri-internal auditory canal pneumatization is present [10]. Administration of IV mannitol (0.5–1 g/kg), started after the scalp incision, and the use of mild hyperventilation will further facilitate brain relaxation for the dural entry. Patients should be kept euvolemic, and the electrolyte status should be monitored during the surgery.

Controlled hypotension (see "Anesthesia induction and maintenance" in "Anesthetic management of otologic surgical procedures" section) is used often to maximize surgical visibility and reduce congestion of the vascular lesion(s) [2]. The use of deliberate hypotension and hypothermia may be limited by the SSEP recording, as both these interventions may affect the cortical SSEP latencies [111]. Pharmacological manipulation of MAP may be necessary if the ICA will be occluded or resected. As a rule, normothermia should be maintained intraoperatively.

The selected anesthetic technique must be able to facilitate the INM. Intraoperative use of NMB is avoided (see "Anesthesia induction and maintenance" in "Anesthetic management of otologic surgical procedures" section). Opioid-based techniques, allowing a safe reduction of the concentration of inhalational agent to ≤ 0.5 minimal alveolar concentration (MAC), are widely used, since opioids have only a modest effect on SSEP parameters [14,111]. Higher concentrations of inhalational agents will tend to decrease the cortical SSEP amplitude and increase the latency; the effects of different inhalational anesthetics are similar in that regard [111]. The combination of N_2O and a volatile anesthetic tends to have a greater depressant effect on SSEP than an equipotent administration of a single agent [111]. Compared with EEG and SSEP, BAER are much more resistant to anesthetic effects [111]. Since the threshold of anesthesia effects on SSEP and EMG responses may vary, any amount of inhalational agent may not be acceptable for proper INM in some patients, necessitating either a "sandwich" anesthetic technique or TIVA (see "Anesthesia induction and maintenance" in "Anesthetic management of otologic surgical procedures" section) [112]. TIVA can also be selected as a primary anesthetic technique from the outset, if appropriate. Intravenous remifentanil infusion is commonly used for the reasons

285

outlined above (see "Anesthesia induction and maintenance" in "Anesthetic management of otologic surgical procedures" section).

Stimulation of the trigeminal or vagus nerves during skull base surgery can cause bradycardia, both hypotension and hypertension, arrhythmias and even transient asystole; therefore, the surgeon should be promptly informed of their occurrence [2,113,114]. Surgical dissection should be immediately suspended, and cardiovascular instability treated, as appropriate [113,114]. The mechanisms underlying bradycardia, hypotension, and asystole induced by the vagus nerve stimulation also involve adrenergic transmission from the medulla, and therefore may not be fully prevented or treated with IV atropine; however, these effects are usually short-lived [113,114].

Emergence from anesthesia

Considerations for smooth extubation and non-stimulating emergence should be carefully observed (see "Emergence from anesthesia" in "Anesthetic management of otologic surgical procedures" section). Coughing and bucking on the ETT may provoke postoperative bleeding, increase cerebral edema, and cause tension pneumocephalus (TP) [107,115]. TP may occur in up to 12% of the cases after classical craniofacial resection, and represents a potentially fatal complication leading to rapid neurological deterioration postoperatively [115]. It may be provoked by a sudden increase in the airway pressure (coughing, sneezing, Valsalva maneuvers), when the air enters the cranial vault through a potential communication between the sinonasal tract and the epidural space, and becomes trapped [115]. PONV prophylaxis must be routine, and multimodal PONV prophylaxis should be strongly considered, especially after acoustic neuroma surgery (see "Emergence from anesthesia" in "Anesthetic management of otologic surgical procedures" section).

Tracheal extubation is carried out in the majority of cases, with the exception of those where the free flap reconstruction of the cranial base was required, and the possible exception of those where cranial nerve deficits existed preoperatively. With regard to the latter, the extubation strategy will be decided on an individual patient basis, depending on the degree of preoperative airway compromise, aspiration risk, and the extent of the procedure performed. The dynamic nature of edema around the cranial nerves in the early postoperative period must be appreciated by both the

anesthesiologist and the surgeon, and nursing staff [107]. New paralysis of the lower cranial nerves with dysphasia remains the most serious complication related to surgery, and delayed extubation and tracheotomy may be required in selected cases [106].

Immediate post-anesthesia recovery period

If extubated, patients should be awake, and able to follow commands and cooperate with the early neurological assessment. The majority of the extubated patients are monitored in the intensive care unit overnight; minimal sedation is administered to allow for adequate neurological monitoring [2]. Airway and aspiration precautions should be observed in patients with possible lower cranial nerve palsies [2].

Postoperative pain is usually mild-to-moderate (VAS 4–6) [2]. With the remifentanil-based anesthesia technique it is not uncommon, in the author's experience, for patients to have moderate-to-severe postoperative pain (VAS 7–8) over the first several hours. This pain should be promptly controlled to prevent postoperative hypertensive responses. Continuous IV administration of vasoactive drugs may be required for adequate blood pressure control to maintain postoperative MAP within the range desired by the neurotologist and/or neurosurgeon.

Even with the extended anterior skull base surgeries, operative mortality is well under 1%, and intracranial bleeding or hematomas are exceedingly rare [105]. Serious central nervous system deficits (including cerebrovascular accidents, unanticipated blindness, postinfection deficits, and autonomic dysfunction) are also rarely observed (2–3% of patients) [105].

Summary

Otologic and neurotologic procedures are highly sophisticated, require precision surgery, and present significant challenges to the anesthesiologist. The anesthesiologist should be very familiar with the nature of the pathological process, understand the critical parts of the surgical procedure, and communicate closely with the surgeon during the perioperative period.

Thorough appreciation of the fundamental principles of the anesthetic management for otologic and neurotologic surgery, discussed in this chapter, and meticulous execution of the properly selected anesthetic techniques and strategies will greatly facilitate the success of surgery and help improve postoperative patient outcomes.

Case study: anesthesia for middle ear surgery

Case description and preoperative evaluation

A 52-year-old female, a professional singing teacher, was scheduled to undergo elective right tympanoplasty for chronic middle ear infection. The recurrent middle ear infections have produced a slight hearing loss in the patient, resulting in voice strain.

Preoperatively, the patient expressed significant concern and anxiety about the adverse effects of tracheal intubation, and specifically possible damage to the vocal cords and larynx. Ten years previously, she was tracheally intubated for elective laparoscopic cholecystectomy, with resultant significant postoperative dysphonia and prolonged vocal recovery.

The patient's past medical history was otherwise unremarkable, review of systems was negative, and the airway and physical exams were normal. The patient was not taking any medications, and preoperative laboratory tests were non-contributory. The patient's baseline vocal cord function and voice quality were comprehensively evaluated by the otolaryngologist preoperatively.

Preoperative vital signs were: NIBP 128/75 mmHg, heart rate 72/min, respiratory rate 16/min, SpO_2 98% on room air; the patient's height was 168 cm, weight 76 kg.

Anesthetic management

The patient was reassured preoperatively, and the options of intraoperative airway management to prevent voice damage were discussed. The patient expressed strong interest in avoiding tracheal intubation, and in the use of the LMA by the anesthesiologist.

On the day of surgery, the patient had been NPO for over 6 hours. After standard premedication (midazolam 2 mg IV), the patient was brought to the OR and standard monitors were applied. After adequate preoxygentaion ($FiO_2 = 1.0$), anesthesia was induced uneventfully with fentanyl IV 100 μg and propofol IV 200 mg given over 30 s. Once adequate depth of anesthesia was confirmed by absence of patient movement to jaw thrust [116], a size 4 LMA Proseal™ was easily inserted using a standard, digital insertion technique. The cuff of the LMA Proseal™ was inflated with 20 ml of air. Correct positioning of the LMA Proseal™ was confirmed [117] by the positive suprasternal notch test, the lack of air leak from the gastric tube, by positioning of more than 50% of the integral bite block beyond the upper incisors, by the absence of gastric insufflation during positive-pressure ventilation (PPV), the presence of a square-wave $EtCO_2$ capnography trace, and by the easy passage of a lubricated 14Fr orogastric tube (OGT) through the drainage tube of the device into the patient's stomach, with subsequent aspiration of the small amount (< 15 ml) of clear gastric contents (Figures 29.7 and 29.8).

The oropharyngeal leak pressure (OLP) was recorded at 30 cmH_2O, with fresh gas flow 3 l/min

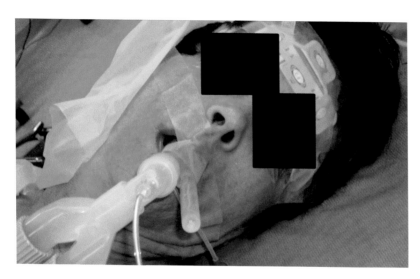

Figure 29.7. Airway management with the LMA Proseal™ as a primary ventilator device in a patient anesthetized for middle ear surgery. Note a small film of a lubricant placed inside the drainage tube, to elicit positive suprasternal notch test and confirm absence of air leak during PPV. Deep LMA Proseal™ positioning, with more than 50% of the integral bite block located beyond the upper incisors serves as an additional confirmation test of the correct LMA Proseal™ positioning. Proper midline fixation of the LMA Proseal™, which also preserves the natural forward curvature of the device, is essential for facilitating maintenance of the LMA seal and separation of the respiratory and gastrointestinal tracts. See text for details.

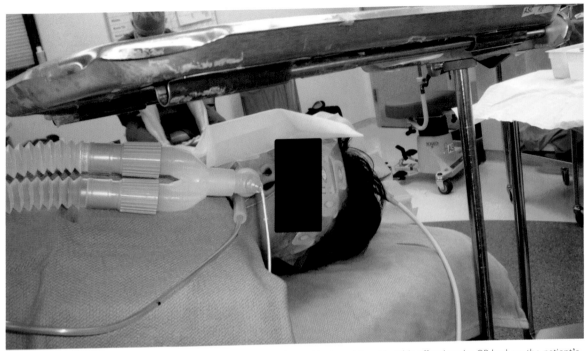

Figure 29.8. The above patient being prepped for surgery. Note the positioning of the side table affixed to the OR bed, on the patient's left. Such arrangement allows for the anesthesiologist to reach the patient's airway under the surgical drapes, and troubleshoot the positioning of the LMA Proseal™, should the need arise. The orogastric tube is passed through the drainage tube into the patient's stomach to facilitate safe administration of positive-pressure ventilation. See text for the details.

and closed pressure-adjusted expiratory valve on the anesthesia machine [121]. The LMA Proseal™ was taped midline, to maintain stable cuff position and optimal airway seal (Figure 29.7).

The patient's lungs were ventilated with a mixture of O_2 and air ($FiO_2 = 0.4$, total fresh gas flow 0.6 l/min), in a pressure-controlled mode (PCV) of 15 cmH_2O, RR of 8 breaths/min, and inspiratory/expiratory (I:E) ratio of 1:2. Adequacy of ventilation was confirmed by achieving an appropriate expired V_t of 600 ml, absent oropharyngeal leak, SpO_2 of 99%, and $EtCO_2 < 40$ mmHg. Adequacy of ventilation was further assessed continuously during the case, by monitoring V_t, $EtCO_2$ value, total leak fraction, total compliance, and by observing the flow–volume and pressure–volume loops and $EtCO_2$ waveform on the display of the anesthesia machine (see "Conventional and alternative airway management options" in "Anesthetic management of otologic surgical procedures" section).

Additional preventive measures aimed at reducing the risk of possible gastric insufflation during PPV, gastric regurgitation, and aspiration included maintaining PIP below OLP, and passively emptying gastric contents into an empty IV bag through the OGT left in the drainage tube of the device (Figure 29.8) [20,118,119]. The *in situ* OGT also served as a functional guide, enabling advancement of the LMA Proseal™ back into the optimal position, had accidental displacement of the device and loss of seal occurred intraoperatively (Figure 29.8) [122].

Anesthesia was maintained with continuous IV infusions of propofol and remifentanil, titrated to the Patient State Index (PSI™) (SEDLine® Brain-Function Monitoring System, Masimo Corp., Irvine, CA, USA) value between 25 and 50, which indicated adequate hypnotic state. Maintenance of moderate controlled hypotension (MAP 60–70 mmHg) was facilitated with intermittent IV boluses of labetalol (total 15 mg). Surgical duration was 1 h 50 min, and the anesthetic course was uneventful. Antiemetic prophylaxis was achieved with dexamethasone IV 8 mg and ondansetron (Zofran®) IV 4 mg. Additional labetalol IV 20 mg was given at the end of surgery, to prevent a rebound hypertension.

TIVA was discontinued during the dressing application, and the patient was allowed to emerge from anesthesia while breathing spontaneously with

$FiO_2 = 1.0$. The patient's stomach and oropharynx were suctioned, the LMA Proseal™ cuff was deflated, and the LMA was removed smoothly and uneventfully, with the patient fully awake. The patient was transported to the recovery room while breathing O_2 delivered at 3 l/min through the nasal cannula. Immediate postoperative recovery room course was uneventful, without PONV. Pain was effectively controlled with fentanyl intermittent IV bolus doses (total 150 µg), and the patient's vital signs remained stable. The patient was discharged home from the recovery room 1.5 hours after the completion of surgery.

No voice changes were observed postoperatively, and the patient gradually resumed singing activity during her postoperative recovery. She was very satisfied with the anesthetic management.

Discussion

Anesthetic management of this patient emphasizes the principles of a safe use of the LMA with PPV. The use of the LMA for otologic surgical procedures offers significant advantages over the ETT, and may be preferred (see "Anesthetic management of otologic surgical procedures" section and Table 29.3). The use of the LMA Proseal™, or its disposable equivalent LMA Supreme™, should be strongly considered, due to the superior ventilation capabilities of these devices, and the ability to confirm a proper LMA placement. Compared to the LMA Proseal™, the use of the LMA Supreme™ results in the same or a slightly higher insertion success rate on the first attempt, but lower OLP [120,123,124].

Patients who are vocal performers or professional voice users present unique challenges, requiring the anesthesiologist to avert even the slightest trauma to the patient's vocal cords and/or cricoarytenoid joints, and to protect laryngeal and vocal function at all times [125]. Preoperatively, these patients are frequently very sensitive and anxious, as inadvertent laryngeal trauma may jeopardize their professional career and psychological health [125]. In this regard, the use of the LMA in this patient was particularly beneficial. Even routine, short-term tracheal intubation is frequently associated with transient post-intubation dysphonia, characterized by decreased voice intensity, increased voice roughness and decreased affect [126]. Rieger et al. [127] prospectively studied over 200 ASA I–III patients presenting for non-airway surgery, and

demonstrated that tracheally intubated patients were almost twice as likely (47% vs. 25%) to develop mild postoperative dysphonia as the patients in the LMA group. In a systematic review of studies comparing airway complications associated with the use of the ETT vs. the LMA, Yu and Beirne [128] showed that the incidence of postoperative hoarseness was more than three times higher when the ETT was used (25% vs. 7.5%). Although the patients' laryngeal complaints usually resolve within 72 h [126,129], both the duration [127,129] and severity [130] of postoperative symptoms are more pronounced when tracheal intubation is employed. Direct trauma to the vocal cords and larynx with LMA use is uncommon, and is typically caused by either malpositioning (direct contact of the tip of the LMA with the vocal cords) or removal of the LMA with an inflated cuff, particularly with forced/twisting traction, which may produce rotation of the larynx and dislocation of the arytenoids [130]. In this patient diligent confirmation of the correct LMA Proseal™ positioning was performed, and full deflation of the LMA Proseal™ cuff before removal of the device was carefully observed. Additional intraoperative measures aimed at minimizing extralaryngeal causes of dysphonia included inflating the LMA Proseal™ cuff with only two-thirds of the maximum recommended volume [118] and the use of low gas flows (0.6 l/min). Inhalation of cold and dry anesthetic gases may produce thinning and dehydration of vocal cord mucosa, increasing the adhesiveness of the vocal folds during phonation [127,131].

Had tracheal intubation been used instead, avoidance of vocal cord and laryngeal injury could have been facilitated by smooth, atraumatic intubation, the use of a small ETT (ID 5.0–6.0 mm), inflation of the ETT cuff to seal pressure only [131], and strict adherence to smooth extubation protocol (see "Emergence from anesthesia" in "Anesthetic management of otologic surgical procedures" section), which would have helped to avoid cough-induced vocal cord injury [132].

Conclusions

The use of the SGAs during otologic surgery offers significant advantages, including avoidance of the administration of the NMB, improved cardiovascular stability and maintenance of a stable plane of anesthesia, facilitatation of the monitoring of adequate hypnotic state, and promotion of smooth emergence from anesthesia without associated coughing, bucking, or straining (see "Conventional and alternative airway management options" in "Anesthetic management of otologic surgical procedures" section). Safe and effective use of the LMA devices, such as the LMA Proseal™ or the LMA Supreme™, which possess great ventilating capabilities and provide gastric access, is strongly preferred for this purpose. Such safeguards as the anesthesiologist's thorough familiarity with these devices' design and technical aspects, knowledge of the confirmation tests of their proper placement and function, and meticulous monitoring of the optimal performance of these devices intraoperatively, are essential for the patient safety.

Clinical pearls

- Essential requirements for precision otologic and neurotologic surgery include a clear, dry surgical field, absence of patient movement, preservation of facial/cranial nerve function, and smooth emergence from anesthesia.
- The operating room (OR) table is typically turned 180° away from the anesthesiologist, making immediate access to the patient's head difficult for the anesthesiologist. The dedicated artificial airway must be diligently taped, and all the anesthesia circuit connections must be checked to prevent accidental disconnection under the surgical drapes.
- Situational awareness is required on the part of the anesthesiologist at all times to avoid any inadvertent action that may result in accidental movement of the OR table.

- Perioperative communication with the patients may be difficult due to their decreased hearing ability, and written communication may sometimes be required. Patients should be allowed to wear hearing aids for as long as possible, which must then be removed before the induction of anesthesia to prevent intraoperative pressure injury to the external ear. The hearing aid can be replaced before emergence to help minimize anxiety and facilitate communication
- Either an ETT or an LMA can be used intraoperatively. With the LMA, pressure support or controlled ventilation is usually required in anesthetized, spontaneously breathing patients to avoid hypoventilation.
- Deeper planes of anesthesia are required to avoid sudden patient motor responses, because maintenance of intraoperative neuromuscular blockade (NMB) is usually contraindicated.
- The use of nitrous oxide (N_2O) should be discouraged, especially during revision otologic surgery, as it may not only interfere with the graft placement, but also provoke graft dislodgement and even disarticulation of stapes.
- Antiemetic prophylaxis should be routine.
- Maintenance of remifentanil IV infusion 0.05–0.06 μg/kg/min during emergence can be effective for achieving smooth emergence.

References

1. Benecke JE, Stahl BA. Otologic instrumentation. In Brackmann DE, Shelton C, Arriaga MA, eds. *Otologic Surgery*. Philadelphia: W. B. Saunders; 1994. pp. 1–26.

2. Blevins NH, Jackler RK, V. Nekhendzy, Guta C. Section 3.0: Otolaryngology – head and neck surgery. Otology and neurotology. In Jaffe RA, Samuels SI, Schmiesing CA, Golianu B, eds. *Anesthesiologist's Manual of Surgical Procedures*, 4th edn. Philadelphia: Wolters Kluwer Health/Lippincott Williams & Wilkins; 2009. pp. 239–49.

3. Glasscock ME. The history of neuro-otology. A personal perspective. *Otolaryngol Clin North Am* 2002;35:227–38.

4. Liang S, Irwin MG. Review of anesthesia for middle ear surgery. *Anesthesiol Clin* 2010;28:519–28.

5. Sheehy JL. Tympanoplasty: outer surface grafting technique. In Brackmann DE, Shelton C, Arriaga MA, eds. *Otologic Surgery*. Philadelphia: W.B. Saunders; 1994. pp. 121–32.

6. Gantz BJ, Redleaf MI. Management of Bell's palsy and Ramsay Hunt syndrome. In Brackmann DE, Shelton C, Arriaga MA, eds. *Otologic Surgery*. Philadelphia: W.B. Saunders; 1994. pp. 385–95.

7. Smith MF, Roberson JB. Avoidance and management of complications. In Brackmann DE, Shelton C, Arriaga MA, eds. *Otologic Surgery*. Philadelphia: W.B. Saunders; 1994. pp. 359–71.

8. Brackmann DE, Arraiga MA. Surgery for glomus tumors. In Brackmann DE, Shelton C, Arriaga MA, eds. *Otologic Surgery*. Philadelphia: W. B. Saunders; 1994. pp. 579–93.

9. House WF, C. Shelton. The middle fossa approach. IIn Brackmann DE, Shelton C, Arriaga MA, eds. *Otologic Surgery*. Philadelphia: W.B. Saunders; 1994. pp. 595–604.

10. Jackler RK, Sim DW. Retrosigmoid approach to tumors of the cerebellopontine angle. In Brackmann DE, Shelton C, Arriaga MA, eds. *Otologic Surgery*. Philadelphia: W.B. Saunders; 1994. pp. 619–36.

11. Wiett RJ, Harvey SA, Bauer GP. Management of complications of chronic otitis media. In Brackmann DE, Shelton C, Arriaga MA, eds. *Otologic Surgery*. Philadelphia: W.B. Saunders; 1994. pp. 259–76.

12. Jellish WS, Owen K, Edelstein S, *et al.* Standard anesthetic technique for middle ear surgical procedures: a comparison of desflurane and sevoflurane. *Otolaryngol Head Neck Surg* 2005;**133**:269–74.

13. Firat Y, Kizilay A, Akarcay M, *et al.* The effect of dexmedetomidine on middle ear pressure. *Otolaryngol Head Neck Surg* 2007;**137**:218–23.

14. Jellish WS, Murdoch J, Leonetti JP. Perioperative management of complex skull base surgery: the anesthesiologist's point of view. *Neurosurg Focus* 2002;**12**(5):e5.

15. Chandra RK, Epstein VA, Fishman AJ. Prevalence of depression and antidepressant use in an otolaryngology patient population. *Otolaryngol Head Neck Surg* 2009;**141**:136–8.

16. Webster AC, Morley-Forster PK, Janzen V, *et al.* Anesthesia for intranasal surgery: a comparison between tracheal intubation and the flexible reinforced laryngeal mask airway. *Anesth Analg* 1999;**88**:421–5.

17. Atef A, Fawaz A. Comparison of laryngeal mask with endotracheal tube for anesthesia in endoscopic sinus surgery. *Am J Rhinol* 2008;**22**:653–7.

18. Ayala MA, Sanderson A, Marks R, *et al.* Laryngeal mask airway use in otologic surgery. *Otol Neurotol* 2009;**30**:599–601.

19. Taheri A, Hajimohamadi F, Soltanghoraee H, *et al.* Complications of using laryngeal mask airway during anaesthesia in patients undergoing major ear surgery. *Acta Otorhinolaryngol Ital* 2009;**29**:151–5.

20. Mandel JE. Laryngeal mask airways in ear, nose, and throat procedures. *Anesthesiol Clin* 2010;**28**:469–83.

21. Uppal V, Fletcher G, Kinsella J. Comparison of the i-gel with the cuffed tracheal tube during pressure-controlled ventilation. *Br J Anaesth* 2009;**102**:264–8.

22. Sharma B, Sehgal R, Sahai C, *et al.* PLMA vs. I-gel: a comparative evaluation of respiratory mechanics in laparoscopic cholecystectomy. *J Anaesthesiol Clin Pharmacol* 2010;**26**:451–7.

23. Theiler LG, Kleine-Brueggeney M, Kaiser D, *et al.* Crossover comparison of the laryngeal mask supreme and the i-gel in simulated difficult airway scenario in anesthetized patients. *Anesthesiology* 2009;**111**:55–62.

24. Jagannathan N, Kozlowski RJ, Sohn LE, *et al.* A clinical evaluation of the intubating laryngeal airway as a conduit for tracheal intubation in children. *Anesth Analg* 2011;**112**:176–82.

25. Galgon RE, Schroeder KM, Han S, *et al.* The air-Q(®) intubating laryngeal airway vs the LMA-ProSeal(TM): a prospective, randomised trial of airway seal pressure. *Anaesthesia* 2011;**66**:1093–100.

26. Joffe AM, Liew EC, Galgon RE, *et al.* The second-generation air-Q intubating laryngeal mask for airway maintenance during anaesthesia in adults: a report of the first 70 uses. *Anaesth Intensive Care* 2011;**39**:40–5.

27. Gelb AW, Southorn P, Rehder K. Effect of general anaesthesia on respiratory function. *Lung* 1981;**159**:187–98.

28. Fujii Y. Clinical strategies for preventing postoperative nausea and vomitting after middle ear surgery in adult patients. *Curr Drug Saf* 2008;**3**:230–9.

29. Soppitt AJ, Glass PS, Howell S, *et al.* The use of propofol for its antiemetic effect: a survey of clinical practice in the United States. *J Clin Anesth* 2000;**12**: 265–9.

30. Tramèr M, Moore A, McQuay H. Propofol anaesthesia and postoperative nausea and vomiting: quantitative systematic review of randomized controlled studies. *Br J Anaesth* 1997;**78**: 247–55.

31. Siddik-Sayyid SM, Taha SK, Kanazi GE, *et al.* Excellent intubating conditions with remifentanil-propofol and either low-dose rocuronium or succinylcholine. *Can J Anaesth* 2009;**56**:483–8.

32. Scheller MS, Zornow MH, Saidman LJ. Tracheal intubation without the use of muscle relaxants: a technique using propofol and varying doses of alfentanil. *Anesth Analg* 1992;**75**:788–93.

33. Erhan E, Ugur G, Alper I, *et al.* Tracheal intubation without muscle relaxants: remifentanil or alfentanil in combination with propofol. *Eur J Anaesthesiol* 2003;**20**:37–43.

34. Erhan E, Ugur G, Gunusen I, *et al.* Propofol – not thiopental or etomidate – with remifentanil provides adequate intubating conditions in the absence of neuromuscular blockade. *Can J Anaesth* 2003;**50**:108–15.

35. Jellish WS, Leonetti JP, Avramov A, *et al.* Remifentanil-based anesthesia versus a propofol technique for otologic surgical procedures. *Otolaryngol Head Neck Surg* 2000;**122**:222–7.

36. Jellish WS, Leonetti JP, Fahey K, *et al.* Comparison of 3 different anesthetic techniques on 24-hour recovery after otologic surgical

procedures. *Otolaryngol Head Neck Surg* 1999;**120**:406–11.

37. Eberhart LH, Eberspaecher M, Wulf H, *et al.* Fast-track eligibility, costs and quality of recovery after intravenous anaesthesia with propofol-remifentanil versus balanced anaesthesia with isoflurane-alfentanil. *Eur J Anaesthesiol* 2004;**21**:107–14.

38. Van den Berg AA, Savva D, Honjol NM, *et al.* Comparison of total intravenous, balanced inhalational and combined intravenous-inhalational anaesthesia for tympanoplasty, septorhinoplasty and adenotonsillectomy. *Anaesth Intensive Care* 1995;**23**:574–82.

39. Loop T, Priebe HJ. Recovery after anesthesia with remifentanil combined with propofol, desflurane, or sevoflurane for otorhinolaryngeal surgery. *Anesth Analg* 2000;**91**:123–9.

40. White PF, Tang J, Wender RH, *et al.* Desflurane versus sevoflurane for maintenance of outpatient anesthesia: the effect on early versus late recovery and perioperative coughing. *Anesth Analg* 2009;**109**:387–93.

41. Gupta A, Stierer T, Zuckerman R, *et al.* Comparison of recovery profile after ambulatory anesthesia with propofol, isoflurane, sevoflurane and desflurane: a systematic review. *Anesth Analg* 2004;**98**:632–41.

42. Philip BK, Kallar SK, Bogetz MS, *et al.* A multicenter comparison of maintenance and recovery with sevoflurane or isoflurane for adult ambulatory anesthesia. The Sevoflurane Multicenter Ambulatory Group. *Anesth Analg* 1996;**83**:314–19.

43. Koksal GM, Sayilgan C, Gungor G, *et al.* Effects of sevoflurane and desflurane on cytokine response during tympanoplasty surgery. *Acta Anaesthesiol Scand* 2005;**49**:835–9.

44. Jellish WS, Leonetti JP, Murdoch JR, *et al.* Propofol-based anesthesia as compared with standard anesthetic techniques for middle ear surgery. *J Clin Anesth* 1995;**7**:292–6.

45. Jellish WS, Leonetti JP, Murdoch J, *et al.* Propofol based anesthesia as compared with standard anesthetic techniques for middle ear surgery. *Otolaryngol Head Neck Surg* 1995;**112**:262–7.

46. Wuesten R, Van Aken H, Glass PS, *et al.* Assessment of depth of anesthesia and postoperative respiratory recovery after remifentanil- versus alfentanil-based total intravenous anesthesia in patients undergoing ear-nose-throat surgery. *Anesthesiology* 2001;**94**:211–17.

47. Ledowski T, Bein B, Hanss R, *et al.* Neuroendocrine stress response and heart rate variability: a comparison of total intravenous versus balanced anesthesia. *Anesth Analg* 2005;**101**:1700–5.

48. Sonne NM, Clausen TG, Valentin N, *et al.* Total intravenous anaesthesia for direct laryngoscopy: propofol infusion compared to thiopentone combined with midazolam and methohexitone infusion. *Acta Anaesthesiol Scand* 1992;**36**:250–4.

49. Montes FR, Trillos JE, Rincón IE, *et al.* Comparison of total intravenous anesthesia and sevoflurane-fentanyl anesthesia for outpatient otorhinolaryngeal surgery. *J Clin Anesth* 2002;**14**:324–8.

50. Larsen B, Seitz A, Larsen R. Recovery of cognitive function after remifentanil-propofol anesthesia: a comparison with desflurane and sevoflurane anesthesia. *Anesth Analg* 2000;**90**:168–74.

51. Visser K, Hassink EA, Bonsel GJ, *et al.* Randomized controlled trial of total intravenous anesthesia with propofol versus inhalation anesthesia with isoflurane-nitrous oxide: postoperative nausea with vomiting and economic analysis. *Anesthesiology* 2001;**95**:616–26.

52. McKeating K, Bali IM, Dundee JW. The effects of thiopentone and propofol on upper airway integrity. *Anaesthesia* 1988;**43**:638–40.

53. Mustola ST, Baer GA, Metsä-Ketelä T, *et al.* Haemodynamic and plasma catecholamine responses during total intravenous anaesthesia for laryngomicroscopy. Thiopentone compared with propofol. *Anaesthesia* 1995;**50**:108–13.

54. Ewalenko P, Deloof T, Gerin M, *et al.* Propofol infusion with or without fentanyl supplementation for microlaryngoscopy. *Acta Anaesthesiol Belg* 1990;**41**:297–306.

55. Jellish WS, Leonetti JP, Buoy CM, *et al.* Facial nerve electromyographic monitoring to predict movement in patients titrated to a standard anesthetic depth. *Anesth Analg* 2009;**109**:551–8.

56. Siler JN, Horrow JC, Rosenberg H. Propofol reduces prolonged outpatient PACU stay. An analysis according to surgical procedure. *Anesthesiol Rev* 1994;**21**:129–32.

57. Tang J, Chen L, White PF, *et al.* Recovery profile, costs, and patient satisfaction with propofol and sevoflurane for fast-track office-based anesthesia. *Anesthesiology* 1999;**91**:253–61.

58. Sommer M, Geurts JW, Stessel B, *et al.* Prevalence and predictors of postoperative pain after ear, nose, and throat surgery. *Arch Otolaryngol Head Neck Surg* 2009;**135**:124–30.

59. Mustola ST, Baer GA, Neuvonen PJ, *et al.* Requirements of propofol at different end-points without adjuvant and during two different steady infusions of

remifentanil. *Acta Anaesthesiol Scand* 2005;**49**:215–21.

60. Pavlin JD, Colley PS, Weymuller EA Jr, *et al.* Propofol versus isoflurane for endoscopic sinus surgery. *Am J Otolaryngol* 1999;**20**:96–101.

61. Vuyk J. Clinical interpretation of pharmacokinetic and pharmacodynamic propofol-opioid interactions. *Acta Anaesth Belg* 2001;**52**:445–51.

62. Ausems ME, Vuyk J, Hug CC Jr, *et al.* Comparison of a computer-assisted infusion versus intermittent bolus administration of alfentanil as a supplement to nitrous oxide for lower abdominal surgery. *Anesthesiology* 1988;**68**:851–61.

63. Kern SE, Stanski DR. Pharmacokinetics and pharmacodynamics of intravenously administered anesthetic drugs: concepts and lessons for drug development. *Clin Pharmacol Ther* 2008;**84**: 153–7.

64. Stanski DR, Shafer SL. Quantifying anesthetic drug interaction. Implications for drug dosing. *Anesthesiology* 1995; **83**:1–5.

65. Twersky RS, Jamerson B, Warner DS, *et al.* Hemodynamics and emergence profile of remifentanil versus fentanyl prospectively compared in a large population of surgical patients. *J Clin Anesth* 2001;**13**:407–16.

66. Wiel E, Davette M, Carpentier L, *et al.* Comparison of remifentanil and alfentanil during anaesthesia for patients undergoing direct laryngoscopy without intubation. *Br J Anaesth* 2003;**91**:421–3.

67. Ozkose Z, Yalcin Cok O, Tuncer B, *et al.* Comparison of hemodynamics, recovery profile, and early postoperative pain control and costs of remifentanil versus alfentanil-based total intravenous anaesthesia (TIVA). *J Clin Anesth* 2002;**14**:161–8.

68. Alper I, Erhan E, Ugur G, *et al.* Remifentanil versus alfentanil in total intravenous anaesthesia for day case surgery. *Eur J Anaesthesiol* 2003;**20**:61–4.

69. Pandazi AK, Louizos AA, Davilis DJ, *et al.* Inhalational anesthetic technique in microlaryngeal surgery: a comparison between sevoflurane-remifentanil and sevoflurane-alfentanil anesthesia. *Ann Otol Rhinol Laryngol* 2003;**112**:373–8.

70. Albertin A, Casati A, Federica L, *et al.* The effect-site concentration of remifentanil blunting cardiovascular responses to tracheal intubation and skin incision during bispectral index-guided propofol anesthesia. *Anesth Analg* 2005;**101**:125–30.

71. Björkman S, Wada DR, Stanski DR. Application of physiologic models to predict the influence of changes in body composition and blood flows on the pharmacokinetics of fentanyl and alfentanil in patients. *Anesthesiology* 1998;**88**: 657–67.

72. Passot S, Servin F, Allary R, *et al.* Target-controlled versus manually-controlled infusion of propofol for direct laryngoscopy and bronchoscopy. *Anesth Analg* 2002;**94**:1212–16.

73. Yeganeh N, Roshani B, Yari M, *et al.* Target-controlled infusion anesthesia with propofol and remifentanil compared with manually controlled infusion anesthesia in mastoidectomy surgeries. *Middle East J Anesthesiol* 2010;**20**:785–93.

74. Troy AM, Hutchinson RC, Easy WR, *et al.* Tracheal intubating conditions using propofol and remifentanil target-controlled infusions. *Anaesthesia* 2002;**57**:1204–7.

75. Ryu JH, Sohn IS, Do SH. Controlled hypotension for middle ear surgery: a comparison between remifentanil and

magnesium sulphate. *Br J Anaesth* 2009;**103**:490–5.

76. Leone M, Rousseau S, Avidan M, *et al.* Target concentrations of remifentanil with propofol to blunt coughing during intubation, cuff inflation, and tracheal suctioning. *Br J Anaesth* 2004;**93**:660–3

77. Takahashi H, Sugimaru T, Honjo I, *et al.* Assessment of the gas exchange function of the middle ear using nitrous oxide. A preliminary study. *Acta Otolaryngol* 1994;**114**:643–6.

78. Graham AM, Myles PS, Leslie K, *et al.* A cost-benefit analysis of the ENIGMA trial. *Anesthesiology* 2011;**115**:265–72.

79. Degoute CS, Ray MJ, Manchon M, *et al.* Remifentanil and controlled hypotension; comparison with nitroprusside or esmolol during tympanoplasty. *Can J Anaesth* 2001;**48**:20–7.

80. Richa F, Yazigi A, Sleilaty G, *et al.* Comparison between dexmedetomidine and remifentanil for controlled hypotension during tympanoplasty. *Eur J Anaesthesiol* 2008;**25**:369–74.

81. Dal D, Celiker V, Ozer E, *et al.* Induced hypotension for tympanoplasty: a comparison of desflurane, isoflurane and sevoflurane. *Eur J Anaesthesiol* 2004;**21**:902–6.

82. Degoute CS. Controlled hypotension: a guide to drug choice. *Drugs* 2007;**67**:1053–76.

83. Yu SK, Tait G, Karkouti K, *et al.* The safety of perioperative esmolol: a systematic review and meta-analysis of randomized controlled trials. *Anesth Analg* 2011;**112**:267–81.

84. Miller DR, Martineau RJ, Wynands JE, *et al.* Bolus administration of esmolol for controlling the haemodynamic response to tracheal intubation: the Canadian Multicentre Trial.

Can J Anaesth 1991;**38**: 849–58.

85. Menigaux C, Guignard B, Adam F, *et al.* Esmolol prevents movement and attenuates the BIS response to orotracheal intubation. *Br J Anaesth* 2002;**89**:857–62.

86. Oda Y, Nishikawa K, Hase I, *et al.* The short-acting beta1-adrenoceptor antagonists esmolol and landiolol suppress the bispectral index response to tracheal intubation during sevoflurane anesthesia. *Anesth Analg* 2005;**100**:733–7.

87. White PF, Wang B, Tang J, *et al.* The effect of intraoperative use of esmolol and nicardipine on recovery after ambulatory surgery. *Anesth Analg* 2003;**97**:1633–8.

88. Coloma M, Chiu JW, White PF, *et al.* The use of esmolol as an alternative to remifentanil during desflurane anesthesia for fast-track outpatient gynecologic laparoscopic surgery. *Anesth Analg* 2001;**92**:352–7.

89. Smith I, Van Hemelrijck J, White PF. Efficacy of esmolol versus alfentanil as a supplement to propofol-nitrous oxide anesthesia. *Anesth Analg* 1991;**73**:540–6.

90. Albera R, Ferrero V, Canale A, *et al.* Cochlear blood flow modifications induced by anaesthetic drugs in middle ear surgery: comparison between sevoflurane and propofol. *Acta Otolaryngol* 2003;**123**:812–6.

91. Preckel MP, Ferber-Viart C, Leftheriotis G, *et al.* Autoregulation of human inner ear blood flow during middle ear surgery with propofol or isoflurane anesthesia during controlled hypotension. *Anesth Analg* 1998;**87**:1002–8.

92. Cai YR, Xu J, Chen LH, *et al.* Electromyographic monitoring of facial nerve under different levels of neuromuscular blockade

during middle ear microsurgery. *Chin Med J (Engl)* 2009;**122**:311–4.

93. Lennon RL, Hosking MP, Daube JR, *et al.* Effect of partial neuromuscular blockade on intraoperative electromyography in patients undergoing resection of acoustic neuromas. *Anesth Analg* 1992;**75**:729–33.

94. Kizilay A, Aladag I, Cokkeser Y, *et al.* Effects of partial neuromuscular blockade on facial nerve monitorization in otologic surgery. *Acta Otolaryngol* 2003;**123**:321–4.

95. Chang T, Dworsky WA, White PF. Continuous electromyography for monitoring depth of anesthesia. *Anesth Analg* 1988;**67**:521–5.

96. Verghese C. Laryngeal mask airway devices: three maneuvers for any clinical situation. Available at: http://www.anesthesiologynews.com/download/3Maneuvers_ANGAM10_WM.pdf. Accessed November 4, 2011.

97. Rees L, Mason RA. Advanced upper airway obstruction in ENT surgery. *Br J Anaesth CEPD Reviews* 2002;**2**:134–8.

98. Machata AM, Illievich UM, Gustorff B, *et al.* Remifentanil for tracheal tube tolerance: a case control study. *Anaesthesia* 2007;**62**:796–801.

99. Nho JS, Lee SY, Kang JM, *et al.* Effects of maintaining a remifentanil infusion on the recovery profiles during emergence from anaesthesia and tracheal extubation. *Br J Anaesth* 2009;**103**:817–21.

100. Liu YH, Li MJ, Wang PC, *et al.* Use of dexamethasone on the prophylaxis of nausea and vomiting after tympanomastoid surgery. *Laryngoscope* 2001;**111**:1271–4.

101. Issioui T, Klein KW, White PF, *et al.* The efficacy of premedication with celecoxib

and acetaminophen in preventing pain after otolaryngologic surgery. *Anesth Analg* 2002;**94**:1188–93.

102. White PF, Tang J, Wender RH, *et al.* The effects of oral ibuprofen and celecoxib in preventing pain, improving recovery outcomes and patient satisfaction after ambulatory surgery. *Anesth Analg* 2011;**112**:323–9.

103. Lerman J, Jöhr M. Inhalational anesthesia vs total intravenous anesthesia (TIVA) for pediatric anesthesia. *Paediatr Anaesth* 2009;**19**:521–34.

104. Abuzayed B, Canbaz B, Sanus GZ, *et al.* Combined craniofacial resection of anterior skull base tumors: long-term results and experience of single institution. *Neurosurg Rev* 2011;**34**:101–13.

105. Kaplan MJ, Fischbein NJ, Harsh GR. Anterior skull base surgery. *Otolaryngol Clin North Am* 2005;**38**:107–31.

106. Ramina R, Maniglia JJ, Fernandes YB, *et al.* Tumors of the jugular foramen: diagnosis and management. *Neurosurgery* 2005;**57**(1 Suppl):59–68.

107. Jensen NF. Glomus tumors of the head and neck: anesthetic considerations. *Anesth Analg* 1994;**78**:112–9.

108. Sen C, Hague K, Kacchara R, *et al.* Jugular foramen: microscopic anatomic features and implications for neural preservation with reference to glomus tumors involving the temporal bone. *Neurosurgery* 2001;**48**:838–47.

109. Jackson LE, Roberson JB Jr. Vagal nerve monitoring in surgery of the skull base: a comparison of efficacy of three techniques. *Am J Otol* 1999;**20**:649–56.

110. Topsakal C, Al-Mefty O, Bulsara KR, *et al.* Intraoperative monitoring of lower cranial

nerves in skull base surgery: technical report and review of 123 monitored cases. *Neurosurg Rev* 2008;**31**:45–53.

111. Lopez JR. The use of evoked potentials in intraoperative neurophysiologic monitoring. *Phys Med Rehabil Clin N Am* 2004;**15**:63–8.

112. Sloan T. Anesthesia and intraoperative neurophysiological monitoring in children. *Childs Nerv Syst* 2010;**26**:227–35.

113. Bauer DF, Youkilis A, Schenck C, *et al.* The falcine trigeminocardiac reflex: case report and review of the literature. *Surg Neurol* 2005;**63**:143–8.

114. Schaller B, Cornelius JF, Prabhakar H, *et al.* Trigemino-Cardiac Reflex Examination Group (TCREG). The trigemino-cardiac reflex: an update of the current knowledge. *J Neurosurg Anesthesiol* 2009;**21**:187–95.

115. Gil Z, Cohen JT, Spektor S, *et al.* Anterior skull base surgery without prophylactic airway diversion procedures. *Otolaryngol Head Neck Surg* 2003;**128**: 681–5.

116. Drage MP, Nunez J, Vaughan RS, *et al.* Jaw thrusting as a clinical test to assess the adequate depth of anaesthesia for insertion of the laryngeal mask. *Anaesthesia* 1996;**51**:1167–70.

117. O'Connor CJ, Borromeo CJ, Stix MS. Assessing ProSeal laryngeal mask positioning: the suprasternal notch test. *Anesth Analg* 2002;**94**:1374–5.

118. Brimacombe J, Keller C. The ProSeal laryngeal mask airway. *Anesthesiology Clin N Am* 2002;**20**:871–91.

119. Cook TM, Nolan JP. The ProSeal™ laryngeal mask airway: a review of the literature. *Can J Anesth* 2005;**52**:739–60.

120. Timmermann A, Cremer S, Eich C, *et al.* Prospective clinical and fiberoptic evaluation of the Supreme Laryngeal Mask Airway™. *Anesthesiology* 2009;**110**:262–5.

121. Keller C, Brimacombe JR, Keller K, *et al.* Comparison of four methods for assessing airway sealing pressure with the laryngeal mask airway in adult patients. *Br J Anaesth* 1999;**82**:286–7.

122. Drolet P, Girard M. An aid to correct positioning of the ProSeal laryngeal mask. *Can J Anaesth* 2001;**48**:718–9.

123. Eschertzhuber S, Brimacombe J, Hohlrieder M, *et al.* The Laryngeal Mask Airway Supreme™ – a single use laryngeal mask airway with an oesophageal vent. A randomised, cross-over study with the Laryngeal Mask Airway ProSeal™ in paralysed, anaesthetised patients. *Anaesthesia* 2009;**64**:79–83.

124. Seet E, Rajeev S, Firoz T, *et al.* Safety and efficacy of laryngeal mask airway Supreme versus laryngeal mask airway ProSeal: a randomized controlled trial. *Eur J Anaesthesiol* 2010;**27**: 602–7

125. Sataloff RT, Hawkshaw MJ, Divi V, *et al.* Voice surgery. *Otolaryngol Clin North Am* 2007;**40**:1151–83.

126. Beckford NS, Mayo R, Wilkinson A 3rd, *et al.* Effects of short-term endotracheal intubation on vocal function. *Laryngoscope* 1990;**100**:331–6.

127. Rieger A, Brunne B, Hass I, *et al.* Laryngo-pharyngeal complaints following laryngeal mask airway and endotracheal intubation. *J Clin Anesth* 1997;**9**:42–7.

128. Yu SH, Beirne OR. Laryngeal mask airways have a lower risk of airway complications compared with endotracheal intubation: a systematic review. *J Oral Maxillofac Surg* 2010;**68**:2359–76.

129. Zimmert M, Zwirner P, Kruse E, *et al.* Effects on vocal function and incidence of laryngeal disorder when using a laryngeal mask airway in comparison with an endotracheal tube. *Eur J Anaesthesiol* 1999;**16**:511–5.

130. Hönemann CW, Hahnenkamp K, Möllhoff T, *et al.* Minimal-flow anaesthesia with controlled ventilation: comparison between laryngeal mask airway and endotracheal tube. *Eur J Anaesthesiol* 2001;**18**:458–66.

131. Hamdan AL, Kanazi G, Rameh C, *et al.* Immediate post-operative vocal changes in patients using laryngeal mask airway versus endotracheal tube. *J Laryngol Otol* 2008;**122**:829–35.

132. Hamdan AL, Sibai A, Rameh C, *et al.* Short-term effects of endotracheal intubation on voice. *J Voice* 2007;**21**:762–8.

Chapter

30

Anesthesia for diagnostic bronchoscopic procedures

Basem Abdelmalak and Mona Sarkiss

Diagnostic bronchoscopic procedures are performed every day by both pulmonologists and thoracic surgeons. Diagnostic bronchoscopy is indicated for airway exam, bronchioalveolar lavage, biopsy of airway lesions, autofluorescence bronchoscopy, and narrow band imaging. Most of the diagnostic procedures are performed in an outpatient setting under moderate (conscious) sedation in conjunction with local anesthesia to numb the airway. Moderate sedation is commonly provided by a trained sedation nurse under the supervision of the bronchoscopist and has become a well-accepted method of providing anesthesia for diagnostic bronchoscopy. The short duration of diagnostic bronchoscopy procedures makes moderate sedation a suitable method of anesthesia [1]. In recent years more prolonged sophisticated diagnostic bronchoscopic procedures have emerged. These include endobronchial ultrasound with fine-needle aspiration (EBUS-FNA) [2], staging of lung cancer, and electromagnetic navigation (EMN) with biopsy of peripheral lung lesions. These procedures require a longer duration and a quiet field for precise targeting of the mediastinal lymph nodes or lung lesions without injury to surrounding large vessels or breach of the pleura. As a result there is increasing demand for general anesthesia under the care of anesthesiologists for advanced diagnostic bronchoscopic procedures.

The demand for the advanced diagnostic bronchoscopic procedures is increasing as these procedures provide a minimally invasive approach. Although it seems intuitive to perform general anesthesia for airway procedures in the operating room, the current practice is that most of these procedures are performed in interventional bronchoscopy suites that have been modified to mimic an operating room

(Figure 30.1) These suites are commonly found in large academic centers with high volumes of patients needing advanced diagnostic bronchoscopic procedures on a daily basis. Several factors have caused the shift of performing such airway procedures to outside the operating room. These include the high safety profile of EBUS-FNA, the increased cost of performing procedures in the operating room, inability to obtain operating room block time on short notice for the pulmonologists, and the cumbersome process of moving the equipment required to perform the procedures to the operating room. The interventional bronchoscopy suites are designed with both safety and excellence in mind [3]. The American Society of Anesthesiology guidelines on establishing out of the operating room anesthesia support have to be implemented during the design of such interventional bronchoscopic suites [4].

In addition to the concern over performing airway procedures outside the operating room, there is a greater concern over patients requiring such procedures. The majority of patients needing diagnostic bronchoscopic procedures are diagnosed with or suspected to have lung cancer with underlying severe morbidities that commonly place them as ASA status 3–5. This represents a challenge for the anesthesiologists, who must simultaneously consider the severity of their lung pathology and their other comorbidities. It must also be emphasized that a continuous discussion between the anesthesiologist and the bronchoscopist needs to be maintained during the procedure as they both share the airway. Consequently, the anesthesiologist has to familiarize him/herself with the procedure, possible complications and their management as well as alternative anesthetic and airway management plans.

Anesthesia for Otolaryngologic Surgery, ed. Basem Abdelmalak and D. John Doyle. Published by Cambridge University Press.
© Cambridge University Press 2013.

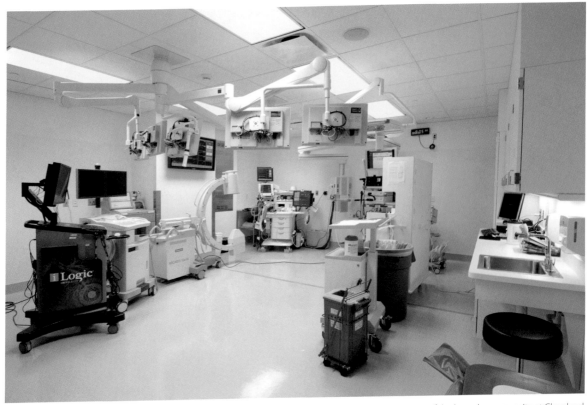

Figure 30.1. An example of the configuration of a modern bronchoscopy surgery room (image courtesy of the bronchoscopy suite at Cleveland Clinic, Cleveland, OH). Reprinted with permission, Cleveland Clinic Center for Medical Art & Photography © 2011–2012. All rights reserved.

Advanced diagnostic bronchoscopic procedures

Endobronchial ultrasound fine-needle aspiration

Definition

EBUS is a minimally invasive procedure that was designed to evaluate mediastinal and hilar lymphadenopathy using a linear array ultrasound probe modified flexible bronchoscope. Once enlarged lymph nodes are detected, real-time transbronchial fine-needle aspiration can be performed under direct vision facilitated by ultrasound guidance. Tissue confirmation by on-site pathology commonly follows. Noteworthy is that the ultrasonic bronchoscope has Doppler capabilities that allow for monocolor flow mapping of mediastinal blood vessels.

Indications

1. Histological diagnosis of mediastinal and/or hilar lymphadenopathy or masses.

2. Staging of known lung cancer.

Procedure description

Due to the large external diameter of 6.9 mm of the EBUS bronchoscope, it is usually introduced through the mouth instead of the nose. Once the EBUS bronchoscope is positioned in the desired location a balloon at the tip of the scope is inflated with normal saline. Saline acts as a coupling medium for the ultrasound and allows the distal end of the bronchoscope to abut the wall of the airway. A two-screen display provides the fiberoptic image of the airway as well as the ultrasound image (Figure 30.2). Vascular landmarks are then identified and the associated lymph nodes described in the Mountain classification are measured. A fine needle ranging in gauge from 22 to 25 is then introduced through the working channel of the EBUS bronchoscope and is advanced through the wall of the airway into the lymph node. Sampling may be repeated until adequate samples are confirmed by rapid on-site pathology evaluation (ROSE).

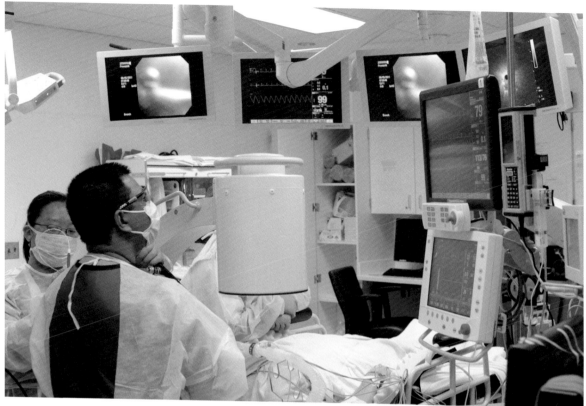

Figure 30.2. Bronchoscopy suite set-up for EBUS-FNA mediastinal staging. Reprinted with permission, Cleveland Clinic Center for Medical Art & Photography © 2011–2012. All rights reserved.

Electromagnetic navigational bronchoscopy (ENB)

Definition

ENB is a bronchoscopic procedure that utilizes the principle of GPS to allow the bronchoscopist to reach peripheral lung lesions adjacent to very small distal bronchi.

Indications

1. Biopsy of peripheral lung nodules.
2. Lymph node biopsy.
3. Guide the insertion of radiotherapy or brachytherapy markers.

Procedure description (Figure 30.3)

Planning phase

A recent chest CT scan of the patient is loaded into software that reconstructs the patient's airways in 3D images. The bronchoscopist marks the targeted area on the 3D image and plans the pathway to the target.

Navigation phase

The bronchoscopist then introduces an extended working channel with a sensor probe through a bronchoscope in the airway. The extended working channel and the sensor probe are then navigated under real-time guidance to the target location. Once the desired location is reached the bronchoscopist locks the extended working channel in place and removes the sensor probe. Consequently, any bronchoscopic tool desired (e.g., needle, radiotherapy markers) can be introduced through the extended working channel to the lesion of interest. It should be noted that in such procedures, specially designed and measured procedure beds are used, with the precaution of excluding all ferromagnetic items from the bed; for example, we have devised a plastic replica of the commonly used circuit holder to be used for these procedures (Figure 30.4).

299

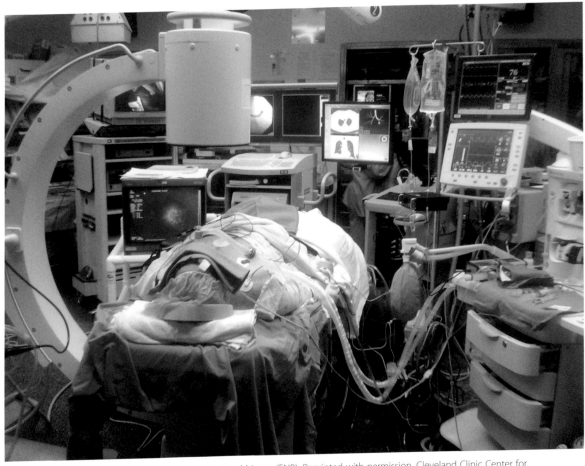

Figure 30.3. OR set up for electromagnetic navigational biopsy (ENB). Reprinted with permission, Cleveland Clinic Center for Medical Art & Photography © 2011–2012. All rights reserved.

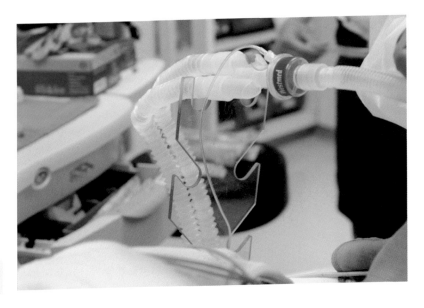

Figure 30.4. Nonferromagnetic circuit holder to be used with electromagnetic navigational biopsies (innovation of Ken Barclay, of Cleveland Clinic Bronchoscopy Suite). Reprinted with permission, Cleveland Clinic Center for Medical Art & Photography © 2011–2012. All rights reserved.

Anesthetic care

Preoperative evaluation

Diagnostic bronchoscopy can be considered an urgent procedure where a definitive diagnosis and/or staging of a known cancer is needed to plan treatment. Preoperative assessment can be conducted in a customary fashion with special attention to airway and respiration.

Symptoms: hoarseness, stridor, dysphagia, hemoptysis, dyspnea on exertion, orthopnea.

Signs: use of accessory muscles, wheezing, rhonchi, crackles.

Imaging: location of enlarged lymph node station in relation to the airway and number of stations to be biopsied, extent of lung and mediastinal involvement, airway and major vessels compression or obstruction, evidence of pneumonia or other lung pathology.

Associated comorbidities: history of tobacco, alcohol use, coronary artery disease, COPD, supplemental oxygen use, chemotherapy or radiation treatment, evidence of metastatic disease

Premedication

Anxiolytics: in patients with compromised airway anxiolytics should be used with care if indicated in very anxious patients. Supplemental oxygen should be provided or be readily available.

Antisialagogue: if the patient can tolerate tachycardia, glycopyrrolate 0.2–0.4 mg can be given to reduce secretions that might dilute topical anesthetics used during bronchoscopy.

Oxygen: preoxygenation with 100% FiO_2 can be vital especially in patients exhibiting various degrees of hypoxemia on room air, or those who are already requiring home O_2 therapy.

Anesthesia technique

Advanced diagnostic bronchoscopy can be performed under moderate sedation, monitored anesthesia care or general anesthesia.

Moderate (conscious) sedation

Interventional bronchoscopists with no access to anesthesia support commonly perform advanced bronchoscopic procedures under moderate sedation. Anxiolytics, e.g., midazolam, and narcotics, e.g., fentanyl, are titrated for sedation. The airway is topicalized with local anesthetics in a spray-as-you-go

fashion. Difficulties with this approach are commonly encountered due to the extended length of the procedure and lower tolerance of the large-diameter EBUS bronchoscope by the patient. As a result higher than commonly used doses of sedating medications are given to allow the patient to tolerate the longer duration and the large bronchoscope. This may result in respiratory depression, unplanned intubation or hospital admission and prolonged recovery time.

Monitored anesthesia care

In a selected group of patients monitored anesthesia care can be the anesthetic technique of choice: for example, procedures of short duration such as when only one lymph node station will be biopsied, especially if it were of a large size, or in patients with no underlying lung pathology or oxygen dependence.

The drugs of choice should be the ultra-short-acting anesthetics that are easily titrated to match the patient tolerance to the procedure as well as the status of respiration, e.g., remifentanil, alfentanil, propofol, dexmedetomidine and fospropofol [5,6]. On the other hand midazolam, fentanyl, and morphine can also be acceptable choices.

General anesthesia

The total intravenous anesthetic technique (TIVA) is the technique of choice [7–9] and is preferred over inhalational anesthetic for the following reasons. Frequent suctioning of the airway secretions during the procedure can result in fluctuating levels of anesthetic gas in the airway that can change the depth of anesthesia. Additionally, frequent opening of the anesthetic circuit to air to introduce and remove the bronchoscope causes pollution of the procedure room air. It is noteworthy that inhalation anesthetics can be used to treat bronchospasm that is refractory to conventional medical treatment such as β-agonists, which may occur during bronchoscopy.

Propofol infusion rates between 100 and 250 μg/kg/min are used and can be titrated to effect based on the bispectral index monitor (BIS). On one hand the use of the BIS monitors can help the anesthesiologist avoid excessive anesthesia and hemodynamic compromise and on the other hand it can alert the anesthesiologist to light anesthesia and possible recall, which could occur as a result of pump failure, line disconnect or occlusion.

Opiates

Despite the fact that advanced bronchoscopic procedures are not associated with somatic pain, the use of low-dose opiates (e.g., fentanyl 50–100 μg) or ultra-short-acting opiates (e.g., remifentanil) can help reduce the sympathetic stimulation associated with airway manipulation during bronchoscopy as well as ameliorate the commonly experienced post-procedure cough. It should be noted, however, that remifentanil use may result in bradycardia and hypotension,which may lead to the administration of an unnecessarily large amount of fluid, as the goal is to keep these patients on the dry side.

Muscle relaxant

Introduction of the bronchoscope through the vocal cords into the airway results in laryngospasm and excessive coughing. This can be easily managed by installation of local anesthetics such as lidocaine 1%. However, care should be taken to avoid exceeding the maximum dose of lidocaine (5 mg/kg plain, 7 mg/kg with added epinephrine). The addition of muscle relaxant during the induction of anesthesia helps prevent laryngospasm and coughing. Muscle relaxants provide the bronchoscopist with a quiet field where small lymph nodes in difficult positions, such as between the aorta and the pulmonary artery, can be safely reached. Additionally EMN requires the patient to be motionless in order to overlap the CT scan image onto the patient's actual tracheobronchial tree. A succinylcholine infusion, rocuronium or cisatracurium, can be used safely. However, care should be taken in patients with lung cancer and associated Eaton–Lambert syndrome, where prolonged paralysis may occur.

Fraction inspired oxygen (FiO$_2$)

Administration of 100% oxygen is commonly needed during advanced bronchoscopic procedures. Patients with underlying lung pathology and low baseline oxygen saturation desaturate frequently during the procedure. Consequently, FiO$_2$ should be titrated to maintain patient saturation above 94%.

Airway devices

Procedures performed under conscious sedation or monitored anesthesia care require no airway devices. However, oxygen should be delivered via nasal cannula and carbon dioxide levels should be monitored by capnography.

Supraglottic airways

Supraglottic airways (SGA) are ideal airway devices for advanced bronchoscopic procedures. The large diameter of the shaft of the SGA makes it easy to insert the large EBUS bronchoscope (diameter 6.9 mm) and to ventilate around the bronchoscope. The SGA also allows the bronchoscopist to inspect the entire length of the airway from the vocal cord to distal large bronchi (Figure 30.5) [10]. Additionally, the LMA allows free mobility of the bronchoscope in the airway in order to bring the ultrasound tip into close proximity to the wall of the tracheobronchial tree. A bite block needs to be inserted around the SGA or the built-in bite block in some brands, as in the i-gel version of the SGA, suffices (Figure 30.6). Disadvantages of the SGA are lack of protection against aspiration and the inability to seat the SGA well in patients with oral, pharyngeal or laryngeal deformity, pathology or radiation.

An ideal SGA for these procedures would have:

(1) a large-diameter short shaft
(2) high seal pressure
(3) built-in bite block
(4) no obstacles for the passage of the bronchoscope such as aperture bars
(5) esophageal access to avoid gastric distension and emptying of gastric contents
(6) the option to intubate through it if needed.

Endotracheal tubes (ETT)

Due to the large diameter of the EBUS bronchoscope (6.9 mm) a large endotracheal tube (ETT) with internal diameter of 8.5 or 9.0 mm has to be used to facilitate ventilation (Figure 30.7) [10]. Once inserted the ETT needs to be positioned above the level of the lymph nodes to be biopsied. For example station 2 paratracheal lymph node may require a very high insertion of the ETT in the airway where the ETT cuff is in close proximity to the vocal cord. Additionally the ETT needs to be cut close (Figure 30.8B) to the patient to allow the insertion of the maximum length of the bronchoscope to reach the most distal lymph nodes, minimize resistance and facilitate bronchoscope navigation. However, in special circumstances when bleeding is anticipated, it is preferable not to cut the tube short to keep it available in case it

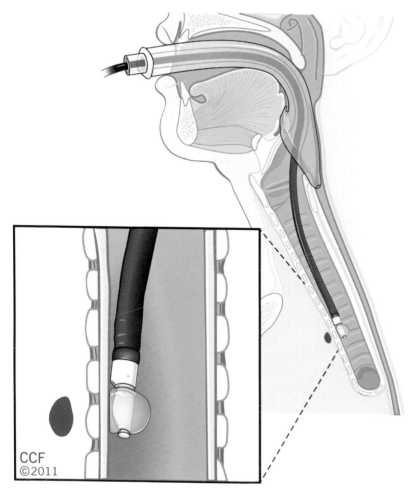

Figure 30.5. The use of supraglottic airway in the context of EBUS TBFNA. Reprinted with permission, Cleveland Clinic Center for Medical Art & Photography © 2011–2012. All rights reserved.

is needed to tamponade a bronchial bleeding or to advance into one of the mainstem bronchi for the purpose of lung isolation (Figure 30.8A). Another situation when the use of an ETT is helpful is when the EBUS bronchoscope is used as an esophagoscope when it is desirable to biopsy nodes that are closer to the esophagus than to the trachea. An airway secured with an ETT will greatly facilitate the esophageal insertion of the EBUS bronchoscope (Figure 30.9).

Independent of the airway device used, a swivel connector adaptor is needed to connect the airway device to the anesthesia circuit to allow simultaneous ventilation and bronchoscopy insertion (Figures 30.6 and 30.8).

Continuous clear communication between the anesthesiologist and the bronchoscopist is essential throughout the procedure as the condition of the airway is constantly changing. For example inflation of the balloon on the EBUS bronchoscope in the trachea can cause an increase in airway pressure and limit ventilation, or excessive bleeding in the airway and suctioning can result in atelectasis and desaturation.

Postoperative care

Patients should be transported to a standard post-anesthesia care unit (PACU) with well-trained nursing staff. Supplemental oxygen should be continued via face mask or nasal cannula and weaned off gradually. Patients should be monitored with standard monitors (EKG, pulse oximetery, noninvasive blood pressure). Due to the use of ultra-short-acting general anesthetic drugs, patients are commonly alert and oriented within a short period of arrival in the PACU.

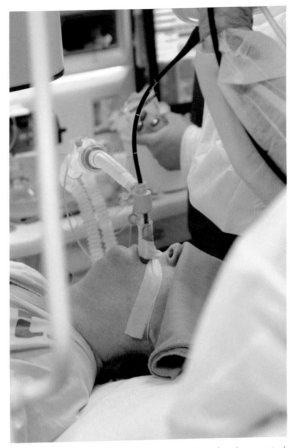

Figure 30.6. An i-gel supraglottic airway inserted and connected to the breathing circuit through a blue Portex swivel adapter and a corrugated Bennet connector. Reprinted with permission, Cleveland Clinic Center for Medical Art & Photography © 2011–2012. All rights reserved.

Patients are observed until they meet PACU discharge criteria (30–45 minutes) before discharge. Detection and management of possible post-procedure complications is described next.

Complications

EBUS and EMN are considered relatively safe procedures. Rare complications and morbidities can occur.

Complications during diagnostic bronchoscopic procedures

Low to no yield: when the pulmonologist is unsuccessful in obtaining tissue at all or obtaining very little tissue for the biopsy. One aspect the anesthesiologist can help with here is to provide a motionless patient through the use of either deep anesthesia alone, or balanced anesthesia with muscle relaxation. Any little movement, such as those associated with coughing secondary to tracheal and carinal irritation by the tube and/or the bronchoscope, especially occurring at the time of obtaining the biopsy, may cause the pulmonologist to miss the target.

Hypercarbia may be noted during the procedure due to ventilator perception of increased airway resistance after insertion of the bronchoscope in the airway. This is especially common with the use of SGA with imposed pressure limit of 20 mmHg to avoid inflation of the stomach. Hypercarbia can be treated by increasing the minute ventilation.

Transient hypoxemia is encountered rarely and can be due to several factors:

(1) lung atelectasis due to excessive bleeding in the airway that migrates to the distal alveoli, or excessive suctioning of the airway creating negative pressure that collapses the alveoli;

(2) inadequate ventilation;

(3) pneumothorax:

Pneumothorax occurs most often with sampling of station 2 lymph node. Pneumothorax can be detected on the ultrasound image or using fluoroscopy during or after the procedure. Pneumothorax can also manifest post procedure as chest pain.

Bleeding: multiple needle puncture sites cause minor bleeding in the airway that can be easily suctioned. Major bleeding from large mediastinal vessels has not been reported. The use of a small-gauge needle for biopsy makes major bleeding an unlikely complication.

Laryngospasm can be encountered mainly around extubation time after the muscle relaxant is reversed. The etiology is unclear but it may be due to the irritation of the vocal cord by the movement of the large bronchoscope during the lengthy procedure. Laryngospasm is easily treated with installation of local anesthetics on the vocal cord under direct vision through the working channel of the flexible bronchoscope.

Bronchospasm: although the etiology is unclear bronchospasm may occur during bronchoscopy. Bronchospasm can be detected by audible wheeze, increase in airway pressure and decreased tidal volume delivered by mechanical ventilation. Inhalation of a β-agonist such as albuterol and conversion

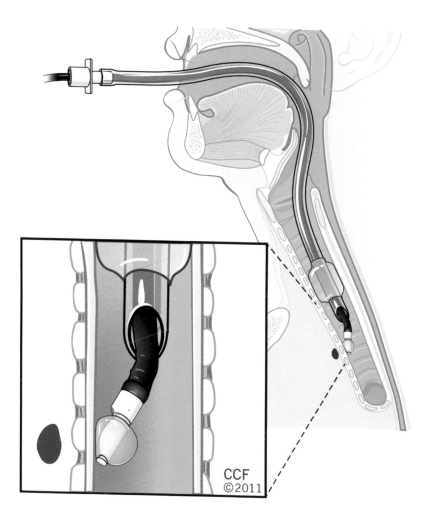

(a)

(b)

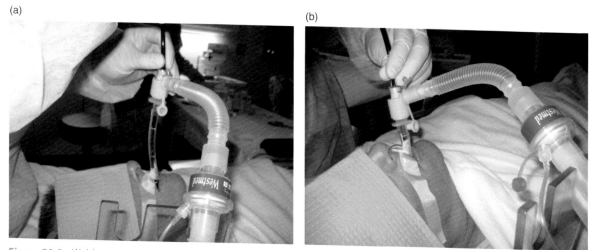

Figure 30.8. (A) A large diameter (8.5) ETT left uncut at the original length, which increases the resistance to the in-and-out motion of the bronchoscope, but can help in cases where endobronchial bleeding is a risk. In such circumstances it can be advanced and used for lung isolation to maintain ventilation. (B) ETT, cut short, allowing for better manuvering and less resistance for the EBUS bronchoscope. In both images the ETT is connected to the circuit with a blue Portex swivel adapter and a corrugated Bennet connector while the fiberoptic bronchoscope is seen entering the ETT via the Portex adapter.

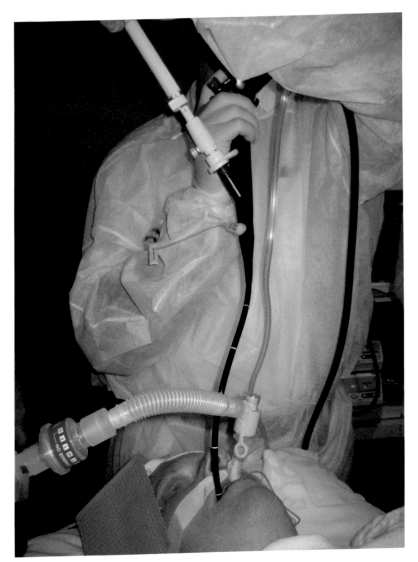

Figure 30.9. The EBUS bronchoscope is used as an esophagoscope when it is desirable to biopsy nodes that are closer to the esophagus than to the trachea. Please note that the EBUS bronchoscope is inserted into the mouth next to the ETT that is securing the airway. Reprinted with permission, Cleveland Clinic Center for Medical Art & Photography © 2011–2012. All rights reserved.

to inhalation anesthetic such as sevoflurane can generally relieve the refractory bronchospasm.

Respiratory failure may occur in the PACU and results in unplanned hospital admission, intubation and possible ICU stay. Although all common causes of respiratory failure should be entertained, residual muscle weakness and increased sensitivity to muscle relaxant in patients with lung cancer and Eaton–Lambert syndrome should be considered.

Cough: coughing after bronchoscopy is a common encounter. Cough may be due to throat irritation from the bronchoscope or airway device used or due to distal airway irritation from needle puncture sites and bleeding.

Delayed infections: there have been case reports of mediastinal abscess, lung abscess, and infected pericardial effusion 1–3 weeks after the procedure.

Summary

Diagnostic bronchoscopy is a rapidly expanding field. Diagnostic bronchoscopic procedures can be complex, the patient population generally has multiple comorbidities, and the procedures are performed mostly out of the operating rooms. Anesthesiologists need to stay up to date with the advances in this field, and the anesthetic challenges that might come with them. Open communication between the anesthesiologist and pulmonologist, understanding the nature of the procedure, and, above all, extreme vigilance and preparedness are mandatory to achieve a favorable outcome.

Case study

The patient was a 48-year-old male, 5′9″ (175 cm) in height and weighing 95 kg, with a history of hypertension, diabetes and an incidental finding of a peripheral right lower lung nodule, lower paratracheal lymphadenopathy, with two nodes measuring 2 × 2 cm each as estimated by chest CT.

He was scheduled for an endobronchial ultrasound (EBUS) biopsy of his paratracheal lymph nodes, and an endobronchial navigational biopsy (ENB) of his right lung nodule.

Preoperative evaluation

- Comorbidities: well-controlled hypertension and diabetes.
- Airway: Mallampati 2 airway, thyromental distance of 3 finger breadths, no overbite, neck circumference of 15.5 inches.

Induction of anesthesia

On the morning of the procedure, the patient had been NPO for more than 8 hours. The anesthesiologist and the pulmonolgist discussed the procedure and airway management plans.

After applying standard monitors, the patient was premedicated with 2 mg of midazolam IV. The patient was then pre-oxygenated with 100% oxygen via a face mask while a BIS monitor (Aspect Medical, Newton, MA) was applied to the forehead to monitor depth of anesthesia for the planned total intravenous anesthesia (TIVA) technique, thus decreasing the risk of unintended intraoperative awareness.

General anesthesia was then induced with 150 μg of fentanyl, 40 mg of lidocaine (to lessen the burning sensation associated with propofol injection), and 160 mg of propofol IV. A continuous IV propofol infusion was started at 140 μg/kg/min, followed by rocuronium 70 mg for muscle relaxation. Bag-mask ventilation was initiated with the aid of an oral airway. In about 2 minutes, when muscle relaxation was confirmed, the patient was intubated with a large 9 mm ID endotracheal tube, using a MAC 4 laryngoscope. Endotracheal (ET) intubation was confirmed by

observing the ET tube (ETT) passing through the vocal cords, chest rise, the presence of bilateral breath sounds, and via capnography. A large ETT was chosen to allow enough space around the US bronchoscope for easy ventilation and to decrease resistance for the movement of the bronchoscope within the ETT.

The ETT was secured at 20 cm as measured at the lip in the midline, and was then cut short (above the take-off of the pilot balloon) to facilitate movement of the bronchoscope. A Portex swivel adapter (Smiths Medical, Dublin, OH) was applied to connect the ETT to the circuit through a Bennet connector instead of the L-shaped circuit connector ordinarily used to connct to the ETT (Figure 30.8). This Portex swivel adapter helps facilitate spontaneous/positive-pressure ventilation during the procedure while the bronchoscope is in the airway.

Note: had the paratracheal lymph nodes been higher in anatomical position, the use of the ETT would have precluded successful completion of the procedure, and a supraglottic airway (SGA) such as the i-gel would have been the airway of choice in this situation. Another scenario where an ETT would not have been particularly appropriate is with upper right lung lesions, as the presence of the ETT in the trachea will make the bending of the bronchoscope to navigate through the endobronchial tree to reach an upper right lung lesion more difficult. On such an occasion, the use of a SGA would be more helpful (Figure 30.5).

Maintenance of anesthesia

General anesthesia was maintained with a titrated IV propofol infusion as per clinical needs and to a BIS ~ 50. Muscle relaxation was maintained at 1–2 twitches. Dexamethasone 8 mg IV was given for PONV prophylaxis and to decrease postoperative airway edema.

Emergence and recovery from anesthesia

At the completion of the case, muscle relaxation was reversed, and the propfol infusion was discontinued. The patient was extubated when he regained muscle power, became fully awake and followed commands. The patient was then admitted to PACU, where a chest X-ray was found to be negative for any acute changes; he spent an uneventful 60 minutes in PACU and was then discharged home once he met the PACU discharge criteria.

Clinical pearls

- In recent years some very sophisticated diagnostic bronchoscopic procedures have emerged: endobronchial ultrasound with fine-needle aspiration (EBUS-FNA), staging of lung cancer, and electromagnetic navigation (EMN) with biopsy of peripheral lung lesions. These procedures require extended periods where a quiet field is needed to allow precise targeting of the mediastinal lymph nodes or lung lesions without injury to surrounding large vessels or breach of the pleura. Thus there is increasing demand for general anesthesia under the supervision of anesthesiologists.

- Total intravenous anesthesia (TIVA) is the technique of choice in such cases, and is preferred over inhalational anesthesia since frequent opening of the anesthetic circuit to introduce and remove the bronchoscope causes pollution of the procedure room air. In addition, frequent suctioning during the procedure can result in fluctuating levels of anesthetic gas in the airway that can change the depth of anesthesia.

- Supraglottic airways (SGAs), e.g., i-gel or a large-diameter ETT (8.5 or 9.0 mm ID), are commonly used as an airway for these procedures.

- Muscle relaxants provide the bronchoscopist with a quiet field where small lymph nodes located in difficult positions can be safely reached with precision. This can improve safety and diagnostic yield.

- Administration of 100% oxygen is commonly needed during advanced bronchoscopic procedures.

- Continuous clear communication between the anesthesiologist and the bronchoscopist is essential throughout the procedure as the condition of the airway is constantly changing.

- Potential complications include, cough, pneumothorax, laryngospasm or bronchospasm.

References

1. Sarkiss M. Anesthesia for bronchoscopy and interventional pulmonology: from moderate sedation to jet ventilation. *Curr Opin Pulm Med* 2011;**17**(4):274–8. Epub 2011/04/27.

2. Yasufuku K, Chiyo M, Koh E, *et al.* Endobronchial ultrasound guided transbronchial needle aspiration for staging of lung cancer. *Lung Cancer* 2005; **50**(3):347–54. Epub 2005/09/21.

3. Beatriz A. What is an interventional pulmonolgy unit in Europe? *Clin Pulmon Med* 2010;**17**(1):42–6.

4. Practice guidelines for sedation and analgesia by non-anesthesiologists. *Anesthesiology* 2002;**96**(4):1004–17.

5. Abdelmalak B, Makary L, Hoban J, Doyle DJ. Dexmedetomidine as sole sedative for awake intubation in management of the critical airway. *J Clin Anesth* 2007;**19**(5):370–3. Epub 2007/09/18.

6. Silvestri GA, Vincent BD, Wahidi MM, *et al.* A phase 3, randomized, double-blind study to assess the efficacy and safety of fospropofol disodium injection for moderate sedation in patients undergoing flexible bronchoscopy. *Chest* 2009; **135**(1):41–7. Epub 2008/07/22.

7. Sarkiss M, Kennedy M, Riedel B, *et al.* Anesthesia technique for endobronchial ultrasound-guided fine needle aspiration of mediastinal lymph node. *J Cardiothorac Vasc Anesth* 2007;**21**(6):892–6. Epub 2007/12/11.

8. Abdelmalak B. Anesthesia for interventional pulmonology. In Urman RGW, Philip B, eds. *Anesthesia Outside of the Operating Room.* New York: Oxford University Press; 2011. pp. 167–74.

9. Doyle DJ, Abdelmalak B, Machuzak M, Gildea TR. Anesthesia and airway management for removing pulmonary self-expanding metallic stents. *J Clin Anesth* 2009;**21**(7):529–32. Epub 2009/12/17.

10. Abdelmalak B, Gildea T, Doyle DJ. Anesthesia for bronchoscopy. *Curr Pharm Des* 2012: in press.

Anesthesia for therapeutic bronchoscopic procedures

Basem Abdelmalak and Mona Sarkiss

The field of therapeutic bronchoscopy started in 1865 when Dr. Killian, a head and neck surgeon, invented the rigid bronchoscope. The rigid bronchoscope was initially used to remove aspirated foreign bodies from the airway [1]. Topical cocaine and subsequently general anesthesia were utilized to enable the patient to tolerate the procedure. By 1968 the flexible bronchoscope was invented by Ikeda. The small diameter and plasticity of the flexible bronchoscope rendered bronchoscopy a well-tolerated procedure, eliminating the need for general anesthesia, and rigid bronchoscopy became obsolete [1]. Flexible bronchoscopy was initially used for diagnostic bronchoscopic procedures such as airway exam, bronchioalveolar lavage, airway biopsy and foreign-body removal. Subsequently, the emergence of multiple small instruments that could fit through the flexible bronchoscope working channel expanded the scope of utilization of the flexible bronchoscope; examples of such instruments are laser, electrocautery, biopsy forceps and balloon dilators. These small probes allowed the bronchoscopist to perform therapeutic procedures in the airway where airway tumors could be ablated and/or debulked. Furthermore several airway stents designed to maintain the patency of airways compromised by benign or malignant disease were invented. Some of the airway stents can be deployed over a guidewire introduced through the flexible bronchoscope working channel with or without fluoroscopic guidance. On the other hand, silicone stents have a large deployment device that mandates stent insertion through the rigid bronchoscope. Similarly, large devices to debulk airway tumors, e.g., the microdebrider, could only be introduced into the airway through the barrel of the rigid bronchoscope. As a result, interest in rigid bronchoscopy and general anesthesia was revived. General anesthesia and rigid bronchoscopy has also become a more suitable option for lengthy therapeutic procedures performed on the compromised airway and requiring more accuracy and precession.

Patients presenting for therapeutic bronchoscopy procedures commonly have multiple comorbidities and advanced lung pathology in addition to their compromised airway. Terminally ill patients are also encountered frequently. The presence of an anesthesiologist to manage the patient comorbidity as well as the compromised airway is invaluable especially when therapeutic airway procedures are performed in terminally ill patients [2]. An added challenge to the anesthesiologist is the need to share the airway with the bronchoscopist. Coordination between the bronchoscopist and the anesthesiologist is needed as the airway dynamics, the ventilatory parameters, and required fractional inspired oxygen FiO_2 are continuously changing throughout the procedure.

As a result, an open discussion and planning among the anesthesiologist and the bronchoscopist has to take place prior to and throughout the procedure. The discussion should include tumor location, e.g., trachea vs. bronchi, degree of airway obstruction, e.g., complete vs. partial obstruction, type of anesthesia needed, e.g., general or sedation, airway device options, e.g., none, endotracheal tube, laryngeal mask airway, rigid bronchoscope, and the most suitable mode of ventilation, e.g., spontaneous ventilation, assisted ventilation, mechanical ventilation or jet ventilation. Additionally the anesthesiologist has to be familiar with the step-by-step plan the bronchoscopist has to follow to manage the airway pathology.

Anesthesia for Otolaryngologic Surgery, ed. Basem Abdelmalak and D. John Doyle. Published by Cambridge University Press. © Cambridge University Press 2013.

Therapeutic bronchoscopic procedures

Therapeutic bronchoscopic procedures can be divided into two categories:

(1) tumor-debulking procedures carried out with the intention to decrease tumor burden and size in the airway, thus minimizing the airway compromise;

(2) procedures aimed at maintaining airway patency such as balloon dilatation and deployment of airway stents.

Tumor debulking

Depending on the tumor location, size, and vascularity and the bronchoscopist's experience, one of the following tools can be used for debulking of airway tumor.

Mechanical tumor debulking can be achieved using one of the following methods

1. The rigid bronchoscope can be used as a coring device where a corkscrew back and forth twisting motion is employed to shave off the tumor inside the airway into the barrel of the bronchoscope. The rigid bronchoscope is then used to tamponade the bleeding.
2. The rigid or flexible forceps can be used to debride tumors in a piecemeal fashion.
3. The microdebrider is an enclosed powered rotary blade that has simultaneous tissue resection and suction for removal of debris. The microdebrider has to be inserted through a rigid bronchoscope.

Thermal tumor ablation

1. A laser can be applied through both flexible and rigid bronchoscopes. The Nd:YAG laser is the most commonly used laser in the airway due to its combined ability to vaporize tumor tissue and coagulate bleeding points.
2. Electrocautery uses electric current to destroy tissue by heating.
3. Argon plasma coagulation (APC) uses argon gas to carry electrons to tissue, causing heating and destruction without directly contacting the tissue.
4. Cryotherapy causes tissue destruction by repetitive cycles of freeze-thaw.

Others

1. Photodynamic therapy causes excitation of a photosensitizer in the tissue by a light of matching wavelength that results in production of oxygen free radicals and cell necrosis.
2. Brachytherapy catheters can be inserted through the nose and positioned in place inside or adjacent to airway or lung tumors. This can be achieved under direct vision provided by a flexible bronchoscopy inserted next to the brachytherapy catheter.
3. Fiducial markers can be implanted close to or inside the lung lesion in order to target the lesion for radiation therapy. The fiducial markers can be placed under bronchoscopic direct vision or using electromagnetic navigation for peripheral lung lesions [3].

Maintaining airway patency

Stents

Indications for airway stent insertion are either to maintain airway patency after debulking of intrinsic airway lesions or to splint open the airway compressed by an external mass. Stents can be placed in both benign and malignant airway diseases [4]. The initial stents invented were silicon stents. Due to the large size of the deployment device for silicone stents a rigid bronchoscope is needed for their insertion and consequently general anesthesia. Silicone stents were found to have a tendency to migrate when inserted in an area with a stricture. As a result vascular metal stents were modified to be inserted in the airway. Metal stents can be deployed easily over a guide wire inserted through the flexible bronchoscope with or without fluoroscopic guidance. Complications of metal stents are frequent granulation tissue at the edges of the stent, tumor growth through or over the stent and epithelialization of the stent interior, making removal of the stent difficult and traumatic [5–7].

Balloon dilatation is indicated in the treatment of airway stricture. Airway balloons can be inserted through the working channel of the flexible bronchoscope (Figure 31.1A). The balloon is then inflated with normal saline or radioopaque material if fluoroscopic guidance is utilized. Airway balloons can be inflated to a diameter of 4–20 mm and a length of 40–80 mm, generating 6–12 atmospheres of pressure. The balloon can be held inflated for 1 minute at a time and reinflation is repeated until the desired airway diameter is reached. Airway tear and recurrent stenosis are reported complications [8]. Figure 31.1B

(A)

(B)

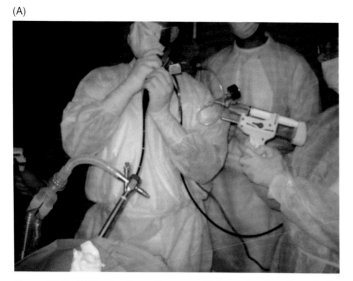
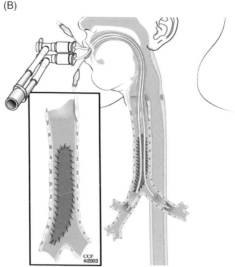

Figure 31.1. (A) Showing the performance of balloon dilatation of a tracheal stenosis through a rigid bronchoscope. (B) A tracheal rent as a complication of balloon tracheal dilatation was repaired with a posterior tracheal wall graft aided by median sternotomy, and for postoperative ventilation each main bronchus was intubated with a small MLT tube; both were connected to the same ventilator after using a double lumen tube (DLT) connector. Reprinted with permission, Cleveland Clinic Center for Medical Art & Photography © 2011–2012. All rights reserved.

shows a repaired tracheal rupture as a complication of balloon dilatation, which was treated with a graft through open thoracotomy, and required the insertion of a double microlaryngeal tube deep into the main bronchi below the level of the repair to allow for healing.

Anesthetic management
Preoperative evaluation

Therapeutic bronchoscopic procedures are considered urgent and in some instances where the airway is compromised the procedure is considered an emergency. Preoperative evaluation is the same as for the diagnostic bronchoscopy as detailed in the previous chapter in addition to special attention to the following.

Hemoptysis

The amount of blood expectorated over the few days prior to the procedure needs to be assessed.

The definition of massive hemoptysis varies from coughing of 100 ml/24 h to 1000 ml/24 h. However, hemoptysis requiring transfusion, hospitalization, intubation or causing aspiration and airway obstruction or hypoxemia could also be defined as massive hemoptysis [9]. Type and screen and blood

availability are important parts of the preparation for the procedure.

Anterior mediastinal mass

Symptoms and signs of positional dyspnea, stridor or desaturation and/or orthopnea should be sought. The position where the patient is most comfortable with minimal respiratory effort should be identified prior to the procedure. Compression of the heart and major vessels detected on CT scan should alert the anesthesiologist to seek symptoms and signs of cardiovascular compromise [10].

Superior vena cava syndrome

Compression of the superior vena cava (SVC) results in congestion of the head and neck, prominent tortuous cutaneous veins on the anterior chest wall and jugular venous distention [11]. If possible an SVC stent should be placed prior to airway procedures.

Pericardial effusion and tamponade

This can result in symptoms and signs similar to SVC syndrome in addition to pulsus paradoxus. The presence of these symptoms with evidence of cardiac compression or pericardial effusion on chest CT scan necessitates a preoperative echocardiogram to assess the effect of the compression on cardiac function and output [12]. A transthoracic echocardiogram can

311

also be used intraoperatively to evaluate and manage intraoperative hemodynamic instability [13]. Depending on the size and the hemodynamic effects of an existing pericardial effusion, preoperative pericardiocentesis might be necessary. The need for cardiopulmonary bypass on a stand-by basis should be discussed.

Flow–volume loops/spirometery

In some reports widening of the mid-expiratory plateau was shown to predict risk of airway compromise under anesthesia [14]. It is noteworthy that blunting of the expiratory limb of the flow-volume loop denoting variable intrathoracic obstruction has not been shown to predict complications. However, the presence of a mixed obstructive and restrictive pattern was shown to be a good predictor of postoperative complications [11]. To date the significance of preoperative spirometery in predicting risk and improvement of anesthetic management has not been confirmed.

Tracheal compression

The degree of tracheal compression detected on CT scan has been linked to risk of airway compromise under general anesthesia [15]. Patients with tracheal cross-sectional area < 50% are usually symptomatic and likely to suffer perioperative complications [11]. The combination of left mainstem obstruction and right pulmonary artery compression has been reported to cause catastrophic ventilation–perfusion mismatch [16].

Tracheoesophageal fistula

Symptoms and signs of aspiration should be sought. Radiographic evidence of aspiration should be documented preoperatively. The location and size of the fistulas as well as the number of fistulas present should be confirmed on preoperative chest CT scan. Plans for airway management, method of ventilation and airway rescue should be discussed with the bronchoscopist prior to the procedure.

Intraluminal obstruction of trachea and main bronchi

Obstruction of the major airway by external compression was discussed in the anterior mediastinal mass section. On the other hand intraluminal obstruction of the trachea and bronchi by a malignant tumor offers a different challenge. The patient symptoms may range from being asymptomatic to suffering from stridor and dyspnea or the patient may present as an emergency acute central airway obstruction with imminent suffocation. Intraluminal bleeding from the tumor mass may acutely increase the degree of airway obstruction by clot formation. Blood clots in the central airway can also result in acute lobar collapse or complete lung collapse. Emergency procedures are required in theses cases in order to reduce the bleeding, debulk the tumor and maintain airway patency [17]. Unfortunately a large majority of these patients are terminally ill with advanced lung cancer and severe comorbidities and the goal of the bronchoscopic therapy is at best palliative.

General anesthesia

Therapeutic bronchoscopic procedures performed through the flexible bronchoscope can be easily performed in the bronchoscopy suite outside the operating room under moderate sedation, monitored anesthesia care (MAC) or general anesthesia. However, procedures with higher risks performed through the rigid bronchoscope mandate the use of general anesthesia and are preferably performed in the operating room [18], unless the bronchoscopy suite is designed to function as a hybrid operating room (Figure 31.2).

As described under advanced diagnostic bronchoscopy (Chapter 30) total intravenous anesthesia (TIVA) is the anesthetic technique of choice [19]. Inhalational anesthetic has multiple disadvantages that include variable levels of anesthetic gas delivered due to frequent suctioning during the procedure and contamination of the operating room air by inhalation agents. However, it is important to emphasize that inhalation agents can be helpful in cases of bronchospasm or in patients with anterior mediastinal mass where maintenance of spontaneous ventilation is mandatory.

Narcotics

Similar to advanced diagnostic bronchoscopic procedures (Chapter 30), therapeutic bronchoscopy is not associated with somatic pain. However, the insertion of the rigid bronchoscope can cause sympathetic stimulation similar to direct laryngoscopy. Such a response is observed mainly during insertion and less so during the remainder of the procedure, in contrast to direct laryngoscopy. This sympathetic stimulation can be attenuated by instillation of lidocaine in the

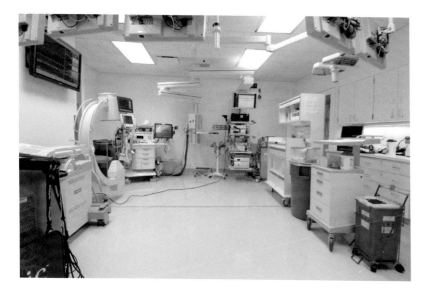

Figure 31.2. An interventional bronchoscopy suite designed to function essentially as a hybrid operating room (image courtesy of Cleveland Clinic Bronchoscopy Suite). Reprinted with permission, Cleveland Clinic Center for Medical Art & Photography © 2011–2012. All rights reserved.

airway, intravenous lidocaine, or the use of low-dose narcotics (e.g., fentanyl 50–100 μg) or ultra-short-acting narcotics (e.g., remifentanil).

General anesthesia for patients with anterior mediastinal mass

Due to the issues regarding the potential for airway obstruction as discussed above, maintaining a spontaneously ventilating patient is mandatory. One successfully utilized technique calls for propofol infusion rates between 100 and 250 μg/kg/min for anesthesia induction while maintaining spontaneous ventilation. The bispectral index monitor (BIS) can be utilized to achieve and sustain an appropriate depth of anesthesia. Once the patient attains adequate depth of anesthesia the ability to bag-mask ventilate has to be assessed. This is a very important step in anesthesia induction in patients with central airway tumors. The inability to bag-mask ventilate should immediately alert the anesthesiologist to avoid the use of muscle relaxation. In this instance direct laryngoscopy and instillation of lidocaine on the vocal cord is a better alternative to the use of muscle relaxation prior to insertion of the rigid bronchoscope or endotracheal tube.

Another technique is described by Abdelmalak et al. [20] where the procedure commenced with awake intubation with dexmedetomidine infusion-induced sedation, followed by deepening the anesthetic through (off label) higher dexmedetomidine infusion rates, supplemented by very low-dose inhalational anesthetic to complement the weak amnestic properties of dexmedetomidine, and to decrease room inhalational anesthetic contamination concerns. Thus, deep anesthetic planes were achieved that enabled insertion of the rigid bronchoscope in exchange for the ETT, while maintaining spontaneous ventilation.

General anesthesia for tracheoesophageal fistula

As in the case of anterior mediastinal mass patients, spontaneous ventilation induction is recommended for patients with tracheoesophageal fistulas, to avoid positive-pressure ventilation and the potential for inflating the stomach, at least till intubation is accomplished and the ETT cuff is positioned distal to the fistula site if feasible.

The use of muscle relaxation

The use of muscle relaxation for therapeutic bronchoscopic procedures has many advantages. These include:

(1) facilitating the insertion of airway devices, e.g., LMA, endotracheal tube;
(2) safer and easier insertion of the rigid bronchoscope; attempting to insert the rigid bronchoscope while the vocal cords are moving can result in vocal cord injury;

313

(3) better lung compliance during positive-pressure ventilation or jet ventilation;

(4) providing the bronchoscopist with a still field where precise laser targeting of lesions adjacent to major vessels and the heart is needed;

(5) maintaining the glottis aperture open during multiple insertion and removal of the bronchoscope and other instruments, thus minimizing trauma to the vocal cord.

Disadvantages of the use of muscle relaxation should also be considered:

(1) loss of the airway patency especially with large anterior mediastinal mass;

(2) positive-pressure ventilation-induced pneumomediastinum or pneumothorax in patients with tracheoesophageal or bronchiopleural fistulas or in the event of airway tears during the procedure;

(3) prolonged unwanted muscle relaxation in patients with lung cancer and paraneoplastic Eaton–Lambert syndrome.

In the experience of the authors we recommend the use of a small dose of muscle relaxant, where the patient becomes weak enough to safely insert the rigid bronchoscope or other airway device but the muscle relaxation could still be reversed promptly when needed. The use of succinylcholine infusion can also produce rapid muscle relaxation that can be terminated if the need arises. Additionally the use of muscle relaxants that are metabolized in the blood independently of organ metabolism should be considered in patients with multiple systemic comorbidities, e.g., atracurium or cisatracurium. If muscle relaxation is determined to be detrimental to the patient, then the use of lidocaine is an appropriate alternative to minimize airway reflexes to instrumentation. Lidocaine can be given through the intravenous cannula or sprayed in the airway in a spray-as-you-go fashion. The maximum tolerated dose of lidocaine should be calculated and not exceeded in each patient (8.2 mg/kg) [21].

Fluid management in bronchoscopic surgery

Fluids should be administered wisely in therapeutic bronchoscopic procedures and based only on patients' requirement. While fluid restriction is advised in patients with heart failure or cor pulmonale, aggressive hydration might be needed in severely dehydrated patients or patients with pericardial effusion. It is important to note that there is no third-space fluid loss in therapeutic bronchoscopic procedures and blood loss is commonly minimal.

Management of the FiO_2

It is common to maintain the fraction of inspired oxygen (FiO_2) at 100% during therapeutic bronchoscopic procedures for multiple reasons.

1. Patients with advanced lung pathology commonly have poor baseline oxygen saturation < 90% and/or use supplemental oxygen. We recommend preoxygenation in these patients with 100% FiO_2 prior to induction.

2. Complete airway occlusion and inability to mechanically ventilate the lung occur during the critical phases of deploying or extracting stents; similarly during balloon dilatation of airway strictures where the lung distal to the balloon is not ventilated.

3. Periods of apnea where positive-pressure ventilation is not feasible can occur during therapeutic bronchoscopic procedures. For example, during extraction of tumor mass positive-pressure ventilation can force the excised tumor down the mainstem bronchi, causing acute obstruction. Another example of a period of apnea is when a different-size rigid bronchoscope has to be exchanged and reinserted in the airway.

In these instances, it is always advisable to return to ventilation with 100% oxygen before anticipated periods of apnea or iatrogenic airway occlusion.

However, low FiO_2 < 40% is required during cautery, laser, argon plasma coagulation and cautery snare in order to avoid airway fire.

Airway and ventilation

Endotracheal tube

Although endotracheal tubes are the definitive and most reliable airway devices in patients undergoing general anesthesia, they have their challenges when inserted in patients with central airway obstruction presenting for therapeutic bronchoscopic procedures. Insertion of the endotracheal tube does not allow the bronchoscopist to examine the vocal cord and upper part of the trachea for pathology. The large external

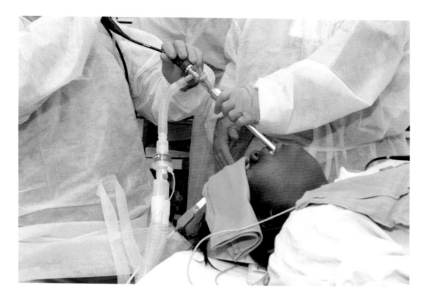

Figure 31.3. Positive-pressure ventilation through connecting the anesthesia circuit to the side port of a rigid bronchoscope. Not obvious in the picture is the wet gauze packing around the rigid bronchoscope barrel to minimize leaks around the scope and facilitate positive-pressure ventilation. Reprinted with permission, Cleveland Clinic Center for Medical Art & Photography © 2011–2012. All rights reserved.

diameter of the therapeutic flexible bronchoscope requires the insertion of an ETT with internal diameter of 8.5 or 9 mm in order to ventilate effectively around the bronchoscope. The length of ETT projecting from the patient's mouth limits the length of the flexible bronchoscope available for insertion in the airway and the ETT proximal end is commonly cut short. Insertion of an ETT in patients with preexisting tracheal or bronchial stents by direct laryngoscopy carries a risk of dislodging or deforming the stents, which can potentially result in airway compromise.

Rigid bronchoscope

The rigid bronchoscope (Figure 31.3) is a stainless-steel tube that ranges in diameter from 8 to 14 mm and in length from 27 to 40 cm. The barrel of the longer rigid bronchoscope is fenestrated in order to allow for ventilation of the contralateral lung, while the shorter rigid tracheoscope barrel lacks fenestrations. The distal end of the rigid bronchoscope is beveled to allow for lifting of the epiglottis and safer insertion through the vocal cord and can also be used for the coring out of tumors. The proximal end of the rigid bronchoscope can remain open to air to allow for simultaneous insertion of multiple instruments. However, in this case jet ventilation or spontaneous ventilation is the only possible mode of ventilation. On the other hand placing a cap that seals the proximal end of the rigid bronchoscope and packing of the patient's oropharynx with

saline-soaked gauze and occlusion of the nostrils can allow for positive-pressure ventilation using an anesthesia breathing circuit (Figure 31.3). A shorter stainless-steel cylinder with multiple side ports is commonly attached to the proximal end of the rigid bronchoscope. The side ports are designed to accommodate a jet ventilator, breathing circuit and insertion ports for bronchoscopic instruments, e.g., suction catheters [22].

The rigid bronchoscope has many advantages over the flexible bronchoscope. They include the ability to provide positive-pressure ventilation during lengthy airway procedures and the ability to insert instruments of large diameter into the airway, such as a microdebrider, a large suction catheter or a deployment device for silicone stents (Figure 31.4). The rigid bronchoscope can also be used as a coring device to debulk airway tumors, dilate stenotic areas, stent the airway open in the case of external airway compression by an anterior mediastinal mass and tamponade airway bleeding [23].

Supraglottic airway

The LMA was first introduced over 20 years ago and remains in use today with a consistently low incidence of complications. The SGA has several advantages over the endotracheal tube when it comes to therapeutic bronchoscopic procedures. The supraglottic position allows for complete inspection of the central airway as well as vocal cord mobility similar to

(A)

(B)

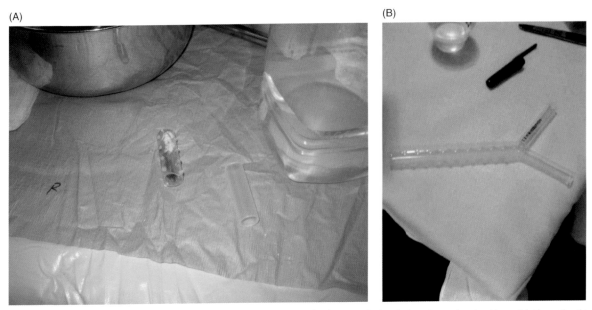

Figure 31.4. Silicone stents; (A) an endobronchial stent, and (B) a Y stent for the carina before being trimmed and cut to match the patient's dimensions Reprinted with permission, Cleveland Clinic Center for Medical Art & Photography © 2011–2012. All rights reserved.

(A)

(B)

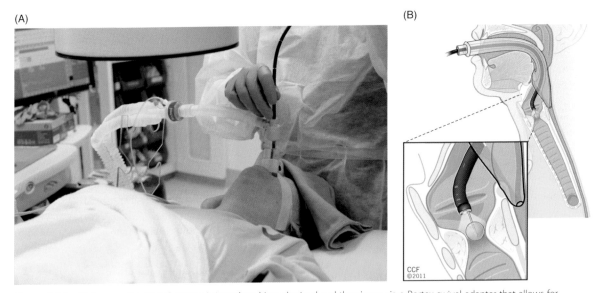

Figure 31.5. (A) An operative bronchoscope is introduced into the i-gel and the airway via a Portex swivel adapter that allows for simultaneous ventilation while examining and performing interventions on the airway such as treatment of subglottic stenosis. (B) The use of supraglottic airway to facilitate access and treatment of subglottic lesions. Reprinted with permission, Cleveland Clinic Center for Medical Art & Photography © 2011–2012. All rights reserved.

bronchoscopic examination performed under conscious sedation, as well as for treatment of subglottic lesions (Figure 31.5) [24]. The large internal diameter of the shaft of the SGA permits the insertion of a large therapeutic bronchoscope or a metal stent deployment device without interference with ventilation. Although the SGAs were originally designed for spontaneously ventilating patients, mechanical ventilation can be performed, with a limitation on maximum airway pressure of 20 cmH$_2$O [25,26].

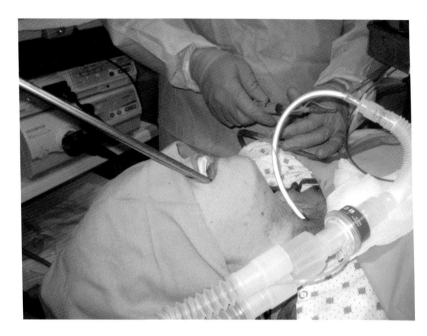

Figure 31.6. Patient with history of prolonged intubation following a severe acute lung injury and ARDS, which required tracheostomy, and was complicated by granulation tissue obstructing the upper trachea and preventing her from talking for about 6 months. An intermittent ventilation technique utilizing an ETT through the existing tracheostomy allowed dual access to the granulation tissue above the tracheostomy, from above with the rigid bronchoscope and from below (tracheostomy) through the flexible bronchoscope, and the application of laser and electrocautery that resulted in establishing the continuity of the tracheal lumen to allow her to talk. Reprinted with permission, Cleveland Clinic Center for Medical Art & Photography © 2011–2012. All rights reserved.

Jet ventilation

Jet ventilation can be performed using a hand-held device, where 100% oxygen is injected into the rigid bronchoscope (the final delivered FiO_2 is dependent on the amount of entrained room air). The pressure of the injected oxygen can be adjusted by a dial and the frequency of ventilation is left to the operator, and frequently ranges from 8 to 20 breaths per minute. Jet ventilation should only be performed when the proximal end of the rigid bronchoscope is open to air in order to avoid barotrauma [27]. Air is entrained at the open proximal end of the rigid bronchoscope, causing variation in the delivered oxygen FiO_2. More recently, the mechanical Monsoon high-frequency jet ventilator (Acutronic Medical Systems, Hirzel, Switzerland) became available [28]. The mechanical jet ventilator has many advantages over the simple hand-held jet ventilators. The user can control the fractional inspired oxygen, frequency of ventilation (up to 150 breaths per minute) and the driving pressure of ventilation (up to 40 mmHg). The inspired oxygen can be humidified up to 100%, allowing for prolonged periods of jet ventilation without the risk of airway mucosa dryness and necrosis or damage to ciliary function [28]. Additionally the mechanical jet ventilator has two alarms to protect from barotrauma and will discontinue ventilation if the set maximum airway pressure limit is reached.

Changing airway and ventilation

In the management of complex airway cases, it is not uncommon to use different airways and different ventilation modes to suit the needs and accomplish the goals of the procedures. Examples of such procedures are the long-term management of tracheobronchial deformity and recurring stenosis post airway fires, as well as the case shown in Figure 31.6, where establishing tracheal continuity between the tracheostomy and the vocal cords required apnea at times, intermittent ventilation through an ETT introduced intermittently through the tracheostomy, and finally through the rigid bronchoscope as the tracheal lumen was re-established.

Postoperative care

Most of the procedures described above are performed as outpatient procedures; patients are discharged on the same day. The use of ultra-short-acting anesthesia medication is vital to achieve prompt discharge.

Complications

Residual muscle relaxation or post-procedure respiratory failures for a variety of reasons are possible complications that mandate unplanned hospital stays and probably ICU admission.

Case study

A 28-year-old 85 kg male who had a history of Wegner's granulomatosis, without any kidney involvement, presented with stridor secondary to recurrent subglottic stenosis. He was scheduled for bronchoscopy, laser and dilatation of his subglottic stenosis.

In the morning of the procedure, the patient had been NPO for 8 hours; he was premedicated with 2 mg of midazolam IV in the OR and, after application of standard ASA monitors and adequate pre-oxygenation, the patient was induced with 150 mg of propofol preceded by 40 mg of IV lidocaine, 100 µg of fentanyl and 40 mg of rocuronium. Immediately following loss of consciousness, bag mask ventilation was established without difficulty. Anesthesia was maintained with continuous infusion of plain propofol at 140 µg/kg/min and depth of anesthesia was monitored via a BIS monitor. Intravenous dexamethasone 10 mg was given to help decrease swelling resulting from treating this endotracheal lesion as well as to serve as a PONV prophylaxis. An i-gel size 4 was then inserted without difficulty, and positive-pressure ventilation was commenced using pressure-controlled ventilation with inspiratory driving pressure of 17 cmH$_2$O; the operating flexible bronchoscope was inserted into the airway through a Portex swivel adapter allowing simultaneous ventilation. Gas flow was always kept at 15 l/min to compensate for the circuit leaks and suction through the bronchoscope.

The lesion was treated with electrocautery, argon laser, and balloon dilatation. During cauterization and laser the FiO$_2$ was reduced to around 30% (also high gas flow was maintained at the maximum airflow of the machine, 12 l/min, and 1–2 l/min O$_2$ to maintain the desired FiO$_2$; high flow would also eliminate the need to use the O$_2$ flush button to inflate collapsing ventilator pillows, or a bag which can ignite a fire during laser or electrocautery). When the saturation fell below 88%, the procedure was temporarily halted to permit effective positive-pressure ventilation and oxygenation with 100% oxygen. Once stabilized, the oxygen concentration was returned to 30% and lasering was resumed. Then the trachea was dilated using a balloon dilator. At the end of the procedure, mitomycin was applied to the lesion; it is believed that this will result in delaying recurrence at the site of application.

Muscle relaxation was reversed, the propofol infusion stopped, and the patient was extubated when he was fully awake and following commands.

The postoperative course was complicated by cough that lasted for about 30 minutes, which was relieved with intermittent doses of 25 µg of fentanyl. The patient was discharged home a couple of hours later in a satisfactory state, with much improved breathing with no stridor.

Clinical pearls

- Therapeutic bronchoscopic procedures can be either tumor-debulking procedures or procedures aimed at maintaining airway patency, such as balloon dilatation and deployment of airway stents.
- These procedures can be done through a flexible or a rigid bronchoscope and are generally done under general anesthesia.
- Total intravenous anesthesia (TIVA) is the technique of choice, and is preferred over inhalational anesthetic since frequent opening of the anesthetic circuit to introduce and remove the bronchoscope pollutes the procedure room and together with frequent suctioning during the procedure can result in a fluctuating depth of anesthesia.
- Airway options include: patient's natural airway, supraglottic airway, large-diameter ETT tube (ID 8.5 or 9.0 mm), and rigid bronchoscope.
- Muscle relaxation is often needed to facilitate safe completion of these procedures. However, spontaneous ventilation needs to be maintained at least for the initial phase of the anesthetic in managing patients with anterior mediastinal masses or tracheoesophageal fistula.
- Continuous communication between the anesthesiologist and the bronchoscopist is essential throughout the procedure as the clinical conditions are constantly changing. In particular, FiO$_2$ changes and changes in airway management are often needed to meet the requirements of the different stages of these procedures,
- Potential complications include cough, pneumothorax, laryngospasm, bronchospasm and complete loss of the airway.

References

1. Becker HD. Bronchoscopy: the past, the present, and the future. *Clin Chest Med* 2010;**31**(1):1–18.

2. Sarkiss M. Anesthesia for bronchoscopy and interventional pulmonology: from moderate sedation to jet ventilation. *Curr Opin Pulm Med* 2011;**17**(4):274–8.

3. Anantham D, Feller-Kopman D, Shanmugham LN, *et al.* Electromagnetic navigation bronchoscopy-guided fiducial placement for robotic stereotactic radiosurgery of lung tumors: a feasibility study. *Chest* 2007;**132** (3):930–5.

4. Rafanan AL, Mehta AC. Stenting of the tracheobronchial tree. *Radiol Clin North Am* 2000; **38**(2):395–408.

5. Saito Y, Imamura H. Airway stenting. *Surg Today* 2005;**35** (4):265–70.

6. Wood D. Airway stenting. *Chest Surg Clin N Am* 2003;**13**(2): 211–29.

7. Doyle DJ, Abdelmalak B, Machuzak M, Gildea TR. Anesthesia and airway management for removing pulmonary self-expanding metallic stents. *J Clin Anesth* 2009;**21**(7):529–32.

8. Folch E, Mehta AC. Airway interventions in the tracheobronchial tree. *Semin Respir Crit Care Med* 2008;**29** (4):441–52.

9. Sakr L, Dutau H. Massive hemoptysis: an update on the role of bronchoscopy in diagnosis and management. *Respiration* 2010; **80**(1):38–58.

10. Blank RS, de Souza DG. Anesthetic management of patients with an anterior mediastinal mass: continuing professional development. *Can J Anaesth* 2011;**58**(9):853–67.

11. Bechard P, Letourneau L, Lacasse Y, Cote D, Bussieres JS. Perioperative cardiorespiratory complications in adults with mediastinal mass: incidence and risk factors. *Anesthesiology* 2004;**100**(4):826–34; discussion 825A.

12. Redford DT, Kim AS, Barber BJ, Copeland JG. Transesophageal echocardiography for the intraoperative evaluation of a large anterior mediastinal mass. *Anesth Analg* 2006;**103**(3):578–9.

13. Brooker RF, Zvara DA, Roitstein A. Mediastinal mass diagnosed with intraoperative transesophageal echocardiography. *J Cardiothorac Vasc Anesth* 2007;**21**(2):257–8.

14. Erdos G, Tzanova I. Perioperative anaesthetic management of mediastinal mass in adults. *Eur J Anaesthesiol* 2009;**26**(8):627–32.

15. Stricker PA, Gurnaney HG, Litman RS. Anesthetic management of children with an anterior mediastinal mass. *J Clin Anesth* 2010;**22**(3):159–63.

16. Huang YL, Yang MC, Huang CH, *et al.* Rescue of cardiopulmonary collapse in anterior mediastinal tumor: case presentation and review of literature. *Pediatr Emerg Care* 2010;**26**(4):296–8.

17. Conacher ID, Curran E. Local anaesthesia and sedation for rigid bronchoscopy for emergency relief of central airway obstruction. *Anaesthesia* 2004; **59**(3):290–2.

18. Eckardt J, Petersen HO, Hakami-Kermani A, *et al.* Endobronchial ultrasound-guided transbronchial needle aspiration of undiagnosed intrathoracic lesions. *Interact Cardiovasc Thorac Surg* 2009; **9**(2):232–5.

19. Sarkiss M, Kennedy M, Riedel B, *et al.* Anesthesia technique for endobronchial ultrasound-guided fine needle aspiration of mediastinal lymph node. *J Cardiothorac Vasc Anesth* 2007;**21**(6):892–6.

20. Abdelmalak B, Marcanthony N, Abdelmalak J, *et al.* Dexmedetomidine for anesthetic management of anterior mediastinal mass. *J Anesth* 2010;**24**(4):607–10.

21. British Thoracic Society guidelines on diagnostic flexible bronchoscopy. *Thorax* 2001; **56**(Suppl 1):i1–21.

22. Ayers ML, Beamis JF Jr. Rigid bronchoscopy in the twenty-first century. *Clin Chest Med* 2001; **22**(2):355–64.

23. Wahidi MM, Herth FJ, Ernst A. State of the art: interventional pulmonology. *Chest* 2007; **131**(1):261–74.

24. Abdelmalak B, Gildea T, Doyle DJ. Anesthesia for bronchoscopy. *Curr Pharm Des* 2012: in press.

25. Abdelmalak B, Ryckman JV, Al Haddad S, Sprung J. Respiratory arrest after successful neodymium:yttrium-aluminum-garnet laser treatment of subglottic tracheal stenosis. *Anesth Analg* 2002;**95**(2):485–6.

26. Hung WT, Liao SM, Su JM. Laryngeal mask airway in patients with tracheal stents who are undergoing non-airway related interventions: report of three cases. *J Clin Anesth* 2004; **16**(3):214–6.

27. Fernandez-Bustamante A, Ibanez V, Alfaro JJ, *et al.* High-frequency jet ventilation in interventional bronchoscopy: factors with predictive value on high-frequency jet ventilation complications. *J Clin Anesth* 2006;**18**(5):349–56.

28. Kraincuk P, Kepka A, Ihra G, Schabernig C, Aloy A. A new prototype of an electronic jet-ventilator and its humidification system. *Crit Care* 1999;**3**(4):101–10.

Chapter

32

Anesthesia for pediatric otolaryngologic surgery

Rahul G. Baijal and Emad B. Mossad

Introduction

Anesthesia for pediatric otorhinolaryngologic procedures represents the largest proportion of elective surgery for not only pediatric anesthesiologists but also general anesthesiologists taking care of children.

Anesthesia for otologic procedures

Myringotomy

Chronic otitis media with effusion (COME) is common in young children secondary to impaired eustachian tube drainage, potentially leading to conductive hearing loss and cholesteatoma formation. Surgical drainage with myringotomy tubes is indicated when conservative medical management fails. Many children with congenital anomalies, such as those with cleft palate, Down's syndrome, and craniofacial abnormalities, require myringotomy tubes secondary to abnormal eustachian tube anatomy.

General anesthesia is required for this brief ambulatory procedure and is often accomplished with an inhalational anesthetic, usually sevoflurane, oxygen and/or nitrous oxide by a facemask. An oropharyngeal airway may help maintain airway patency while sharing the airway with the otolaryngologist and minimize head movements as perceived by the otolaryngologist through the microscope. Additionally, this procedure may also be surgically challenging and longer in children with narrow ear canals, such as children with Down's syndrome and craniofacial abnormalities, and a supraglottic airway (SGA) or an endotracheal tube (ETT) should be considered for maintenance of anesthesia. Intravenous access is usually not needed unless significant airway obstruction or hemodynamic instability is expected; for example, children with Down's syndrome may develop significant bradyarrythmias with sevoflurane inhalational induction, and children with hypotonia may develop airway obstruction following inhalational induction.

Analgesia may be administered by various routes. Acetaminophen is administered orally preoperatively (10 to 20 mg/kg) or rectally intraoperatively (30 to 40 mg/kg). Oral acetaminophen is absorbed rapidly preoperatively whereas rectal acetaminophen has an onset time of 60 to 90 minutes and a peak effect of 2 to 3 hours. Children receiving a preauricular block with 0.2 ml of 0.25% bupivicaine versus 2 µg/kg intranasal fentanyl had similar pain scores, need for rescue medications postoperatively, and time to discharge [1]. Intramuscular morphine 0.1 mg/kg and ketorolac 0.5 mg/kg may also be administered with no irritation like intranasal fentanyl, but the 30 minutes onset of duration may preclude immediate postoperative benefit as many children are discharged within 30 minutes from the PACU with simply acetaminophen (Tylenol) or acetaminophen (Tylenol) with codeine.

Preschool children receiving unsupplemented sevoflurane anesthesia may exhibit emergence delirium of unknown etiology postoperatively. Since intravenous access is not usually needed for this brief procedure, intranasal fentanyl 1 to 2 µg/kg was shown to reduce emergence delirium postoperatively from sevoflurane anesthesia for myringotomy tubes [2]. A recent study comparing intranasal dexmedetomidine 1 to 2 µg/kg to intranasal fentanyl 1 to 2 µg/kg showed no difference in emergence delirium and postoperative pain scores but revealed increased time to discharge with dexmedetomidine [3].

Children with COME may also have recurrent upper respiratory tract (URI) infections that do not resolve until myringotomy tubes are inserted to improve middle ear drainage. Children with an active or recent URI may be at risk for up to 6 weeks, for perioperative respiratory complications including airway obstruction, laryngospasm, bronchospasm, and breath-holding [4]. The anesthesiologist is faced with the decision of proceeding with the procedure given these risks, knowing that the child may be re-exposed to an inciting pathogen, or the symptoms may not improve without surgical intervention. Airway reactivity may persist for up to 8 weeks even for children with a recent, uncomplicated URI. However, there was no difference in perioperative respiratory complications in those children presenting with an acute uncomplicated upper respiratory tract infection for minor surgery not requiring airway instrumentation [4].

Tympanoplasty and mastoidectomy

Tympanoplasty reconstructs the tympanic membrane with or without a graft in children with a chronic tympanic membrane perforation or cholesteatoma, an epithelial perforation in the middle ear. Mastoidectomies are performed in children with mastoiditis and/or a cholesteatoma.

Children undergoing tympanoplasty and mastoidectomy are positioned supine with the head laterally rotated from the affected side 90° or 180° from the anesthesiologist. The airway must be carefully secured secondary to limited access and the neck must be carefully rotated to reduce the risk of atlantoaxial subluxation. Besides standard monitoring, electromyography is used to monitor and prevent facial nerve injury given the close proximity of the facial nerve to the surgical site; subsequently, neuromuscular blockade is avoided during the procedure. Nitrous oxide is contraindicated during and following graft placement to avoid graft dislodgement. The middle ear is an air-filled, not distensible cavity, and an increase in volume within this cavity also increases the pressure within the cavity. Nitrous oxide may accumulate in this closed space as it diffuses along a concentration gradient more rapidly than nitrogen moves out since nitrous oxide is 34 times more soluble than nitrogen in the blood. The most common complication following tympanoplasty and mastoidectomy is postoperative nausea and vomiting from vestibular labyrinth stimulation. Prophylactic antiemetics, such as dexamethasone and a serotonin antagonist, and total intravenous anesthesia (TIVA) with propofol reduce the risk of postoperative nausea

and vomiting compared to inhalational anesthetics and opiods alone. A preemptive great auricular nerve block does not decrease postoperative analgesic requirements compared to children who received this block 1 hour prior to procedure completion but did decrease the incidence of postoperative opioid requirements, nausea, and vomiting [5]. A smooth emergence is desired to prevent graft disruption and may be achieved with an extubation performed while the child is still in a deep plane of anesthesia, (the so called "deep" extubation) and opiods titrated to produce a slow, regular respiratory pattern.

Cochlear implants

Early insertion of cochlear implants is occurring in children with profound hearing loss to allow for better development of speech and language skills. Children as young as 6 months may receive a cochlear implant. The cochlear implant stimulates the auditory nerve, and intraoperative limits of implant stimulation are set by evoked stapedius reflex thresholds (ESRT). Volatile anesthetics abolish the stapedius reflex in more than 50% of children and can result in a dose-dependent increase in the ESRT, possibly overestimating a child's comfort level. Since propofol does not affect the ESRT, TIVA may be preferred during cochlear implantation [6].

Anesthesia for rhinologic procedures
Reduction of nasal fractures

Nasal fractures are seen more frequently in older children, resulting from direct trauma. Since the nasal mucosa is very vascular, acute nasal fractures may produce significant bleeding, and a large volume of blood may be swallowed into the stomach. Acutely, an ETT following rapid sequence induction is required to prevent aspiration. However, closed reduction is often delayed for a few days to allow inflammation to subside and for the bleeding risk to decrease An LMA may then be substituted for ETT.

Choanal atresia

Choanal atresia is a congenital malformation with an absent connection between the nasal cavity and the aerodigestive tract. The atresia is bony and/or mixed membranous. Choanal atresia is usually not associated with other craniofacial abnormalities but may be part of a constellation of congenital anomalies known as CHARGE (coloboma, heart malformations, atresia choanae, retardation of growth and development, genitourinary defects, and ear anomalies). If the obstruction is bilateral, children may present with acute respiratory failure, particularly neonates who are obligate nose breathers. Bilateral choanal atresia usually manifests with airway obstruction at rest, which resolves with crying or an oral airway. A large hole may also be cut into the pacifier to maintain airway patency. Unilateral choanal atresia is not a medical or surgical emergency and may present as only persistent unilateral nasal discharge several years later. Surgical correction for bilateral choanal atresia depends on the neonate's ability to compensate with oral breathing and receive adequate nutrition. Some surgeons advocate a "rule of tens" for timing of the repair: the child must be 10 weeks of age, weigh 10 pounds, and have a hemoglobin of 10 gm/dl.

Both inhalational and intravenous induction and maintenance with an inhaled anesthetic, muscle relaxant, and opioid are appropriate. Neonates undergoing bilateral repair may have airway obstruction postoperatively and should be observed in a monitored setting. Following the surgical correction of the atresia, restenosis may occur but can be reduced with topical application of mitomycin C, an aminoglycoside and alkylating agent that prevents fibroblast growth and migration.

Endoscopic sinus surgery

When medical management with broad-spectrum antibiotics fails for the treatment of chronic sinusitis, endoscopic sinus surgery is the primary surgical management. The operation involves direct telescopic visualization of the nasal mucosal membranes for microdebridement. Many children with chronic sinusitis have coexisting morbidities, particularly asthma and cystic fibrosis, that must be optimized prior to surgery. Both inhalational and intravenous induction and maintenance with an inhaled anesthetic, muscle relaxant, and opiods are appropriate. A cuffed preformed ETT (RAE tube) is required to allow unobstructed access to the maxilla and sinuses and prevent an air leak that may fog the endoscopic instruments. Bleeding is common with this procedure and the nasal cavity is packed with pledgets soaked with a vasoconstrictor. The most commonly used vasoconstrictors are oxymetazoline 0.025% to

0.05%, phenylephrine 0.25% to 1%, lidocaine 0.5% to 1% with epinephrine (1:100 000 solution), and cocaine 4% to 10%. Topical vasoconstrictors may cause severe hypertension, reflex bradycardia, and possibly cardiac arrest. Severe hypertension is usually transient and may not require treatment. Corticosteroids such as dexamethasone (0.5 to 1 mg/kg) are administered intraoperatively to reduce inflammation. Additionally, the surgeon may leave an absorbable stenting material at the end of the procedure, which makes the child an obligate nose breather and increases the possibility of emergence delirium.

Adenotonsillectomy

Adenotonsillectomy (T&A) is one of the most commonly performed pediatric surgical procedures, with recurrent tonsillitis or pharyngitis and adenotonsillar hypertrophy as the major indications. Surgical management is indicated for recurrent tonsillitis or pharyngitis when medical therapy fails and for adenotonsillar hypertrophy when it leads to sleep-disordered breathing. Although adenoidectomies are routinely performed with tonsillectomies, an adenoidectomy may be done independently for recurrent adenitis, chronic sinusitis, and recurrent otitis media with effusion.

Surgical techniques

Surgical techniques for T&A include cold and hot knife dissection, suction, coblation (a non-heat-driven process using radiofrequency energy), and unipolar and bipolar electrocautery techniques. Electrocautery techniques are associated with less perioperative hemorrhage but increased perioperative pain and reduced postoperative oral intake.

Obstructive sleep apnea

Sleep-disordered breathing is a spectrum of illness ranging from primary snoring to severe obstructive sleep apnea (OSA). Although it is important to distinguish children with obstructive sleep apnea, it may be difficult simply based on clinical symptoms without a documented sleep study as both disease processes may present with similar symptoms. Documented severe obstructive sleep apnea places children at higher risk of perioperative respiratory complications, along with some other characteristics and

Table 32.1. Classification and severity of pediatric sleep disorder breathing

	AHI	SpO$_2$ nadir (%)	PETCO$_2$ > 50 mmHg (% testing)
Normal	≤1	>94	<10
Primary snoring	≤1	>94	<10
Upper airway resistance syndrome	≤2	>92	10–15
Obstructive alveolar hypoventilation	≤2	>92	>20
Obstructive sleep apnea			
Mild	2–4	88–92	10–15
Moderate	5–10	80–88	15–20
Severe	>10	<80	>20

AHI, apnea/hypopnea index.

comorbidities such as age less than 3 years, craniofacial syndromes, cranial base disorders, neuromuscular disorders, trisomy 21, infiltrative disorders and storage diseases, and obesity [7].

Obstruction may result not only in chronic hypoxia and hybercarbia but also in cardiovascular abnormalities, such as right ventricular hypertrophy, biventricular dysfunction and pulmonary hypertension, failure to thrive, recurrent upper and lower respiratory infections, and neurocognitive deficits, such as poor learning, behavior problems, and lower grades. Many of these sequelae are fortunately reversible following a T&A.

Polysomnography

The severity of obstruction can only be assessed by a sleep study. The severity of the obstruction varies during sleep but is worse during REM sleep in the early morning hours. The sleep study assesses end-tidal CO$_2$, an electroencephalogram, chest wall movement, leg movement, and oxygen saturation. Several indices are reported, including the apnea/hypopnea index (AHI), which is the number of apneas (complete cessation of airflow) and hypopneas (50% reduction in airflow) per hour, peak end-tidal CO$_2$, and oxygen saturation nadir (see Table 32.1) [8]. Apneas and hypopneas may be central, obstructive and mixed, where there is no respiratory effort with central apnea and inspiratory effort against limited upper airway patency with obstructive apnea. Although there is no consensus on the criteria for diagnosing OSA in children, each index helps categorize the severity of the obstruction, which is important in determining the perioperative plan. Increasing AHI is associated with increased risk of perioperative respiratory complications. Additionally, true documentation of obstructive sleep apnea should be based only on obstructive episodes, as central apnea may be normal in children without associated respiratory compromise. Furthermore, various scores have been modeled to help predict the risk of perioperative respiratory complications, but no one score has been shown to be convincingly reliable and reproducible. Even though the severity of the obstruction can only be assessed by a sleep study, many children are not tested given the dearth of sleep-study laboratories and the inconvenience and difficulty of completing the sleep study in a young child. Other diagnostic tests, such as videotaping and nocturnal pulse oximetry, may help predict perioperative respiratory complications, but they do not completely stratify the severity of obstruction and the necessary follow-up. A preoperative oxygen saturation nadir of less than 80% is associated with an increased risk of perioperative respiratory complications [9]. The American Academy of Otolaryngology recently issued recommendations for polysomnography for sleep-disordered breathing prior to tonsillectomy in children. The academy made the following recommendations: (1) before determining the need for tonsillectomy, the clinician should refer children with sleep-disordered breathing for polysomnography if they exhibit certain complex medical conditions such as obesity, Down's syndrome, craniofacial abnormalities, neuromuscular disorders, sickle cell disease, or mucopolysaccharidosis. (2) The clinician should advocate polysomnography prior to tonsillectomy for sleep-disordered breathing in children without any of the comorbidities listed in statement 1 for whom the need for surgery is uncertain or when there is discordance between tonsillar size on physical examination and the reported severity of sleep-disordered breathing. (3) Clinicians should communicate polysomnography results to the anesthesiologist prior to the induction of anesthesia for tonsillectomy in a child with sleep-disordered breathing. (4) Clinicians should admit children with obstructive sleep apnea documented on polysomnography for inpatient, overnight monitoring after tonsillectomy if they are younger than age 3 or have severe obstructive sleep apnea (AHI of 10 or more obstructive events/hour, oxygen saturation nadir less than 80%, or both). (5) In children for whom polysomnography is indicated to assess sleep-disordered breathing prior to tonsillectomy, clinicians should obtain laboratory-based polysomnography, when available [10].

Perioperative anesthetic concerns

A thorough history and physical examination is essential, focusing on obstructive symptoms including snoring, gasping or pausing, restless sleep, daytime somnolence, and enuresis. The loudness of the snoring, however, does not correlate with the severity of the obstruction. A sleep study should be reviewed, if available, to assess the severity of obstruction. Although the oropharynx may be examined to qualitatively classify tonsillar size, there is no evidence that the incidence of perioperative respiratory complications is directly associated with tonsillar size [11]. There is no evidence that routine preoperative CBC or coagulation studies are necessary unless indicated by a thorough history for bleeding diathesis. A routine chemistry panel to evaluate for a compensatory metabolic alkalosis for hypercarbia is not routinely indicated as well. Cardiology evaluation with a baseline EKG assessing for right ventricular hypertrophy and a subsequent echocardiogram if the EKG indicates right ventricular hypertrophy should only be performed if clinical history and physical examination indicate right ventricular strain or failure, such as a loud second heart sound, exercise intolerance, or hepatomegaly.

A number of unique situations may be encountered in children presenting for T&A. Children with trisomy 21 have craniofacial abnormalities with midface hypoplasia. Hypopharyngeal hypotonia with the midface hypoplasia increases the risk of airway obstruction during induction of anesthesia, potentially making mask ventilation difficult. Children with mucopolysaccharidosis I (Hurler's syndrome) and II (Hunter's syndrome) have diffuse infiltration of the upper airway with mucopolysaccharidosis, also predisposing them to airway obstruction and difficult mask ventilation and intubation.

Anxious children may receive oral sedation preoperatively with midazolam (0.5 mg/kg). A premedication has not been shown to increases the incidence of perioperative respiratory complications even in those patients with severe obstruction [12].

During induction of anesthesia, early pharyngeal obstruction may require a jaw thrust maneuver, insertion of an oral or nasopharyngeal airway, and moderate CPAP (10 to 20 cmH$_2$O) may be necessary to prevent airway obstruction from loss of pharyngeal tone. The closing pressure of the pharynx increases with OSA severity, so greater levels of CPAP are required with severe OSA than mild OSA. This serves as a subjective assessment on the degree of airway obstruction for children who do not obtain a preoperative sleep study. A T&A at most centers is a short procedure from 15 to 45 minutes, and neuromuscular blockade is not usually necessary. The patient is intubated with a preformed-cuffed oral RAE (Ring–Adair–Elwyn) to reduce the risk of aspirating blood and secretions. A tube size 0.5 to 1 smaller than the age-appropriate size is used to avoid airway trauma. The ETT is placed during deep inhalational anesthesia, which may be supplemented with a laryngeal spray of topical lidocaine or an intravenous bolus of propofol of 2–3 mg/kg. The ETT is held in place by the grooved tongue depressor that is part of the Brown–Davis mouth gag. The FiO$_2$ should be reduced to the lowest level possible to allow adequate oxygenation while minimizing the risk of airway fire. Maintenance may be achieved with inhaled anesthetics or TIVA and supplemented with opiods, usually initially titrated with 1–2 µg/kg of fentanyl, 100–200 µg/kg of morphine, or 10–20 µg/kg of hydromorphone. Children with severe OSA have lower perioperative morphine equivalent requirements and are 50% more likely to have apnea with fentanyl than healthy children [13]. Furthermore, young children and those with lower preoperative oxygen saturation nadir also have lower postoperative morphine equivalent requirements [14]. The use of spontaneous respiration during maintenance enables an assessment of the response to small incremental doses of opiods.

Although opioids are the mainstay for analgesia, the use of opioid-sparing adjuncts such as anti-inflammatory agents, acetaminophen, dexmedetomidine, and ketamine have been advocated. Non-steroidal anti-inflammatory drugs for T&A are controversial, with a recent meta-analysis showing an increased risk of post-tonsillectomy bleeding but a Cochrane database review showing no significant correlation with post-tonsillectomy bleeding [15]. Acetaminophen may be administered orally preoperatively (10–15 mg/kg), rectally (30–40 mg/kg), and now intravenously (10–15 mg/kg). A randomized controlled trial assessing duration of analgesia following intravenous or rectal acetaminophen after T&A showed an increased time to opioid rescue for both rectal and intravenous acetaminophen, with a longer duration of analgesia for the rectal administration [16]. A recent meta-analysis found that administration of ketamine is associated with decreased postoperative PACU pain scores and non-opioid analgesic requirement but failed to exhibit a postoperative opioid-sparing effect [17]. Dexmedetomidine, an α_2-agonist, with mild analgesic properties, at doses of 0.75–1 µg/kg increased the time to postoperative opioid rescue but did not decrease the total postoperative morphine equivalents when compared to patients who only received morphine intraoperatively [18].

High-dose dexamethasone (0.5–1 mg/kg) decreases the incidence of postoperative inflammation and nausea and vomiting. There has been recent discussion about the reported increased risk of bleeding with larger doses of dexamethasone, but this report was criticized for the high incidence of primary hemorrhage and the need to return to the OR on the day of surgery [19].

At the end of the procedure, the surgeon suctions the oropharynx and the stomach to remove residual secretions and blood. The surgeon may electively infiltrate the tonsillar fossa with local anesthetic for postoperative pain control. There is no evidence which local anesthetic, if any, and which concentration of local anesthetic improves postoperative pain control. Extubation for low-risk children may be accomplished under a deep or awake plane of anesthesia. Deep extubation is defined as extubation in the absence of laryngeal reflexes. Blunting of laryngeal reflexes may be achieved with a higher concentration of inhaled anesthetics (MAC extubation, ~1.2 MAC) or local anesthetics. Lidocaine may be administered intravenously 1–2 mg/kg 5 minutes before the end of the procedure, sprayed topically on the larynx during laryngoscopy (1–3 ml of 2–4%), injected through the ETT at the end of the procedure (1–2 ml of 1–2%), or placed in the ETT cuff (1–2 ml of 1–2%) following laryngoscopy. Deep extubation decreases the incidence of coughing and bucking at extubation, reducing the possibility of post-tonsillectomy bleeding, but may increase the possibility of laryngospasm in the absence of airway reflexes and the presence of secretions and blood in the oropharynx. Deep extubation for high-risk children may increase the incidence of airway obstruction and postoperative respiratory complications. Another common practice is to position the child in the lateral position with head slightly down at the time of extubation to allow drainage of blood and secretions out of the oropharynx. Unfortunately, there are no conclusive studies correlating extubation techniques and perioperative respiratory complications in children undergoing T&A. The anesthetic setting is also important in determining extubation decisions since most perioperative respiratory complications will occur in the post-anesthesia care unit (PACU). Many outpatient surgery centers do not have a backup anesthesiologist available and recovery nurses often have limited pediatric experience, so admitting a pediatric patient to PACU without laryngeal reflexes following deep extubation should be done very cautiously.

LMA and T&A

The use of the LMA for adenotonsillectomies was described in the early 1990s but did not become widespread until a flexible-spiral metallic reinforced tube was developed. Insertion of the LMA with adenotonsillar hypertrophy may be challenging and various maneuvers may have to be used for appropriate placement; however, the LMA is rarely dislodged when the neck is placed in extreme extension for the procedure, assuming appropriate position with adequate ventilation and oxygenation were present before the neck extension. Advantages of the LMA over an ETT include a possible decrease in postoperative stridor and immediate recovery in a child with a spontaneous regular ventilatory pattern [20]. However, it remains controversial whether an LMA changes the incidence of perioperative respiratory complications.

Postoperative management

Perioperative respiratory complications are defined as major and minor respiratory complications. Major respiratory complications include those that require invasive and noninvasive airway interventions, such as BIPAP, CPAP, and reintubation, and pharmacologic intervention, such as succinylcholine for laryngospasm. Minor respiratory complications include mild to moderate hypoxia with and without O_2 dependence. Airway obstruction does not resolve immediately in the postoperative period and may be exacerbated by the administration of sedative agents. Blood and secretions in the oropharynx may further precipitate laryngospasm.

Postoperative nausea and vomiting is common due to pharyngeal mucosal irritation and swallowed bloody secretions and should be prophylactically treated with antiemetics such as a serotonin antagonist or a promotility agent like metoclopramide. A single intraoperative dose of dexamethasone also reduces the incidence of emesis in the first 24 hours postoperatively. The smallest effective dose is, however, unclear.

The child who must be monitored as an inpatient postoperatively is difficult to identify. Children with even mild OSA continue to have documented airway obstruction the night following adenotonsillectomy [21]. Obstruction with associated hypoxia postoperatively is four times more likely in children with severe OSA than in children with mild OSA. There is, however, no evidence to help determine whether children should be monitored in an intensive care unit, intermediate care unit, or telemetry floor bed, and for how long children should be monitored postoperatively. At the authors' institution, the practice is to observe low-risk children for 2 hours postoperatively prior to discharge, assuming they are tolerating oral intake and maintaining SpO_2 >93%.

Post-tonsillectomy hemorrhage

Post-tonsillectomy bleeding can be primary or secondary. Primary bleeding occurs within 24 hours postoperatively and is more brisk than secondary bleeding. Secondary bleeding usually occurs beyond 24 hours postoperatively (usually between 7 and 10 days postoperatively) when the surgical eschar falls off the tonsillar bed. Post-tonsillectomy bleeding is more common in children older than 10 years of age.

Anesthetic management in both circumstances can be challenging. Intravenous access should be established preoperatively for volume resuscitation and possible blood transfusion to compensate for significant hemorrhage preoperatively. The child should be adequately volume-resuscitated before induction of anesthesia. The surgeon should be at the bedside during induction as the bleeding may obstruct the airway and a surgical airway may be necessary. An awake fiberoptic intubation may be challenging in an anxious child and an airway obscured by blood. The child should be treated as full stomach and aspiration risk. Rapid sequence induction with propofol (2 mg/kg), etomidate (0.3 mg/kg), or ketamine (1–2 mg/kg), with selection and dosage guided by the patient's hemodynamic status, and succinylcholine (1–2 mg/kg) or rocuronium (1.2 mg/kg) are appropriate. Two large suctions should be available to help visualize the airway. A cuffed ETT should be used to prevent aspiration of blood. The ETT should be directed to the site where bubbles are seen escaping from the glottic opening when an assistant presses on the chest wall to produce a forced exhalation if the vocal cords are not visible during laryngoscopy. Management and maintenance of anesthesia focuses on maintaining the patient's hemodynamic and volume status, guided by fluid therapy or blood transfusion. Suctioning of the stomach at the end of the procedure may not remove all the swallowed blood as much of the blood may be clots that are too large to be suctioned. The child should be extubated awake at the end of the procedure.

Anesthesia for pharyngeal and laryngeal surgery

Laser surgery

A laser (**l**ight **a**mplification by **s**timulated **e**mission of **r**adiation) generates electron activity in the form of light. The laser beam can be focused on a small area, allowing for controlled coagulation, incision, and vaporization of the target tissue without affecting neighboring tissues. The CO_2 laser, which is the most commonly used laser, is absorbed by all biologic tissues and rapidly vaporizes intracellular water present in the tissue, increasing temperature and denaturing proteins in the target tissue. The CO_2 laser produces focused vaporization of the target tissue with minimal damage to surrounding tissues and subsequent postoperative edema. The CO_2 laser has been used to treat oropharyngeal and larynotracheal papillomas, subglottic stenosis, subglottic hemangiomas, glottic webs, post-intubation granulomas, and vocal cord nodules. The argon and the neodymium: ytrrium–aluminum–garnet (Nd:YAG) lasers are used in ophthalmologic surgery and in treating gastrointestinal bleeding. The CO_2 laser cannot penetrate the cornea and may cause corneal injury whereas the argon and Nd:YAG lasers can penetrate the cornea, causing retinal injury. Therefore, all operating room personnel should wear safety goggles that provide protection from reflected beams, and the patient's eyes should be covered with saline-soaked eye pads or metal eye shields. Flammable objects, such as surgical drapes, PVC or non-metallic rubber tubes, and unprotected skin should be removed from the path of the laser to reduce the risk of fire.

Anesthetic management of laser surgery consists of intubation and nonintubation techniques. Standard PVC tubes are flammable and can be ignited by the laser whereas red-rubber tubes cannot be ignited but deflect the laser when wrapped with metal. Metal-wrapped tubes may irritate the tracheal mucosa causing postoperative edema, obstruct the airway if the metal separates from the tube, and allow the laser to penetrate and ignite unprotected portions of the tube. Special nonflammable, non-reflective flexible ETTs have been manufactured for laser surgery; however, the outer diameter of these ETTs is greater than an equivalent PVC or red-rubber ETT, making them inappropriate for small airways. A syringe or bucket should always be available to douse ignited ETTs or surrounding tissue. A non-intubation technique following a routine inhalational induction may also be used for laser surgery to allow for an unobstructed view during the procedure and eliminate a potentially flammable ETT. Furthermore, the depth of anesthesia can be controlled by the patient's minute ventilation. A review of spontaneous ventilation has shown this to be a safe and efficacious technique [22]. After the patient is positioned with a suspension laryngoscope the larynx is anesthetized with topical lidocaine, and anesthesia is maintained with a TIVA technique of propofol (200–400 µg/kg/min) and remifentanil (0.1–0.25 µg/kg/min) or passively delivered inhaled anesthetic via the side-port of the bronchoscope. Some anesthesiologists advocate the use of anticholinergics to prevent reflex bradycardia and decrease

secretions. This technique allows ventilation and passive oxygenation during the procedure. The mixture of gases delivered into the ETT or through the bronchoscope affects the risk of combustion. Helium impedes combustion from the CO_2 laser, whereas nitrous oxide and oxygen are additive in sustaining combustion. Oxygen concentration should be less then 30% to reduce the risk of airway fire, and the patient's ventilation and oxygenation are monitored visibly or with a precordial stethoscope and pulse oximeter. Intermittent mask ventilation or alternatively intermittent intubation by the surgeon may be required to treat episodes of hypoxia. Mask ventilation is preferable as repeat trauma from intermittent intubation may increase the risk of postoperative edema. A modification of this technique uses a jet ventilator during periods of apnea. Supraglottic jet ventilation via a catheter through the bronchoscope allows air to be entrained and large airways to be intermittently ventilated by the jet. This technique provides a relatively immobile surgical field by eliminating large diaphragmatic excursions during the procedure but may not provide effective ventilation for children with small airway disease. Dexamethasone (0.5–1 mg/kg) is administered during the procedure to reduce postoperative laryngeal edema, and racemic epinephrine may be needed for postoperative stridor.

The most catastrophic complication from laser surgery is airway fire. If the ETT ignites, oxygen flow should be discontinued, and the ETT should be disconnected from the gas source and removed from the airway. The fire should be doused with saline and the airway reexamined with a bronchoscope to determine the extent of tracheal and lung injury.

Tracheotomy

A tracheotomy may be performed as an emergency, urgently, or electively. Since the airway is shared between the anesthesiologist and the surgeon, a plan should be established preoperatively. The tracheostomy tube should conform to the trachea and neck without causing skin or tracheal mucosal injury. Plastic tracheostomy tubes are often used to prevent tissue injury. Plastic tracheostomy tubes are manufactured in metric sizes that correspond to ETT sizes whereas metal tracheostomy tubes are still measured in French sizes.

Elective tracheotomies are usually performed in children with an *in situ* ETT, who have failed extubation secondary to persistent hypoxemia, hypercarbia, or airway obstruction. Emergency or urgent tracheotomies are usually performed in children who initially maintain oxygenation and ventilation but are at risk of acute respiratory failure from upper airway or laryngeal trauma, corrosive ingestion, infections, and tumors.

For urgent tracheotomies the anesthesiologist must determine whether the child can maintain an airway under general anesthesia and can be intubated by standard laryngoscopy or fiberoptic bronchoscopy. Spontaneous ventilation should be maintained with an inhaled anesthetic induction. Ketamine, or TIVA technique with propofol (200–400 μg/kg/min), remifentanil (0.1–0.25 μg/kg/min), or dexmedetomidine (1–2 μg/kg/h) may also be used for children with impending respiratory failure. Muscle relaxants should be avoided to prevent airway obstruction if an unobstructed airway cannot be maintained. After the child is induced, topical lidocaine (1–3 ml of 2–4%) may be sprayed on the larynx to blunt laryngeal reflexes. If intubation is not possible, the airway may be maintained with an LMA or facemask. An ETT may be preferred to help the surgeon identify the trachea.

Elective tracheotomies are performed in children with an *in situ* ETT and anesthesia may be maintained with an inhaled anesthetic, opioid, and muscle relaxant. The child is positioned with a shoulder roll, so the neck is hyperextended, and the head is taped to the end of the bed. Before the tracheostomy tube is inserted, the ETT is pulled out to accommodate the tracheostomy tube, but the ETT should not be removed completely until ventilation is confirmed with the tracheostomy tube. Stay sutures are placed at the end of the procedure, so the surgeon may identify the tracheal incision and lumen if the tracheostomy tube is removed accidentally. At the authors' institution, children are sedated and paralyzed in the ICU for 5 days postoperatively to allow stoma healing and prevent accidental loss of the airway if the tracheostomy tube becomes dislodged.

The reader is directed to Chapter 33 on reconstructive airway surgery in pediatrics for details.

Anesthesia for laryngoscopy, bronchoscopy, and endoscopy

Rigid and flexible bronchoscopy allows both anatomic and dynamic evaluation of the upper and lower airways. Lesions commonly evaluated include laryngotracheomalacia, external anomalies causing tracheobronchial compression, congenital or acquired subglottic stenosis, laryngeal papillomas, hemangiomas, granulomas, and airway foreign bodies.

Anesthesia for rigid and flexible bronchoscopy and endoscopy requires constant cooperation and communication between the surgeon and the anesthesiologist since they must both share the airway. Preoperative evaluation should focus on the degree of airway obstruction at rest and with activity and positions or maneuvers that aggravate or improve the symptoms. The anesthesiologist should evaluate all imaging studies, pulmonary function tests, and arterial blood gases as part of the evaluation. Preoperative sedatives and opiods should be administered with caution, so as not to cause respiratory depression and worsen airway obstruction.

The rigid bronchoscope consists of the bronchoscope, a glass rod telescope, a side arm for ventilating with the anesthesia circuit, a light source for the telescope, and in instrument channel for grasping and incising (see Figure 32.1). The entire system is closed, permitting ventilation while the telescope is in place. Pediatric rigid bronchoscopes are available in three lengths and various diameters. The smallest optical telescope should be used to prevent increases in airflow resistance for ventilation as the optical telescope may occupy the entire lumen of the smaller bronchoscopes [23]. A persistent increase in intrathoracic pressure may occur when the telescope impedes airflow, increasing the risk of barotrauma and cardiovascular compromise. For example, when a 2.8 mm telescope is used with a 3.5 mm bronchoscope, adequate exhalation occurs. However, when a smaller bronchoscope is used, adequate exhalation may not occur and the telescope should be intermittently removed, particularly for longer procedures, to allow ventilation and passive exhalation.

An alternative method of ventilation during bronchoscopy is the Sanders jet ventilation technique (see Figure 32.2) [24]. The principle involves bursts of oxygen up to 50 psi from a hand-held pressure-reducing valve via a 16-gauge catheter attached to the rigid bronchoscope. Current jet ventilators have adjustable pressure valves that may decrease the risk of barotrauma. Oxygen is released through the catheter, creating a Venturi effect that entrains room air in the rigid bronchoscope, inflating the lungs. A FiO$_2$ of considerably less than 100% is administered since the

(A)

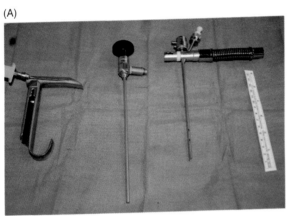

(B)

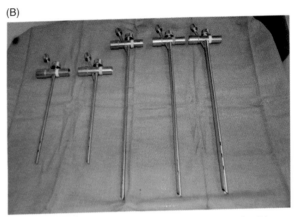

Figure 32.1. (A) The rigid bronchoscope consists of (from left to right) the laryngoscope, glass rod telescope, bronchoscope, and a side arm for ventilating with the anesthesia circuit. (B) Different bronchoscope sizes (3.5 to 6.0) and lengths from left to right are shown.

Figure 32.2. Sanders jet ventilator.

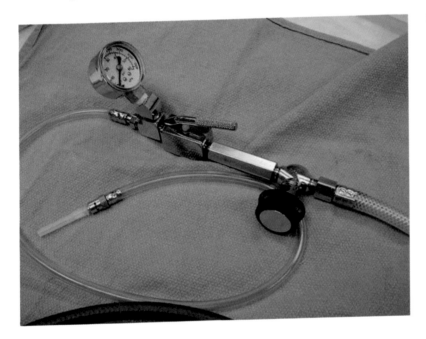

entrained air dilutes the oxygen delivered. Exhalation is passive following elastic recoil of the lungs and chest. The high inflation pressures may cause barotrauma, pneumothorax, pneumomediastinum, and gastric insufflation. Hypoxia from room air entrapment and hypercapnea from incomplete exhalation may also occur. Children with significant underlying pulmonary or chest wall disease are not candidates for jet ventilation. Anesthesia is usually maintained with a TIVA technique as mentioned below.

The anesthesiologist must maintain oxygenation and ventilation, prevent aspiration, and minimize laryngeal motion during bronchoscopy while the surgeon controls the airway. Both inhalational and intravenous induction are appropriate, but spontaneous ventilation should be maintained to allow the surgeon to evaluate upper airway or tracheobronchial dynamics. An anticholinergic may be administered to decrease secretions and prevent a vagally mediated bradycardia. Topicalizaion of the vocal cords with lidocaine 1–3 ml of 2–4% blunts laryngeal reflexes to prevent coughing and bucking during instrumentation and allows a lighter plane of anesthesia to help evaluate airway dynamics. Maintenance of anesthesia with either an inhaled anesthetic or a TIVA with propofol and/or opioid must be balanced to ensure a "quiet" surgical field but prevent apnea to allow evaluation of airway dynamics. A propofol-based TIVA technique (200–400 μg/kg/min) can be given continuously during the bronchoscopy, producing a more stable depth of anesthesia than an inhalational anesthetic delivered through the side port of the bronchoscope. Remifentanil (0.1–0.25 μg/kg/min) has the advantage of increasing the depth of anesthesia and blunting additional sympathetic stimulation, and its short-acting property minimizes the risk of respiratory depression when the surgical stimulus is removed. Because ventilation may be intermittent or occluded by the bronchoscope, 100% O_2 should be delivered during the bronchoscopy. High fresh gas flow rates and high concentration of inhaled anesthetic are necessary to compensate for leaks around the rigid bronchoscope. Only the telescope without a ventilating side channel may be used in a neonate, necessitating the use of an ETT placed in the mouth or nose for insufflation of oxygen. At the end of the procedure, the surgeon may size the larynx with an uncuffed ETT to determine an air leak with positive pressure between 15 and 25 cmH_2O. Dexamethasone 0.5–1 mg/kg is administered to reduce airway edema postoperatively. The child should be spontaneously ventilating with a natural airway at the end of the procedure when the bronchoscope is removed.

Continuous $EtCO_2$ monitoring is not always possible with bronchoscopy, and clinical observation of chest wall movement or a precordial stethoscope is useful. Hypercapnea is inevitable but usually well tolerated in most children. Hypoxia, however, is usually not well tolerated and the bronchoscopy may have to be stopped while the child is reoxygenated with either a facemask or intermittent intubation. Persistent hypoxia or rapid cardiovascular deterioration should make one suspicious for the diagnosis of tension pneumothorax.

Stridor

Stridor is a term generally used to describe noisy breathing and to refer specifically to a high-pitched crowing sound associated with various respiratory etiologies. The etiology of stridor may be extrathoracic or intrathoracic, acquired or congenital, and fixed or dynamic. Inspiratory stridor occurs from anomalies above the thoracic inlet whereas expiratory stridor typically occurs from anomalies below the thoracic inlet. A preoperative history should focus on the onset and duration of symptoms, position with symptoms (e.g., supine or upright), activity with symptoms (e.g., at rest or exertion), and previous tracheal intubations. A nasal flexible bronchoscope in an awake neonate may help evaluate the neonate's laryngeal dynamics without stressing the child. An anticholinergic agent may be administered to prevent a vagally mediated bradycardia, and the nasal mucosa can be topicalizaed with lidocaine to prevent discomfort during the transnasal approach. Alternatively, a rigid bronchoscope with general anesthesia not only allows visualization of the lower tracheobronchial tree but also maintains control over oxygenation and ventilation as described previously.

Acute epiglottitis

Acute epiglottitis is a potentially life-threatening supraglottic bacterial infection. Epiglottitis was more common before the *Haemophilus influenzae* type b vaccine became available. Children are toxic-appearing with high fever, sore throat, dysphagia, dysphonia, and inspiratory stridor. Classically, the child is sitting up with the chin forward, mouth open and drooling, and hands in a tripod posture. The child may deteriorate rapidly unless a definitive airway is established. Lateral neck radiographs may show a swollen epiglottis but should not be performed if causing a delay in definitive airway establishment. The child should not be disturbed from this position, to prevent complete airway obstruction, and immediately transferred without disturbance, usually in a parent's arms, to the operating room by an anesthesiologist, otolaryngologist, or intensivist with the goal of securing the airway in a controlled manner. ETT is the preferred method of supportive airway care.

An inhaled induction maintaining spontaneous ventilation and airway tone should be performed gently with the child, usually in the parent's arms, to avoid causing acute airway obstruction. Intravenous access should only be performed when the child is obtunded. Moderate CPAP may be added to prevent airway collapse, but spontaneous ventilation should be maintained for airway tone. Intubation is usually performed with ETT one or two sizes smaller than the age-appropriate size. A classic cherry-red epiglottis may be visible under direct laryngoscopy, but significant inflammation of the epiglottis and other supraglottic structures may distort oropharyngeal anatomy, making direct laryngoscopy difficult. Emergency airway equipment such as videolaryngoscopes and bronchoscopes should be readily available, and the surgeon may also perform an emergency tracheostomy under mask ventilation.

The child is mechanically ventilated postoperatively in the ICU until an air leak is audible, usually 24 to 48 hours following the initiation of antibiotics.

Croup

Croup has a more insidious onset than epiglottitis, usually following an upper respiratory infection. Children may have a bark-like cough with inspiratory stridor at rest or activity but are not toxic-appearing, unlike children with epiglottitis. Anteroposterior radiographs of the neck reveal the classic "steeple church" sign with symmetric narrowing of the subglottis. Most cases of croup resolve spontaneously, but children may occasionally present with respiratory failure. Humidification of inspired gases prevents drying of secretions. Supplemental oxygen may be needed for hypoxia. Racemic epinephrine is the most effective therapy, while corticosteroids, such as dexamethasone and budesonide, are also effective [25]. Antibiotics are usually not indicated as clinical improvement usually occurs in 12 to 24 hours.

Peritonsillar abscess

Peritonsillar abscess is the most common deep neck infection treated by an otolaryngologist. Children may present preoperatively with fever, pharyngeal swelling, sore throat, dysphagia, dysphonia, and trismus. Preoperative evaluation should focus on the degree of airway obstruction. Computed tomography preoperatively helps identify airway deviation and obstruction. Although intravenous induction may be appropriate since airway obstruction from the abscess is less likely as the abscess is in a fixed location in the lateral pharynx, inhalational induction maintaining spontaneous ventilation may be preferable to prevent loss of airway tone during induction. An oropharyngeal airway should be avoided and care must be taken during laryngoscopy to prevent rupture of the abscess and aspiration of purulent material.

Vocal cord visualization should not be impaired since the pathology is supraglottic and above the laryngeal inlet although a right-sided abscess may interfere with the normal sweeping of the tongue to the left during laryngoscopy. Occasionally, laryngoscopy may be difficult if pharyngeal swelling distorts normal oropharyngeal anatomy. A cuffed ETT should be used to prevent aspiration of purulent material.

Airway foreign body

Airway foreign bodies are most common in children between 1 and 3 years of age. Aspirated objects are usually peanuts, food, and plastic or metal objects. Symptoms depend on the location, size, and acuity of the aspirated object. Children may present with hoarseness, stridor, dyspnea, unilateral decreased air entry, or an acute history of choking. Children may also have chronic cough, wheezing, or lower respiratory infections that are not responsive to medical therapy. Normal physical examination cannot eliminate the possibility of an aspirated foreign object, as up to 45% of children with an abnormal bronchoscopic exam will have a normal preoperative physical examination [26]. Foreign-body aspiration is diagnosed within 24 hours in only half of children whereas the remaining patients are diagnosed following failure of medical management for chronic cough, wheezing, stridor, or recurrent lower respiratory tract infections. Some aspirated objects, such as plastic toys, are radiopaque and may be detected on chest radiograph; unfortunately, the majority of aspirated objects, including food items, are radiolucent and are unlikely to be detected by chest radiograph.

The effect of the aspirated foreign body depends on the pattern of obstruction [27]: (1) bypass valve, where both respiratory phases are involved, but the radiograph is normal since there is enough aeration beyond the obstruction; (2) check valve, where inhalation is normal but exhalation is impeded, creating hyperinflation on expiratory radiographs; a mediastinal shift towards the normal side may be seen if there is a significant volume difference; (3) ball valve, where inhalation is impeded, leading to atelectasis on the affected side; and (4) stop valve, where air flow is completely impeded during inhalation and exhalation. Consolidation of the involved area occurs, followed by collapse.

The urgency to proceed with anesthesia and bronchoscopic removal of the foreign body is dictated by the severity of respiratory distress and the location and type of aspirated material. For example, unroasted peanuts should be removed immediately as the unsaturated oils may cause a severe inflammatory response. Additionally, peanuts may fragment over time, making en bloc removal challenging. Children who aspirate foreign bodies while eating present with the additional risk of a full stomach and aspiration. Waiting for the appropriate NPO time may not be possible, particularly with signs of airway obstruction. Given the risk of airway obstruction, the airway takes precedence over the risk of gastric content aspiration. The major unresolved controversy with airway foreign bodies is whether to maintain controlled ventilation or spontaneous ventilation. Although an intravenous induction may be possible in children who do not present with airway obstruction, an inhalational induction while maintaining spontaneous ventilation is preferable to reduce the risk of further obstruction and minimize movement of the foreign body with positive-pressure ventilation. Anesthesia is maintained similar to bronchoscopy with an inhalational anesthetic or TIVA technique with propofol with/without remifentanil. Spontaneous ventilation should be preserved until the location and degree of obstruction are identified, noting that the position of the foreign body may change intraoperatively. Nitrous oxide is relatively contraindicated as it reduces the inspired concentration of oxygen, but more importantly may significantly increase lung volumes if air trapping occurs. The foreign body is usually removed easily through the bronchoscope, but occasionally it may have to be pushed peripherally to relieve significant airway obstruction or broken into smaller pieces to facilitate removal. The size of the foreign body may also exceed the internal diameter of the bronchoscope. The foreign body, forceps, and the bronchoscope must be removed together through the vocal cords. If the foreign body is lost during attempted removal the bronchoscope may have to be re-introduced several times to facilitate removal, increasing the risk of mucosal edema. Dexamethasone 0.5–1 mg/kg should be administered intraoperatively to reduce the risk of airway edema postoperatively. Postoperative croup may be treated with nebulized racemic epinephrine.

Endoscopy for esophageal foreign body ingestion

The most commonly ingested esophageal foreign body is a coin, followed by food and bones. Frequently, esophageal foreign bodies pass through the gastric outlet and the gastrointestinal tract, rarely requiring surgical intervention. Children with a mid-esophageal foreign body may present with dysphagia, drooling, retching, and vomiting, but children with an upper esophageal foreign body may present with respiratory distress from anatomic compression of the airway. Major complications are rare, but a coin lodged for more than 24 hours may cause esophageal erosion. A chest radiograph, which should be obtained in all cases of suspected esophageal foreign body ingestion, usually shows lodgement at the proximal esophagus, the thoracic inlet, or the mid-esophagus. A coin will appear transverse on a radiograph since the esophagus is widest in the transverse position.

If the child is not in respiratory distress, the foreign body may be removed following an appropriate fasting period. Either an intravenous or inhalational induction is appropriate, and an ETT for airway protection should precede removal. The ETT should be taped to the left side to allow space in the oropharynx for the surgeon to insert the esophagoscope. The ETT may be dislodged when the esophagoscope is withdrawn. Finally, the foreign body may be dislodged in the hyopharynx and slip into the larynx during removal, completely occluding the airway and requiring urgent retrieval.

Anesthetic complications in pediatric otolaryngologic procedures

As presented in this chapter, otolaryngologic procedures require proper preoperative evaluation, intraoperative planning and anticipation of postoperative complications to ensure a favorable outcome. Although many of the children presenting for these procedures are healthy, and the procedures are done as outpatient/ambulatory interventions, some are done on children with complex medical history, syndromes and with extensive surgical trauma.

Complications following otolaryngologic procedures are either patient or procedure related. Pediatric patients are more prone to separation anxiety and difficulty with induction, postoperative emergence delirium and lower pain tolerance with recovery.

Teenage girls have a higher incidence of postoperative nausea and vomiting, and most airway instrumentation procedures require prophylaxis or therapy for such complication. Children with enlarged adenoids and tonsils have increased risk of intra- and postoperative airway obstruction, laryngospasm, and desaturation. Pediatric patients with syndromes or chromosomal abnormalities have a higher risk of obstructive airway disease and post-operative compromise, requiring prolonged recovery, especially in those less than 3 years of age.

Laser procedures have the risk of airway fires as well as occupational hazards to healthcare providers in the operating room. Unique complications to such procedures as adenotonsillectomy, with early or late postoperative tonsillar bleeding, and ear and mastoid surgery, with potential for nerve injury, require anticipation and appropriate preparation for therapy. Laryngeal surgery can result in postoperative airway compromise, secondary to swelling or laryngo-tracheomalacia.

Summary

In conclusion, anesthesia for otolaryngologic procedures in children is one of the most challenging and rewarding fields in anesthesia. It requires a careful understanding of the underlying pathophysiology, the planned surgical procedure, and the anesthetic risks. It also requires a concerted effort and clear communication with our surgical colleagues with whom we share the airway in many of these interventions. A safe and smooth postoperative recovery can be achieved by anticipation of potential complications and careful planning for prophylaxis, and effective therapy.

Case study of anesthesia for pediatric otolaryngologic surgery

Preoperative evaluation

A 3-month old female presents for an elective T&A. The parents report a history of extremely loud snoring, self-resolving pauses (~2–3 seconds), restless sleep, daytime somnolence, and hyperactivity at pre-school according to her providers. She has baseline chronic congestion presumed secondary to allergic rhinitis and had a recent exacerbation of her chronic congestion with upper respiratory tract infection. She had 1 day of vomiting at that time, which required a visit to an urgent care center. She was given oral hydration therapy at the urgent care center; a chemistry panel drawn at that time was unremarkable except for an HCO_3 of 30, and she was discharged home. She has had no previous surgeries or general anesthetics. Parents report no history of anesthetic complications in the family. She has no known food or drug allergies and is currently taking fexofenadine (Allegra), montelukast (Singulair), and albuterol as needed, last used

approximately 4 weeks prior to her upper respiratory tract infection. Physical examination reveals an extremely anxious and clingy child with clear nasal secretions that are baseline according to her parents. Vital signs are temperature 98.2°F, respiratory rate (RR) 20, heart rate (HR) 132, and a weight of 19 kg. Blood pressure (BP) and SpO_2 cannot be obtained since the child is crying. Cardiorespiratory exam is difficult to elicit through her crying.

Intraoperative course

She is given midazolam 6 mg (0.5 mg/kg) PO 20 minutes prior to the procedure, and is transported to the OR sedated but able to communicate with the operating room team when prompted verbally. Standard ASA monitors are placed prior to induction with initial vital signs as HR 120, BP 102/65, SpO_2 93% on room air. Inhalational induction with 70%/30% N_2O/O_2 and 8% sevoflurane produces moderate obstruction requiring CPAP 10 cmH_2O, repositioning of the head, and an oral way. Propofol 30 mg, morphine 1.2 mg, dexamethasone 6 mg, and ondansetron 2 mg are given following placement of a peripheral IV. A 4.5 oral RAE ETT is placed following direct laryngoscopy with a grade I view. The 15-minute surgical procedure is uneventful as hemorrhage is controlled from the tonsillar bed, and an orogastric tube is passed with minimal gastric contents recovered. The child is extubated awake, but develops airway obstruction immediately following extubation, requiring CPAP 10 cmH_2O. SpO_2 at this time was 90% with no change in HR and BP. She resumes spontaneous ventilation with a regular respiratory pattern and SpO_2 increases to 99%

Postoperative course

The child is transported to the PACU in the head-up position and has a non-obstructive respiratory pattern on arrival at the PACU. Initial vital signs in the PACU are SpO_2 98% on blow-by O_2, HR 112, RR 10, BP 102/54. Approximately 10 minutes following arrival at the PACU, she develops significant airway obstruction with SpO_2 80% on blow-by O_2, HR 104, RR no air entry noted with a paradoxical respiration, and BP 124/84. BIPAP and a jaw thrust are required by the PACU nurse and the anesthesiologist to improve airway obstruction. Vital signs are now SpO_2 94% on 6l via Jackson-Rees circuit, RR 10 with moderate airway obstruction, HR 120, and BP 126/76. She is still asleep with minimal response to the jaw thrust. Naloxone 15 µg for four doses is given at 3-minute intervals. The child is now more awake and following commands with SpO$_2$ 95% on blow-by O2, RR 10 with mild airway obstruction, HR 120, and BP 126/82. She redevelops significant airway obstruction approximately 30 minutes following her last naloxone dose, again requiring BIPAP and a jaw thrust by the PACU nurse and the anesthesiologist to improve the airway obstruction; she is again asleep with minimal response to the jaw thrust. An arterial blood gas is obtained with a pH 7.20, pCO$_2$ 120, pO$_2$ 80, HCO$_3$ 34. The child is reintubated and admitted to the PICU.

She is extubated on postoperative day 2 and discharged home on postoperative day 4. She has a sleep study 2 months postoperatively that shows an RDI 4.5, SpO$_2$ nadir 88%, and peak EtCO$_2$ 50, with the mother reporting occasional snoring at night with pauses, but improvement in hyperactivity at preschool.

Sleep-disordered breathing is a disease continuum. Although there are no definitive guidelines for the anesthetic management for T&A, it is important to attempt to identify high-risk patients preoperatively or intraoperatively as the analgesic requirements and postoperative monitoring may need to be modified.

Clinical pearls

- Preschool children receiving unsupplemented sevoflurane anesthesia for myringotomy tube placement may exhibit emergence delirium of unknown etiology. Since intravenous access is not usually needed for this brief procedure, intranasal fentanyl 1–2 µg/kg can be used to reduce postoperative emergence delirium from sevoflurane anesthesia.
- Children with an active or recent upper respiratory tract infection may be at risk of perioperative respiratory complications, including airway obstruction, laryngospasm, bronchospasm, and breath-holding, for up to 6 weeks. Increased airway reactivity may persist for up to 8 weeks even for children with a recent, uncomplicated URI. However, no increases in perioperative respiratory complications were found in those children presenting with an acute uncomplicated upper respiratory tract infection for minor surgery not requiring airway instrumentation.
- Unilateral choanal atresia is not a medical or surgical emergency and may present as only persistent unilateral nasal discharge years later. If the obstruction is bilateral, children may present with acute respiratory failure; surgical correction depends on the neonate's ability to compensate with oral breathing and receive adequate nutrition. Some surgeons advocate a "rule of tens" for timing of the repair: the child must over 10 weeks of age, weigh over 10 pounds, and have hemoglobin over 10 gm/dl.
- Documented severe obstructive sleep apnea (OSA) places children at higher risk of perioperative respiratory complications, along with other factors: age less than 3 years old, craniofacial syndromes, cranial base disorders, neuromuscular disorders, trisomy 21, infiltrative disorders and storage diseases, and obesity.
- Children with mucopolysaccharidosis I (Hurler's syndrome) and II (Hunter's syndrome) have diffuse infiltration of the upper airway with mucopolysaccharidosis, predisposing them to airway obstruction, difficult mask ventilation and difficulty with intubation.
- Deep extubation for high-risk children may increase the incidence of airway obstruction and postoperative respiratory complications.
- In managing acute epiglottitis, an inhaled induction maintaining spontaneous ventilation and airway tone should be performed gently with the child, usually in the parent's arms. Intravenous access is ordinarily only performed when the child is obtunded. Moderate CPAP may be added to help prevent airway collapse. Intubation is usually performed using an ETT one or two sizes smaller than the usual age-appropriate size.

References

1. Vornov P, Tobim MJ, Billings K, *et al.* Postoperative pain relief in infants undergoing myringotomy and tube placement: comparison of a novel regional anesthetic block to intranasal fentanyl – a pilot analysis. *Pediatr Anesth* 2008;**18**:1196–201.

2. Galinkin JL, Fazi LM, Cuy RM, *et al.* Use of intranasal fentanyl in children undergoing myringotomy and tube placement during halothane and sevoflurane

anesthesia. *Anesthesiology* 2000;**93**:1378–83.

3. Pestieau SR, Quezado ZM, Johnson YJ, *et al.* The effect of dexmedetomidine during myringotomy and pressure-equalizing tube placement in children. *Pediatr Anesth* 2011;**21**:1128–35.

4. Tait AR, Malviya S. Anesthesia for the child with an upper respiratory tract infection: still a dilemma? *Anesth Analg* 2005;**100**:59–65.

5. Suresh S, Barcelone SL, Young NM, *et al.* Postoperative pain relief in children undergoing tympanomastoid surgery: is a regional block better than opioids. *Anesth Analg* 2002;**94**:859–62.

6. Crawford MW, White MC, Propst EJ, *et al.* Dose-dependent suppression of the electrical elicited stapedius reflex by general anesthetics in children undergoing cochlear implant surgery. *Anesth Analg* 2009;**18**:1480–7.

7. Rosen GM, Muckle RP, Mahowald MW, *et al.* Postoperative respiratory compromise in children with obstructive sleep apnea syndrome. Can it be anticipated? *Pediatrics* 1994;**93**:784–8.

8. Karlson KH Jr. What's new in pediatric obstructive sleep apnea? *Clin Pulm Med* 2008;**15**:226.

9. Brown KA. Outcome, risk, and error and the child with obstructive sleep apnea. *Pediatr Anesth* 2011;**21**:771–80.

10. Roland PS, Rosenfeld RM, Brooks LJ, *et al.* Clinical practice guideline: polysomnography for sleep-disordered breathing prior to tonsillectomy in children. *Otolaryngol Head Neck Surg* 2011;**145**(1 Suppl):S1–15.

11. Nolan J, Brietzke SE. Systematic review of pediatric tonsil size and polysomnogram-measured obstructive sleep apnea severity. *Otolaryngol Head Neck Surg* 2011;**144**:844–50.

12. Francis A, Eltaki K, Bash T, *et al.* The safety of preoperative sedation in children with sleep-disordered breathing. *Int J Pediatr Otorhinolaryngol* 2006;**70**:517–21

13. Brown KA, Laferrière A, Lakheeram I, *et al.* Recurrent hypoxemia in children is associated with increased analgesic sensitivity to opiates. *Anesthesiology* 2006;**105**:665–9.

14. Brown KA, Laferrière A, Moss IR. Recurrent hypoxemia in young children with obstructive sleep apnea is associated with reduced opioid requirement for analgesia. *Anesthesiology* 2004;**100**:806–10.

15. Cardwell M, Siviter G, Smith A. Non-steroidal anti-inflammatory drugs and perioperative bleeding in paediatric tonsillectomy. *Cochrane Database Syst Rev* 2005;**2**:CD003591.

16. Capici F, Ingelmo PM, Davidson A, *et al.* Randomized controlled trial of duration of analgesia following intravenous or rectal acetaminophen after adenotonsillectomy in children. *Br J Anaesth* 2008;**100**:251–5.

17. Dahmani S, Michelet D, Abback PS, *et al.* Ketamine for perioperative pain management in children: a meta-analysis of published studies. *Pediatr Anesth* 2011;**21**:636–52.

18. Olutotye OA, Glover CD, Diefenderge JW, *et al.* The effect of intraoperative dexmedetomidine on postoperative analgesia and sedation in pediatrics patients undergoing tonsillectomy and adenoidectomy. *Anesth Analg* 2010;**111**:490–5.

19. Czarnetizki C, Elia N, Lysakowski C, *et al.* Dexamethasone and risk of vomiting and postoperative bleeding after tonsillectomy in children: a randomized trial. *JAMA* 2008;**300**:2621–30.

20. Peng A, Dodson KM, Thacker LR. Use of laryngeal mask airway in pediatric adenotonsillectomy. *Arch Otolaryngol Head Neck Surg* 2011;**137**:42–6

21. Helfaer MA, McColley SA, Pyzik PL, *et al.* Polysomnography after adenotonsillectomy in mild pediatric obstructive sleep apnea. *Crit Care Med* 1996;**24**:1323–7.

22. Quintal M, Cunningham M, Ferrari L. Tubeless spontaneous respiration technique for pediatric microlaryngeal surgery. *Arch Otolaryngol* 1997;**123**:209–14.

23. Woods AM, Gal TJ. Decreaseing airflow resistance during infant and pediatric bronschoscopy. *Anesth Analg* 1987;**66**:457–9.

24. Miyasaka K, Sloan IA, Froese AB. An evaluation of the jet injector (Sanders) technique for bronchoscopy in paediatric patients. *Can Anaesth Soc* 1980;**27**:117–24.

25. Russell KF, Liang Y, O'Gorman K, *et al.* Glucocorticoids for croup. *Cochrane Database Syst Rev* 2011;**1**:CD001955.

26. Even L, Heno N, Talmon Y, *et al.* Diagnostic evaluation of foreign body aspiration in children: a prospective study. *J Pediatr Surg* 2005;**40**:1122–7.

27. Zur KB, Litman RS. Pediatric airway foreign body: surgical and anesthetic perspectives. *Pediatr Anesth* 2009;**19**:109–17.

33

Anesthesia for reconstructive airway surgery in pediatrics

Megan Nolan and David S. Beebe

Introduction/background

Reconstructive surgery for the airway first began being performed in children in the early part of the twentieth century. At that time the chief cause of laryngeal or tracheal pathology was diphtheria. In the 1920s and 1930s a variety of surgical techniques were developed by Jackson and Arbuckle to correct laryngotracheal stenosis resulting from diphtheria. Using resection of diseased tissue as well as skin grafts, this allowed many of these children to no longer require a tracheostomy. With the diphtheria vaccine, the incidence of infectious laryngeal stenosis declined. However, in the 1930s to the 1960s airway injuries from automobile accidents increased. Techniques to correct posttraumatic stenosis using rib cartilage grafts were developed during this time. In the 1960s premature babies began being managed by prolonged intubation for ventilatory support. Subglottic stenosis from prolonged intubation soon became a serious problem as these babies survived to childhood. Often these children required a permanent tracheostomy. However, airway operations such as the anterior cricoid split were developed by otolaryngologists that allowed an infant with subglottic stenosis to have an adequate airway and often forgo a tracheostomy. Cricoid resection is now also utilized in infants and children with severe subglottic stenosis as well, as are resections of short segments of the trachea for acquired or congenital stenosis. In recent years tracheoplasty techniques that allow the reconstruction of the airway in infants or small children who have long segments of stenosis have been developed, often using a cardiopulmonary bypass. In the past these lesions were often fatal [1,2].

Infants and children undergoing reconstructive airway surgery present many challenges to the anesthesiologist. If they are not yet tracheally intubated at the time of surgery they may have stridor or some degree of airway obstruction from their stenotic lesion, making induction of general anesthesia hazardous. Anesthesiologists and surgeons must be prepared to handle a difficult airway when anesthetizing these patients. Both flexible and rigid bronchoscopy are often performed prior to beginning reconstructive airway surgery. These procedures require close cooperation between the anesthesiologist and surgeon when managing a shared airway. Often these infants require tracheal intubation for a week or two following operations on their airway. This is a challenge for the pediatric intensivist. Adequate but not excessive sedation must be provided so that tracheal intubation is tolerated without long-term complications. Extubation and post-extubation care can be a challenge as well because postoperative edema can lead to airway obstruction. Finally, many infants and children undergoing airway reconstructive procedures require frequent laryngoscopies and bronchoscopies under anesthesia to assess their progress and determine whether further procedures are necessary. These patients often have challenging airways and become well known to the treating anesthesiologists.

Surgical procedures

Subglottic stenosis is the primary indication for reconstructive airway surgery in infants and small children. Subglottic stenosis is a reduction in the lumen of the airway below the level of the glottic opening. Cotton in 1984 introduced a simple classification system for subglottic stenosis based on the degree of obstruction. Grade 1 is any degree of stenosis less that 70%. Grade 2 is a reduction of the lumen of 70% to 90%. Grade 3 is a 90% stenosis with an

Anesthesia for Otolaryngologic Surgery, ed. Basem Abdelmalak and D. John Doyle. Published by Cambridge University Press.
© Cambridge University Press 2013.

identifiable lumen. Grade 4 is complete obstruction. Children with greater than 70% stenosis will require surgery to allow ventilation without a tracheostomy. The most common cause of subglottic stenosis is prolonged intubation, and neonates are the most common patient population affected. Congenital subglottic stenosis not resulting from prolonged intubation only occurs about 5% of the time. Today, the incidence of subglottic stenosis in neonates ranges from 0.63% to 2.0% [3].

Acquired subglottic stenosis is thought to result from airway injury causing an excess of granulation tissue. This granulation tissue consists of fibroblasts, macrophages, loose connective tissue, and new capillaries. The fibroblasts act to pull the edges of the injured site together and decrease the size of the airway. Even without trauma at the time of intubation, any long-term intubation (greater than 14 days duration) is irritating to the delicate tissue of the airway and can result in edema, ulcerations, tissue erosion, and scarring, with the development of subglottic stenosis. Chronic aspiration and infection can also cause or aggravate subglottic stenosis. In addition, acquired subglottic stenosis can result from external trauma such as a motor vehicle accident. In the past subglottic stenosis was managed by long-term tracheostomy below the site of the stenotic lesion. Currently there are several operations available that allow decannulation of a tracheostomy in children with subglottic stenosis, or elimination of the need for a tracheostomy in the management of subglottic stenosis altogether [3].

One common operation developed for neonates with subglottic stenosis is the anterior cricoid split. The surgical criteria to perform an anterior cricoid split are: (1) failed extubation on two or more occasions; (2) a weight greater than 1500 g; (3) extubation failure secondary to laryngeal pathology; (4) no assisted ventilation for ten days prior to the procedure; (5) supplemental oxygen less than 35%; (6) no congestive heart failure for at least 1 month prior to the procedure; (7) no upper respiratory tract infection; and (8) no antihypertensive medications for 10 days prior to the procedure [3,4].

Following rigid bronchoscopy to identify the site of the stenosis, the infants are tracheally intubated with the tip of the tracheal tube placed just below the site of the lesion. The head and neck are extended and a horizontal incision is made in the skin over the cricoid cartilage. An incision is made through the

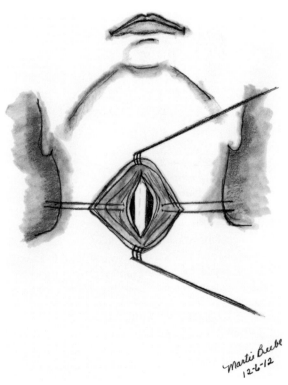

Figure 33.1. Anterior cricoid split. An incision is made through the cricoid cartilage, lower third of the thyroid cartilage, first two tracheal rings and the underlying mucosa. The skin and subcutaneous tissue are then loosely closed. The patient is left intubated for approximately 1 week so the endotracheal tube can act as a stent through the stenotic area. Artwork created by Martie Beebe.

cricoid ring and underlying mucosa, the lower third of the thyroid cartilage and the first two tracheal rings (Figure 33.1). The endotracheal tube used is removed and replaced, often nasally under surgical guidance, with a tracheal tube one size larger (0.5 mm) than predicted for the child's age and weight. The skin and subcutaneous tissue are loosely closed. The infant is left intubated for approximately 1 week so the tracheal tube can stent the subglottic aperture [4].

The classic anterior cricoid split has now largely been succeeded by laryngotracheoplasty and, in selected cases, cricotracheal resection. Laryngotracheoplasty is similar to the anterior cricoid split. However, both an anterior and posterior cricoid split may be performed. Cartilage usually harvested from the thyroid cartilage is sutured into place in the anterior and occasionally the posterior splits to provide a wider subglottic opening. The patients are managed with tracheal intubation for approximately 1 week to allow healing to occur [4].

(A)

(B)

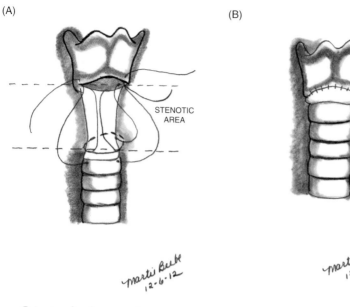

STENOTIC
AREA

Figure 33.2. Cricotracheal resection. The anterior cricoid arch is resected and the posterior cricoid plate thinned with preservation of a posterior mucosal flap. The transected normal trachea is telescoped and sutured to the submucosal flap and the thyroid cartilage. Artwork created by Martie Beebe.

Cricotracheal resection is another surgical option to treat subglottic stenosis in children. It is technically more challenging than larnygotracheoplasty and has the potential complications of anastomotic dehiscence and recurrent laryngeal nerve damage. However, it has allowed successful decannulation of children who had such severe subglottic stenosis that laryngotracheoplasty was not likely to be successful. It has also proved useful as a salvage technique following failed laryngotracheoplasty [5].

The technique involves resection of the anterior cricoid arch and thinning of the posterior cricoid plate with preservation of a posterior mucosal flap (Figure 33.2). The transected normal trachea is telescoped and sutured to the submucosal flap and thyroid cartilage. Usually a tracheostomy is in place for the procedure and can be left intact postoperatively. Stenting of the anastomosis may be accomplished either with tracheal intubation for 7 to 14 days as with laryngotracheoplasty or with a T tube. Some surgeons also place sutures between the chin and chest to keep the anastomosis without tension from head extension [5].

One type of challenging airway lesion that was often fatal in the past but now can be treated surgically is severe congenital tracheal stenosis. These fortunately are very rare lesions and represent only between 0.3% and 1% of all laryngotracheal stenosis. Complete tracheal rings that have no posterior membranous portion of the trachea cause the most severe stenosis. These patients typically present in infancy with "washing machine breathing". This describes the characteristic bi-phasic noise made by secretions being moved by respiration through an area of distal tracheal stenosis. Anesthesiologists also commonly discover these children when they come to the operating room for an unrelated procedure and a narrow airway that is "unintubatable" due to its small size is found. Often these children suffer other congenital defects such as cardiac defects, pulmonary artery slings, VATER syndrome and Down's syndrome. Short segments (< 30% of the tracheal length) can be managed with primary tracheal resection with end-to-end anastomosis. Longer segments or segments extending to the bronchus are more problematic. One type of surgical repair used commonly in the past involved splitting the stenotic trachea longitudinally and sewing a graft of cartilage or more commonly pericardium in place to give the trachea a bigger lumen. These grafts were often plagued by the development of granulation tissue in the new lumen with recurrent stenosis. Graft disruption and mediastinitis also frequently developed [2,6].

In 1989 Tang *et al.* first described the technique of the slide-tracheoplasty [7]. In this repair the trachea is bisected and the midpoint of the stenotic segment is then split longitudinally superiorly and inferiorly. The slide tracheoplasty overlaps stenotic segments of the trachea, shortening the trachea but doubling the circumference and diameter of the stenotic area. The segments are then telescoped and sewn together

339

(A)   (B)   (C)

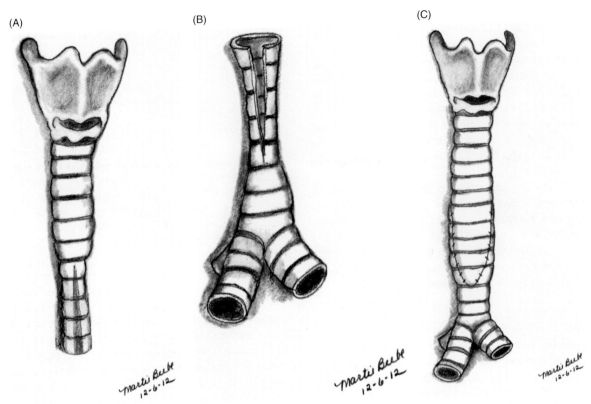

Figure 33.3. Slide tracheoplasty. The trachea is bisected at the midpoint of the stenotic segment then split longitudinally superiorly and inferiorly. The segments are then telescoped and sutured together, shortening the trachea but doubling the area of the stenotic segment. Artwork created by Martie Beebe.

(Figure 33.3). The advantage of this technique is that the tracheal mucosa is preserved on the suture line so that primary healing can occur without the development of granulation tissue. The operation is quite complex and usually cardiopulmonary bypass is required to provide gas exchange during this operation. This challenging operation can allow survival of infants with types of severe tracheal stenosis that were once uniformly fatal [2,6,7].

Anesthetic management

Preoperative evaluation

Pediatric patients undergoing reconstructive surgery on the airway require a thorough preoperative evaluation by the anesthesiologist. The type of lesion being repaired and type of repair must be determined. Pediatric patients requiring airway reconstruction often have other congenital defects such as congenital heart disease, particularly if the airway lesion is congenital in origin. These conditions should be evaluated thoroughly by the pediatrician prior to beginning airway reconstructive surgery. If there is a stenotic lesion, the degree of stenosis should be determined from previous studies such as CT or MRI scans or by reviewing the results of flexible endoscopy. If the patient is a neonate or child who is still tracheally intubated, the ventilator settings and oxygen requirements should be determined. In extubated or ambulatory patients the oxygen requirements should be determined from the parents or nurses as well as the necessity for other aids to ventilation such as nebulized bronchodilators. The parents and/or nurses should be asked about the presence of stridor or respiratory distress. The presence or absence of an upper respiratory tract infection should also be ascertained. The presence of a significant upper respiratory infection will often warrant delay of surgery if it is not urgent.

Physical examination of the pediatric patient undergoing airway surgery should start with the examination of the airway. A large tongue or limited mouth opening may make tracheal intubation difficult. The presence of stridor suggests a stenotic lesion that may make induction of anesthesia hazardous. The patients may also have a tracheostomy tube or airway stent in place from previous surgery that will affect the anesthetic management. The lungs should be examined for the presence of wheezing that may indicate the need for bronchodilators, and the heart should be listened to for murmurs suggesting an undiagnosed congenital cardiac defect.

Finally it is important to discuss the plan for the operation with the surgeon prior to entering the operating room. The type of tracheal tube necessary, whether spontaneous ventilation is required, and if nerve monitoring forbidding the use of muscle relaxants is planned are all common questions that should be discussed with the surgeon.

Intraoperative management

Prior to induction of general anesthesia it is often helpful to administer oral midazolam 0.5 mg/kg to infants and children greater than 1 year of age who are not stridorous to calm the child during the induction process. If the patient is stridorous or in respiratory distress, the premedicant should be withheld. Standard monitors, in particular the pulse oximeter, should be placed prior to induction of general anesthesia. In most infants and children requiring airway reconstructive surgery who are not already tracheally intubated, anesthesia is induced with sevoflurane and 100% oxygen and spontaneous ventilation. Often, it is necessary to administer 5–8 cmH$_2$O of positive end expiratory pressure to overcome upper airway obstruction if there is a stenotic lesion as the child becomes anesthetized. In all cases of airway stenosis the surgeon should be standing by to provide a surgical airway or perform rigid bronchoscopy to establish ventilation should complete airway obstruction occur. An intravenous catheter is then established and the patient is administered glycopyrrolate (10 µg/kg) as a drying agent prior to beginning the surgical procedures

Often before starting the actual reconstruction the surgeon performs flexible and rigid bronchoscopy to examine the airway and determine the location of any obstructing lesion. Usually spontaneous ventilation is required so that the proper movement of the vocal chords can be visualized. There are numerous

techniques that can provide these conditions. One technique utilized at the authors' institution is to begin an infusion of intravenous propofol at a relatively high dose (200–250 µg/kg/min) as well as small, intermittent bolus doses of fentanyl (0.5–1 µg/kg) during periods of intense stimulation. Oxygen is applied through a nasal cannula at 4–6 l/min. The end-tidal CO$_2$ concentration is measured using the built-in side port of the nasal cannula or with a separate catheter placed in one of the nares if the side port is not available. The surgeon also applies topical lidocaine to the airway prior to inserting the rigid bronchoscope. Using this technique the airway can be examined while maintaining spontaneous ventilation in most patients. Occasionally succinylcholine (0.5 mg/kg) may need to be administered if laryngospasm occurs with insertion of the bronchoscope.

Following examination of the airway the trachea is intubated with the appropriately sized tracheal tube by either the surgeon or the anesthesiologist. The size of tube is guided by the airway exam. Often cuffed tracheal tubes are utilized for airway surgery in larger infants or children. Cuffed tracheal tubes are more stable during surgery, require fewer intubations and prevent operating room contamination from anesthetic gases. However, in neonates and small infants undergoing airway surgery the external diameter of the cuffed tubes may be too large for their small airways. Also the long-term effects of even the modern, low-pressure cuffs in neonates have not yet been determined.

In most cases skeletal muscle relaxants can be utilized following completion of the bronchoscopy, both to facilitate tracheal intubation and provide muscle relaxation for the case. At this point a balanced technique using an inhaled agent such as sevoflurane, a non-depolarizing skeletal muscle relaxant (rocuronium or cis-atracurium), and fentanyl (1–2 µg/kg/h) is utilized. Controlled ventilation using an air–oxygen mixture of less than 50% is usually utilized and adjusted appropriately based on the oxygen saturation. Nitrous oxide is currently rarely if ever used because it can support combustion and increase the risk of airway fires from electrocautery. For the same reason the FiO$_2$ is kept as low as possible. Both pressure mode and volume modes of ventilation may be utilized with the rate, tidal volumes and inspiratory airway pressures adjusted based on the oxygen saturation and end-tidal CO$_2$.

During reconstructive airway surgery it is common that the patient may need to be reintubated at some time, either by the anesthesiologist or under direct vision by the surgeon, or that a tracheotomy may need to be performed. If a tracheotomy is performed an armored sterile cuffed tube is placed through the tracheostomy site and either taped or sutured into place then reconnected with a sterile breathing circuit to the anesthesia machine. Both flexible and rigid bronchoscopy may also be performed at any time during the operation. Anesthesiologists should discuss the types of tracheal tubes that may be necessary with the surgeon so such tubes can be readily available.

The slide tracheoplasty has some unique considerations for the anesthesiologist. Typically an inhalation induction is performed with the endotracheal tube placed just cephalad to the complete rings. Arterial and central venous catheters are placed prior to start of surgery. Full heparinization is required if, as is usually the case, cardiopulmonary bypass is utilized for the repair. The endotracheal tube must be free of blood and mucous and ventilation must be adequate prior to discontinuing cardiopulmonary bypass and reversal of heparinization. The surgeon also checks the anastomosis bronchoscopically prior to the completion of surgery.

Infants and small children usually need some period of tracheal intubation or airway stenting for 1 week or more postoperatively; it is rare in our institution that children undergoing reconstructive airway surgery are extubated at the end of surgery. Instead the patients are transported to the pediatric intensive care unit and initially placed on mechanical ventilation. The postoperative management is then turned over to the pediatric intensivist.

Postoperative care/recovery

Pediatric patients undergoing reconstructive airway surgery often require 1–2 weeks of tracheal intubation to provide a stent and an airway while healing occurs. Providing adequate but not excessive sedation to allow these children to tolerate tracheal intubation for this period is often difficult. Success has been reported using minimal sedation in patients greater than 2 years of age if they were nasotracheally intubated. Minimizing sedation can prevent symptoms of withdrawal when the sedative agents are discontinued, and avoiding muscle relaxants may help prevent the muscle weakness and atrophy often seen with long-term skeletal muscle relaxant use [8].

A variety of sedative agents can be used to allow adequate immobility following tracheal reconstruction in children. Commonly, narcotics such as fentanyl or morphine are utilized as well as benzodiazepines such as midazolam. Propofol by infusion is also commonly used. However, propofol may not be the first choice as an agent to provide sedation following tracheal reconstruction because of the possible development of propofol infusion syndrome. This is typically seen with infusions lasting greater than 48 hours with propofol infusion rates in excess of 67 µg/kg/min [9]. The symptoms include metabolic acidosis, bradycardia, arrhythmias, rhabdomyolysis, and cardiac failure. Recently dexmedetomidine has been used as a sedative agent following tracheal reconstruction because it can provide effective sedation without clinically significant respiratory depression, although it can result in hypotension and bradycardia. Dexmedetomidine has proved particularly valuable at our institution as an aid to the weaning process as narcotic sedatives are withdrawn. Intermediate-acting non-depolarizing skeletal muscle relaxants such as vecuronium or cis-atracurium are also often required. If skeletal muscle relaxants are utilized, the train-of-four should be monitored and the least amount of drug necessary utilized to reduce the incidence of muscle weakness following prolonged administration of neuromuscular blocking agents that has been reported [9].

Extubation following tracheal reconstruction is often performed in the operating room so that reintubation can be easily performed if failure occurs, either from airway edema or problems with the mechanical repair. A course of steroids (dexamethasone) is often administered for several days prior to extubation to minimize airway edema. Bronchoscopy is also often performed at that time to evaluate the repair. Following many reconstructive operations, bronchoscopies are often performed at weekly intervals initially to evaluate the repair, and periodically as the child grows to determine whether further procedures are necessary.

Complications

Complications can occur at numerous points during pediatric airway surgery and the often long recovery process. Infants and children requiring airway reconstructive procedures often present with the symptoms of airway obstruction. In some cases induction of general anesthesia may result in complete airway obstruction requiring emergency tracheal intubation

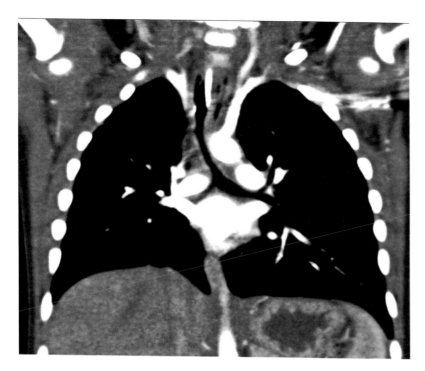

Figure 33.4. Case study. CT angiogram of patient with congenital tracheobronchial anomalies including tracheal stenosis with two complete tracheal rings as well as an aberrant takeoff of the right mainstem bronchus and a hypoplastic right lung. This patient underwent a slide tracheoplasty.

or tracheostomy. Accidental extubation may occur during the surgery, and obstruction of the tracheal tube with blood and/or secretions is common. Right mainstem intubation or tube kinking can occur secondary to changes in the patient's position or repositioning of the tracheal tube by the surgeon. With positive-pressure ventilation, extravasation of air can occur into the mediastinum or pleura, causing a pneumothorax or pneumomediastinum. Hemorrhage from thymic, innominate or thyroid vessels can occur. During the recovery period accidental extubation may occur prior to the planned extubation. This may result in the need for emergency reintubation and possible disruption of the repair. Following planned extubation airway obstruction may also occur from airway edema, vocal chord dysfunction or problems with the surgical repair. Even if the surgery and recovery are uneventful children undergoing these operations may suffer from the adverse effects of narcotic and sedative agents and their withdrawal or muscular atrophy from the use of skeletal muscle relaxants [9].

Surgical complications include scar tissue formation from granulation tissue, recurrent laryngeal nerve injury and airway obstruction from disruption of graft material. Abnormal healing may occur at the resection or anastomotic sites and result in stenosis or areas of deformity in the airway. Finally the airway reconstructive surgery may affect the function and position of the arytenoids. This may require further surgery and impact voice development [2–7].

Summary

Surgical procedures have been developed that now allow most infants and children suffering from acquired or congenital defects in the airway to be corrected and no longer need to be managed with tracheostomy for their entire life. Some defects that were uniformly fatal can now be successfully managed surgically. Although the surgical and perioperative care can be very demanding, with proper management most pediatric patients can undergo airway reconstructive surgery with a good outcome.

Case study

A 22-month-old 13.3 kg male was admitted for slide tracheoplasty to repair congenital tracheobronchial anomalies including two complete tracheal rings and aberrant takeoff of the right mainstem bronchus. (Figure 33.4) He had a history of being a "noisy breather" and ultimately was diagnosed with complete tracheal rings at the age of 14 months by bronchoscopy. He was also noted to have a hypoplastic right lung and aberrant takeoff of the right mainstem bronchus. He had a normal upper airway and normal heart sounds, but had stridor on examination.

Anesthesia was induced via inhalation induction with sevoflurane in 100% oxygen. A 20-gauge peripheral IV was then inserted and 0.1 mg glycopyrrolate, 1 mg of vecuronium, and 25 μg of fentanyl were administered. The patient was then intubated easily with a Miller number 2 blade. A Cormack–Lehan (CL) grade I view was seen and a 4.5 Microcuff® endotracheal tube (Kimberly Clark, Roswell GA, USA) was placed and taped at 13 cm at the teeth. Anesthesia was maintained with isoflurane 0.5–1.0%, vecuronium and fentanyl. An arterial line and central venous catheter were inserted. The patient was then cannulated for cardiac bypass, 5200 units of heparin were administered, and vecuronium and fentanyl infusions were started. The total bypass time was 4 hours and 25 minutes. After surgical correction, fiberoptic visualization of the anastomosis was performed. When the anastomosis was deemed stable, the oral endotracheal tube was removed and a 4.0 cuffed endotracheal tube was placed nasally with fiberoptic confirmation of placement. After confirmation of the nasotracheal tube proper position, discontinuation of cardiopulmonary bypass was attempted. Ventilation was difficult because of the presence of a tissue ball valve obstruction at the right mainstem bronchus. Following discontinuation of bypass rigid bronchoscopy was performed to further clear the obstruction. The patient was reintubated with a 4.0 nasotracheal tube. This was very difficult due to airway edema. The patient was then transferred to the pediatric intensive care unit.

Throughout the first night the patient had marked respiratory acidosis in spite of excellent oxygenation, due to obstruction from airway edema. The patient was then placed on an oscillating ventilator. Bronchoscopy was performed several times and the tracheal tube was increased to a size 4.5 Microcuff® nasotracheal tube. Heliox was also utilized.

The patient gradually improved and extubation was attempted 3 weeks following surgery. The attempt at extubation failed 2 days later. The patient required reintubation and eventually a tracheostomy. Subsequently the patient developed tracheal stenosis at the distal one-third of the trachea that required repeated trips to the operating room for rigid bronchoscopies and dilatations. He eventually recovered respiratory function well enough to be weaned from mechanical ventilation. He did, however, suffer from narcotic withdrawal during this process. He was discharged to home approximately 3 months later although still with a tracheostomy in place and requiring intermittent oxygen administration at night. He is expected to require further endoscopic examinations and possible dilatations in the future.

Clinical pearls

- Pediatric patients requiring airway reconstruction often have other congenital anomalies such as heart defects, particularly if the airway lesion is congenital in origin. These conditions should be evaluated thoroughly prior to surgery.
- Subglottic stenosis is the primary indication for reconstructive airway surgery in infants and small children.
- Severe congenital tracheal stenosis typically presents in infancy with "washing machine breathing", a characteristic bi-phasic noise made from secretions being repeatedly moved through an area of distal tracheal stenosis via respiration. Anesthesiologists may discover these children when they come to the operating room for an unrelated procedure and find a narrow airway that is "unintubatable".
- During reconstructive airway surgery it is common that the patient may need to be reintubated at some time, either by the anesthesiologist or under direct vision by the surgeon, or that a tracheotomy may need to be performed. If a tracheotomy is performed an armored sterile cuffed tube is placed through the tracheostomy site and either taped or sutured into place.
- Extubation following tracheal reconstruction is often performed in the operating room, sometimes using a tube exchanger, so that reintubation can be easily performed if failure occurs.

References

1. Santos D, Mitchell R. The history of pediatric airway reconstruction. *Laryngoscope* 2010;**120**: 815–20.

2. Hein EA, Rutter MJ. New perspectives in pediatric airway reconstruction. *Int Anesthesiol Clin* 2006;**44**: 51–56.

3. Cotton RT. Management of subglottic stenosis. *Otolaryngol Clin North Am* 2000;**33**:111–30.

4. O'Connor TE, Bilish DD, Choy D, *et al.* Laryngotracheoplasty to

avoid tracheostomy in neonatal and infant subglottic stenosis. *Otolaryngol Head Neck Surg* 2011;**144**:435–9.

5. Rutter MJ, Hartley BEJ, Cotton RT. Cricotracheal resection in children. *Arch Otolaryngol Head Neck Surg* 2001;**127**:289–92.

6. Rutter MJ, Cotton RT, Azizkhan RG, *et al.* Slide tracheoplasty for the management of complete tracheal rings. *J Pediatr Surg* 2003;**38**:928–34.

7. Tsang V, Murday A, Gilbe C, Goldstraw P. Slide tracheoplasty for congenital funnel shaped tracheal stenosis. *Ann Thorac Surg* 1989;**48**:632–5.

8. Jacobs BR, Salman BA, Cotton RT, *et al.*

    Postoperative management of children after single-stage laryngotracheal reconstruction. *Crit Care Med* 2001;**29**:164–8.

9. Hammer GB. Sedation and analgesia in the pediatric intensive care unit following laryngotracheal reconstruction. *Pediatr Anesth* 2009;**19**(Suppl S1):166–79.

Index

acetaminophen 321, 326
acoustic neuromas *see* vestibular schwannomas
acromegaly 134, 136
adenotonsillectomy (T&A) 323–7
  anesthetic management 325–6
  case study 334–5
  postoperative management 327
  surgical techniques 323
advance directives 32
airway
  bleeding 91
  difficult *see* difficult airway
  edema 46, 181, 250–1, 268
  fires 105–11
  foreign bodies 332–3
  infections 91, 94–5
  pathologic conditions 94–8
  pediatric anatomy 30–1, 263
  preoperative evaluation 27–8, 41, 50–6
  sensory innervation 67–8
  tumors 94, 95, 96
airway obstruction 36, 90, 91
  awake intubation 58, 61
  bronchoscopic surgery 312
  instrumentation 18, 20
  pediatric airway reconstruction 342–3
alfentanil 62, 280
American College of Cardiology Foundation/American Heart Association (ACCF/AHA)
  perioperative guidelines 31, 144
American Society of Anesthesiologists (ASA)
  difficult airway algorithm 36, 37, 39–40, 50, 51, 58
  operating room fire algorithm 105, 106
  physical status classification 28–9
  preanesthesia evaluation advisory 28
  preoperative fasting guidelines 29
anatomy, clinical 1–7
angioedema 91
ankyloglossus 6
anterior cricoid split 337, 338
anterior ethmoidal nerve 67

block 68–9
anterior mediastinal mass 96–7, 311, 313
anticholinergic agents 60
anticoagulation, after free flap surgery 160
antiemetic prophylaxis 129, 233, 282, 327
antisialagogues 60, 301
apneic ventilation 230, 232
arytenoid adduction 247, 248–9
arytenoid cartilage 10
arytenopexy 246–7
ASA *see* American Society of Anesthesiologists
aspiration prophylaxis 29, 61, 180
atomizers, disposable plastic 66
atropine 60
awake intubation 40, 41–6, 58–78
  case study 77
  nerve blocks 66–74
  orotracheal vs. nasotracheal route 75
  panendoscopy 229
  post-tonsillectomy hemorrhage 327
  premedication 60–1
  preoperative endoscopic airway examination 52, 54
  preoperative preparation 58–60
  sedation 42–3, 61–4
  staff, monitors and equipment 59–60
  techniques 75–7
  topicalization of airway 64–6
  trauma 84
  Zenker's diverticulectomy 197–8, 200–1
awake tracheotomy 144, 230, 258

Bailey maneuver 165, 171, 282
Ben-jet tube 232
Bennett connectors 123, 304, 305, 307
benzocaine, airway topicalization 65
Berman airway 75
Bispectral Index (BIS) monitoring 22–3, 124–5, 233
bleeding
  airway-related 91
  bronchoscopic procedures 304

ear surgery 273
endoscopic sinus surgery 122–3
mandibular surgery 214, 218
maxillary surgery 211
nasal surgery 115, 119–20
obstructive sleep apnea surgery 182
post-tonsillectomy 327
tracheotomy surgery 259, 260
transsphenoidal pituitary surgery 137
β-blockers 117, 233, 281
blood transfusions 158, 189, 224
bone flaps, vascularized 152
Bonfils Retromolar Intubating Fiberscope™ 76–7
bronchial obstruction, intraluminal 312
bronchoscope
  fiberoptic (FOB) 66, 90, 309
  rigid 18, 20, 309
    examination under anesthesia 228, 229
    jet ventilation via 317
    pediatric 329, 330
    therapeutic bronchoscopy 310, 315
bronchoscopy
  awake intubation 75–6
  diagnostic 228, 229, 297–308
    advanced procedures 298–9, 300
    anesthetic care 301–3, 304, 305
    case study 307
    complications 304–6
    postoperative care 303–4
  pediatric 329–33
  suite 297, 298, 312, 313
  therapeutic 309–18
    anesthetic management 311–17
    case study 318
    postoperative care 317
    types of procedures 310–11
bronchospasm 304–6

calcium channel blockers 117
cancellation of surgery, indications for 29

capacity, decision-making 31–2
carbon dioxide (CO$_2$), airway fire
    prevention 107
carbon dioxide (CO$_2$) laser 237, 238,
    327–8
cardiac risk, major head and neck
    surgery 31, 144
cardiopulmonary bypass (CPB) 96,
    268, 342, 344
cardiovascular assessment,
    preoperative 31, 144
carotid artery occlusion, intraoperative
    188, 189, 190–1
carotid body 186
carotid body tumors (CBTs) 186–7
    functioning 186, 188, 189
    resection 187–93
        case study 192
        complications 191
        intraoperative management
            188–91
        preoperative management 187–8
cerebellar hemorrhage, remote (RCH)
    126–7, 128
cerebellopontine angle (CPA) 273,
    274, 283
cerebral protection, carotid body
    tumor surgery 190–1
cerebrospinal fluid (CSF)
    drains 133
    leaks 125–6, 137, 273–4
cervical fascia 8
cervical spine
    "clearance" methods 86
    injuries 83, 86
    protection, trauma 83–4, 86
cetacaine, airway topicalization 65
CHARGE association 323
choanal atresia 322–3
cholesteatoma 272
chronic facial pain, after maxillary
    surgery 211
chronic obstructive pulmonary disease
    145
chronic otitis media with effusion
    (COME) 321
cocaine 61, 65, 116–17
cochlear implants 272–3, 322
congenital cardiac anomalies 27
congenital tracheal stenosis 263, 338,
    339–40
    associated defects 339, 340
    case study 343–4
consent, informed 30
continuous positive airways pressure
    (CPAP) 175, 176, 183, 325
Cotton grading, pediatric subglottic
    stenosis 265, 337–8
cricoarytenoid joint 10

cricoid cartilage 10
cricoid resection 337
cricopharyngeal myotomy, endoscopic
    199
cricopharyngeus muscle 13
cricothyroid joint 10
cricothyroid membrane 10
cricothyroidotomy (cricothyrotomy)
    85, 255
cricotracheal resection 265
    pediatric patients 337, 339
    see also tracheal resection
croup 332
cuff test 129
Cushing's disease 134, 136

deep cervical plexus block 190, 199
delirium, emergence 321
dexamethasone
    panendoscopy 233
    postoperative antiemesis 129, 326
    stridor 102, 104
dexmedetomidine
    awake intubation 42–3, 63
    bronchoscopic surgery 313
    laryngoplasty 248
    pediatric patients 321, 326, 342
diabetes insipidus 137
difficult airway 36–47
    ASA algorithm 36, 37, 39–40, 50, 51,
        58
    awake intubation see awake
        intubation
    case report 47
    causes 38
    failed intubation 46
    form 41, 44
    laryngoscopes 40–1
    management techniques 41
    mask ventilation 36–9
    panendoscopy 229–30
    predicting difficult intubation 40, 41
difficult extubation 46
difficult mask ventilation (DMV) 38–9
diphtheria 337
do-not-resuscitate (DNR) orders 32
Dohlman procedure 196
Down syndrome (trisomy 21) 28, 321,
    325
droperidol, awake intubation 64

ear, anatomy 3
EEG monitoring, intraoperative 190
electrocautery, fire risk 105, 107, 110
electromagnetic navigational
    bronchoscopy (ENB) 297, 299,
    300, 304–6, 307
electromyography (EMG)
    facial nerve 204, 206, 281

laryngeal 246, 284
embolization, preoperative tumor 283,
    284
emergencies, ENT 90–2
    case study 92
    equipment 90
emphysema, subcutaneous 97, 259
endobronchial ultrasound with fine
    needle aspiration (EBUS-FNA)
    297, 298, 299
    anesthetic care 302–3, 305, 306
    case study 307
    complications 304–6
endoscopes 18–20, 22, 55
endoscopic cricopharyngeal myotomy
    199
endoscopic sinus surgery (ESS)
    121–31
    anesthetic emergence 123, 127–9
    clinical goals 121–2
    complex procedures 124–5
    complications 129
    equipment set-up 20–3
    functional see functional endoscopic
        sinus surgery
    pediatric patients 323
    repeat, and emergencies 125–7
endoscopic staple diverticulectomy 196
endoscopy
    esophageal foreign bodies 333
    pediatric 329–33
    preoperative see preoperative
        endoscopic airway
        examination
    see also bronchoscopy;
        esophagoscopy; laryngoscopy;
        panendoscopy
endotracheal tubes (ETT) 39
    diagnostic bronchoscopy 302–3,
        305, 307
    difficult extubation 46
    exchange catheters 46
    intralaryngeal EMG recording 168,
        169
    laryngotracheal surgery 18, 19
    laser-safe 240, 328
    management during fires 105
    nasal intubation 215
    nasal surgery 114, 115, 116
    pediatric surgery 341
    pharyngeal and esophageal surgery
        18, 22
    therapeutic bronchoscopy 314–15
    topical anesthesia application via
        128–9
    tracheal resection 267, 269
    tracheotomy procedure 258
    vs. laryngeal mask airway
        278

epidural anesthesia, cervical 190, 268
epiglottis 10
epiglottitis, acute 94–5, 331–2
epiglottoplasty 178
epinephrine 91, 102, 104, 114
epistaxis 91, 115, 119–20
Eschman stylet 40
esmolol, otologic surgery 281
esophageal obturator airways, trauma 85
esophagoscope, rigid 18–20, 22
esophagoscopy 228, 303, 306
esophagus 13
    dilatation systems 20, 23
    foreign bodies 333
    surgical instruments 18–20, 22
examination under anesthesia (EAU) 228–35
    see also panendoscopy
external auditory canal surgery 271
external ear 3, 5
extubation, difficult 46
eye protection, laser surgery 239, 328

face
    anatomy 1–2
    fractures 1–2, 85–6
face transplantation 220–6
    anesthetic team 225
    donor management 220
    intraoperative management 222–5
    preoperative assessment 220–2
    subsequent surgery 225
facial expression, muscles of 2, 4
facial nerve 2
    ear surgery 3, 277
    monitoring, intraoperative 204, 206, 281
    salivary gland surgery 203, 204, 206, 213
fasciocutaneous flaps 152
fasting, preoperative 29, 197
fentanyl 62, 158, 321
Feyh–Kastenbauer (FK) laryngo-pharyngoscope 18–20, 22
fires
    airway 105–11
        case studies 110
        chicken model 107
        flooding surgical site with CO_2 107
        management 105, 107, 110
        safety precautions 105, 107, 114, 241
        tracheotomy surgery 105–7, 108, 109, 259
    ASA algorithm for operating room 105, 106

laser-related risks 110, 238, 328
flap reconstructive surgery 151–62
    anesthetic management 157–9
    case study 161–2
    complications 160–1
    operating room setup 154–5, 156, 157
    postoperative care 159–60
    preoperative preparation 153
    surgical aspects 151–3
flumazenil 62
Fontaine's sign 186
foreign bodies 332–3
free flaps 151, 152, 223–4
    see also flap reconstructive surgery
Frey's syndrome 206
functional endoscopic sinus surgery (FESS) 121–2, 130
    case study 130, 131
    intraoperative management 122–4
    preoperative aspects 122
    see also endoscopic sinus surgery

gastroesophageal reflux disease 264, 265
genioglossus advancement (GA) 177–8
geriatric patients, preoperative evaluation 31–2
GlideScope® videolaryngoscope 40–1, 42, 43–6, 76
glomus jugulare tumors (GT) 272, 283–4
glossopharyngeal nerve 67
    blocks 69–70, 71
glottic tumors 11, 12, 14
glottis 10–11
glycopyrrolate 60, 301
great auricular nerve (GAN) 203
gum elastic bougie 40

hearing aids 278
hearing loss 272–3
Heliox, 101–2, 103
hematoma, postoperative 166, 192, 206, 249–50
hemoptysis 311
hemorrhage see bleeding
high-frequency jet ventilation (HFJV) 232, 267
history, patient 26
Hunsaker monjet tube 232
hyoid suspension 178
hypercalcemia 169
hypercarbia 304
hyperparathyroidism 169–70
hyperthyroidism 163–4
hypocalcemia, postoperative 168–9
hypopharyngeal tumor 13, 14

hypopharynx 11–13
hypotension
    complicating free flap surgery 160
    controlled
        carotid body tumor resection 188–9
        ear surgery 274, 280–1, 285
        mandibular surgery 214
        nasal surgery 117
hypothermia, free flap surgery 156, 160–1
hypothyroidism 164
hypoxemia, transient 304

i-gel supraglottic airway 278–9, 302, 304, 316
implants see prostheses
infections
    airway 91, 94–5
    postoperative 260, 306
    upper respiratory (URI) 29, 122, 321–2
inhalational anesthesia
    face transplantation 223–4
    nasal surgery 117
    otologic/neurotologic surgery 280, 285
    panendoscopy 232–3
    tracheal resection 267
inhalational injuries 86–7
inner ear 3
instruments, otolaryngology 18–24
intracranial pressure (ICP), raised 188, 283, 284, 285
intraoperative neurophysiological monitoring (INM) 285
introducers, tracheal tube 40, 42
intubating oral airways 75
Intubation Difficulty Scale (IDS) 40

Jehovah's Witnesses 210
jet ventilation
    bronchoscopic surgery 317
    laryngeal surgery 18, 19
    panendoscopy 229–30, 231–2, 235
    pediatric patients 328, 329–30
    tracheal resection surgery 267
jugular foramen surgery 272, 275, 283

ketamine 63–4, 326
Kiesselbach's plexus 4

laboratory tests, preoperative 28
laryngeal cancer 143–4
laryngeal framework surgery (LFS) 245
laryngeal mask airway (LMA)
    adenotonsillectomy 326
    endoscopic sinus surgery 123, 124

laryngoplasty 249
otologic surgery 278–9, 281–2,
    287–90
trauma 85
vs. endotracheal tube 278
see also supraglottic airways
laryngeal papillomatosis 96, 97
laryngeal surgery
    instruments 18
    pediatric 327–8
laryngectomy 143–9
    case study 147–9
    complications 146
    intraoperative management 145–6
    neck anatomy after 16
    partial 143
    preoperative evaluation 144–5
    total 143, 144
laryngoplasty (LPL) 245–52
    case study 251–2
    complications 249–51
    general anesthesia 248–9
    monitored anesthesia care 247–8
    preoperative evaluation 246
    surgical procedure 246–7, 248
laryngoscopes 18
    panendoscopy 228, 229
    suspension devices/systems 18, 21
    tracheal intubation 38, 40–1
laryngoscopy
    awake look technique 56
    examination under anesthesia 228
    pediatric 329–33
    video 43–6, 76, 246, 247
    virtual 56
laryngospasm 304
laryngotracheal reconstruction (LTR)
    265
laryngotracheal stenosis 11, 263–70
    classification 265
    pediatric 337
    see also subglottic stenosis
laryngotracheoplasty 338
larynx
    anatomy 9–11
    intubation-mediated damage 287,
        289
    pediatric 30–1, 263
    preoperative endoscopic
        examination 55, 56
    sensory innervation 67–8
    topical anesthesia 65–6
    trauma 85
laser surgery 237–43
    anesthetic technique 240–1
    atmospheric contamination 241,
        242
    case study 242–3
    clinical applications 237

endotracheal tubes 240, 328
fire risks 110, 238, 328
pediatric patients 327–8
postoperative concerns 241
safety issues 238–40
subglottic stenosis 265
tumor debulking 310
lasers 237, 238
Le Fort classification, maxillary
    fractures 2, 85–6
lidocaine 61, 64, 65–6, 128–9, 314
LMA *see* laryngeal mask airway
local anesthesia 113–14, 246, 258
local anesthetics 55, 64–5
Ludwig's angina 6, 92, 95

MADgic® Mucosal Atomization
    Device 66
Mallampati scale 27
mandible 213
mandibular fractures 1–2, 85
mandibular surgery 213–15
    case study 216–18
    complications 214, 217–18
mask ventilation 36–9
    after rhinoplasty 118
    difficult (DMV) 38–9
mastoidectomy 272, 322
maxillary fractures 2, 85–6
maxillary surgery 210–12
maxillectomy 210–12
maxillomandibular advancement
    (MMA) 178
maxillomandibular expansion 178
McCaffrey grading, subglottic stenosis
    265
McGrath® videolaryngoscope 76
methylprednisolone (Solumedrol) 102,
    104
microlaryngeal instruments 18, 21
microlaryngeal tube (MLT) 229, 230,
    231
midazolam, awake intubation 62
middle ear
    anatomy 3, 276
    surgery 271–2, 287–90
middle fossa approach, acoustic
    neuroma 272, 275
mivacurium, parotid surgery 205
morphine, pediatric patients 325
mouth, anatomy 5–14
mucopolysaccharidoses 325
Muller maneuver 180
multiple endocrine neoplasia (MEN)
    syndromes 165
muscle flaps 152
muscle relaxants *see* neuromuscular
    blockade
myocutaneous flaps 152

myringoplasty 271–2
myringotomy 271, 321–2

naloxone 63
nasal septum 3–4
nasal surgery
    instruments 20–4
    obstructive sleep apnea 113, 176–7
    pediatric patients 322–3
    see also septoplasty/rhinoplasty
nasopharyngeal airways, trauma 84
nasopharynx, sensory innervation 67
nasotracheal intubation 4–5
    awake 75, 76
    mandibular surgery 214, 216, 217
    temporomandibular joint surgery 215
    trauma 84
nebulizers 66, 67
neck
    anatomical levels 14–16, 145
    anatomy 14–16
    hematoma, postoperative 166, 192,
        206
    radiation changes 144
neck dissection 16, 143–9
    case study 147–9
    complications 146
    intraoperative management 145–6
    preoperative evaluation 144–5
    procedures 143–4, 145
neodymium:
    yttrium–aluminum–garnet
    (Nd:YAG) laser 237, 238, 328
nerve blocks, awake intubation 66–74
neuroleptanalgesia, awake
    intubation 64
neurological assessment,
    preoperative 27
neuromuscular blockade (NMB)
    bronchoscopic procedures 302,
        313–14
    ear surgery 279, 281, 285
    face transplantation 225
    laser surgery 241
    panendoscopy 233
    parotid surgery 205, 206
    pediatric surgery 341
neuronavigation 135
neurotologic surgery 271–90
    anesthesia objectives 274–7
    anesthetic management 282–6
    intraoperative complications 273–4
    surgical procedures 271, 272–3, 274,
        275
nitroglycerin 117
nitroprusside, sodium 117
nitrous oxide (N_2O)
    fire risk 105, 110
    otologic surgery 280, 322

nose 3–5
  fractures 322
  patency assessment 215
  sensory innervation 67
  topical anesthesia 65

obstructive sleep apnea (OSA) 175–84
  comorbidities 175, 178–9
  diagnosis 175–6, 324–5
  medical treatment 176
  pediatric patients 323–7
  preoperative airway evaluation
      27–8, 179, 180
  surgery 176–84
    case study 182–3
    complications 181, 183
    intraoperative management
        180–1
    postoperative management 181–2
    preoperative management
        178–80
    procedures 113, 176–8
occlusion 1
opioids
  adverse effects 62–3, 282
  awake intubation 62–3
  bronchoscopic procedures 302,
      312–13
  carotid body tumor resection 189
  face transplantation 224
  obstructive sleep apnea surgery 180,
      181
  otologic/neurotologic surgery 280,
      281–2, 285
  pediatric patients 321, 325
optical stylets, awake intubation 76–7
oral airways, intubating 75
oral appliances (OA), obstructive sleep
      apnea 176
oral cavity
  anatomy 5–6
  large tumors 14
orbital fractures 2
oropharyngeal airways, trauma 84
oropharynx
  anatomy 6–9
  topical anesthesia 65
orotracheal intubation
  awake 75–6
  trauma 84
ossicular chain reconstruction 272
osteocutaneous flaps 152
otalgia, referred 5, 6
otologic surgery 271–90
  anesthesia objectives 274–7
  anesthetic management 277–82
  case study 287–90
  complications 273–4, 282
  pediatric 321–2

procedures 271–2
outpatient procedures, patient
      selection 29
Ovassapian airway 75
oxygen administration
  awake intubation 60
  bronchoscopic procedures 302, 314
  fire risks 105, 107, 110, 114
  nasal surgery 20, 114
oxymetazoline 115–16

palate
  hard 5
  primary tumor 5, 6
  soft 7, 8, 9
palatine nerves 67
panendoscopy 228–35
  case study 234–5
  complications 234
  emergence phase 234
  equipment 228
  intraoperative management 229–33,
      234
  preoperative assessment 228–9
paragangliomas 283–4
  see also carotid body tumors;
      glomus jugulare tumors
paranasal sinuses 5
  surgical instruments 20–4
  tumors 283
parathyroid glands 16
parathyroid surgery 169–70
parotid gland 203–4
  pathology 203–4, 206–7
parotid gland tumors 203–4, 212
  case study 207–8
  difficult airway 40
parotid surgery 203–8
parotidectomy 204–6
  anesthesia management 204–6
  case study 207–8
  complications 206
  facial nerve monitoring 204,
      206
  superficial, procedure 204
peanuts, aspirated 332–3
pediatric patients
  acute epiglottitis 94–5, 331–2
  adenotonsillectomy 323–7
  airway anatomy 30–1, 263
  anesthetic complications 333–4
  case study 334–5
  endoscopic sinus surgery 323
  informed consent 30
  laryngoscopy, bronchoscopy and
      endoscopy 329–33
  otolaryngologic surgery
      321–35
  otologic surgery 321–2

pharyngeal and laryngeal surgery
      327–8
  preoperative evaluation 26–8, 29,
      30–1
  reconstructive airway surgery
      337–44
  rhinologic procedures 322–3
  stridor 102, 103, 331
  subglottic stenosis 263, 265, 337–40
  tracheotomy 328–9, 342
pedicled flaps 151, 152
Pentax-AWS® videolaryngoscope 76
pericardial effusion/tamponade
      311–12
peritonsillar abscess 332
pharyngeal surgery
  instruments 18–20, 22
  pediatric 327–8
pharyngeal web 51
pharynx 9–13
  muscles 7, 9
  sensory innervation 67
phenylephrine 61, 115
phonosurgery (PS) 245
photodynamic therapy 310
physical examination, preoperative
      26–8
piriform sinus tumor 14
pituitary tumors 133, 134–5
platysma muscle 14
pleomorphic adenoma 203–4
pneumocephalus, tension (TP) 286
pneumomediastinum 259, 314
pneumothorax 259, 304, 314
polyps, airway 95
polysomnography (PSG) 175–6, 324–5
positioning, patient
  after obstructive sleep apnea surgery
      182
  flap reconstructive surgery 154–5
  nasal surgery 117–18
  otologic/neurotologic surgery
      274–7, 284–5
  panendoscopy 228
  transsphenoidal pituitary surgery
      136, 138, 139
positive airways pressure (PAP) 176
post-thyroidectomy tracheomalacia
      (PTTM) 167
post-tonsillectomy hemorrhage 327
posterior fossa 272, 273
postponement of surgery, indications
      for 29
premature infants 29
preoperative endoscopic airway
      examination (PEAE) 50–6
  information sought 52, 53–4
  procedure 54–6
preoperative evaluation 26–34

airway 27–8, 41
  case study 32–4
prolactinomas 135
propofol
  after pediatric airway reconstruction 342
  awake intubation 63
  diagnostic bronchoscopy 301
  face transplantation 223–4
  panendoscopy 233
prostheses
  laryngoplasty 245, 246–7, 252
    complications 250, 251
  voice 16, 143, 144
  see also cochlear implants
psychological evaluation and preparation, preoperative 27
pulmonary assessment, preoperative 27

radiation therapy 144, 153, 310
reconstructive airway surgery, pediatric 337–44
  case study 343–4
  complications 342–3
  intraoperative management 341–2
  postoperative care 342
  preoperative evaluation 340–1
  surgical procedures 337–40
  see also tracheal resection
recurrent laryngeal nerve (RLN) 11, 68
  intraoperative monitoring 167–8, 169
  palsy 167–8
refusal of care 30
regional anesthesia 189–90, 199
remifentanil
  awake intubation 62
  flap reconstructive surgery 157–8
  nasal surgery 114–15
  otologic surgery 280, 281–2
  panendoscopy 233
respiratory complications, adenotonsillectomy 327
respiratory distress, postoperative 166, 192, 241, 250
respiratory disturbance index (RDI) 175, 176
respiratory failure 306
respiratory papillomatosis 96, 97, 242
retromolar trigone 5
retropharyngeal abscess 95
retropharyngeal space 7–9
retrosigmoid posterior fossa craniotomy 272, 274
retrosternal goiter (RSG) 164–72
rhinoplasty see septoplasty/rhinoplasty
ROTIGS device 75–6

salivary glands 212–13
  surgical resection 212–13
  tumors 212
  see also parotid gland
Sanders jet ventilation technique 329–30
scopolamine 60
sedation
  after face transplantation 225
  after pediatric airway reconstruction 342
  awake intubation 42–3, 61–4
  awake tracheotomy 258
  diagnostic bronchoscopy 297, 301
  laryngoplasty 247–8
  nasal surgery 113–14
Sensascope™ 77
septoplasty/rhinoplasty 113–20
  anesthetic management 113–18
  case report 119–20
  postoperative care 118–19
sevoflurane anesthesia, preschool children 321
sialolithiasis 204, 206–7
skull base surgery 23–4, 273
  anesthesia objectives 274–7
  anesthetic management 282–6
  surgical procedures 271, 272–3, 274, 275
skull base tumors 283–4
sleep apnea
  central 175
  obstructive see obstructive sleep apnea
sleep-disordered breathing, pediatric 323–7, 334–5
slide tracheoplasty 339–40, 342, 343–4
somatosensory evoked potentials (SSEPs) 190–1, 285
sphenopalatine ganglion block 68, 69
stapedectomy (stapedotomy) 272, 282
stents, airway 266, 309, 310, 316
sternocleidomastoid muscle (SCM) 14
stridor 91–2, 101–4
  case presentation 103
  causes 102, 103
  diagnosis 103
  Heliox treatment 101–2, 103
  management options 102
  pediatric patients 102, 103, 331
  thyroid surgery patients 164
subglottic jet ventilation 232
subglottic stenosis 11, 263–70
  anesthetic management 14, 266–8
  case studies 269, 318
  classification 265, 337–8
  congenital see congenital tracheal stenosis

etiology 259, 260, 263, 264, 338
  pathophysiology 263–4
  pediatric 263, 265, 337–40
  postoperative management 268
  stenting 266
  surgical management 265
  tracheal dilatation see tracheal dilatation
subglottic tumor 11, 13
subglottis 11
submandibular gland surgery 212–13
succinylcholine 205, 279
sugammadex 206, 241
superficial cervical plexus block 190, 199
superior laryngeal nerve (SLN) 67–8
  block 70–3
superior vena cava (SVC) syndrome 97, 164–5, 311
supraglottic airways (SGA)
  diagnostic bronchoscopy 302, 303, 304, 307
  difficult airway 38, 46
  endoscopic sinus surgery 123, 124
  nasal surgery 114, 115
  otologic surgery 278–9, 281–2, 287–90
  panendoscopy 229
  preoperative endoscopic airway examination 53
  therapeutic bronchoscopy 315–16
  trauma 85
  see also laryngeal mask airway
supraglottic jet ventilation 231–2
supraglottic tumors 10, 11, 147–9
supraglottis 10
surgical airways, trauma 85
syndrome of inappropriate antidiuretic hormone (SIADH) 137

teamwork 32
teeth 1, 27, 28
temporal bone 273–4, 276
temporomandibular joint (TMJ) 213
  arthroscopy 215, 216
  dysfunction 214, 215
  surgery 215–16
tension pneumocephalus (TP) 286
thermoregulation, flap reconstructive surgery 156
throat see pharynx
thyroid cancer 32–4, 163
thyroid cartilage 9–10
thyroid gland 16
  enlarged 170, 164–71
thyroid storm (thyrotoxic crisis) 163, 166–7
thyroid surgery 163–73

thyroid surgery (cont.)
  anesthesia technique 165–6
  case study 170–1, 172
  complications 166–9
  preoperative assessment 163–5
thyromental distance 179
thyroplasty (TPL) 245, 246–7,
    248–9
  see also laryngoplasty
thyrotoxicosis 163–4
tongue 5–6, 8
  advancement/stabilization surgery
    177–8
  base 9
    tumors 9, 14
  reduction surgeries 177, 178
  sensory innervation 67
tonsillectomy see adenotonsillectomy
tonsils 9
  lingual 9
topical anesthesia, airway
  application techniques 65–6
  awake intubation 64–6, 198
  bronchoscopic surgery 314
  local anesthetics 64–5
  panendoscopy 233
  postoperative extubation 128–9
  preoperative endoscopic airway
    examination 55
total intravenous anesthesia (TIVA)
  bronchoscopic procedures 301–2,
    312–13
  endoscopic sinus surgery 123, 124–5
  face transplantation 223–4
  laser surgery 240–1
  nasal surgery 114–15
  otologic/neurotologic surgery 280,
    285–6, 288
  panendoscopy 232–3
  tracheal resection 267
trachea
  compression 164–72, 312
  iatrogenic perforation 97
  iatrogenic rupture 310–11
  intraluminal obstruction 312
  topical anesthesia at end of surgery
    128–9
  see also transtracheal anesthesia
tracheal dilatation 13, 265, 310–11
  case studies 269, 318
  prior to tracheal resection 267
tracheal intubation 39
  after pediatric airway reconstruction
    337, 342
  awake see awake intubation
  distal technique, tracheal surgery
    267
  endoscopic sinus surgery 124, 125
  failed, management options 46

fiberoptic (FOI) 41–6, 75–6, 84
flap reconstructive surgery 154
laryngectomy and neck dissection
    144
laryngoscopes 38, 40–1
postoperative neck hematoma 166
prediction of difficulty 40, 41
retrograde 84–5
subglottic stenosis complicating
    263–4, 338
subglottic stenosis repair surgery
    267
total laryngectomy patient 16
transsphenoidal pituitary surgery
    135–6
trauma 84–5
vocal cord damage 287, 289
see also difficult airway;
    endotracheal tubes
tracheal resection 263–70
  anesthetic management 266–8
  case study 269
  complications 268
  pediatric patients 337
  postoperative management 268
  see also cricotracheal resection;
    subglottic stenosis
tracheal stenosis see subglottic stenosis
tracheal surgery, instruments 18
tracheoesophageal fistula
  bronchoscopic surgery 312, 313
  complicating tracheotomy 259, 260
tracheoesophageal puncture (TEP) 143
tracheoplasty 337
  slide technique 339–40, 342, 343–4
tracheotomy/tracheostomy 255–62
  airway fires 105–7, 108, 109, 110,
    259
  anesthetic management 256–9
  awake 144, 230, 258
  case study 260–1
  complications 259–60
  face transplantation 222
  flap reconstructive surgery 154,
    159–60
  obstructive sleep apnea 178
  pediatric patients 328–9, 342
  percutaneous dilatational 255, 256,
    258, 260
  permanent tube-free 256
  surgical procedure 255
  terminology 255
  trauma 85
tracheotomy tubes
  blockage 259–60
  displacement 258, 259
  pediatric 328
transcranial Doppler, carotid body
    tumor resection 191

transglottic tumor 11, 12, 14
transjugular craniotomy 272,
    275
translabyrinthine posterior fossa
    craniotomy 272, 273
transsphenoidal pituitary surgery
    133–41
  anesthetic management 133–5
  case study 137–40
  complications 137
  intraoperative management 135–6,
    138, 139
  operating room setup 135, 140
  postoperative/recovery 137
  surgical procedure 133
transtracheal anesthesia 73–4
transtracheal jet ventilation 229–30,
    232
trauma, head and neck 83–7
  airway management 83–5
  case study 87
  facial fractures 1–2, 85–6
  flap reconstructive surgery 153
  primary survey (ABCDE) 83
  types of injury 85–7
trigeminal nerve, surgical stimulation
    286
triple endoscopy see panendoscopy
trisomy 21 (Down syndrome) 28, 321,
    325
tumors
  airway 94, 95, 96
  bronchoscopic debulking 310
  flap reconstructive surgery 152–3,
    153
tympanomastoidectomy 272, 322
tympanoplasty 271–2, 287–90, 322

upper respiratory infections (URI) 29,
    122, 321–2
uvulopalatal flap (UPF) 177
uvulopalatopharyngoplasty (UPPP)
    177
uvuloplasty, laser-assisted 177

vagus nerve
  monitoring, intraoperative 284
  surgical stimulation 286
  see also recurrent laryngeal nerve
vascular access
  carotid body tumor resection 188
  face transplantation 222–3
  flap reconstructive surgery 154–5
  tracheal resection 266
  tracheotomy 257, 259
vascular catheter dislodgment, free
    flap surgery 160
vasoconstrictors, nasal mucosal 4–5,
    55, 61, 114, 115–17, 323

vasopressors 158, 224–5
venous air embolism (VAE) 137, 189, 259, 273
vertigo, postoperative 282
vestibular schwannomas 272, 275, 283
videolaryngoscopy 43–6, 76, 246, 247
videostroboscopy, laryngeal 246
vocal cords (folds) 10–11
    intubation-mediated damage 287, 289
    unilateral paralysis (UVFP) 245–6, 251
vocal ligament 10

voice
    postoperative changes 287, 289
    prosthesis 16, 143, 144
    users, professional 287, 289
Voice Handicap Index (VHI) 246

Warthin tumor 203, 204
"washing machine" breathing 339
Weerda diverticuloscope 18–20, 22
Wegener's granulomatosis 263, 269, 318
Williams airway 75
World Health Organization (WHO), Safe Surgery Checklist 32

Xomed NIM™ EMG Endotracheal Tube 168, 169

Zenker's diverticulectomy 195–201
    anesthetic management 197–9
    case study 200–1
    postoperative issues 199–200
    preoperative management 197
    surgical approaches 195–6
Zenker's diverticulum 195, 196, 197
    cricoid pressure 198, 201
    inadvertent perforation 199
    other surgery in patients with 200